Mayo Clinic Examinations in Neurology

Mayo Clinic Examinations in Neurology

Seventh Edition

Members of the Mayo Clinic Department of Neurology

Mayo Clinic and Mayo Foundation
Rochester, Minnesota

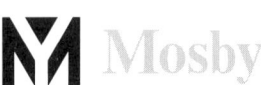

St. Louis Baltimore Boston Carlsbad Chicago Minneapolis New York Philadelphia Portland
London Milan Sydney Tokyo Toronto

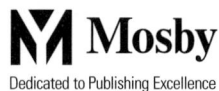

Mosby
Dedicated to Publishing Excellence

A Times Mirror Company

Vice President and Publisher: Anne S. Patterson
Editor: Michael Brown
Developmental Editor: Becca Gruliow
Project Manager: Chris Baumle
Production Editor: Eric Van Gorden
Design Manager: Nancy J. McDonald
Manufacturing Manager: William A. Winneberger, Jr.
Cover Photo: Custom Medical Stock

SEVENTH EDITION

Copyright 1998 Mayo Foundation.

Nothing in this publication implies that Mayo Foundation endorses any product mentioned in this book.

All rights reserved. This book is protected by copyright. No part of it may be reproduced, stored in a retrieval system, or transmitted in any form by any means, electronic, mechanical, recording, or otherwise, without written permission from Mayo Foundation, Rochester, Minnesota.

Editors

David O. Wiebers, M.D.
Chair, Division of Cerebrovascular Diseases,*
Professor of Neurology†

Allan J. D. Dale, M.D.
Consultant, Division of Cerebrovascular Diseases,*
Associate Professor of Neurology†

Emre Kokmen, M.D.
Consultant, Division of Behavioral Neurology,*
Professor of Neurology†

Jerry W. Swanson, M.D.
Consultant, Division of Cerebrovascular Diseases,*
Associate Professor of Neurology†

*Mayo Clinic and Mayo Foundation, Rochester, Minnesota.
†Mayo Medical School, Rochester, Minnesota.

Contributors

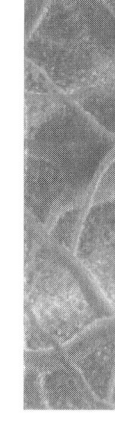

Andrea C. Adams, M.D.
Head of a Section of Neurology,*
Assistant Professor of Neurology†

J. Eric Ahlskog, M.D., Ph.D.
Chair, Division of Movement
Disorders,* Associate Professor of
Neurology†

Allen J. Aksamit, M.D.
Consultant, Division of
Neuroimmunology,* Associate
Professor of Neurology†

Arnold E. Aronson, Ph.D.
Senior Speech Consultant,*
Professor of Speech Pathology†

Raymond G. Auger, M.D.
Consultant, Section of
Electromyography,* Associate
Professor of Neurology†

J. D. Bartleson, M.D.
Consultant, Department of
Neurology,* Assistant Professor of
Neurology†

Paul W. Brazis, M.D.
Consultant, Department of
Neurology and Department of
Ophthalmology,‡
Associate Professor of Neurology†

Jeffrey W. Britton, M.D.
Consultant, Division of Epilepsy,*
Assistant Professor of Neurology†

Robert D. Brown, Jr., M.D.
Consultant, Division of
Cerebrovascular Diseases,* Assistant
Professor of Neurology†

Gregory D. Cascino, M.D.
Chair, Division of Epilepsy,*
Professor of Neurology†

Terrence L. Cascino, M.D.
Head of a Section of Neurology,*
Professor of Neurology†

Richard J. Caselli, M.D.
Chair, Division of Behavorial
Neurology,§ Associate Professor of
Neurology†

Shelley A. Cross, M.D.
Consultant, Department of
Neurology, Neuro-ophthalmology,*
Assistant Professor of Neurology†

Jasper R. Daube, M.D.
Chair, Department of Neurology,*
Professor of Neurology†

Robert P. Dinapoli, M.D.
Consultant, Division of Neuro-
oncology,* Associate Professor of
Neurology†

Joseph R. Duffy, Ph.D.
Head, Section of Medical Speech
Pathology,* Professor of Speech
Pathology†

Peter James Dyck, M.D.
Director, Neuromuscular Pathology
(Nerve) Laboratory,* Roy E. and
Merle Meyer Professor of
Neuroscience†

Alison M. Emslie-Smith, M.D.
Consultant, Department of
Neurology,* Assistant Professor of
Neurology†

Andrew G. Engel, M.D.
Director, Muscle Research
Laboratory,* Professor of Neurology†

Bruce A. Evans, M.D.
Consultant, Division of
Cerebrovascular Diseases,* Assistant
Professor of Neurology†

vii

Robert D. Fealey, M.D.
Consultant, Division of Cerebrovascular Diseases,* Assistant Professor of Neurology†

W. Neath Folger, M.D.
Consultant, Division of Cerebrovascular Diseases,* Assistant Professor of Neurology†

Neill R. Graff-Radford, M.D.
Chair, Department of Neurology,‡ Professor of Neurology†

Robert V. Groover, M.D.
Emeritus Consultant, Section of Child and Adolescent Neurology,* Emeritus Associate Professor of Neurology†

Julie E. Hammack, M.D.
Consultant, Division of Neuro-oncology,* Assistant Professor of Neurology†

C. Michel Harper, Jr., M.D.
Director, Section of Electromyography,* Associate Professor of Neurology†

Robert C. Hermann, Jr., M.D.
Consultant, Section of Electromyography,* Assistant Professor of Neurology†

David W. Kimmel, M.D.
Head of a Section of Neurology,* Associate Professor of Neurology†

Donald W. Klass, M.D.
Emeritus Senior Consultant, Section of Electroencephalography,* Emeritus Professor of Neurology†

William J. Litchy, M.D.
Formerly, Head, Section of Electromyography,* Associate Professor of Neurology†

Phillip A. Low, M.D.
Chair, Division of Clinical Neurophysiology,* Professor of Neurology†

Irene Meissner, M.D.
Consultant, Division of Cerebrovascular Diseases,* Associate Professor of Neurology†

Bahram Mokri, M.D.
Consultant, Divisions of Neuro-oncology and Cerebrovascular Diseases,* Professor of Neurology†

B. P. O'Neill, M.D.
Chair, Interinstitutional Division of Neuro-oncology,* Professor of Neurology†

Marc C. Patterson, M.D.
Consultant, Section of Child and Adolescent Neurology,* Assistant Professor of Neurology†

Ronald C. Petersen, Ph.D., M.D.
Consultant, Division of Behavioral Neurology,* Professor of Neurology†

George W. Petty, M.D.
Consultant, Division of Cerebrovascular Diseases,* Associate Professor of Neurology†

Moses Rodriguez, M.D.
Consultant, Division of Neuroimmunology,* Professor of Neurology†

Frank W. Sharbrough, M.D.
Head, Section of Electroencephalography,* Professor of Neurology†

Michael H. Silber, M.B.,Ch.B., F.C.P. (SA)
Consultant, Sleep Disorders Center,* Assistant Professor of Neurology†

J. Clarke Stevens, M.D.
Chair, Department of Neurology,§ Professor of Neurology†

Barbara F. Westmoreland, M.D.
Program Director, Division of Clinical Neurophysiology,* Professor of Neurology†

Jack P. Whisnant, M.D.
Emeritus Consultant, Division of Cerebrovascular Diseases,* Emeritus Professor of Neurology†

Eelco F. M. Wijdicks, M.D., Ph.D.
Co-Director, Neurology-Neurosurgery Intensive Care Unit,* Professor of Neurology†

Anthony J. Windebank, M.D.
Director, Molecular Neuroscience Program,* Professor of Neurology†

*Mayo Clinic and Mayo Foundation, Rochester, Minnesota.

†Mayo Medical School, Rochester, Minnesota.

‡Mayo Clinic Jacksonville, Jacksonville, Florida.

§Mayo Clinic Scottsdale, Scottsdale, Arizona.

Preface

Within the field of neurology, the past decade has brought widespread major advances in the fundamental understanding of many diseases and therapeutic approaches to their management. Yet despite such advances and the ever increasing influence of other high technology within medicine, the clinician continues to have a clear, fundamental need to develop a practical, systematic approach to the neurologic evaluation and to the use of diagnostic procedures in clinical practice. These clinical tools form the basis for the appropriate application of any advances in treatment to individual patients.

As in the previous six editions, the purpose of the seventh edition of *Mayo Clinic Examinations in Neurology* remains to provide the medical clinician with a comprehensive set of clinical tools to facilitate the optimal approach to the clinical and laboratory evaluation of neurologic patients. The first section of the book is devoted to components of the neurologic history and examination and the second section to laboratory aids and diagnostic procedures that assist with patient evaluation. Since the last edition, the book has been updated throughout. In particular, the sections on neuroradiology, neurophysiology, movement disorders, examination of the comatose patient, and laboratory aids in the neurologic diagnosis of disorders of muscle and neuromuscular transmission, disorders of peripheral nerves, and encephalopathies have been extensively updated and rewritten. Two sections pertaining to the evaluation of patients with sleep disorders have also been added to this edition.

The editors are greatly indebted to numerous individuals who made possible the completion of this book. We express deep gratitude to all our colleagues who contributed to this book for their hard work, outstanding cooperation, and sense of purpose in the preparation of this edition. We also gratefully acknowledge the invaluable contributions of Roberta Schwartz, LeAnn Stee, John Prickman, Sharon Wadleigh, Jeanette Schlotthauer, and Mary Schwager for their editorial support at the Mayo Clinic; Michael Brown, Rebecca Gruliow, Marla Sussman, Kim Davis, Eric Van Gorden, Laura DeYoung, Jennifer Byington, and Alicia Moten for their editorial support at Mosby-Year Book; and Marcia Jannatpour and Denise Gravenhof for their secretarial support. Finally, we extend a special thanks to our collective patients and students for their roles in inspiring the contributors to write this book and for providing us with the opportunity to experience the profound satisfaction of assisting them.

David O. Wiebers, M.D.

Allan J. D. Dale, M.D.

Emre Kokmen, M.D.

Jerry W. Swanson, M.D.

Editors, Seventh Edition

Dedication from the First Edition

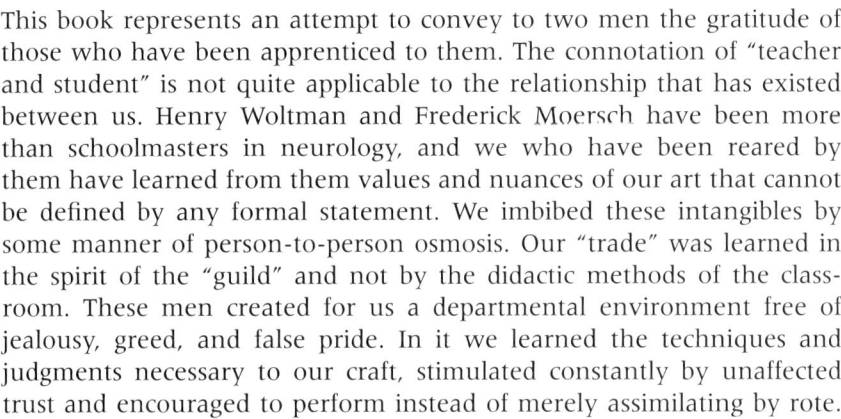

Dedicated to

Henry W. Woltman, M.D.
and
Frederick P. Moersch, M.D.

Pioneers in Neurology—Mayo Clinic
Inspiring Teachers—Mayo Foundation
Generous Associates of the Authors

This book represents an attempt to convey to two men the gratitude of those who have been apprenticed to them. The connotation of "teacher and student" is not quite applicable to the relationship that has existed between us. Henry Woltman and Frederick Moersch have been more than schoolmasters in neurology, and we who have been reared by them have learned from them values and nuances of our art that cannot be defined by any formal statement. We imbibed these intangibles by some manner of person-to-person osmosis. Our "trade" was learned in the spirit of the "guild" and not by the didactic methods of the classroom. These men created for us a departmental environment free of jealousy, greed, and false pride. In it we learned the techniques and judgments necessary to our craft, stimulated constantly by unaffected trust and encouraged to perform instead of merely assimilating by rote.

Paradoxically, we now venture a work that was never a formal part of our training—a factual outline of the practical components of the neurologic examination. This effort of ours will succeed or fail as we succeed or fail to impart to others something of the essence of our indoctrination. We intend this book as a series of working blueprints and not a course of lectures delivered from a remote podium. And so, we who are now journeymen write about the prosaic aspects of our branch of medicine, about the tools to be used and the manner of their using. We hope that these two masters of the "guild" may read into this primer our common gratitude for the uncommon things that happened to us through our association with them.

Alexander R. MacLean, M.D.

Contents

Part One   The Neurologic Examination

1 The Neurologic History 3
   General Aspects 3
      The Chief Complaints and History of the Present Illness 5
      Past Medical Events 6
      Review of Neurologic Symptoms and Review of Systems ... 6
      Family History 7
      Social History 8
   Specific Inquiry About Some Common Neurologic Problems.... 8
      1. Pain 8
      2. Headache 15
      3. Seizure Disorders 19
      4. Sleep Disorders 25

2 General Observations and Order of Procedure 29
   Order of Procedure 30
   Examination of the Scalp and Skull 31
   Facies 32
   Peripheral Nerves 33

3 Mental Function 35
   Introduction 35
   History 37
      Questions To Be Answered During History-Taking 37
      Behavioral Observations During History-Taking 38
   Examination 38
      Attention 39
      Language 41
      Memory 42
      Visuospatial and Perceptual Tasks 44
      Agnosias 44
      Apraxia 44
      Constructional Tasks 45
      Abstract Reasoning and Conceptual Functions 45
      Other Cortical Functions 46
      Summary 47
   Short Test of Mental Status 48
      Orientation 48
      Attention 48

xv

Learning	49
Arithmetic Calculation	49
Abstraction	49
Information	49
Construction	49
Recall	50
Total Score	50
Conclusions	51

4 Language and Motor Speech — 53

Motor Speech Disorders	53
Definition of Motor Speech Disorders	53
The Dysarthrias	54
Apraxia of Speech	68
Language Disorders	70
Basic Concepts	70
Localization of Language	71
Examination of Language	72
The Disorders	80

5 The Cranial Nerves (Except II, III, IV, and VI) — 87

Cranial Nerve I—Olfactory Nerve	87
Clinical Examination	88
Interpretation	89
Cranial Nerve V—Trigeminal Nerve	89
Anatomy	89
Clinical Examination	90
Cranial Nerve VII—Facial Nerve	91
Anatomy	91
Clinical Examination	93
Cranial Nerve VIII—Acoustic Nerve	94
Anatomy	94
Clinical Examination	95
Cranial Nerve IX—Glossopharyngeal Nerve	99
Anatomy	99
Clinical Examination	100
Cranial Nerve X—Vagus Nerve	100
Anatomy	100
Clinical Examination	101
Cranial Nerve XI—Accessory Nerve	101
Anatomy	101
Clinical Examination	101

Cranial Nerve XII — Hypoglossal Nerve 102
    Anatomy 102
    Clinical Examination 102

6 Neuro-Ophthalmology (Including Cranial Nerves II, III, IV, and VI) 103

    Cranial Nerve II (Optic Nerve) and Visual Pathway 103
        Anatomy 103
        Visual Acuity 104
        Color Vision 109
        The Field of Vision 109
        Interpretation of Visual Field Defects 116
        Ophthalmoscopy 121
    Cranial Nerves III, IV, and VI (Oculomotor, Trochlear, and Abducens Nerves), Ocular Motility, and Autonomic Functions 125
        Anatomy 125
        External Examination 129
    Ocular Movements 136

7 Motor Function. Part I: Central Integration 151

    Muscle Tone 154
        Symptoms and Signs of Disturbances of Muscle Tone 154
        Examination of Muscle Tone 155
    Coordination 157
        Testing of Coordination 158
    Alternate Motion Rate 159
        Tongue Wiggle 160
        Finger Wiggle 160
        Foot Pat 161
    Abnormal Involuntary Movements 161
        Abnormal Movements Provoked by an Uncontrollable Urge 162
        Abnormal Movements Initiated Outside Conscious Awareness 163
    Gait and Station 169
        Gait 169
        Station 175

8 Motor Function. Part II: Specific Study of Muscle 177

    Disorders of Muscle Size 177
        Atrophy 177
        Hypertrophy 178
    Intrinsic Muscle Movements 178
        Fasciculations 178
        Cramps 180

　　　　Myokymia 180
　　　　Fibrillation 180
　　Response to Percussion 181
　　　　Normal 181
　　　　Myotonic Reaction 181
　　　　Myoedema 182
　　Palpation of Muscle 183
　　　　Tenderness 183
　　　　Consistency 184
　　　　Contracture 184
　　Muscle Strength 185
　　　　Symptoms 185
　　　　Grading and Recording of Muscle Strength 187
　　　　Normal Strength 188
　　　　General Survey of Motor Function 189
　　　　Testing Muscle Strength 190
　　　　Hysterical Motor Dysfunction ("Weakness") 192
　　　　Scheme Employed in Examining Muscles 193
　　　　Outline of Anatomic Information Required for Tests
　　　　　　of Strength of Specific Muscles 193

9 Reflexes 241
　　Muscle-Stretch Reflexes 242
　　　　Technique of Elicitation 242
　　　　Interpretation and Grading of Reflexes 245
　　　　Specific Muscle-Stretch Reflexes 246
　　Superficial Reflexes 250
　　　　Specific Superficial Reflexes 250
　　Pathologic Reflexes 252
　　　　Specific Pathologic Reflexes 253

10 The Sensory Examination 255
　　Types of Sensation 255
　　　　Superficial Sensation 256
　　　　Deep Sensation 256
　　　　Cortical Function in Sensation 256
　　　　Thalamic Function in Sensation 256
　　General Methods of Examination 257
　　Specific Methods of Examination 258
　　　　Tests for Superficial Sensation 259
　　　　Tests for Deep Sensation 263
　　　　Tests for Combined Sensation (Two-Point Distinction,
　　　　　　Traced-Figure Identification, and Stereognosis) 266
　　Sensory Supply (Segmental and Neural) 268

11 Autonomic Function 275
Respiration 278
Temperature Control 280
Regulation of Skin Blood Flow and Vasomotor Function 281
The Bladder 283
Gastrointestinal Tract 284
Clinical Evaluation of Autonomic Nervous System Function 285
    The Autonomic History 285
    The Autonomic Examination 285

12 Clinical Examinations for Selected Neurologic Problems 287
Examination of the Comatose Patient 287
    1. Level of Consciousness 289
    2. Pupils 290
    3. Ocular Movements 291
    4. Motor Responses 291
    5. Respiratory Patterns 291
The Neurovascular Examination 294
    Blood Pressure 295
    Palpation 295
    Auscultation 296
    Ocular Fundus 297
Clinical Examinations in Selected Pain Problems 298
    Tests for Diagnosis of Pain Problems in the Lower Back
      and Lower Extremities 298
    Tests for Diagnosis of Pain Problems in the Cervical Region
      and Upper Extremities 300

13 Examination of Infants and Children 303
History 303
    Prenatal Period 303
    Birth and Neonatal Period 304
    Development 304
Examination of Infant 307
    Posture, Tone, and Muscle Strength 308
Motor Responses 309
    Extremities 309
    Neck 310
    Ambulation 310
    Reflexes 311
    The Cranial Nerves 314
    Examination of the Head 315
Examination of Children More Than 2 Years of Age 317

Spontaneous Motor Activity 318
　　　Praxis 319
　　　Lateral Dominance or Preference 320
　　　Drawing 321
　　　Articulation of Sounds 321
　　　Language 323
　　　Auditory Discrimination and Memory 324
　　　Reading and Spelling 325
　　　Calculation 325
　　　Corporeal Orientation 325
　　　Extracorporeal Space Orientation 327
　Summary 327

Part Two Diagnostic Procedures

14 Neuroradiologic Procedures 331
　Plain Roentgenography 332
　　　Spine Roentgenography 332
　　　Roentgenography of the Skull 336
　Myelography 338
　　　General Aspects 338
　　　Complications 339
　　　Pathologic Findings 340
　Cerebral Angiography 341
　　　Methods, Contrast Media, and Complications 342
　　　Cerebrovascular Disease 342
　　　Mass Lesions 344
　　　Craniocerebral Trauma 344
　Computed Tomography 345
　　　Theory 345
　　　Contrast Enhancement 345
　　　Clinical Applications 346
　Magnetic Resonance Imaging 350
　　　Clinical Applications 351
　MRI Angiography 355
　Radionuclide Imaging 356
　Future Perspectives 356

15 Clinical Neurophysiology 357
　Section I: Electroencephalography 357
　　　Recording Procedure and Preparation of Patient 357

Special Electrodes 359
Normal EEG Activity 359
Abnormal EEG Activity 361
The EEG Report 364
EEG and Clinical Correlates 365
Ancillary Techniques in EEG 376
The EEG in Infants and Children—Normal Patterns 378
EEG Abnormalities in Infants 381
EEG Abnormalities in Children 382
Prolonged Monitoring 385
Ambulatory EEG Monitoring 385
Quantitative Analysis of Spontaneous EEG 387
EEG Monitoring During Surgery 388
Section II: Electromyography 389
Survey of Clinical Uses of EMG 389
The Electromyograph 391
Origin of Electric Activity of Muscle 392
Procedure of the Examination 393
Criteria of Abnormality in the EMG 396
Sequence of Abnormalities of the EMG After
    Nerve Injury 407
Location of Lesions Affecting the Lower Motor Neuron 409
Differentiation of Primary Muscle Disease From
    That Secondary to Denervation 410
Single Fiber Electromyography 411
Recording Abnormal Movements 416
Section III: Nerve Conduction Studies 416
Conduction in Motor Nerve Fibers 416
Excitability of the Peripheral Neuromuscular System 418
Conduction Velocity of Motor Nerves 418
Late Responses 420
Motor Unit Number Estimates 422
Repetitive Stimulation 423
Conduction in Sensory Nerve Fibers 426
Cranial Nerve Conduction Studies 427
Section IV: Surgical Monitoring 428
Surgical Monitoring Techniques 429
Applications of Surgical Monitoring Techniques 435
Section V: Somatosensory System Testing 443
Averaging 443
Nomenclature 444
Stimulation Methods 444
Origin of SEP Waveforms 444
Criteria of SEP Abnormality 446
SEP Abnormalities 447

Section VI: Auditory-Vestibular System Testing 449
  Brain Stem Auditory Evoked Potentials 449
  Testing Hearing 453
  Testing Vestibular Function 454
Section VII: Visual System Testing 455
  Electroretinogram 456
  Pattern Reversal Evoked Potentials 456
Section VIII: Evaluation of Patients With Sleep Disorders 457
  Physiologic Changes With Sleep 458
  Polysomnography 460
  Multiple Sleep Latency Test 462
  Pupillography 462
Section IX: Autonomic Function Tests 463
  Some Tests of Distal Sympathetic Autonomic Function 463
  Tests Usually Used To Detect Generalized
      Autonomic Failure 464
  Testing Gastrointestinal Autonomic Function 466
  Urinary Bladder Function Tests 467

16 Examination of the Cerebrospinal Fluid 469
Indications for CSF Examination 469
Contraindications for Lumbar Puncture 470
Technique of Lumbar Puncture 470
  Preparation and Positioning of the Patient 471
  Anesthesia 471
  Insertion of the Lumbar Puncture Needle 472
  Pressure Studies 473
Bloody Tap 473
Dry Tap 474
Amount of CSF Required for Tests 475

17 Other Laboratory Aids in Neurologic Diagnosis 477
Cerebrovascular Disease 477
  Noninvasive Neurovascular Studies 477
  Measurement of Cerebral Blood Flow 481
  Radioisotope Cisternography 481
Encephalopathies 482
  Toxic Encephalopathies 482
  Metabolic Encephalopathies 483
  Hereditary Metabolic Disorders 487
Disorders of Muscle and Neuromuscular Transmission 498
  Myasthenia Gravis 498
  Serum Creatine Kinase 500
  Muscle Biopsy 501

Disorders or Diseases of Peripheral Nerves 507
    Differential Diagnosis of Peripheral Neuropathy 507
    Quantitative Sensory Testing (QST) 509
    Sural Nerve Biopsy 511

Index 515

PART ONE

The Neurologic Examination

Chapter 1

The Neurologic History

GENERAL ASPECTS

The medical and neurologic history is the window into the patient's world and is often the first interaction that leads to the formation of the caregiver-patient relationship. One may describe history-taking as an art in the subtle directing of a conversation with a patient. The importance of this history to a clinical neurologist cannot be overestimated. After the interview, the skilled clinician should be well on the way to answering the following questions, which will be clarified with a higher level of certainty after the neurologic examination, guided in part by the historical data, and then confirmed by any required ancillary testing.

1. Does the patient have neurologic disease?
2. If so, what is the localization of the lesion or lesions?
3. What is the pathophysiology of the process?
4. What is the preliminary differential diagnosis?

To facilitate the clarification of these questions, the caregiver must learn the art of eliciting history from many types of challenging patients, including a poor observer, an uneducated person, a person who may delight in twisting the meaning of things, and sometimes a person who has cognitive difficulties. The task can be long; if time has to be limited, subsequent interviews are imperative, particularly if the problem is complex. In difficult problems, a second interview is of value, since the patient's recollection may have been stimulated during the interval and important events may then be told with ease and accuracy. Caregivers frequently complain that the patient misled them, that the history was changed, and that, therefore, the patient is an unreliable witness. Sometimes this is true, but frequently the person taking the history has misunderstood the patient and written down his or her own interpretation of the patient's statements or the patient had trouble recalling all details during the stress of the initial interview.

The amount of time required to take a history varies both with the personality of the caregiver and with the patient's particular problem.

The extent to which the caregiver may guide and interrupt the patient as the story is told depends in part on the person's experience and ability. One frequently needs to ask for clarification of the meaning of certain words used to describe symptoms, and it is reasonable to do this as the history evolves chronologically. Too often, however, it is believed that time can be saved by direct questioning, and such interrogation begins early in the interview. This technique may work reasonably well for the experienced caregiver and for the inexperienced in evaluating simple problems. In difficult diagnostic problems, such a method is not efficient or satisfactory for anyone. The method must also be modified according to the education and cultural background of the patient.

The recording of the history is important; if it can be remembered that one is documenting evidence, the record is likely to be clear and complete. Within reasonable limits, one should make use of the patient's own words, since these give a picture of the patient in a cultural background. Attempts to abbreviate remarks of the patient by using technical terms or by interpreting the remarks usually result in an inaccurate history. If the patient possesses reasonable mental competence, it is often worthwhile to record almost verbatim the patient's chief complaint and part or all of the symptoms in the present illness. The importance of an accurate and detailed account of events if the patient has a compensation or insurance problem cannot be overemphasized. In such instances, a verbatim report may be essential in making a correct diagnosis and giving evidence in court. A record of the interview should be made at the time of the interaction or immediately afterward.

The order in which information is obtained about the family, past illnesses, review of systems, and the social situation may vary from one caregiver to another and may depend on the problem. Although the emphasis is not always the same, the inquiry should be pursued systematically; otherwise, the history is likely to be incomplete. The history of the illness is part of a life story and not something unrelated to home, work, and community. The correct perspective and emphasis on these aspects are essential in making an accurate diagnosis and in providing optimal care for the patient and his or her family.

Evaluation of the clinical problem begins with an interview with the patient. This approach is advisable, and the exceptions to it are few, even with patients who are cognitively impaired or have psychiatric illness. However, relatives and friends should not be ignored. In fact, they should be given every opportunity to report information and ask questions. Often, the patient cannot recall the details of specific symptoms or may not even realize that a certain symptom or deficit exists. A relative or friend who has been in close contact with the patient may be critical in providing details that clarify the presence and type of a neurologic process. Sometimes information about changes in behavior, memory, hearing, vision, speech, coordination, and gait can be obtained only by interviewing the relatives. For example, in convulsive disorders, the observations of the relatives may be of the utmost importance in establishing the existence of the disorder, the seizure subtype, and the origin of the discharge focus that initiates the spell. Furthermore, it is important to understand the attitudes of the patient and the relatives in the general management of the medical or surgical disorder.

The method of taking and recording a history is the same for the caregiver who uses a form as it is for the one who prefers to take a blank sheet of paper and write notes. Our form, used as a guide for students, residents, staff, and nurses, serves as a template for recording the chronologic history, encourages a comprehensive review of neurologic symptoms and review of systems, and reminds the history-taker of important aspects of the family and social history that should be recorded for all neurology patients. A form may permit the recording of certain negative and positive findings graphically, but at the same time it must allow for the free description of observations that cannot be reduced satisfactorily to symbols.

The Chief Complaints and History of the Present Illness

The chief complaint or complaints and their duration should be documented carefully. One should allow the patient the opportunity to tell the story for several minutes without interruption. Otherwise, important details may be pushed aside in the patient's mind. Sometimes it is necessary to bring the patient back to the onset of the illness by asking such a question as "When were you last well?" or "How did these symptoms begin?" Circumstances surrounding the onset of symptoms, such as time of day or night, patient activity, and the relation of symptoms to other events, should be elicited. The actual analysis of different symptoms follows a rather similar plan; the suggested order of inquiry about each symptom is as follows:

1. Date of onset.
2. Character and severity.
3. Location and extension.
4. Time relationships.
5. Associated complaints.
6. Aggravating and alleviating factors.
7. Previous treatment and effects.
8. Progress, noting remissions and exacerbations.

The history is then developed chronologically. Knowledge about the sequence of events is used in localizing lesions and in determining the nature of the pathologic process producing symptoms. During this part of the interview, questions are asked about other possible symptoms often associated with the main complaints. Later, a systematic review of neurologic symptoms, or what may be called the "functional inquiry of the nervous system," is carried out. It is often advisable to ask the patient what is meant by the particular words used. There is a surprising variation in what people mean by such symptoms as "dizziness," "headaches," and "numbness." "Headache" to some patients means a drawing sensation and to others, an ache or pain or even numbness or dizziness. At the end of this part of the interview, if the information has not already been volunteered, the patient should be asked whether he or she has stopped working. This datum is of special importance in compensation and insurance problems, but actually in any illness some idea of the functional disability is imperative.

Past Medical Events
There are many reasons for taking the history of the present illness before beginning questions about past events unrelated to the current chief complaints. The patient should have an opportunity to talk about what he or she considers important before these questions are asked. Furthermore, one may better direct the inquiry into the past history, family history, review of systems, and review of neurologic symptoms once one is acquainted with the present situation.

Careful evaluation and recording of past events are important. A common error is to accept the patient's use of a diagnostic term as a statement of fact during the reporting of a past illness. It is wise to make some inquiry into the symptoms and situations that caused a certain diagnosis to be made, for terms such as "stroke," "migraine," and "seizure" may be used without clear supporting historical data. In addition to reviewing previous medical diagnoses, one should ask the patient about any blood transfusions. History of travel outside the United States is also important in selected patients. A comprehensive list of current medications and known allergies is useful, since neurologic side effects are possible with most drugs.

Review of Neurologic Symptoms and Review of Systems
It is important to allow time for a review of other neurologic symptoms that may not have been mentioned as the history unfolded. For example, in the history of headaches, inquiry is made about nausea, vomiting, and visual disturbances. However, a more detailed and systematic review is necessary after the history of present illness is completed. This neurologic review may reveal additional symptoms germane to the presenting complaint or other important issues that the patient did not mention earlier or was not aware of until the clinician mentioned the symptom. Although some believe it most useful to review neurologic symptoms during the history, others find a certain ease and naturalness in asking some of these questions as the physical examination is being done. For example, some find it efficient to ask the patient questions about vision and then to test the function of the eyes, repeating this

approach for each neurologic function as it is examined. This plan of questioning and examining does not overemphasize the question in the patient's mind. More important, the caregiver thinks functionally as well as anatomically in evaluating a clinical problem. Students and residents may try both approaches and decide which better suits their individual style.

In addition to the review of neurologic symptoms and functional inquiry, a medical review of systems should be performed. Because many neurologic illnesses are co-occurring with medical disorders or caused by certain systemic processes, the general review may be crucial in clarifying whether some other disorder is affecting the nervous system. The review should be comprehensive, including inquiry about skin, endocrine, ear, nose, and throat, respiratory, cardiovascular, gastrointestinal, genitourinary, musculoskeletal, hematologic, and psychiatric issues. Additional specific questions should be asked of female patients, such as menstrual history, any breast lumps noticed, and number of pregnancies, whether culminating in live births, miscarriages, or abortions.

Family History
The family history may be of special importance to the neurologist. The health history of the parents and the siblings should be carefully recorded. If the patient's condition or preliminary family history suggests that a hereditary disorder may be present, a more detailed family history is required. Although charts and symbols commonly used by a geneticist may be adopted, sufficient detail may not be available at the first interview with the patient, and time may not allow a comprehensive family review at the initial visit, particularly if the pedigree is complex. A minimal family history should include name, age, state of health, and cause of death for each parent. Similar information is then obtained for the patient's siblings, the siblings of each parent, and other relatives as appropriate. At a later date, this information may be reduced to a diagrammatic format.

Questions about other relatives are frequently indicated, particularly in the case of headache, epilepsy, hyperkinesia, nystagmus, muscular atrophy and dystrophy, cerebellar disorders, ataxia, and neuropathy. Many other examples might be given, but in a broad way one should think to ask such questions as "Have any of your relatives had an illness such as you have?" or, as in convulsive disorder, one may need to frame the questions in a meaningful way for the patient and ask, "Have any of your relatives had fainting spells, spasms, or blackouts?" The questions should be asked more than once when there is a reason to expect a positive answer. Sometimes during a second interview, the patient may come with a family tree carefully prepared as the result of some research at home or of correspondence with relatives in other parts of the country.

Social History

A patient's social history allows the additional clarification of factors that may be important in determining the cause of a neurologic disorder and aids the caregiver in understanding the response of the patient to the disease and its impact on his or her life. Issues to discuss in the social history include the patient's education and previous vocations. Developmental history may be important in selected patients, particularly young patients. Any history of substance use, including tobacco, alcohol, caffeine, and recreational or street drugs, should be noted by recording current use, previous use, and, if applicable, type, amount, frequency, and duration. Risk factors for sexually transmitted disorders and human immunodeficiency virus infection should also be considered.

Data should also be obtained on the patient's home environment. In addition to clarifying the type of home setting, one may ask about social support and any important social issues affecting the family. Inquiry should be made about the patient's personality development and previous reaction to stress and illness. Information about current marital status, any marital difficulties, and behavior of the patient's children may also be important in clarifying the cause of symptoms and delivering optimal care.

SPECIFIC INQUIRY ABOUT SOME COMMON NEUROLOGIC PROBLEMS

It is only natural that the experienced neurologist is more adept than the novice at quickly eliciting pertinent data from the patient. Experience is acquired slowly, but the skill of the beginner can be augmented by guidance. Consequently, a brief discussion of the symptoms relative to the more common neurologic problems, namely, pain, headache, convulsions, and sleep disorders, is inserted here to aid the novice in taking the neurologic history.

1. Pain

Pain is one of the most common complaints brought to the physician's attention. The initial goal of the neurologist is to ascertain whether the pain represents disease of the nervous system (neuropathic pain), disease of visceral or somatic structures (nociceptive pain), or a sensation without a definite organic cause (idiopathic pain). The most common pains of neurologic origin, exclusive of headache, are those that originate from lesions of the peripheral nerves and spinal roots. Less frequent, but no less important, are pains resulting from injury to or dysfunction of the sensory neurons of the central nervous system (central pain syndromes).

Nociceptive pain is produced by activation of normal peripheral nerve fibers when the structures they innervate are injured. The nociceptive stimuli travel through fibers innervating somatic structures (bone, muscle, dura, fascia, skin, blood vessels) or visceral structures (pleura, peritoneum, organ capsules, hollow viscera) when these structures are injured, stretched, or obstructed. Neuropathic pain results from direct injury to the central or peripheral nervous system, with subsequent aberrant pain fiber transmission, deafferentation, and reorganization of central sensory processing.

A logically sequenced system of inquiry supplemented by appropriate clinical examination and laboratory investigation assists in differentiating neuropathic from nociceptive and idiopathic pain syndromes. Once a neuropathic origin is determined, the specific locus within the nervous system is sought. As with any other symptom, one should ascertain the onset, quality, intensity, location, duration, frequency, associated symptoms, and precipitating and ameliorating factors of the pain. Severity alone does not permit one to judge the underlying mechanism of pain, although many neuropathic pain syndromes produce severe pain. Many patients with chronic severe pain do not manifest the usual affective and autonomic features of those with acute pain (for example, crying, writhing, moaning, and tachycardia). Patients with severe chronic pain may instead appear withdrawn and depressed.

The quality of neuropathic pain is unique. It may be described as "sharp electric-like flashes" *(lancinating)*, burning, or "pins and needles" *(paresthesia)*. Some patients describe a feeling as if the painful area were being squeezed in a vice or were swollen. Itching is a common feature of neuropathic pain, as is *allodynia* (pain due to a stimulus that does not normally provoke pain). A related symptom is *hyperalgesia*, which is severe pain in response to a mild noxious stimulus. Depending on the locus of involvement within the nervous system, neuropathic pain usually follows the dermatomal pattern of a specific peripheral nerve, plexus, root, or central sensory pathway. There are often other signs and symptoms of neurologic disease, including sensory loss, weakness, reflex changes, and autonomic dysfunction, associated with the pain.

Pain in peripheral nerve lesions

Injury to the peripheral nervous system produces increased and abnormal firing of nociceptive fibers associated with sprouting as the damaged nerve attempts to regenerate, sometimes with formation of a neuroma. The resulting dysesthetic sensation is described as burning, prickling, itching, and, occasionally, lancinating. Dysesthetic pain is typically located distally in the dermatomal distribution of the nerve and may be elicited by percussion over the injured nerve (Tinel's sign), especially at the site of injury. Tinel's sign is a reflection of the enhanced mechanosensitivity of regenerating nerve sprouts and neuromas. Nerve injury also stimulates the nociceptive afferents that supply the epineurium (nervi nervorum), producing a more familiar dull, aching, or gnawing pain that is experienced more proximally and is referred to as "nerve trunk" pain.

The pain and paresthesia produced by lesions of the peripheral cutaneous nerves are usually limited to the region supplied by the affected nerve or nerves. Thus, compression of the median nerve at the wrist (carpal tunnel syndrome) produces a dull, aching pain at the wrist or thenar eminence (nerve trunk pain) and dysesthetic pain in the palm and palmar aspect of the thumb and first three and a half fingers. Tinel's sign is often present at the wrist. In meralgia paresthetica, which results from compression of the lateral femoral cutaneous nerve, the subjective sensory experience is likewise limited to the skin on the lateral surface of the thigh that is supplied by this nerve. Tinel's sign may be present at the inguinal ligament. Inestimable help in diagnosis is obtained by consulting the charts depicting areas supplied by the principal cutaneous nerves (see Fig. 10-5 through 10-9). Thus, the location of the pain may be compared with the area of skin supplied by the cutaneous nerves, although the clinical description may not conform exactly to the graphic representation.

In lesions of sensory nerves, one must depend on sensory phenomena alone for localization. In lesions of mixed nerves (those composed of motor, sensory, and autonomic fibers), the diagnosis may be confirmed by the detection of weakness, wasting, decrease in the deep tendon reflex, and electromyographic findings of denervation in the muscles supplied by the affected nerve peripheral to the site of the lesion. Signs of autonomic fiber involvement include alterations in the skin's sweating, color, texture, temperature, and distribution of hair growth. The distribution of these abnormalities is key to determining the location of nerve injury. Peripheral polyneuropathies typically produce signs and symptoms in a glove-and-stocking distribution, usually most prominent in the distal lower extremities. In mononeuropathies or mononeuritis multiplex, the lesions are in the distribution of single or multiple peripheral nerves.

The pain of some peripheral nerve lesions, particularly that of diabetic polyneuropathy, is often worse at night. It differs from the nocturnal aggravation commonly reported by patients who have nerve root lesions, because the nocturnal intensification is independent of position and is not related to assumption of the horizontal position as such.

Disease of the brachial or lumbosacral plexus is usually associated with dull, aching "nerve trunk" pain that is maximal in the proximal limb or limb girdle, with variable extension of dysesthetic pain into the involved extremity. The pattern of radiation may resemble that of root pain. However, the Valsalva maneuver, position changes, and spinal motion may have no aggravating effect. A precipitous onset may suggest an ischemic or compressive cause, whereas slow progression warrants concern about a neoplasm. Any associated clinical or electromyographic deficit usually does not correlate with a monoradicular pattern but rather conforms to the affected region of the plexus (see Fig. 8-19 and 8-20). Furthermore, electromyographic studies may confirm that the lesion is distal to the dorsal root ganglion and motor root.

Pain resulting from lesions involving the sensory nerve roots (root pain)

Lesions involving the spinal root should be considered when one or more of the following characteristics are present.

1. The pain is localized in the dermatome supplied by the affected nerve root. Although often widely distributed throughout the dermatome, the pain occasionally is limited to a small area within it. It is well to remember this point, since it frequently accounts for failure in diagnosis. The charts depicting dermatomes (see Fig. 10-4 and 10-10) serve an important function in determining whether the pain under consideration is of radicular origin. Although dermatomal in distribution, nerve root pain in the limbs seldom extends beyond the wrist or ankle. However, any associated dermatomal dysesthesia is usually most prominent distally and may be described in the hand or foot as originating where the pain apparently ends. Furthermore, in most instances, pain in the vertebral column is temporally associated with pain or dysesthesia in a limb.

    Pain from lesions involving deep somatic or visceral structures, such as the bone, muscles, and ligaments of the spinal column or the thoracic and abdominal viscera, may be felt in superficial regions some distance from the site of the lesion and, consequently, is designated "referred pain." As a rule, the pain extends to regions that approximate the dermatomal distribution of the nerve root supplying the irritated viscus or deep somatic structure. Because the distributions of root pain and referred pain may be similar, the two can be difficult to distinguish. The quality and other characteristics of root pain (see below) may be of value in the differential diagnosis of such problems. The well-known effects of cough, strain, and sneeze must be interpreted carefully, as these may also induce painful movement of the diseased spinal column. The most reliable features of root pain are aggravation by the chin-chest maneuver, intensification after several hours in a horizontal position, and amelioration soon after the patient assumes an upright position.

2. Root pain is frequently produced or aggravated by any activity that abruptly increases intrathoracic and intra-abdominal pressure, such as coughing, sneezing, or straining. Such increases in pressure block the venous outflow from the epidural space and cause distention of the valveless intervertebral veins. This in turn forces

the dura, which envelops the nerve roots, toward the spinal cord. Since the nerve roots are fixed to the spinal cord proximally and peripherally at the intervertebral foramen, the displacement of the dura results in stretching of the involved root, which may result in pain if the root is diseased. In addition, distention of the intervertebral veins may result in direct nerve root compression.
3. Root pain may awaken the patient at night after several hours of sleep and may be relieved from 15 to 30 minutes after the upright position is assumed. The patient may learn to prevent the pain by sleeping in a reclining chair. However, in contrast to painful peripheral neuropathy, the position is the important determining factor. If the patient with peripheral neuropathy were to lie long enough in a similar position during the day, the pain would occur just as it does at night. This feature of root pain has its basis in the lengthening of the spinal column that takes place when the horizontal position is assumed and in its shortening in the upright position. Since the length of the spinal cord remains the same regardless of the position assumed by the patient, the lengthening of the spinal column results in traction on the roots that emerge from the thoracic, lumbar, and sacral segments of the cord. From these segments, the roots course downward and outward to emerge from their respective intervertebral foramina (Fig. 1-1).
4. Root pain often is intensified by other maneuvers that stretch the involved roots. Lower lumbar and sacral roots are stretched from the periphery by the straight-leg raising test (Lasègue's sign) or by bending forward, which puts traction on the sciatic nerve. If the cauda equina is tethered, as with a large extruded spinal disk or tumor, even raising the contralateral leg may exacerbate radicular pain down the symptomatic leg (crossed straight-leg raising test). Reverse straight-leg raising (extending the hip with the patient prone) in a patient with an L-3 or L-4 radiculopathy may elicit pain from traction on the femoral nerve. Cervical roots may be stretched by downward displacement of the shoulder girdle. The chin-chest maneuver of passively flexing the neck so that the chin rests on the chest induces an ascension of the spinal cord within the spinal canal. Thus, the nerve roots, particularly those of the lower thoracic, lumbar, and sacral segments, are placed under tension, which elicits pain in the dermatomes of injured roots. If this test is performed without inducing motion of the spinal column, with the patient recumbent and relaxed, a positive result is one of the most reliable signs in the detection of disease of nerve roots.
5. Root pain may be aggravated by spinal movements that narrow the intervertebral foramen through which the diseased nerve root passes. In cervical root disease, simultaneous extension and lateral flexion of the neck to the affected side (Spurling's sign) may result

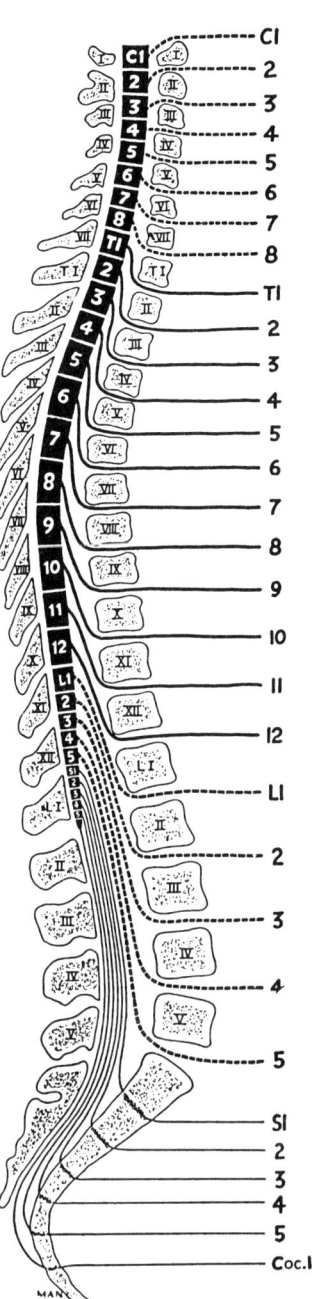

Figure 1-1
Relationship of spinal cord segments, intraspinal roots, and spinal nerves to the vertebral bodies and spines and intervertebral interspaces. *(From Haymaker W, Woodhall B: Peripheral nerve injuries: principles of diagnosis, ed 2, Philadelphia, 1953, WB Saunders Co. By permission of the publisher.)*

in sudden aggravation of neck and dermatomal arm pain or paresthesia. In the lumbar spine, lateral flexion toward the affected side further narrows the neural foramen and may result not only in aggravation of the spinal pain but also in dermatomal limb pain and paresthesia.

Weakness and reflex changes may occur in muscles supplied by the affected root. Loss of cutaneous sensation is rare with disease or transection of a single nerve root, however, because there is typically considerable dermatomal overlap of adjacent spinal roots.

Pain of trigeminal neuralgia and other diseases of nerve

The diagnosis of trigeminal neuralgia depends almost entirely on the history related by the patient. The pain of trigeminal neuralgia is usually limited to the skin and mucosa supplied by one or more branches of the trigeminal nerve. Typically, the pain is severe and paroxysmal (of abrupt onset and lasting a few seconds). Some patients experience a series of individual paroxysms lasting several minutes or more. The pain has a lancinating or electric shock-like quality and is often described as "shooting," "flashing," or "jumping." Between paroxysms, the patient is usually asymptomatic. Pain that is continuous, lacks a shock–like quality, or is associated with objective evidence of cranial nerve dysfunction should raise the suspicion of diseases other than trigeminal neuralgia, such as injury to the gasserian ganglion or trigeminal root by tumor, inflammation, or a vascular anomaly.

Trigeminal neuralgia may be spontaneous, but it is frequently precipitated by touching a trigger point on the face, lips, tongue, or gums. Talking and eating may also trigger pain and force the patient to refrain from these activities. Even a gentle breeze can trigger pain in some patients.

Injury to the glossopharyngeal and vagal nerves (as in patients with tumors of the head and neck) may produce paroxysmal lancinating pain in the back of the throat or in the external auditory meatus. Typically, other signs of cranial nerve dysfunction, such as dysphagia and dysarthria, accompany pain in this disorder. Vasodepressor syncope may also occur.

Tabes dorsalis and other lesions of the spinal cord and sensory roots may be associated with paroxysmal, lancinating pain. Lhermitte's sign is a sudden shocklike sensation radiating down the back or into the arms and legs with forward flexion of the neck. It is most commonly noted by patients with multiple sclerosis but may also be experienced by patients with other lesions involving the dorsal columns, including tumors, herniated cervical or thoracic disks, and vascular malformations.

Central pain syndromes

Injury to the central pain conducting pathways of the brain and spinal cord may produce pain by a number of mechanisms: (1) loss of pain inhibitory neurons, (2) denervation hypersensitivity of nociceptive neurons that have lost afferent input (deafferentation), (3) aberrant discharge of injured central nociceptive neurons, (4) reorganization of central somatosensory pathways, with formation of "central generators," and (5) abnormal efferent activity in the sympathetic nervous system, with stimulation and sensitization of neurons in the dorsal horn of the spinal cord (sympathetically maintained pain).

The thalamus is a relay point for sensory fibers supplying the contralateral side of the body. Large lesions of the thalamus may produce pain and anesthesia in the entire contralateral half of the body, including the head. There is often associated hyperalgesia and allodynia. In smaller lesions, the pain and anesthesia may be limited to large contiguous portions of the body, such as the whole lower extremity and lower trunk or one-half of the head, upper extremity, and chest. Characteristically, thalamic pain appears as the patient is recovering from a thalamic infarct. The pain is persistent and is aggravated by emotional upset and fatigue. It is often severe and described as burning, squeezing, swelling, or prickling; above all, it has a peculiar, highly distressing quality.

Spinal cord (spinothalamic tract) and, rarely, parietal cortical lesions can produce a neuropathic pain syndrome that may be severe. The site of the pain depends on the level or distribution of the lesion.

Postherpetic neuralgia results from reactivation of herpes zoster in the dorsal root ganglion of one or more nerve roots (usually thoracic). Pain from the acute vesicular eruption usually resolves several weeks or months after the rash heals. In a small percentage of patients, however, a chronic neuropathic pain syndrome develops that is often difficult to treat. The pain is localized to the affected dermatome and may be described as burning, lancinating, squeezing, or itching. Allodynia and hyperalgesia are almost always present, sometimes making even the light touch of a garment excruciatingly painful. The pain is most likely caused by deafferentation resulting in hypersensitive dorsal horn neurons. There may be a component of a sympathetically maintained pain as well, because sympathetic blockade of the affected roots may produce sustained relief.

2. Headache

The complaint of headache is one of the most common symptoms encountered in medical practice. From the history alone, the nature of these headaches can be suspected in most cases. Subsequent neurologic evaluation, however, is important to establish the absence of neurologic abnormalities (as in most instances) or to seek evidence for localization.

The general problem

The approach to taking a history about headache is usually straightforward. Several questions need to be answered, especially when the patient has a chronic condition. It is usually best to begin by asking the patient to tell about the pain or simply to ask what kind of help the patient seeks. Usually the patient speaks only briefly if allowed to speak uninterrupted. This helps to establish rapport with the patient, and directed but open questions can then be asked.

How many types of headaches are experienced?
Many persons with long-standing headaches have more than one type. It is of value to elicit this information at the beginning of the interview so that each type of headache can be delineated. For example, some patients experience both tension-type and migraine headaches. Each type of headache may require a different approach to management. It is also imperative to remember that in a patient with a chronic headache disorder, a new type of headache may develop that heralds the onset of a new disease process, such as subarachnoid hemorrhage, intracranial mass lesion, or intracranial infection.

The specific headache
For each of the headache types, the following questions should be addressed.

When and how did the headache begin?
A headache of many years' duration and with little or no progression is probably of benign origin. Both migraine and tension-type headaches usually begin by early adulthood. In contrast, a headache of new onset has many potential causes. Certainly, an increasingly severe headache suggests the possibility of an expanding intracranial lesion. A new headache in an elderly person is always of concern and should lead to consideration of an expanding intracranial lesion or giant cell arteritis.

Are the headaches periodic? If so, what is their frequency and periodicity?
Migraine is episodic; it does not appear as a daily headache for long periods. It can occasionally occur up to several days a week. More commonly, it occurs a few times a year to a few times a month. Cluster headaches usually occur daily for weeks to months and are usually followed by a headache-free period. In its chronic form, however, cluster headache may occur daily for years. A chronic, constant daily headache usually is of tension type. Sometimes this headache is accompanied by frequent migraine headaches. This combination of headaches was previously referred to as "tension-vascular headache." If there is no regular periodicity, it is helpful to ask about the range of freedom between headaches, that is, the shortest and longest periods between attacks.

How long does it take for headaches to reach maximal intensity? How long do they last?
Migraine usually peaks in minutes to an hour or two and usually lasts a few hours to a day or two. Cluster headache is usually maximal when it awakens a patient from sleep. If onset is during wakefulness, it usually peaks within a few minutes. The duration of cluster headache is usually 30 to 90 minutes. Tension-type headaches commonly increase in intensity and may last from hours to years. A headache of sudden, severe onset suggests the possibility of an intracranial hemorrhage. When not accompanied by focal neurologic symptoms, this headache usually represents a subarachnoid hemorrhage. Stabbing, jabbing, or "ice-pick" head pains are usually momentary and occur in a small localized area. Occipital neuralgia that occurs over the posterior head region is characteristically brief and shocklike. It can usually be precipitated by percussion over the occipital nerve.

When do the headaches occur? Are there precipitating factors?
Cluster headaches characteristically awaken patients from sleep. They tend to occur at the same time each day in an individual. Migraine can occur at any time during the day or night but often begins in the morning. A headache that disturbs sleep should be considered serious until proven otherwise. Tension-type headaches usually persist throughout much of the day, oftentimes worsening late in the day.

Patients with recurrent headaches sometimes recognize factors that trigger an attack. Migraine can be triggered by bright light, menses, excessive sleep, sleep deprivation, and ingested substances (some foods and alcohol). Headaches precipitated by bending, lifting, coughing, or other Valsalva maneuvers are usually due to a benign cause. However, an intracranial lesion may underlie such headaches in a significant minority of patients. Intermittent headaches that occur when the patient is upright and are relieved by recumbency are characteristic of headaches caused by low cerebrospinal fluid pressure. Although most of these occur on the background of a lumbar puncture, spontaneous low-pressure headaches are possible. Headache associated with sexual activity is usually benign, especially if recurrent on multiple occasions. A single headache in this circumstance, however, may be due to a subarachnoid hemorrhage.

Where does the headache begin? How does the headache evolve?
It is helpful to ask the patient to outline the location of the pain. Migraine is often unilateral but may be bilateral. Sometimes it evolves from a unilateral location to become generalized. Cluster headaches are unilateral, most commonly localized behind or in the eye or in the temporal region. Tension-type headaches can be generalized or localized to the

frontal or to the occipitonuchal regions. Some tension headaches seem to begin in the nuchal muscles and spread into the occiput. When pain is localized intraorally to an eye or ear, a process affecting this structure needs to be excluded.

What is the quality and severity of the pain?
Migraine usually has a pulsatile quality that may be superimposed on a more constant pain. Cluster headache is usually characterized as severe, boring, and steady—sometimes said to be "like a hot poker." Tension-type headaches may produce tightness or pressure, and the terms "vise-like" and "bandlike" are often applied.

Do symptoms precede or accompany the headache?
Prodromal symptoms, such as hunger and psychologic changes, may precede migraine by several hours. Focal neurologic symptoms known as aura can also occur between or during migraine headaches. Visual symptoms, especially scintillating scotoma, are the most commonly described. Symptoms consistent with other hemispheric dysfunction are occasionally experienced and consist of weakness, somatosensory disturbance, and even aphasia. When sensory symptoms are present, the patient often describes them as a slow march over several minutes. Symptoms referable to the brain stem or cerebellum, rarely described, help to characterize basilar migraine. Miosis and ptosis (oculosympathetic paresis or partial Horner's syndrome), tearing, conjunctival injection, and nasal stuffiness may accompany cluster headache. In patients with new onset of a unilateral headache with an oculosympathetic paresis, an ipsilateral carotid dissection should be considered.

Nausea and vomiting, phonophobia, and photophobia are frequent accompaniments of migraine. Headache accompanied by jaw claudication, tenderness of the scalp, scalp nodules, or polymyalgia rheumatica should lead to consideration of a diagnosis of giant cell (temporal) arteritis.

What aggravates or relieves the pain?
Physical activity may aggravate migraine and may worsen or relieve tension headache. Migraine is usually ameliorated by rest and sleep. Tension-type headache is sometimes ameliorated by massage. During cluster headache, patients are often agitated and prefer to be upright, sometimes pacing.

Is there a family history of headaches?
Migraine is usually accompanied by a positive family history of similar headaches. Tension-type headaches may also be familial. Cluster headaches are usually sporadic.

What medications have been used to treat the headaches?
Response to medications used to treat individual headache attacks and those used to prevent headaches should be outlined. Dosage, route of administration, duration of treatment, response, and side effects should be recorded. The frequent use of narcotics or other analgesics may predispose the patient to analgesic rebound headaches or dependency. A history of caffeine intake should also be sought, since this substance may cause or aggravate headaches, especially when ingested in large amounts.

What concerns the patient about the headaches?
Why is the patient seeking help now?
Headaches can provoke fear and anxiety about serious underlying disease processes; the patient should be allowed to express these concerns so that they can be appropriately addressed. Furthermore, if the problem is chronic, it can be helpful to ask why the patient is seeking help at this time. The response to this query may reveal that the patient is functioning poorly at work or in the family.

Diagnostic tests and observations
Neurologic diagnostic measures, such as computed tomography, magnetic resonance imaging, electroencephalography (EEG), and angiography, are not considered here or reviewed in relation to pheochromocytoma. These tests are discussed in subsequent chapters.

If a patient is suffering from headache at the time of the examination, a number of observations may be helpful. Are the temporal vessels enlarged? Is the scalp reddened or tender (locally or diffusely)? What, if any, change is brought about in a unilateral headache by compressing the corresponding superficial temporal artery just anterior to the tragus or by cautiously compressing the common carotid artery on the corresponding side or on the opposite side? What effect is produced by hanging the head between the knees? Does coughing or bearing down affect the headache? Can you hear a bruit with the patient in the sitting, lying, or head-between-the-knees position? If the headache is a "throbbing" one, have the patient indicate the beat with his or her hand. Some neurotic "throbs" are not synchronous with the pulse.

When the superficial vessels are distended, when the scalp is unusually tender, and when a throbbing pain is eased by compression of the superficial temporal artery, it seems reasonable to suspect that the extracranial vessels are primarily involved, and the chances of an intracranial lesion seem correspondingly remote.

3. Seizure Disorders
Epilepsy or a seizure disorder is characterized by recurrent and unprovoked seizure activity. An electrographic seizure is an abnormal, sudden,

and excessive discharge of a population of neurons in the brain. Clinically, a seizure is defined as the symptoms and outward manifestations of an electrographic seizure. It should be apparent that the clinical pattern of any seizure depends on the size, location, and organization of the population of neurons initially involved in the electrographic seizure as well as on the manner and extent of spread to involve other populations of neurons. Thus, there are almost limitless patterns for seizures. Some electrographic seizures may have no recognized clinical manifestation. They are silent, or subclinical.

Epilepsy is a condition in which seizures tend to recur chronically because of a persistent morphologic or physiologic abnormality of brain tissue. Seizures, even recurrent ones, may complicate transient abnormalities of brain function with drug intoxication or withdrawal, anoxia or hypoglycemia, infection, or fever, to name a few.

Whether isolated or chronically recurrent, a seizure should be regarded as a symptom rather than a disease. The clinician should always search for the underlying cause, which, if found, may be responsive to specific therapy.

There have been many proposed classifications of seizures and epilepsy, most of which are based on combined clinical and EEG criteria. There are practical reasons for attempting to classify seizures. First, classification may point the way to the diagnosis of the underlying disease. Second, antiepileptic drug therapy appropriate to the seizure type may result. Without the working knowledge of proper classification, the physician may mistakenly diagnose a simple partial (focal) seizure as "petit mal" (now called "absence") because it is "small." The result may be selection of a drug appropriate for absence but not for partial seizures. The physician's search for a cause and counseling of the patient and family about prognosis and potential hereditary risk may also be inappropriate without proper classification and diagnosis.

History-taking from the patient with seizures

Seizures may be associated with an alteration in memory or alertness. Not uncommonly, the patient may be unaware that a seizure has been experienced. It follows that there may be both recalled and not recalled features to the seizure. For this reason, we suggest that both the history-taking and the recording in any patient with seizures be rigidly separated into that part the patient relates from personal recall and that part a witness relates directly to the physician.

The patient should be asked if he or she has had more than one kind of seizure and, if so, to name each and describe it separately. The patient should be asked about the frequency of each kind, the time of day or night it occurred, and the relation to time of falling asleep or waking, to time of menstrual cycle (if female), anovulatory drugs, or pregnancy, and to possible triggering mechanisms, such as stress (hyperventilation), sleep deprivation, alcohol intake, fasting, and sensory stimulation, such as flickering light, sounds, and smells. Does the patient recognize a prodrome? Can the patient stop a seizure once it starts? Has the pattern changed? Have antiepileptic drugs been taken? Which worked best? If discontinued, why?

In searching for a possible underlying structural lesion, the physician should ask about head injuries, infections of the nervous system, cerebrovascular accidents, and symptoms of progressing focal or diffuse cerebral dysfunction.

The patient should describe the seizure itself, from its onset (beginning of the aura, which is actually a part of the seizure) until awareness is lost or the seizure is over. If there is a loss of awareness (memory), the patient should be asked about the first thing that was recalled on coming out of the amnestic interval. Was the patient in the same place or had he or she moved or been moved? What is the best estimate of the time of the amnestic interval? Was there injury or pain of the body, back, head, tongue, buccal mucosa, or lips? Was there headache? Was there sensory, motor, or language deficit (Todd's postictal paralysis)? Was there evidence of incontinence?

The witness is then questioned in the same way. It is almost always faster and more economical to call an observer long-distance and clarify a spell of loss of consciousness than to rely only on hearsay and perhaps to pursue inappropriate avenues of investigation. The witness should also be asked whether there was a period of partial or complete unresponsiveness. Did events occur that the patient did not later recall? Some patients are unaware that there was an amnestic interval until it is substantiated by a reliable witness. What was observed postictally? Was there evidence of aphasia or hemiparesis?

Classification of seizures
The following is an outline of salient historical and descriptive features of various types of seizures patterned from the classification proposed by the International League Against Epilepsy.

Partial (focal or localization-related) seizures
There is generally clinical or EEG evidence of focal onset, and the clinical pattern reflects the site of origin.

Simple partial seizures with motor signs. A focal seizure may have as its first manifestation tonic or clonic unilateral movements of one part of the body, such as the lips, fingers, foot, head (lateral turning), or eyes (conjugate movement). The head and eye movements are usually adversive (away from the side of the seizure focus) but may be ipsiversive. The movements, once started, may remain localized or may spread (march), usually in an orderly progression, to involve other parts of the same side of the body, following the somatotopic representation of body parts on the motor cortex (homunculus). By definition, simple partial seizures are not associated with an alteration in mentation.

Simple partial seizures with sensory symptoms. There may be somatosensory (tingling), visual (flashes, lights, or patterns), auditory (tones, bells), olfactory (usually unpleasant and unidentifiable), gustatory, or vertiginous hallucinations.

Partial seizures with autonomic symptoms. The symptoms may consist of an epigastric sensation (often rising), pallor, sweating, flushing, piloerection (gooseflesh), pupillary dilation, or sexual sensations.

Partial seizures with psychic symptoms. These seizures fall into several categories. Dysphasia (language dysfunction) may result from a seizure discharge from speech areas of the dominant hemisphere. Other categories are dysmnesic (déjà vu—a new or unique experience seems strangely familiar; jamais vu—a familiar experience seems strange or new), cognitive (dreamy states), affective (fear, anger), illusions (things seen appear large or small, sounds seem to boom or echo, digits or limbs seem large), and structured hallucinations (faces, scenes, music, voices). The patient who has one of these experiences may question his or her own sanity and be hesitant to relate the experience. The physician almost always can differentiate the psychic experiences of partial seizures from those of emotional disorders on the basis of history. The seizure has sharp boundaries—a clearly defined beginning and end—described consistently by the intelligent observer. Psychic experiences in the emotionally ill patient are described vaguely and are open-ended, merging with daily experience. Problems in differential diagnosis arise in persons with both kinds of disorder.

Complex partial seizures. Partial seizures with loss or impairment of consciousness often begin with simple symptoms, particularly psychic ones. The period of impaired consciousness is almost always characterized by an amnestic interval, and witnesses may observe simply a cessation of activity or staring or falling. There may be more complex activity (automatism), such as sucking, chewing, lip-smacking, or rubbing, patting, buttoning, fumbling with the hands, or walking about in a dazed state. The activity is semipurposeful, repetitive, stereotyped, and automatic in appearance. The combination of partial complex seizure with psychic symptoms and automatism was once called "psychomotor."

Partial seizures evolving to secondarily generalized seizures. Any seizure of partial onset has the potential to evolve into a generalized seizure. Again, consciousness is lost, and the witness describes the elements of the seizure during the amnestic interval. The physician sometimes labels the part described by the patient the "aura" and the amnestic part described by the witness the "seizure." The dichotomy is obviously erroneous, since both are simply stages of a seizure in evolution.

Generalized seizures (convulsive or nonconvulsive)
The EEG pattern is usually bilateral and generalized at onset, and consciousness is lost at or near onset.

Absence seizures. In these seizures, once called "petit mal," motor activity is usually minimal, and there is simply a loss of consciousness with preserved posture and cessation of activity of a few seconds' duration. Postictally, the patient takes up the activity where it was left off. The patient may be aware of having missed something if actively engaged in conversation, for example, and ask the discussant to repeat the words. On other occasions, the patient may be unaware the episode has occurred unless it is pointed out by others. In some absence seizures, there may be associated slight clonic movements, most often of the eyelids or face, less often of the limbs. In others, postural tone may be lost, and the patient may fall limply (atonic) or, contrariwise, tone may be increased, and the victim may fall rigidly (tonic). A brief automatism may accompany absence seizure, differing from partial complex automatism only in duration, absence of postictal confusion, and, of course, associated EEG pattern.

Myoclonic seizures. Single or multiple jerks may occur, usually bilateral and symmetrical. Myoclonus may occur within minutes of awakening, while the patient attends to morning toilet, resulting in the dropping or flinging of an object, such as a glass or toothbrush, held in the hand. The jerks may become continuous (clonic seizures) and then evolve to tonic-clonic.

Tonic-clonic seizures. Although tonic-clonic seizures, once called "grand mal," may be thought of as the potential "final common pathway" of any lesser seizure, whether partial or generalized at onset, some patients have only generalized tonic-clonic seizures. The astute physician often can deduce from the history related by the patient alone that a particular episode of loss of consciousness was a tonic-clonic seizure. If the origin was focal, the episode may be recalled and described. If not, the patient may simply indicate that during some activity awareness was lost and that when the senses returned 30 minutes later, he or she had a bitten tongue, wet or soiled undergarments, headache, soreness of the back or extremities, and fatigue. The patient's first postictal memory may be of the arrival of the ambulance summoned by others, the ambulance ride, or the emergency room scene. A documented amnestic interval of less than 10 minutes is unusual in a bona fide tonic-clonic seizure.

Differentiating the epileptic seizure from other spells

Vasodepressor syncope is loss of consciousness as part of a vasodepressor reaction. Persons who are particularly susceptible may be labeled "fainters." The episodes characteristically occur in response to psychic trauma, such as the sight of blood, pain, venipuncture, observing surgery, the first time in gross anatomy laboratory, or standing in church. Usually there are associated symptoms and signs of cold sweat, pallor, nausea, light-headedness, and faintness, which may both precede and follow the loss of consciousness and last for several minutes. The loss of consciousness is brief and usually unassociated with any convulsive movements. If the episode is severe, and especially if circumstances prevent the patient from assuming the reclining position, consciousness may be lost for longer periods, and a few clonic movements of the limbs may be observed (convulsive syncope). Observers describe the pallor and limp loss of consciousness preceding relatively brief and unimpressive clonic movements.

Syncope may result from a variety of other circumstances, such as micturition (during or after; thought to be a vagal reflex), postural hypotension (neuropathic or drug-induced), and cardiac arrhythmia. In each instance, there may be minor convulsive movements. The picture may be complicated if the anoxic insult to the brain is severe or prolonged or if a concussion is suffered in an associated fall.

Transient ischemic attacks may resemble partial seizures but can usually be distinguished by sudden onset of deficit phenomena (absence of motor or sensory function) without a march. The symptoms are maximum at onset and slowly resolve.

Migrainous aurae may also resemble partial seizures, consist of positive or negative phenomena (or both), and often march. Included are either negative or fortification scotomata, aphasia, spreading tingling, and hemiparesis. The march is often much slower and less orderly than the march of partial seizures, with symptoms often clearing in one area as they appear in others. The migraine aurae typically last for 10 to 30 minutes.

Transient global amnesia is a well-recognized condition usually occurring once or a few times over several years in a middle-aged person. Memory of events at the time of the episode is lost, and there is some degree of retrograde amnesia. The episodes last several hours. There are no focal neurologic symptoms or signs. Except for repetitive questions and disorientation to current circumstances and events, behavior is normal. The patient later recognizes the event as simply a well-defined hole in the memory; it is described consistently and without embellishment. There is no established relationship to seizures or occlusive cerebrovascular disease. The condition is assumed to be due to transient dysfunction of the limbic system bilaterally and perhaps is related to migraine.

Pseudoseizures are either factitious or related to conversion reaction.

They may create a difficult problem in differential diagnosis, especially in patients familiar with organic seizure patterns or in patients who also have organic seizures. The description given by the patient is often vague, lacking clear-cut, stereotyped features. Often, a variety of symptoms that although taken individually are typical of seizure phenomena seem under careful scrutinization to represent an unlikely and varying pattern of cerebral loci. Bilateral "convulsive" movements with retained awareness, rare in organic seizures, are common in pseudoseizures. Documented incontinence is rare in pseudoseizures. The "convulsive" seizure pattern, often atypical, consists of pelvic flexion-extension movements or thrashing movements with side-to-side movement of the head and forced closure of the eyelids. Often, one must rely on the EEG findings to make the distinction. We have usually followed the rule that although an atypical spell may be organic, it is not diagnosed as organic if the EEG does not disclose specific epileptiform activity. In the patient with known epilepsy, pseudoseizures may be an additional problem. In this instance, the EEG findings again may be helpful. Prolonged recording may disclose a normal pattern during a clinical seizure, virtually excluding the possibility that the seizure is organic.

In summary, as in most neurologic diagnoses, the history is the most important element in the diagnosis of seizures and other transient spells with which they may be confused.

4. Sleep Disorders

Sleep disorders are common, and increasingly patients are expecting their physicians to be competent in solving them. They include disorders of excessive sleepiness (such as sleep apnea syndrome and narcolepsy), insomnia, circadian rhythm abnormalities, and parasomnias (such as sleepwalking and rapid eye movement sleep behavior disorder). Sleep disorders have a profound effect on society; sleepiness is a common cause of motor vehicle accidents, and sleep deprivation played a role in all the major industrial accidents of our age, such as Three Mile Island, Chernobyl, Bhopal, and Exxon Valdez.

Taking a sleep history

A sleep history involves more than a history of a patient's sleep. It is really a sleep-wake history, the compilation of a picture of a 24-hour day from the viewpoints of alertness, occupation, other activities, rest, and sleep. Collateral history from a sleeping partner, if available, should always be obtained.

Overview of a typical night's sleep
The examiner should ascertain if the sleep-wake cycle is regular. If it differs on weekends or with varying work shifts, each condition should be described separately. If it has changed recently, the premorbid sleep

pattern should also be ascertained. The patient should be asked what time she would go to bed and what time she would wake if she could set her own schedule with no societal restraints.

Sleep initiation. What time does the patient go to bed? What does he do in bed before sleep? What time does he switch off the light? How long does it take him to fall asleep? If sleep latency is prolonged, what are the reasons? What is his perceived commonest sleep position?

Sleep maintenance. How often does the patient wake during the night? What wakes her: external noise, restless sleep partner, snoring, dyspnea, cramps, other pain, indigestion, dreaming, leg kicking, sweating, need to urinate (differentiate from urination after waking from another cause)? How long does she remain awake? What does she do while she is awake: worry, clock-watch, remain in bed or get up? What does she estimate her total sleep time to be?

Sleep termination. What time does the patient wake in the morning? Does he wake spontaneously or with the help of an alarm clock? Does he feel refreshed or tired? Any early morning headache, dry mouth, sore throat, blocked nose, or confusion?

Specific nocturnal symptoms

Respiration. On how many pillows does the patient sleep? Is she dyspneic at night? Does she snore? If so, for how long? Has the severity changed? Can the snoring be heard outside the bedroom? Has her sleeping partner had to leave the bedroom because of the severity of the snoring? In which position does she snore the most? Is the patient herself aware of snoring or snorting arousals? Have episodes of stopped breathing been noticed during sleep? If so, how long do they last? Do they best fit a description of obstructive or central events? Does nocturnal stridor occur?

Movements. Is the patient a restful or a restless sleeper? Is there a history of restless legs before sleep or during the night? Has the sleeping partner noticed periodic limb movements of sleep? Does bruxism occur? Is there a current or past record of sleepwalking or sleep terrors? Does he talk, shout, or scream in his sleep? Does he have excessive jerking of his arms, legs, or trunk? If so, has he injured his sleeping partner or himself? Are the movements associated with dreaming? At what time during the night do they occur? Does he eat during the night?

Miscellaneous. Is there a history of sleep paralysis before sleep or on awakening? Have hallucinations occurred before sleep or on awakening?

Daytime symptoms
   General. The patient should be asked to describe the activities of a typical working day and nonworking day. Details of occupations are especially important. Is there a specific time of day when she is maximally alert, such as late at night ("owl") or early in the morning ("lark")?

   Excessive daily sleepiness. Collateral history is vital, because self-evaluation of sleepiness is extremely difficult. Is the patient excessively sleepy? One should attempt to differentiate mental and physical fatigue from true sleepiness. What circumstances precipitate sleepiness: working at a desk, waiting for an appointment, sitting in a conference, religious service, or theater, relaxing with friends, talking to a single person, eating, watching television, reading, driving? If sleepiness is precipitated by driving, after how long? Has a motor vehicle accident occurred due to sleepiness? Has he fallen asleep at a red traffic light? Does he take planned naps? If so, how often and for how long? Does he feel refreshed after napping?

   Cataplexy. Does the patient have spells of weakness with emotions, including laughter, fear, excitement, pleasure, and sadness? Does she have minor spells, such as sagging of the face, drooping of the jaw, or buckling of the knees?

Background history
   Psychosocial. Does the patient have a history of psychiatric disease, especially depression and anxiety disorders? Are there current or past psychosocial stressors, including a history of abuse? What are his family circumstances? Does he smoke? Does he use alcohol, and if so, what time of the day? Is there a history of other substance abuse? Does he drink caffeinated beverages? Does he exercise? Does he have adequate exposure to sunlight?

   Medical. Any past or current record of hypertension, cardiorespiratory disease, or neurologic disease (especially epilepsy or neurodegenerative diseases)? Has he undergone tonsillectomy? Has he a history of nasal trauma or disease? Is he overweight? Does he have symptoms of sexual dysfunction?

   Family History. Any family history of snoring, obstructive sleep apnea syndrome, insomnia, excessive sleepiness, narcolepsy, restless legs syndrome, sleepwalking or sleep terrors, epilepsy, psychiatric disease, or substance abuse?

Examination of the patient with a sleep complaint
There is no single examination for sleep problems. If there is even a suspicion of obstructive sleep apnea syndrome, the oropharynx should be

carefully examined, with special reference to the tonsils, uvula, soft palate, and anteroposterior and lateral diameters. The jaw should be examined for retrognathia, and the size of the tongue noted. The neck should be palpated and the external nares examined. Height, weight, and blood pressure should be measured. Pulmonary, cardiac, neurologic, or psychiatric examination should be performed as appropriate, guided by the individual problem.

Assessment

At the end of the clinical assessment, the physician should be able to give provisional answers to the following questions:

1. Is the patient excessively sleepy? If so, what are the most likely causes?
2. Does the patient have a disorder of sleep initiation or maintenance? If so, what are the most likely causes?
3. Are unusual motor or other events occurring during sleep? If so, what are the most likely causes?
4. Would the patient benefit from a laboratory sleep study or a consultation with a sleep medicine specialist?

Chapter 2

General Observations and Order of Procedure

The neurologic examination starts with the introduction to the patient and continues throughout the time spent with him or her. The patient's handshake, character of clothes, manner of seating, and general deportment may not be matters that deserve written description but may provide clues or hunches that will be helpful guides in history-taking and examination. In the following paragraphs, an attempt will be made to provide some guides to conducting the examination. In doing so, various common or typical abnormalities will be used as examples. The lists of these conditions are not meant to be complete. Rather, they are described and discussed to suggest patterns of procedure that will apply to a larger number of similar conditions.

A general survey of the patient's physical condition is of importance aside from the special tests directed toward examination of neurologic function in particular. Such a survey resembles the general physical examination except that attention is directed more specifically toward conditions that may have neurologic significance. Many systemic diseases or diseases of organ systems other than the central nervous system may have neurologic overtones. To miss the significance of the signs of these diseases might lead to a serious error in estimating the cause of the neurologic signs. The observations referred to here need not be time-consuming and can be accomplished during the course of carrying out the neurologic examination.

Some obvious physical deformities become apparent as soon as the patient has disrobed, for example, the "stork legs" of Charcot-Marie-Tooth disease or the high arch of the foot, pes cavus, and "cocked-up" toes in Friedreich's ataxia. Neurofibromas may be striking because of their large size and disfiguring appearance. More often they are small rounded elevations that, when pressed, may seem to disappear through a buttonhole in the deeper structures. They may be single or multiple and may be associated with café au lait spots. These latter are often oval and slanted along the lines of the dermatome involved. Noteworthy deformities of the spinal column or extremities may suggest the cause of attendant neurologic signs or may adequately explain symptoms that might otherwise be considered to have their basis in some defect in the nervous system. The presence of enlarged lymph nodes may be a clue to an underlying neoplasm that has spread, involving not only these nodes but parts of the nervous system as well. The presence of a brown, hairy nevus, a hairy pad of fat, or a dimple in the skin over the sacral region may be a surface clue to underlying trouble such as spina bifida or myelodysplasia.

Finally, it is essential to perform a rectal examination, particularly in patients who have any trouble with the lower extremities or low back. In doing so, it is important to note the muscle tone and the strength of the rectal sphincter. Any rectal or extrarectal masses suggestive of neoplasm are of particular interest. The hollow of the sacrum should be carefully palpated for evidence of any tumor such as chordoma.

ORDER OF PROCEDURE

When a neurologic examination is performed, it is advisable to develop an orderly method of procedure to ensure thoroughness and to reduce the examiner's effort to a minimum by making the task a matter of habit. Each examiner will develop a routine and vary it to suit his or her needs. In an effort to aid in the establishment of such a routine, the following order of proceeding with an examination is suggested. This is not a pattern to be followed rigidly but, rather, an example of one of several possible solutions to the problem.

A few minutes may well be spent in getting acquainted with the patient. Questions concerning home locality and manner of travel to the office may help to put the patient at ease. Following this, letters from the referring physician and the history, as recorded thus far, are read and verified by discussing the important portions with the patient. This leads naturally into the taking of the neurologic history.

After completion of the formal portion of the history, the more formal portion of the neurologic examination is begun. Of course, it is carried out while the patient is disrobed. First, however, it is advisable to study gait and station while the patient is wearing shoes and is unencumbered by sheets, capes, or whatever covering is supplied after disrobing. In many cases, these observations are repeated after the clothing has been removed. It is also advisable to complete the mental status and language examinations early in the course of the neurologic examination, before the patient becomes fatigued. It is sometimes advisable to watch the patient dress and undress so that difficulties with finer motions, such as those required in buttoning and unbuttoning, can be detected.

Either before or after the study of gait, but at least early in the course of examination, the region of primary interest to the patient, if there is one, should be considered by the examiner. For example, if pain or motor dysfunction of one upper extremity is the chief concern of the patient, the affected extremity should be scrutinized carefully, palpated, moved about, and otherwise examined while questions concerning it are asked in demonstration of the examiner's interest.

From then on, most experienced examiners proceed in an orderly fashion to perform the various components of the neurologic examination. A common practice is to test the cranial nerves except for sensation and then to test muscles, motor function, and stretch reflexes in the upper extremities. Thus, the examination begins to assume a regional pattern. For example, while the upper extremities are examined, the range of joint motion is observed and the arteries and nerves are palpated. At the time of tests of cranial nerves, the scalp may be scrutinized, palpated, and percussed and the head and neck auscultated. After the upper extremities have been checked, the lower extremities are considered in a similar fashion. The numerous tests of sensation may follow next.

Many examiners have evaluated the patient in the sitting and standing positions up to this point. They may now have the patient lie down so that they can check sensation on those parts of the body not accessible in the sitting position. While the patient is lying, prone or supine as the case may be, tests of muscle strength may be completed, the abdominal reflexes evaluated, the chin-chest maneuver applied, and the heel-to-heel and toe-to-finger tests performed. Any other observations best made while the patient is lying down, such as the test for Beevor's sign, are carried out. Often it is necessary to recheck the patient in the sitting or standing position before the examination is considered completed.

EXAMINATION OF THE SCALP AND SKULL

Mere inspection of the scalp of a bald person may be quite revealing, whereas beneath the abundant hair of a woman there may hide striking abnormalities. Careful palpation of the scalp and skull may reveal nothing more abnormal than the banal wen, or it may reveal a localized thickening of the skull or a cluster of abnormal blood vessels suggestive of an underlying meningioma or arteriovenous malformation. Any remarkable abnormalities of the contour and symmetry of the skull should be noted. Depressions in the skull may represent the results of fracture. Tilting of the head to one side may be the result of muscle spasm associated with a posterior cranial fossa tumor or with a herniated cervical disk. In a person who has undergone craniotomy, the scar should be examined to determine whether it is well healed or shows signs of malunion due to infection or a foreign body. In the presence of increased intracranial pressure, the bone flap may become elevated.

Percussion over the skull may reveal regions of tenderness. Such tenderness may be the result of chronic tension in the muscles of an anxious person or may be due to diseased bone overlying a tumor or abscess. In infants and young children with increased intracranial tension, percussion over the skull may give rise to a peculiar tympanic "cracked-pot" resonance. In adults, percussing over the skull for the purpose of eliciting abnormal resonance is usually unrewarding. There is considerable variation in the percussion note, depending on the region of the skull percussed and the amount of hair covering the head. These variations are usually far greater than those that can be ascribed to disease.

FACIES

During the course of history-taking, the patient's head and face may be studied unobtrusively. At times the spontaneous movements made by the patient in talking and gesturing may bring out abnormalities that are less apparent during the course of the more formal part of the neurologic examination. The so-called myopathic facies of myotonic or facioscapulohumeral types of dystrophy and the characteristic facies of myasthenia gravis are examples of abnormalities that may be detected.

The face of a patient with Parkinson's syndrome tends to be expressionless. The ordinary mobility of the features is diminished or lost. The eyes seem to have a fixed stare because of infrequent blinking. This lack of expression along with a monotony of speech may give an erroneous impression of mental dullness. What emotional expression is retained is characterized by its delayed onset and slow spread.

Adenoma sebaceum, although not constantly seen in tuberous sclerosis, is so characteristic that it is worth stressing. The skin lesions are small yellowish or reddish brown nodules and are prominently distributed in a butterfly-shaped region over the cheeks and nose. Except for being disfiguring, the lesions cause no symptoms. *Vascular nevi* of the face, in some portions of the skin supplied by the trigeminal nerve, are associated with pial angiomas and atrophy and calcification of the underlying cerebral cortex in Sturge-Weber syndrome. *Proptosis* of one eye may result from an intraorbital tumor, a meningioma of the sphenoid ridge, exophthalmic goiter, and so forth. A pulsating exophthalmos may be the result of an arteriovenous fistula of the cavernous sinus. Numerous scars over the face may represent the residuals of injuries suffered by a patient with a convulsive disorder.

Some endocrine disorders that may have neurologic accompaniments present characteristic facial changes. In *acromegaly,* the prominent supraorbital ridges, the enlarged nose and lips, and the jutting lower jaw are striking and typical. *Myxedema* may alter the face in a remarkable manner. The swelling of the skin tends to obliterate the normal lines of expression, producing a coarse, heavy face. The nostrils and lips are broad. A person with *exophthalmic goiter* may present a distinct contrast. The staring expression caused by protrusion of the ocular globes and retraction of the lids gives the impression of overalertness. This is augmented by the patient's restless and quick movements.

PERIPHERAL NERVES

In addition to an examination of the function of peripheral nerves by sensory and muscle tests, some nerves may be examined directly by inspection and palpation. If there are signs and symptoms suggestive of some disease of a peripheral nerve, it is well to look and feel carefully along the course of the nerve. Abnormal masses may be seen or felt, or there may be unusual tenderness to palpation or percussion. Some nerves may be readily palpated at the more exposed portions of their course: the radial nerve as it passes laterally around the humerus, the ulnar nerve at the elbow, and the peroneal nerve just inferior to the head of the fibula. Under such circumstances, the size and consistency of the nerve should be noted.

The character of the skin in the distribution of an injured nerve may be altered. These alterations are often described as vasomotor or trophic changes. Their nature and degree depend on the nerve injured and the extent of the injury and result from disturbed function of the sympathetic fibers within them. The changes tend to be more marked distally than proximally. They include increased warmth or coolness, redness, pallor, cyanosis, increase or decrease of sweating, atrophy of the skin or hyperkeratosis, and irregular growth of the hair and nails.

Chapter 3

Mental Function

INTRODUCTION

The study of mental function includes evaluation of cognition, behavior, level of alertness (consciousness), memory, language, and related functions. Changes in mental status are common not only in patients who come to the attention of neurologists but also in those seen by virtually all specialties of medicine, including neurosurgery, psychiatry, and general internal medicine. Changes observed generate a significant number of consultations received by the neurology service in a general hospital or in an outpatient practice. A thorough evaluation of mental function is the most important first step in general neurologic examination, and it must be conducted systematically. A traditional classification of mental status examination is found in Table 3-1.

As with all medical evaluations, the degree of detail to be pursued depends on the nature of the problem. In a patient being evaluated for lower extremity pain and no other complaints, a screening mental status examination should suffice. However, a suspected central nervous system disease of any kind, including but not limited to epilepsy, parkinsonism, dementia, and mass lesion, warrants a more detailed and more precise evaluation of mental function.

The mental status examination needs to be approached in a manner similar to that used in a general neurologic examination. The goals are to determine whether there are any deviations from expected normal values for the patient's age, education, occupational status, and social status; to try to localize the lesion or lesions causing these deviations; and to determine the mechanism of disease. Specific localization of lesions is frequently possible, but, much the same as in other neurologic diseases, in some situations precise localization is difficult to ascertain.

One must be aware of the difference between assessing competence and assessing performance. *Performance* includes the integrity of the specific cognitive function being tested but very importantly also includes the integrity of the input and output channels required to perform the function in question. The examiner must not erroneously conclude that

Table 3-1 Mental Function Subparts to Be Evaluated

1. Level of responsivity, alertness (consciousness)
2. Motivation, spontaneity, mood
3. Thought and behavior patterns
4. Attention (including directed attention and neglect)
5. Orientation
6. Memory
   A. Learning
   B. Retention and immediate recall
   C. Delayed recall
7. Calculations
8. Abstract reasoning
9. Praxis (construction and gestural)
10. Spatial skills (visuospatial and right-left orientation)

the patient has primary constructional deficit when, in fact, constructional skills are intact but the patient is deaf, blind, aphasic, inattentive, or paretic. Each of the component functions should be assessed separately to be certain it is intact before one concludes that the central integration process is impaired. Objectives of the mental status examination are, therefore,

1. To identify an isolated disturbance in a specific modality, for example, memory, attention, or language
2. To identify an impairment in general cognition, such as a confusional state or dementia, that may be produced by a systemic or neurologic condition
3. To locate and to correlate with behavioral aberrations anatomic lesions or physiologic derangement, utilizing, if necessary, ancillary studies such as neuroimaging or electrophysiologic testing
4. To establish measurable baseline values for longitudinal study of the patient

The neurologist must master a clinical routine that can be applied to all patients within a reasonable time and in all sites of patient-physician interaction, including the emergency department, hospital bedside, and outpatient office. For an adequate evaluation, the following procedures are necessary:

1. Neurologic and general medical history
2. Behavioral observations
3. Mental status examination (including the Short Test of Mental Status)

HISTORY

Many patients who have mental status changes cannot, by the very nature of the changes, give an ordered and detailed history. Therefore, the history should be obtained from both the patient and another observer (spouse, sibling, friend, etc.) who is knowledgeable about the patient's current behavior and past condition.

Questions to Be Answered During History-Taking
The following questions are essential:

1. What are the age, educational, sex, and occupational data for the patient (if the patient is retired, one should record the modal occupation, that is, the occupation in which the patient spent the most working years, as well as the last occupation from which the patient retired)?
2. Is the patient right- or left-handed? Has the patient ever switched handedness? Are there first-degree relatives who are left-handed?
3. What is the maximum number of years of formal education attained?
4. What changes have occurred in the patient's memory, behavior, and thinking? Patients and relatives often find it very difficult to describe the changes they observe. They should be encouraged to give specific examples. For example, if the patient's memory is poor, what sort of information does the patient tend to forget? People's names? Recent conversations? Does the patient misplace items frequently?
5. What was the mode of onset of the symptoms? Was it abrupt, occurring over minutes or hours? Was it subacute, occurring over days or weeks? Or was it insidious, occurring over a long period, measurable in months or years? Again, patients and their relatives, especially in instances of chronic progressive disease such as Alzheimer's, find it difficult to define the precise onset. Often, a detailed discussion between the informants and the physician can yield at least the year in which the observed changes were first noted.
6. What has been the rate of progression of the symptoms? Has progression been steady or stepwise? Have there been episodes of improvement or a long period when symptoms did not seem to progress (a plateau) before progression resumed?
7. Have there been any changes in the patient's interest in and involvement with family and outside-the-home activities? Does the patient follow the news, watch television, read newspapers, pursue hobbies, and keep up with family events such as birthdays and other celebrations?
8. What are the patient's current abilities in carrying out everyday activities, specifically

    - Personal care (bathing, toileting, dressing, undressing, grooming, and feeding self)

- Finances and business (ability to work in customary job and ability to take care of bills, checkbook, shopping, and financial planning)
- Personality changes (initiative, sensitivity, irritability, self-control, and social graces)
- Mood (sadness, hopelessness, hilarity, mania, agitation, inappropriateness, swings of mood, and changes in sleep, libido, and appetite)
- Thought and behavior pattern (paranoia, phobia, obsessions, delusions, hallucinations, and fixed ideas)
- Language and communication abilities (difficulty with proper nouns, common nouns, completing thoughts and sentences, and intelligibility; ability to understand and carry out instructions; and ability to read and write)?

Behavioral Observations During History-Taking

The evaluation of mental status begins as soon as the examiner opens the interview by an introduction. One must observe whether the patient is appropriately dressed, proper in demeanor, and attentive. Is the patient's language fluent and appropriate for the occasion and for the level of education and social status? Patients with memory difficulties often turn to their accompanying spouse or other person for help in answering questions. Patients with a memory disorder (amnesia) may not remember their problems, and those with right hemisphere lesions may be unaware of their difficulties (anosognosia) during the evaluations. Preoccupations, hallucinations, or delusions may become apparent. Depressed patients may be slow to respond, negativistic, and bland. Manic patients may be boisterous and logorrheic. Patients with schizophrenia may show bland affect and do not establish eye contact or formal communication. Some patients with frontal lobe disturbances may be *abulic* or may show inappropriate hilarity or aggressiveness. Many patients with mental status problems may have motor impersistence. They also may wander out of the examining room. Some patients may show extreme lability of affect, going from tears to laughter with minimal contextual reason. This lability may indicate lesions of the pathways that project from the prefrontal cortex to the brain stem, and it is sometimes called *pseudobulbar affect.*

EXAMINATION

The mental status examination should be carried out in a setting where the patient is least likely to be distracted by extraneous noise, activity, beepers, telephone, or loudspeaker announcements. Frequently, having a familiar person such as the spouse in the room helps reassure the patient. In some instances, such a person is a distraction, and the patient should be examined alone. To ensure maximal efficiency, the patient should have available his or her usual eyeglasses and hearing aids. For extremely hearing-impaired patients, a communication device such as a sound enhancer should be available to the examiner. An unruled piece of paper on which to draw figures, pencils and pens, and good lighting must be available.

Before intellectual function is assessed, the patient's level of *alertness* (consciousness) must be established. If arousal is diminished, interpretations of the mental status examination will be more difficult. Assessment of an altered level of consciousness and examination of the comatose patient are discussed in Chapter 12. After the level of arousal has been assessed, the examiner should order the mental status examination in such a way that most information can be gathered in the most timely fashion. Specific cognitive function can always be tested, but one must keep in mind the strategy outlined previously about integrity of input and output channels.

Attention

Attention and language need to be assessed early in the examination because, if they are impaired, interpretation of the remainder of the mental status examination must be qualified. A patient may perform poorly in learning and memory not because of specific impairment but because of defective attention. The two essential components of attention are alertness and directed attention.

Alertness

Arousal, or alertness, refers to a patient's overall ability to attend to environmental stimuli. Disturbances of this function result in impersistence, diminished resistance to interference, inability to inhibit inappropriate responses, and perseveration. These functions, which may be manifested in a variety of ways, can be assessed by testing for attention span, perseverance, and resistance to interference.

Attention span
The following assessments can be done to test attention span.
   1. Forward and backward digit spans. The examiner reads a list of random digits to the patient, pausing 1 second between digits and usually starting at a span of four digits and going upward. The patient needs to exactly reproduce the forward or backward span, whichever is asked for. If the patient fails two successive attempts at the same digit span or is able to give nine digits forward, the test can be stopped. Generally, the reverse digit span for a normal person should be no more than two digits fewer than the forward digit span.

2. Continuous performance tasks. The patient is required to attend to a continuing set of stimuli and make a response as instructed. For example, the patient may listen to a series of orally presented letters for 10 minutes and respond every time a target letter is heard. The test also can be presented visually.

Perseverance
Patients with difficulty in holding attention are able to begin the task but unable to sustain its performance. Perseveration can be tested by such tests as

1. Recitation of months of the year forward and backward.
2. Days of the week forward and backward.
3. Alphabet forward and backward.
4. Controlled oral word association test. The patient is asked to give common nouns starting with the letter "F," "A," or "S," with 60 seconds allowed for each letter. The patient is told not to use proper nouns, such as people or place names, or to repeat the same word with a different ending, such as "look," "looking," and "looker."
5. Category fluency test. The patient is asked to name, during a span of 60 seconds each, all animals, vegetables, and fruits he or she can think of.

During recitation of the months backward and forward, the patient should be timed. Most normal persons should be able to recite the months of the year forward accurately and quickly and backward within 20 seconds. In the controlled oral word association test or the category fluency test, intrusion of one category on another and repetitions should be noted. Most patients should produce about 10 words in each category in 60 seconds without repetition or intrusion from one category to another.

Resistance to interference
Some patients with impaired attention are unable to inhibit inappropriate responses. They make embarrassing comments in certain social contexts or behave inappropriately in other ways. Formal tests are available that require the patient to inhibit a "natural" tendency to successfully complete the task. Many of these tests involve more than a single cognitive function, but all require good attention. Consequently, a fine localization of these functions is not possible. Some regions of the brain, however, participate more extensively than others, for example, the ascending reticular activating system in the upper brain stem, thalamus, and frontal regions. Certain subcortical structures that project to the frontal lobes also participate in the maintenance of attention. Typically, bilateral involvement is necessary for a serious disruption of function,

but occasionally unilateral frontal lesions can impair subtle aspects of attention.

Directed attention
The other major dimension of attention refers to directed allocation of attention to extrapersonal space, allowing a person to focus on selected environmental stimuli. Disorders of this function lead to neglect. A variety of tasks may be used.

1. Double simultaneous stimulation of tactile, visual, and auditory sensations
2. Verbal and nonverbal stimulus cancellation tasks
3. Line bisection tasks
4. Manual exploration tasks hidden from sight

The alteration of directed attention appears to be a function of the nondominant hemisphere, although the ability to distribute attention to the right hemispace is partially a bilateral function; hence, a right hemisphere lesion may produce a significant left hemisphere neglect, whereas bilateral lesions may be required to produce right neglect. Left neglect is more common than right neglect, possibly because these functions are unequally distributed in the hemispheres. In general, parietal regions are more intimately involved in the allocation of attention, but prefrontal structures and subcortical structures also contribute to the execution of these functions.

Language
A detailed description of the evaluation of language can be found in Chapter 4. In the context of an appropriate mental status examination, at least a preliminary language evaluation is necessary because, just as in severe problems of attention, severe problems of language interfere with the execution and interpretation of the rest of the mental status examination. During the mental status examination, it is necessary to obtain and record some information on *fluency, comprehension, naming,* and *repetition.*

Fluency
Fluency is defined as the rate and accuracy of expression of thoughts and ideas. In many instances, patients seem to have normal language output when all they are doing is engaging in "automatic," nonpropositional language, such as exchanging pleasantries and greetings. For adequate assessment of fluency, the patient is asked to look at a picture, describe it orally, and write a few sentences about the picture. The appropriate use of language, correctness of grammatical construction, and verbal and literal *paraphasias* can be detected with this procedure.

Comprehension
The patient is asked to do a series of maneuvers. These could be one-stage, such as "Open your mouth," or two-stage, such as "First look at the ceiling, and then point to the floor," or conditional, such as "If there is a bicycle in this room, stand up." The requests to perform these actions can be given orally or in writing to test both aural and written comprehension. Sometimes, the patient is given a sentence to complete, such as "The lawyers' concluding argument failed to convince. . . ." Sometimes the patient is given a passive voice construction, such as "The wolf was eaten by the bear," and then the patient is asked, "Who stayed alive?"

Naming
The patient is asked to identify common pictures. These could be photographs or line drawings. If the patient fails, one needs to understand whether the patient has no idea about the use of the object or has difficulty remembering the actual name. Many patients resort to circumlocutions; for example, while trying to name a key, they might say, "You know, it is used to open things." Patients may be given actual objects, such as a fork, a comb, or a knife, and be asked to demonstrate their actual use if they cannot name them.

Repetition
The patient is asked to repeat sentences such as "No ifs, ands, or buts" or "She came home in a blue Cadillac and a flood of tears."

This very brief screening language examination will give an idea of the nature of the language difficulty and also its effect on the performance of the rest of the mental status examination.

Memory
The accurate assessment of memory is perhaps the most important component of mental status testing. Patients with cognitive disturbances most frequently come to attention because of their or their families' complaints of memory dysfunction. Learning, retention, and recall are complex functions. Exhaustive evaluation can be quite time-consuming. Nevertheless, several procedures can be used to screen memory function. In general, learning and remembering can be described as acquisition and retrieval of the memory traces to be learned.

Memory terminology can be confusing. Different examiners disagree when they use terms such as "short-term memory," "recent memory," "remote memory," and "long-term memory." Consequently, these designations are best avoided; rather, the examiner should describe the evaluation operationally, that is, by the amount and type of material presented to the patient, the recall interval, and the instructions given to the patient to reproduce this material. Typical examples are series of words or pictures, the number of trials required to learn the material, and the delay before the material is recalled. At the time of recall, the patient should be asked to remember the material unaided. If the patient fails, the examiner may give cues or prompts, again operationally defining and describing these. If the cues and prompts fail, the patient should be told to select the target word or picture from the entire list. This is a *recognition* test. In this way, the examiner can assess the essential components of learning and remembering.

1. *Acquisition* is assessed by learning trials.
2. *Retention* is assessed by recall after a delayed interval.
3. *Retrieval* is assessed by noting the difference between the amount of material recalled without cues or prompts and the amount identified on the recognition task.

Some patients with early dementia manifest a retrieval failure only. They are able to learn material, but after a delay of approximately 20 minutes, they are unable to recall it without prompting. However, when given the recognition test, they identify all the items correctly. The implication is that they continue to retain the material but are unable to retrieve it unaided.

It usually is desirable to test both verbal and nonverbal learning; occasionally, memory deficits are detected with only one form of material. To compare verbal and nonverbal learning, one could use the three-word, three-shape test of Mesulam. The patient is shown three words and three shapes and asked to copy the six items. The materials are taken away for 30 seconds, and the patient then is asked to reproduce the six items. If the patient fails, the test items are shown again, and the procedure is repeated until either all six items are recalled correctly or four additional learning trials have been completed. After completing the remainder of the mental status testing, the patient is asked to reproduce the six items. If this attempt ends in failure, the patient is asked to identify the six items from a set of 10 shapes and 10 words.

Localization of the components of memory can be specified with some precision. The temporal lobe, particularly the mesial and temporal structures, including the hippocampus and parahippocampal gyri, is important for acquisition and retrieval of information. Some subcortical structures, such as the basal forebrain, the substantia innominata, the mammillary bodies, the medial dorsal nuclei of the thalamus, and, in particular, the limbic system, are involved in the acquisition of new information. This is not to say, however, that memories are actually stored in these structures. These structures participate in the storage or retrieval processes. Prefrontal structures may be involved in generating learning and recall strategies. In some patients, verbal memory deficits are associated with dominant hemisphere lesions, and nonverbal deficits are correlated with the nondominant hemisphere. Generally, however, bilateral lesions are necessary for profound memory deficits.

Visuospatial and Perceptual Tasks
Perceptual functions are relatively nonverbal and deal with transferring sensory inputs into meaningful interpretations. Much of this behavior is mediated by the nondominant parietal lobe, and damage to the region impairs these functions.

A variety of tasks can be presented to patients to assess visuospatial-perceptual functions, and some require a minimum of testing equipment. These tests are readily available and can be considered by the examiner. A means of assessing visuospatial localization at the bedside is to ask the patient to name the states bordering his or her state of residence, or the patient can be asked to name the states through which one would pass when traveling from Chicago to New York or within any other area familiar to the patient. If the patient has adequate education, these tasks allow one to assess the ability to visualize and interpret visuospatial relations.

Agnosias
Agnosias exist in specific senses: visual, auditory, and tactile. The patient can be asked to identify pictures, line drawings, or actual objects in a visual naming task. If there is anomic aphasia, performance of the task may be impaired. The patient then may be asked to demonstrate the use of actual objects. Tactile agnosia should be differentiated from astereognosis. In tactile agnosia, all basic somatosensory functions are intact, yet the patient has difficulty recognizing familiar objects by touch alone. In astereognosis, objects are not identified because of basic somatosensory imperception. Tactile agnosia results from a focal lesion of the inferior parietal lobe and generally affects only the contralateral hand.

Apraxia
The inability to perform a complex motor task despite the integrity of primary motor, sensory, cerebellar, basal ganglia, and other functions and otherwise normal cognition is called "apraxia." Apraxia is a complex disorder generally involving execution of commands with both the limbs and the midline body parts. To adequately assess apraxia, one should ask the patient to perform a variety of tasks on command, by imitation, or with actual objects in hand. The patient may be asked to demonstrate how to cough, kiss, smile, or blow out the cheeks and then be asked to use, first, the dominant hand and, next, the nondominant hand to demonstrate how to salute, use a toothbrush, hammer a nail, flip a coin, comb one's hair, and beckon to another person. If the patient is unable to perform some of these tasks, the examiner may demonstrate the task and ask the patient to imitate the motion. If the patient is unable to do

this, an actual object, such as a comb, a key, a knife, a fork, or scissors, may be given to the patient, and performance can be assessed with the object. The patient may be asked to do a sequential task, such as hanging a picture on the wall, finding a number in the telephone book and making a telephone call, or writing a letter, sealing it, and mailing it.

Generally speaking, praxis functions require the integrity of the left hemisphere, where motor programs may be stored. Functions performed with the nondominant hand also require the transfer of these programs to the nondominant hemisphere, largely through the corpus callosum, and integrity of nondominant hemisphere structures is necessary.

Constructional Tasks
Constructional tasks expand on perceptual abilities and add skilled motor functions. These functions are assessed by asking the patient to make a drawing, such as a clock face indicating 20 minutes after 11 or a house, or to copy a design, such as a cube. A more complex task is the copying of the Rey-Osterrieth complex figure (Fig. 3-1). The completeness of the execution and the strategy involved in executing the complex figure, such as making an outline first and then filling in the details rather than starting from one corner and continuing onward, can be noted. Once the copy is completed, the patient may be asked to reproduce the figure from memory after an elapse of time. Inability to complete constructional tasks may be due to poor planning, poor sequencing, poor attention, or abnormal directed attention. Some patients neglect one side of the figure.

It has been postulated that the nondominant parietal lobe allows one to provide the overall outline of a figure and that the dominant parietal lobe contributes to the addition of internal detail. In general, most constructional tasks rely more heavily on intact functioning of the nondominant parietal lobe.

Abstract Reasoning and Conceptual Functions
Some higher cortical functions are so complex that many areas of the cortex and subcortical structures participate in the execution. Consequently, they have little localizing value in the mental status assessment. They are important, however, because they may be the only functions affected in mild cognitive impairment. Essentially, these tasks require the patient to draw upon acquired knowledge and apply it to a task in a novel or, at least, unfamiliar fashion. One task commonly used to assess these functions is the interpretation of *proverbs*, which requires the patient to explain what the phrase means. The proverbs can be common, such as, "People who live in glass houses should not throw stones," or uncommon, such as "You can knock down an iron gate with a golden hammer." The responses can be graded by the degree of abstraction. One

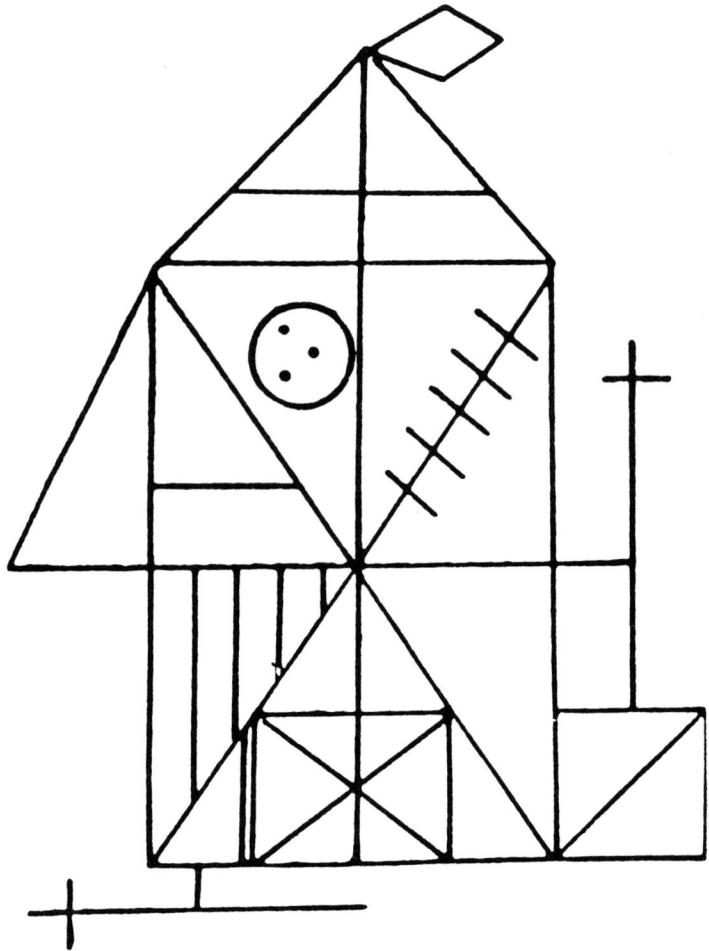

Figure 3-1
Rey-Osterrieth complex figure. (From Osterrieth PA: Le test de copie d'une figure complexe; contribution à l étude dela perception et de la memoire, *Arch Psychol*, 30:205–353, 1945.)

also can evaluate the interpretation of *similarities,* such as an orange and a banana, a dog and a horse, or a table and a bookcase. The inability to see any similarity at all or to interpret similarities on the basis of concrete attributes such as color and shape is noted.

Other Cortical Functions
Calculations
Calculation is a complex cognitive task that involves a variety of different functions, including the use of memorized mathematical tables, proper alignment of numbers in performing written calculation, and the

arithmetic operation itself. In the evaluation of calculations, one should test for

1. Addition, subtraction, multiplication, and division. The tasks given the patient should require true arithmetic manipulations rather than simple rote memory. For example, asking a patient to multiply 5×7 may simply be a memory task, but asking the patient to multiply 5×17 tests true arithmetic function.
2. "Algebra" problem. The patient is given a problem such as "I have a total of 18 books. I want to arrange them in such a fashion that one shelf has twice as many books as the other. How many books shall I put on each shelf?" The correct answer is 6 and 12, of course.
3. Arithmetic "word problem." The patient may be asked to give the correct answer to the following question: "Eggs are 60¢ a dozen. I have $1.00. How many eggs can I purchase for $1.00?" The correct answer is 20.

Right-left orientation

Right and left orientation has some localizing value in the assessment of cognitive function. The task requires that the person identify right from left for his or her own body and for the examiner's body. The task can be further refined by asking the person to identify a specific body part, such as the right index finger or the left earlobe. Focal lesions in the dominant angular gyrus can produce difficulties with right and left orientation but not exclusively so.

Summary

1. Frontal lobe functions are assessed by attention and high-order reasoning tasks.
2. Dominant hemisphere functions are assessed by language and verbal memory tasks that require the temporal limbic system and language function to be intact. Other functions, such as right-left orientation, finger gnosis, and calculations, also have been used to assess more posterior dominant hemisphere functions.
3. The nondominant hemisphere is evaluated by nonverbal memory performance, which assesses temporal limbic system function and visuospatial skills, and by constructional performance.

Thus, performing a systematic mental status examination allows one to survey cortical and subcortical structures from anterior to posterior in the dominant and nondominant hemispheres and to help localize lesions, to a certain degree, that cause cognitive impairment.

A detailed mental status examination can be time-consuming. To achieve an understanding of a patient's mental function in a relatively short time (minutes), one can use a standardized screening examination.

The most commonly used is the Mini-Mental State Examination, which has a maximum of 30 points. A specific test developed at the Mayo Clinic, the Short Test of Mental Status, has been used in a large number of patients.

SHORT TEST OF MENTAL STATUS

The Short Test of Mental Status should be performed early in the neurologic examination to minimize the effects of fatigue and inattention. The test is designed to give semiquantitative information on the patient's functioning on the subtests outlined in Table 3-2.

Orientation
The patient is asked to give his or her (1) full name; (2) address; current location, that is, (3) building, (4) city, and (5) state; and the current date — (6) either the day of the week or the day of the month, (7) the month, and (8) the year. Each correct response is worth 1 point. The maximal score is 8.

Attention
The second subtest is forward digit span. The patient is told, "I will give you a series of numbers. Please pay close attention to them, wait until I

Table 3-2 Short Test of Mental Status

Subtest	Maximal Possible Score
Orientation	8
Attention	7

Learning
  Number of words learned (maximum of 4)
  Number of trials (maximum of 4) for acquisition
	4

Arithmetic calculation	4
Abstraction	3
Information	4
Construction	4
Recall	4
Total score*	38

* Total score = sum of subtest scores − (number of trials for acquisition − 1). For example, if a patient learned all four words on the first trial, nothing was subtracted from the sum of the subtest scores. If a patient required four trials to learn some or all four words, 3 was subtracted from the sum of the subtest scores.

From Kokmen E, Naessens JM, Offord KP: A short test of mental status: description and preliminary results, Mayo Clin Proc 62:281–288, 1987. By permission of Mayo Foundation.

am finished, and then repeat the numbers back to me in the same order as I have given them." Usually, a span of five digits is given to the patient. If the patient responds correctly, the span is increased to six and then to seven. The patient's best performance is then recorded. If the patient is able to repeat seven digits forward, the test is terminated. The number of digits correctly repeated is the score; the maximal score is 7, and the minimal score is 0.

Learning
The patient is told, "I shall now give you four words. I would like you to learn them, keep them in mind, and repeat them to me from time to time when I ask you to do so." The four words are always "apple," "Mr. Johnson," "charity," and "tunnel." The patient is asked to repeat the words. If he or she learns the words on the first trial, the next subtest is given. If the patient is unable to learn all four words, the investigator repeats them for a maximum of four trials and records the number of trials the patient requires to learn all four words. If the patient is unable to learn all four words by the end of the fourth trial, the patient's best performance is recorded (the number of words learned and the number of trials required). A point is earned for each word learned (a maximum of 4 points). The number of trials (a maximum of four) required to learn the words is recorded separately.

Arithmetic Calculation
The patient is asked to multiply 5 by 13, to subtract 7 from 65, to divide 58 by 2, and to add 11 and 29. Each correct answer earns 1 point, and the maximal score is 4.

Abstraction
Interpretation of similarities in word pairs is used as a test of abstraction. The word pairs are as follows: orange/banana, horse/dog, and table/bookcase. One point for each word pair is given only for definitely abstract interpretations (for example, horse/dog = animal). Concrete interpretations or inability to see a similarity earns 0 points for that word pair. The maximal score is 3.

Information
The patient is asked to name the current president of the United States and the first president of the United States, to state the number of weeks in a year, and to define an island. Each correct answer earns 1 point, and the maximal score is 4.

Construction
The patient is asked to draw the face of a clock showing 11:15 and to copy a three-dimensional cube (Fig. 3-2). The patient is able to view the

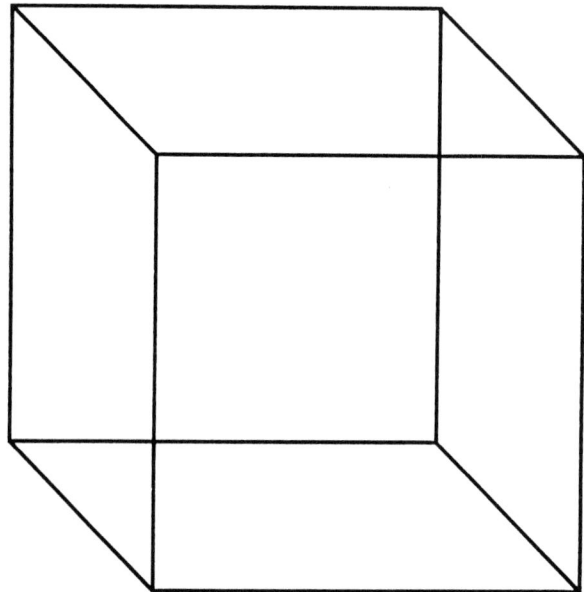

Figure 3-2
Cube that patient is asked to copy in construction portion of Short Test of Mental Status.

diagram of the cube while drawing his or her own version. For each construction, an adequate conceptual drawing is scored as 2, a less than complete drawing as 1, and inability to perform the task as 0. The maximal score for the construction task is 4.

Recall
At the end of the test, the patient is asked to recall the four words from the learning subtest: "apple," "Mr. Johnson," "charity," and "tunnel." No cues or reminders are given. The patient earns 1 point for each word recalled, and the maximal score is 4.

Total Score
The total score for each patient is the sum of the scores on the eight subtests. If more than one trial was required in the learning task, the number of trials in excess of one is subtracted from the total score (thus, a number from 0 to 3 may be subtracted). The highest possible score on the test is 38. The results of the Short Test of Mental Status in normal subjects are summarized in Table 3-3.

The Short Test of Mental Status gives a general idea of the cognitive abilities of the patient. Any patient who scores less than 29 should have

Table 3-3 Mean and Median Values for Component and Total Scores of the Short Test of Mental Status and Characteristics of 93 Patients Without Dementia andf 67 Patients With Alzheimer's Dementia*

Subtest and Patient Characteristics	Patients Without Dementia		Patients With Alzheimer's Dementia	
	MEAN ± SD	MEDIAN	MEAN ± SD	MEDIAN
Orientation	7.9 ± 0.3	8	5.0 ± 2.2	6
Attention	6.1 ± 0.8	6	5.2 ± 0.9	5
Learning	4.0 ± 0	4	3.4 ± 1.0	4
No. of trials	1.2 ± 0.5	1	3.0 ± 1.1	3
Calculation	3.3 ± 0.9	4	1.5 ± 1.5	1
Abstraction	2.0 ± 1.1	2	1.2 ± 1.2	1
Information	3.7 ± 0.7	4	2.1 ± 1.3	2
Construction	3.0 ± 1.1	3	1.3 ± 1.3	1
Recall	3.2 ± 1.0	3	0.9 ± 1.2	0
Total score	33.1 ± 3.0	33	18.5 ± 8.0	20
Age, yr	51.5 ± 16.1	54	71.1 ± 8.4	72
Education, yr	12.9 ± 2.6	12	12.8 ± 3.4	12
Duration of disease, yr	—	—	2.9 ± 1.9	2.8

* Result of Wilcoxon's rank sum test for education was not significant ($P = 0.664$). Results of Wilcoxon's rank sum tests for all other measures were significant ($P < 0.001$).

From Kokmen E, Naessens JM, Offord KP: A short test of mental status: description and preliminary results, Mayo Clin Proc 62:281–288, 1987. By permission of Mayo Foundation.

a more detailed evaluation for dementia and related disorders. It must also be emphasized that a single short test like this one *should not be the sole basis* of a diagnosis of dementia or any other cognitive disturbance. Some demented patients may score high, and some nondemented patients may score low. Performance of patients on the various subtests may also constitute important clues; the profile of individual scores may be more informative than the total score, which must be regarded with caution because the subtests measure different abilities.

CONCLUSIONS

At the end of the mental function examination, the following questions ought to have been answered.

1. Is there a generalized central nervous system dysfunction, such as dementia or a confusional state?

2. Is there an identified condition, such as agnosia, apraxia, aphasia, or selected memory or learning deficits?
3. What is the severity of the patient's problem?
4. What are the implications of observed aberrations of mental function for localization, for example, anterior (frontal) or posterior (parietotemporo-occipital), right (nondominant) or left (dominant), and deep (brain stem, thalamus, and others) or surface (cortex) regions of the brain?
5. What are the implications of the history and examination findings for a pathologic process affecting the central nervous system, for example, hereditary, congenital, "degenerative," cerebrovascular, neoplastic, inflammatory, metabolic-nutritional, or other mechanism?
6. If cognitive impairment is suspected, what is the implication for a lifelong cognitive continuum? Is the observed impairment explicable by the patient's age, education, occupation, or socioeconomic status? Is the impairment minimal and localized, that is, not affecting age, situation, and activities of daily living? Is the impairment the beginning of a progressive dementing illness?

Chapter 4

Language and Motor Speech

A change in language or motor speech can be the first or only sign of neurologic disease, or it can be one of many signs and symptoms. The purposes of this chapter are to identify different types of motor speech and language defects that can occur from lesions of the nervous system, to describe their characteristics, to show how they can enrich the neurologic examination, and to describe how examination of speech and language can contribute to localization of lesions and, in some instances, to identification of a specific neurologic disease. This chapter focuses primarily on three major subtypes of neurologic communicative disorders: *dysarthria, apraxia of speech,* and *aphasia.*

There is a direct and logical relationship between specific deviant auditory-perceptual speech features on the one hand and lesion location and pathophysiology on the other. It needs to be emphasized that it is not the particular disease itself that determines the speech characteristics but the *location* of the disease in the nervous system; for example, although their temporal courses may differ, stroke and neoplasm may produce the same motor speech and language disorders so long as their neuroanatomic locations are the same.

MOTOR SPEECH DISORDERS

Definition of Motor Speech Disorders
Dysarthria
The peripheral motor speech mechanism is a musculoskeletal system comprised of four major components:

1. *Respiration:* the diaphragm and thoracic and abdominal muscles.
2. *Phonation:* the intrinsic and extrinsic laryngeal muscles.
3. *Resonation:* the pharyngeal and velopharyngeal muscles.
4. *Articulation:* the lingual, facial, and mandibular muscles.

"Dysarthria" is a generic term that applies to a family of motor speech disorders that reflect muscular weakness, incoordination, slowness, or excess or variable speed of movement of the muscles of respiration, phonation, resonation, or articulation and that are due to lesions of sensorimotor mechanisms within the central or peripheral nervous system. "Dysarthria" describes speech disorders of *neurologic* origin and not disorders due to anatomic deformities or psychopathology. Dysarthria is a defect of the physiology of motor speech. Although it interferes with the expression of language, it is not a language disorder per se.

Apraxia of speech
Apraxia of speech is a motor speech disorder that results from impaired programming or planning of learned movement patterns, sequences, and placements of speech structures as a result of damage to portions of the dominant cerebral hemisphere. It can impair respiration and phonation but is primarily a disorder of articulation and prosody.

It is important to distinguish between dysarthria and apraxia of speech. The speech musculature in apraxia of speech is normal in strength and basic coordination; the speech deficits arise not from the patient's inability to move muscles physically but from an impaired ability to plan or program *how* they should be moved. Like dysarthria, apraxia is not a language disorder, although it can profoundly impair language expression by blocking its outflow.

Synonyms often used in place of apraxia of speech are "motor aphasia," "oral-verbal apraxia," and "aphemia." The term "aphasia" in referring to apraxia of speech is a historic carryover into current literature and is misleading because by definition aphasia is a language and not a motor speech disorder.

The Dysarthrias
Dysarthria is a plural disorder, one associated with several subtypes. Each type of dysarthria is distinct from other types because (1) it sounds distinctively different, (2) the location of the lesion producing it is different, and (3) the resulting neuromuscular dysfunction producing it is different from other subtypes. As a result, recognizing the characteristics of a specific type of dysarthria can lead to logical inferences about probable location of the offending lesion.

Examination for dysarthria
Before the different speech characteristics of the subtypes of dysarthria and apraxia of speech are described, examination of the patient for these disorders will be reviewed.

History
The following questions are important.
1. When did you first notice a change in your speech?
2. What was the first thing you noticed about it?

3. Did it come on by itself, or did you have other symptoms along with it?
4. Did the speech change come on suddenly or gradually?
5. Has it worsened, stabilized, fluctuated, or improved?
6. Has your speech ever returned to normal?
7. If so, how long did periods of normal speech last?
8. Have you had trouble with swallowing during the course of your speech difficulty?
9. Have you had a tendency to laugh or cry more easily than you used to since your speech problem began?
10. Have other people noticed the change in your speech?
11. Does your speech get noticeably worse during prolonged talking?
12. How difficult is it for others to understand you?
13. Have you had any therapy for your speech disorder?
14. Has therapy been beneficial?
15. Are you taking any medications that seem to affect your speech?

Oral mechanism examination

The oral mechanism is examined to assess the strength, speed, and symmetry of the peripheral speech musculature. The mouth, tongue, velopharynx, and larynx are observed. Tongue blade, flashlight, and mirror are necessary equipment.

1. Mouth. The mouth should be observed under the following conditions:
    a. Rest. Are the angles of the mouth bilaterally symmetrical, or does one side rest lower than the other?
    b. Smiling. Do both angles of the mouth elevate equally, or does one side do so more than the other? Are the angles of the mouth drawn up to a normal height, or are they just pulled laterally in a "horizontal smile"?
    c. Rounding. Do the lips close completely, or does an opening remain between them?
    d. Puffing. When the patient is asked to puff up the cheeks and to impound the air, does air easily leak out between the lips without or with the examiner pressing in on the patient's cheeks?
2. Tongue.
    a. Rest. The patient is asked to open the mouth and to allow the tongue to rest quietly on the floor of the mouth.
        (1) Does it appear normal in size bilaterally?
        (2) Does the tongue as a whole remain quiet on the floor of the mouth, or does it move unpredictably in lateral or anteroposterior directions? Does it have a tendency to twist on its longitudinal axis, or does the tip or back of the tongue tend to rise and fall?

(3) Are there dimpling movements (fasciculations) on the dorsum or along the sides of the tongue?
  b. Protrusion. The patient is asked to protrude the tongue and to hold it at rest.
    (1) Are there signs of loss of tongue mass, such as atrophy or furrowing, or indentations on one or both sides of the tongue?
    (2) Are there fasciculations on the dorsum or along the sides of the tongue?
    (3) Does the tongue protrude symmetrically, or does it deviate to one side?
  c. Wiggle. With the tongue protruded, the patient is asked to wiggle it from side to side as rapidly and evenly as possible.
    (1) Are these movements slow?
    (2) Are the movements more rapid than normal or even tremulous?
    (3) Does the range of tongue movements extend to the angles of the mouth, or is it confined to the center? Are the movements from side to side regular, or are they intermittently fast and slow? Are they uniform or variable in range?
  d. Strength
    (1) Protrusion. The patient is asked to protrude the tongue and resist the pressure of a tongue blade as it is pushed backward against the tip of the tongue.
      (a) Does the tongue fully resist the examiner's inward pressure, or does it buckle under pressure?
      (b) Does the tongue normally resist the pressure at first but then suddenly give way completely?
    (2) Lateralization. The patient is asked to place the tongue in the cheek, bulging it out as much as possible, resisting the examiner's effort to press against the cheek with the index finger. This act is performed on both sides.
      (a) Does the tongue collapse inwardly as the examiner maintains the pressure?
      (b) Does the tongue resist more on one side than on the other? Does it resist normally at first and then give way suddenly and unexpectedly?
3. Velopharynx.
  a. Rest. The patient is asked to open the mouth. With the light illuminating the oropharynx and the tongue depressor gently pressing the tongue downward and out of the way, the examiner observes the soft palate during complete rest.
    (1) Are the faucial arches of the soft palate symmetrical? Does the soft palate appear to rest lower on one side than on the other?

(2) Do both sides appear to rest lower and closer to the dorsum of the back of the tongue than normal?
(3) Is the soft palate completely still, or are there rhythmic upward and downward movements?
   b. Phonation. The patient is asked to say "ah."
      (1) Do both sides of the soft palate elevate symmetrically and fully, or is there little or no movement?
      (2) Does one side elevate more than the other, the pale median raphe of the velum deviating to the side of greater elevation?
      (3) Does the side that appeared higher at rest pull to that side on phonation?
   c. Gag reflex. With the tongue blade, the faucial arches are stroked upward from the lateral borders of the tongue to the midline of the soft palate.
      (1) Do both sides of the soft palate elevate fully and symmetrically as the patient gags, or does the palate move only slightly or not at all?
      (2) Does the soft palate pull to one side on gagging—the side that rested higher than the other?
4. Larynx. Dysarthria more often than not includes laryngeal muscle defects warranting laryngoscopic examination and usually requiring referral to an otolaryngologist for this purpose. The questions that need to be answered are as follows:
   a. On phonation, do the vocal folds adduct symmetrically to the midline, closing the glottis completely, or do they adduct only partially?
   b. Are the vocal folds bowed during phonation?
   c. On inhalation, do the vocal folds abduct symmetrically and fully, or do they appear restricted in extent of abduction?
   d. Do both vocal folds fail to abduct on inhalation and appear to be fixed in the midline?
   e. Does one vocal fold partially or completely fail to move during phonation?
   f. Does the larynx appear to be twisted to one side or the other during phonation?

Speech examination

The speech examination is organized to isolate the sound-producing capabilities of the major muscular anatomic structures of the peripheral speech mechanism.

1. Phonation and respiration.
   a. Vowel prolongation. Ask the patient to inhale deeply and on exhalation to sustain the vowel "ah" for as long, steadily, and clearly as possible.

(1) Is the tone clear, or does it sound hoarse, strained, "wet," breathy, or whispered?
(2) Is the patient able to hold the tone fairly steadily, or is there jerkiness, tremor, or flutter of the voice?
(3) Are there intermittent voice arrests, as if the airstream were suddenly cut off? Are these arrests regular or irregular?
(4) Is the pitch of the voice excessively high or low for the patient's age and sex?
(5) During conversational speech, does the voice sound flat or monopitched?
(6) Does the pitch break upward and downward uncontrollably?
(7) Can two different pitch levels be heard?
 b. "Coup de glotte." Coup de glotte describes a maneuver in which the patient is asked to produce a sharp grunting sound. Its purpose is to test the adductor strength of the vocal folds.
 (1) Is the grunt produced normally sharply, or is it mushy or even absent?
2. Resonation. Holding a mirror or other shiny, moisture-collecting surface under the nares, ask the patient to repeat the phrases "We see three geese" and "The big black dog caught the stick." Because these phrases do not contain any nasal sounds (/m, n, ng/), normally there should be complete velopharyngeal closure and no nasal air escape.
 a. Does the mirror become cloudy during the production of these phrases?
3. Articulation.
 a. Alternate motion rate (AMR). Ask the patient to inhale deeply and on exhalation to repeat the syllable /pa/ as rapidly and evenly as possible. Do the same for /ta/ and /ka/.
 (1) Are these sounds produced at a normal rate (5 to 7 Hz), or are they slow or excessively rapid?
 (2) Are they sometimes indistinct because of tremulous repetitions?
 (3) Are they produced with irregular intervals and degrees of loudness?
 (4) Are they produced with tonic blocking?
 (5) Do they become more rapid, tremulous, or blocked when the patient tries to increase their rate?
 b. Contextual speech. The objective is to obtain a sample of contextual speech by asking the patient to read. The following paragraph, called the "Grandfather Passage," is commonly used for this purpose.

> You wish to know all about my grandfather. Well, he is nearly 93 years old, yet he still thinks as swiftly as ever. He dresses himself in

an old black frock coat, usually several buttons missing. A long beard clings to his chin, giving those who observe him a pronounced feeling of the utmost respect. Twice each day he plays skillfully and with zest upon a small organ. Except in the winter when the snow or ice prevents, he slowly takes a short walk in the open air each day. We have often urged him to walk more and smoke less, but he always answers, "Banana oil!" Grandfather likes to be modern in his language.

(1) Are consonant or vowel sounds distorted?
(2) Does the patient omit, add, reverse, repeat, or prolong individual speech sounds?
(3) Are there speech arrests?
(4) Does the patient make trial-and-error articulatory movements during attempts to produce sounds?
(5) Is the speaking rate excessively slow or fast?
(6) Is there a loss of stress or accent on portions of multisyllabic words within sentences?
(7) Are syllables excessively stressed?
(8) Are jaw, face, or tongue movements made with restricted range of motion?
(9) Are there exaggerated or distorted jaw, face, or tongue movements?
(10) How intelligible is the paragraph overall?

4. Stress test for muscle fatigue. Ask the patient to count vigorously to 150 at a rate of about one number per second.
   a. Is there a noticeable increase in breathy or hoarse voice quality, hypernasality, or articulatory imprecision over time, or does the speech remain essentially the same at the conclusion of counting?

Types of dysarthria

The subtypes of dysarthria are those distinctive motor speech disorders that differentiate themselves from one another on the basis of how they sound, how they look, and the location of their lesions. These dysarthrias are analyzed according to the schema just described, that is, according to the major anatomic sites of sound production and modulation by the peripheral speech mechanism: laryngeal/respiratory, velopharyngeal/resonatory, and labial-lingual-mandibular/articulatory.

The terms used to designate the subtypes of dysarthria basically reflect their presumed underlying neuropathophysiology. A summary of the dysarthria types according to location of lesion and primary distinguishing speech characteristics is given in Table 4-1.

Flaccid dysarthria

Flaccid dysarthria applies to abnormal motor speech resulting from an lesion of lower motor neurons that innervate the speech musculature.

Table 4-1 Types of Dysarthria and Their Primary Speech Characteristics

Type of Dysarthria	Phonation	Resonation	Articulation
1. Flaccid, XII	Normal	Normal	Lingual consonant and vowel imprecision
2. Flaccid, X (RLN)	Breathy-hoarse, diplophonic	Normal	Normal
3. Flaccid, X (high)	Breathy-whispered	Hypernasal	Normal
4. Flaccid, VII	Normal	Normal	Labial consonant and vowel distortion
5. Flaccid, V	Normal	Normal	Labial and lingual consonant and vowel distortion
6. Flaccid, XII, X, VII, V	Breathy-whispered	Hypernasal	Labial and lingual consonant and vowel distortion
7. Flaccid, spinal nerves	Reduced loudness, phrase length, and pitch/loudness variability	Normal	Normal
8. Unilateral UMN	Normal	Normal	Consonant and vowel distortion, irregular articulatory breakdowns
9. Spastic	Strained-hoarse	Hypernasal	Slow rate, consonant and vowel distortion
10. Hypokinetic	Breathy, monopitch, reduced loudness	Normal	Fast rate, consonant distortion
11. Atactic	Normal, voice tremor, excess loudness	Normal	Irregular articulatory breakdowns, consonant and vowel distortion
12. Dystonic	Slow, fluctuating strained hoarseness, voice arrests	Normal	Slow, fluctuating consonant and vowel distortion
13. Choreic	Quick, fluctuating strained hoarseness, voice arrests	Normal	Quick, fluctuating consonant and vowel distortion
14. Organic (essential) tremor	Tremor (4-7 Hz)	Normal	Normal
15. Palatopharyngolaryngeal myoclonus	Regular voice arrests (1-4 Hz)	Normal	Normal
16. Mixed	Variable	Variable	Variable

RLN, recurrent laryngeal nerve; UMN, upper motor neuron.

The lesion may affect the neuron or nerve anywhere along the final common pathway to produce the dysarthria: cell body, axon, myoneural junction, or muscle. The denervating effect of the lesion produces muscle flaccidity, weakness, atrophy, and fasciculations.

Flaccid dysarthrias are produced by lesions of the cranial nerves supplying the bulbar speech muscles or by defects of spinal nerves responsible for abnormal respiration. The cranial nerves that, when damaged, produce flaccid dysarthria are (1) the twelfth nerve, supplying the muscles of the tongue, (2) the tenth nerve, supplying the muscles of the larynx and velopharynx, (3) the seventh nerve, supplying the muscles of the mouth, and (4) the fifth nerve, supplying the mandibular musculature.

It is important to note that because neurologic disease can damage these cranial nerves either singly or in any combination, the specific speech deficits depend on which one or more cranial nerves are involved.

Hypoglossal nerve (XII). A unilateral or bilateral lesion of the twelfth nerve alone produces weakness, atrophy, and fasciculations of the tongue. Its effect on speech is to produce articulatory imprecision of all speech sounds made by the tongue, which are the lingual consonants and vowels, although the latter are affected only in very severe flaccid weakness of the tongue. The lingual consonants are exemplified by the following words: *th*read, *t*op, *d*og, *s*wap, *z*ebra, *sh*oe, mea*s*ure, *ch*ase, *j*ump, *c*ap, *g*o.

Unilateral twelfth nerve lesions produce milder articulatory distortion than bilateral, and the greater the number of motor units damaged, the more severe the distortion of the consonants and vowels. In severe cases, the recognizability of the lingual speech sounds can be entirely obliterated. As Table 4-1 shows, if only the twelfth nerve is damaged, phonation and resonation are normal.

Vagus nerve (X). The vagus nerve supplies the laryngeal and velopharyngeal musculature. The specific branches of the tenth nerve relevant to this discussion are the pharyngeal, superior laryngeal, and recurrent laryngeal nerves.

A unilateral lesion of the recurrent laryngeal nerve produces vocal fold paralysis in the paramedian position. The flaccid dysphonia that results is characterized by hoarseness and often diplophonia because of unequal frequency of vibration between the two vocal folds. Paradoxically, if both recurrent laryngeal nerves are damaged, fixation of the vocal folds in the paramedian position produces very little dysphonia but seriously compromises the airway and produces inhalatory stridor.

More rostrally, a unilateral lesion of the superior laryngeal nerve, which paralyzes the cricothyroid muscle, produces little or no dysphonia, but a bilateral lesion destroys pitch control of the voice.

Still higher along the nerve, unilateral damage to the pharyngeal branch produces unilateral soft palate paralysis and mild to moderate hypernasality and nasal emission of the airstream. If damage is bilateral, these resonatory defects are much more severe.

An intramedullary or extramedullary lesion at the brain stem level affecting the main trunk of the tenth nerve produces a unilateral or bilateral vocal fold paralysis in the abducted position, causing considerable glottic air escape and a severely breathy voice quality combined with hypernasality and nasal emission from accompanying velopharyngeal paralysis. The coup de glotte is profoundly weak.

Facial nerve (VII). Paralysis of the facial nerve produces weakness of the circumoral musculature and thus impairs production of sounds that require closure of the lips—the bilabial consonants, as in the words *"pot"* and *"boy,"* and the nasal semivowel, as in the word *"may."* A second group of sounds affected, because of difficulty in positioning the lower lip against the maxillary incisors, are the labiodental sounds, as in the words *"fright"* and *"vase."* Although unilateral facial nerve weakness has a relatively milder effect on these sounds because the ability to move the lips on one side is retained, bilateral paralysis, if complete, can totally destroy the ability to produce these sounds.

Trigeminal nerve (V). The motor division of the fifth nerve supplies the muscles that elevate and depress the mandible. Although a unilateral lesion of this nerve preserves the ability to elevate the mandible, a bilateral lesion prevents this from happening. If the mandible cannot be elevated, neither the tongue nor the lips can be positioned for articulatory contacts, and the effect is virtually complete inability to articulate.

Spinal nerves. Spinal nerves primarily subserve respiratory functions for speech. They are spread from the cervical through the thoracic divisions of the spinal cord, but the most important respiratory muscle for speech—the diaphragm—is supplied by the phrenic nerves. Diffuse impairment of respiratory muscles or bilateral diaphragmatic paralysis is generally necessary to interfere significantly with speech. When this occurs, vocal loudness, length of spoken phrases, and normal pitch and loudness variability may be reduced; the voice sometimes has a strained quality, reflecting a compensatory effort to make efficient use of the limited air supply for speech.

Unilateral upper motor neuron dysarthria
A unilateral upper motor neuron dysarthria results from a lesion of the right or the left corticobulbar tract at any point along its pathway.

The effect on the speech muscles is to produce a contralateral lower facial and tongue weakness. The jaw, soft palate, and larynx are relatively spared because of their rich bilateral upper motor neuron innervation.

The effect of a unilateral upper motor neuron lesion on speech is to produce a relatively mild distortion of bilabial and lingual consonants. A subcortical lesion, especially in the internal capsule, usually produces more pronounced weakness and dysarthria than a cortical lesion. Phonation may be normal, and resonance is normal or only mildly hypernasal. It is of interest that articulation during conversation or reading and during AMRs for /pa-ta-ka/ is sometimes produced with an irregularity of precision that bears a strong resemblance to ataxic dysarthria from a cerebellar lesion.

Spastic (pseudobulbar) dysarthria
Spastic dysarthria, presumably reflecting spasticity and upper motor neuron weakness of the bulbar speech muscles, results from bilateral lesions of the corticobulbar tracts anywhere along their course. The oral mechanism examination may reveal a positive sucking reflex and slow lateral tongue wiggle. The gag reflex may be hyperactive. The speech musculature is almost always impaired at all three levels: laryngeal, velopharyngeal, and articulatory.

Laryngeal. The voice on vowel prolongation and during conversational speech is typified by a strained-strangled hoarseness and monopitch. Many patients, although by no means all, have a reduced threshold for crying and laughing, which are easily triggered by sad or humorous stimuli that ordinarily would not have produced these reactions before the neurologic disease. In more flagrant instances of "pseudobulbar crying," the cry may take on the characteristics of a long, rising and falling wail.

Velopharyngeal. Because of slow velopharyngeal movements during connected speech, hypernasality and nasal emission are common.

Articulatory. Articulation can be severely impaired in spastic dysarthria. Slow rate of speech is a hallmark of spastic dysarthria. AMRs on repetitions of /p-t-k/ are below normal in rate, depending on severity, and can sometimes drop to as low as 2 Hz (normal, 5 to 7 Hz). Imprecise consonant production, the second major articulatory defect, results from not only reduced force of labial and lingual contact but also loss of intraoral pressure brought about by nasal air escape due to velopharyngeal insufficiency.

Ataxic dysarthria
Lesions of the cerebellum or its connections produce ataxic dysarthria.

Laryngeal. The phonatory signs of ataxic dysarthria are variable. Voice can be normal. If abnormal, it will have irregular loudness variations, especially on vowel prolongation. Bursts of loudness occur in severe forms of the dysarthria. A coarse voice tremor sometimes is noticeable only on vowel prolongation.

Velopharyngeal. Normal.

Articulatory. The hallmark of this dysarthria in both contextual speech and on AMRs for /p-t-k/ is irregular breakdowns in articulatory precision.

Hypokinetic dysarthria
Lesions of the basal ganglia or related structures can produce hypokinetic, or parkinsonian, dysarthria.

Laryngeal. The dysphonia of hypokinetic dysarthria most often consists of breathy voice quality from failure of complete adduction of the vocal folds as well as reduced loudness from both incomplete adduction of the vocal folds and reduced exhalatory air pressure and flow. Monopitch is the third major dysphonic component.

Velopharyngeal. Normal or mild hypernasality.

Articulatory. Persons with hypokinetic dysarthria have rapid articulation and articulatory imprecision, often to the point of producing a tremorous fusion of sounds during speech. Not uncommonly, patients produce rapid rushes of speech, stop suddenly, and, after a moment of silence, continue on in the same accelerated manner. Some patients produce stuttering-like repetitions of initial sounds or syllables of words, of whole words, or even of complete phrases. These usually rapid or accelerated repetitions are called "palilalia." AMRs on /p-t-k/ are especially revealing; syllables are produced rapidly with minimal mouth and tongue movements, and the AMRs disintegrate into an undifferentiated tremulousness of the lips and tongue.

The hyperkinetic dysarthrias
This category refers to a cluster of dysarthrias characterized by excessive or extraneous movements of the speech musculature during speech. They are associated with lesions of the basal ganglia or cerebellar control circuits or of the indirect (extrapyramidal) motor system. The subtypes

of hyperkinetic dysarthria are numerous. A brief description of some of the more common subtypes follows.

Dystonic dysarthria (slow hyperkinesia). Dystonia produces many different speech effects because of relatively slow, unpredictable, and adventitious muscle contractions. When these so-called slow hyperkinesias include the speech musculature, the dystonic movements interfere with the positioning of the articulators and have a tendency to produce hyperadduction of the vocal folds.

Laryngeal. Adventitious hyperadduction of the vocal folds produces momentary hoarseness that takes on the characteristics of what is generally described as "spastic or spasmodic dysphonia." Vowel prolongation produces waxing and waning strained hoarseness. Studies of dystonic patients provide evidence that movement disorders can be confined almost exclusively to the larynx. When this is the case, the diagnosis of spasmodic dysphonia is often made, a diagnosis that technically reflects a laryngeal dystonic dysarthria.

Velopharyngeal. Velopharyngeal closure is either normal or dyssynchronous; when dyssynchronous, it results in fluctuating hypernasality and nasal emission.

Articulatory. Slow, adventitious movements of the lips, tongue, or mandible separated by moments of normal articulation produce distortion of consonants and vowels. Patients with dystonic dysarthria differ from one another in the vectors of movement of their articulators. In certain cases, the main tendency is to uncontrollably spread the lips; in others, to round them; and in still others, to do both. Tongue movements may consist of rolling or humping the tongue within the mouth during attempts to speak. Some patients move the tongue in and out between the teeth or, in extreme forms, keep it fully and continuously out of the mouth as they try to speak. Irregular AMRs on /p-t-k/ are produced because of interference by the unpredictable lip, tongue, and mandibular movements. Momentary, tonic articulatory arrests are common during these maneuvers.

Choreic dysarthria (quick hyperkinesia). The demarcation between the slow hyperkinesia of dystonia and the quick hyperkinesia of chorea is not always clear. The patient with choreic dysarthria tends to produce rapid, jerky, adventitious phonatory and articulatory movements.

Laryngeal. As the patient is speaking, sudden voice arrests can be heard because of quick adduction movements of the vocal folds. These also occur during vowel prolongation.

Velopharyngeal. Dyssynchrony of velopharyngeal movements can produce fluctuating, usually mild, hypernasality and nasal emission.

Articulatory. The patient's conversational speech is intermittently normal interrupted by sudden vocal arrests and articulatory imprecision coincident with sudden bilabial compression, spreading, and lip smacking. The tongue may suddenly protrude straight out between the lips or to one side. Irregular AMRs on /p-t-k/ are caused by these adventitious movements, and sudden complete arrests of articulation may take place during these maneuvers.

Dysarthria of palatopharyngolaryngeal myoclonus. Caused by lesions of the brain stem, palatopharyngolaryngeal myoclonus consists of sudden myoclonic-like synchronous contractions of the laryngeal, pharyngeal, and, at times, lingual musculature. They occur at a semiregular rate of 2 to 4 Hz and are identified by their presence at rest as well as during speech.

This dysarthria can be elusive, however, because the effects are usually masked by conversational speech. They are most easily detected during the oral mechanism examination. For this reason, the routine oral examination should always include a brief period of study of the oropharynx while the patient is completely at rest. If palatopharyngolaryngeal myoclonus is present, ballistic, regular movements of the soft palate and pharynx are evident. The laryngeal myoclonic component can be physically identified in three ways: (1) by observing the skin covering the larynx for rhythmic movements of the larynx beneath it; (2) by placing the fingers over the larynx and feeling the rhythmic movements; and (3) by seeing, during indirect laryngoscopy, the vocal folds adduct and abduct in synchrony with the pharyngeal musculature surrounding them.

Laryngeal. Although a dysphonia is rarely detectable during conversational speech except in severe cases, vowel prolongation usually brings out the myoclonic movements quite audibly. These consist of brief, gentle pulsatile interruptions of the vowel at the same rate as myoclonic movements of the pharynx and soft palate. If severe, the periodic adductions of the vocal folds are sufficiently forceful to cause complete, sharp, and more prolonged vocal arrests taking on the character of adductor laryngospasms.

Velopharyngeal. The periodic undulations of the soft palate are so brief that nasal resonatory changes are rarely heard. However, if a mirror is placed under the nares while the patient is asked to sustain a humming sound, its surface may become intermittently rather than continuously cloudy because of periodic closures of the velopharynx.

Articulatory. Rarely, if ever, is articulation defective unless the palatopharyngolaryngeal myoclonus is combined with another dysarthria, usually from a more extensive lesion within the posterior fossa. If articulation is defective, the defect may reflect any combination of flaccid, spastic, or ataxic dysarthria.

Dysarthria of organic (essential or heredofamilial) voice tremor. Organic voice tremor is another illustration of a dysarthria that can be confined to the larynx. Organic voice tremor consists of rhythmic adduction and abduction of the vocal folds occurring most often within the range of 4 to 7 Hz, although in a minority of cases the tremor may be slower or faster than these values. These are intention or action tremors; they do not occur unless the patient is in the process of phonation. They can be confined exclusively to the larynx or may include tremor of the pharynx, tongue, lips, mandible, head, or extremities. They can be heredofamilial but often are not.

Laryngeal. In moderate-to-severe examples of the disorder, tremor of the voice is heard during conversational speech. If less severe, tremor may be apparent only during vowel prolongation. Here, variations in rhythmic pitch and loudness can be heard, and when viewed laryngoscopically, the vocal folds are seen to adduct and abduct in synchrony with the voice tremor.

In very severe cases of organic voice tremor, the vocal folds hyperadduct so forcefully that they momentarily abut against one another and cause voice arrests or adductor laryngospasms. Also, on vowel prolongation, instead of voice tremor, staccato voice arrests are heard. Conversational speech sounds like a variant of spastic dysphonia. In fact, it can be considered to be an adductor spastic dysphonia of organic voice tremor.

Some patients have intermittent breathy air release during contextual speech, and on vowel prolongation they have voice tremor along with visible tremorous hyperabduction of the vocal folds at the same rate as patients with tremorous hyperadduction of the vocal folds. Hyperabduction gives rise to the disorder known as abductor spastic dysphonia of organic voice tremor.

Velopharyngeal. Normal.

Articulatory. Articulation is normal except when tremor of the articulators also occurs, which has a mildly distorting effect on articulatory precision, especially on AMRs for /p-t-k/, during which the tremors interfere with the syllabic repetitions.

Mixed dysarthrias

Not uncommonly, patients have two or more types of dysarthria simultaneously, and mixed dysarthrias tend to occur more frequently than any single type of dysarthria. Virtually any combination of dysarthria types can occur.

Certain diseases are especially inclined to produce mixtures of two or more dysarthrias. Sometimes, the mix is "classic," because it occurs in a disease with very predictable effects on portions of the motor system. For example, mixed spastic-flaccid dysarthria is very common in amyotrophic lateral sclerosis (ALS) because of the effect of ALS on the upper and lower motor neuron systems bilaterally. More commonly, the mix of dysarthria types is less predictable, because the disease with which it is associated may less predictably affect one or more portions of the motor system. For example, progressive supranuclear palsy, olivopontocerebellar atrophy, and Wilson's disease may be associated with hypokinetic, spastic, or ataxic dysarthria, either singly or in combination; Shy-Drager syndrome may be associated with hypokinetic, spastic, ataxic, or flaccid dysarthria, either singly or in combination; multiple sclerosis may be associated with any type of dysarthria, but ataxic and spastic dysarthrias are probably most common.

The recognition of mixed dysarthrias may aid neurologic differential diagnosis by establishing, for example, whether a mixed dysarthria, or a particular mixed dysarthria, is compatible with a suspected condition. For example, only flaccid dysarthria should be encountered in myasthenia gravis, only hypokinetic dysarthria in Parkinson's disease, and only flaccid or spastic dysarthria (or the combination) in ALS; a mixed dysarthria in myasthenia gravis or Parkinson's disease or a dysarthria other than flaccid or spastic in ALS should raise questions about the neurologic diagnosis or suspicions about whether an additional condition is present.

Apraxia of Speech

Apraxia of speech is a motor speech disorder characterized by substitutions, additions, repetitions, and prolongations of speech sounds, often accompanied by searching, groping, and trial-and-error articulatory movements. These errors are due not to muscular weakness or incoordination but rather to impairment in the organization or programming of previously learned patterns of movement. Although articulation is most often disturbed in apraxia of speech, apraxia of phonation is not uncommon. When apraxia of phonation is accompanied by articulatory apraxia, the patient can be aphonic or mute.

Apraxia of speech is often associated with lesions of the inferior frontal convolution of the language-dominant cerebral hemisphere, but it can also be associated with dominant parietal or even subcortical lesions. Like all disorders, apraxia of speech can occur along a severity continuum. Some patients have only mild hesitancy of speech. Sometimes, hesitancies reflect blocking or repetitions of initial consonants or syllables of words and have a stuttering-like character. Sometimes, substitutions of incorrect sounds are perceived. Many apraxic patients, in an effort to correct their errors, start, stop, and abort sounds in midstream. The patient may try one sound and then another until the right one is produced, all the while reacting with facial grimacing, sighing, and other signs of frustration.

Certain speaking requirements can worsen apraxia of speech. The more complex the articulatory demands, the more frequent and severe the errors; for example, consonants are more prone to errors than vowels, consonant clusters more than single consonants, multisyllabic words more than monosyllabic words, and rapid speech more than slow speech. Automatic speech, such as counting, days of the week, or months of the year, is produced more fluently than spontaneous speech. Profanity and the ability to carry a tune are often well preserved.

Examination for apraxia of speech
Sequential motor rate
The patient is asked to repeat /p-t-k/ in rapid succession, making the transition from "p" to "t" to "k" as smoothly and as effortlessly as possible. The mildly apractic patient hesitates only on shifting from sound to sound. The patient with a more severe disorder blocks or cannot accurately sequence the syllables. Those with very severe apraxia may not be able to begin the task at all.

Multisyllabic words
Asking the patient to repeat multisyllabic words having an increasingly greater number of syllables often precipitates articulatory disintegration:

snowman	several umbrellas
animal	statistical analysis
gingerbread	Methodist Episcopal Church
artillery	please-pleasing-pleasingly
catastrophe	sit-city-citizen-citizenship

Nonverbal oral apraxia
Some patients with apraxia of speech also have difficulty organizing nonspeech oromotor acts. They hesitate, produce trial-and-error movements, or show complete inability to perform the act.
   Test items used to elicit oral nonverbal apraxia can include

Stick out your tongue.
Blow.
Show me your teeth.
Pucker your lips.
Bite your lower lip.
Whistle.
Cough.

Curiously, patients with nonverbal oral apraxia who are asked to cough often appear momentarily confused, take in a breath, open their mouths, and instead of coughing say "cough." Apractic patients are known for their ability to perform an act spontaneously when they are unable to perform the very same act volitionally or on command.

LANGUAGE DISORDERS

The previous section established that careful examination of speech can contribute to the identification and localization of neurologic disease. The examination of language is of equal value. In this section, language is defined in sufficient detail to provide a rationale for its meaningful examination and a framework for recognizing the implications for localization of breakdowns in its various components. Because differential diagnosis of disturbances in communication can contribute to localization and identification of underlying disease, we also attend to disturbances that may be similar to—but must be differentiated from—focal language disturbances.

Basic Concepts
Definition of language

Language involves the understanding and production of individual words and grouping of words for the communication of ideas and feelings. Words are abstract symbols that the speakers of a language agree have a certain meaning. Language symbols are differentiated from nonsymbolic meanings conveyed by facial expression, vocal inflections, and body movements, which communicate affective information about attitudes, emotions, and feelings. The distinction between symbolic and nonsymbolic communication is of more than academic interest, because each is organized differently within the nervous system and may be disturbed independently.

The language modalities

The sensory and motor avenues through which language is comprehended and expressed are known as language modalities: listening, reading, speaking, and writing. Listening (or verbal comprehension) and reading are frequently referred to as receptive language functions, speaking and writing as expressive language functions. The division of language into receptive and expressive functions is convenient for organizing the examination and for isolating unique patterns of breakdown. Such categorizations do not imply, however, that the language modalities have clearly separable neuroanatomic correlates. Verbal comprehension, verbal expression, reading, and writing are intertwined with each other within what may be called a *central language processor*. This integrative process explains why most persons with aphasia have deficits in all language modalities.

The central language processor contains a specialized information base that can be subdivided into the basic components of language, commonly referred to as phonology, vocabulary, semantics, and syntax. *Phonology* refers to the sounds of language and the rules for combining them into meaningful syllables and words. In English there are about 40 sounds, or phonemes. *Vocabulary* refers to the words of a language and their associated meanings. *Semantics* refers to knowledge about the meaning of word combinations that goes beyond the literal meaning of the words that have been combined (for example, "Don't cry over spilled milk" has concrete and abstract meanings, both of which mean something more than, and different from, the individual words in the proverb). *Syntax* refers to rules for ordering and altering words in utterances to establish the subject or object of a sentence, the tense of verbs, whether a noun is single or plural, and so on.

For language to be used effectively, certain general central nervous system processes are essential: attention, retrieval, and short-term recall. *Attention* includes alertness and concentration directed to a particular task and resistance to interference from irrelevant ideas, sensations, and movements. Deficits of attention are more obvious and prominent in generalized intellectual disturbances and confusion than they are in focal disturbances of language (that is, aphasia).

Retrieval, or access to language, is essential, and deficits in this realm are common to nearly all aphasic individuals. For example, a frequent and diagnostically significant complaint of aphasic persons is "I know what I want to say, but I just can't find the words to say it."

Short-term recall is essential to normal language use, especially comprehension. Whether spoken or written, a phrase, sentence, or paragraph often does not have an unambiguous meaning until its completion. Ongoing language, therefore, must be retained long enough to be understood. Deficits in short-term memory for verbal materials are present in most patients with aphasia.

Localization of Language
Lateralization

Language is organized predominantly within the left cerebral hemisphere in more than 90% of the population. Approximately 95% of right-handers and 70% of left-handers (and ambidextrous persons) have left hemisphere language dominance. It is likely that half or more of the right- and left-handers who are not left hemisphere language dominant have "mixed dominance," that is, a relatively equal sharing between the hemispheres of control over speech and language functions. Thus, only a very small percentage of the population is truly right hemisphere language dominant, and unilateral right hemisphere lesions account for only about 2% of all cases of aphasia. It is also noteworthy that recovery from aphasia is generally better when the disorder results from a right hemisphere lesion, when the individual is left-handed, or when the right-handed patient has left-handed first-degree relatives. Finally, left hemisphere lesions during infancy or early childhood may result in transfer of language function to the right hemisphere; right hemisphere language dominance may be as high as 75% among such patients.

Intrahemispheric organization

Localization of language within the dominant hemisphere is a source of continuing uncertainty, but it is well established that the *left perisylvian region,* including portions of the temporal, parietal, and frontal lobes, is crucial for language. Thus, from the vascular standpoint, language is localized within the distribution of the left middle cerebral artery.

Within the perisylvian area, the superior, middle, and posterior portions of the temporal lobe and adjacent areas of the parietal lobe are most important. This zone encompasses but extends beyond *Wernicke's area* and is sometimes referred to as the *posterior speech area.* Also important to language (and motor speech programming) is *Broca's area,* located at the foot of the third frontal convolution. Broca's area, along with some additional surrounding cortex, is sometimes referred to as the *anterior speech area.*

Large lesions in the perisylvian area usually produce severe aphasia affecting all language modalities, and even small lesions in this central area typically produce multimodality impairments. Small lesions producing severe and lasting aphasia are most often located in the posterior speech area and include Wernicke's area. Small lesions at the periphery of the perisylvian language area may produce prominent or even isolated difficulties in one modality of language; they may or may not reflect a true language disturbance. When an isolated modality disturbance occurs, it most often can be ascribed to a relatively pure sensory or motor deficit (for example, cortical deafness or apraxia) or to a disconnection between a sensory or motor modality and the perisylvian language area.

Aphasia can also result from lesions in *subcortical areas* of the dominant hemisphere. The subcortical structures most often associated with aphasia are the basal ganglia and thalamus. Their specific contribution to language and the mechanism through which aphasia results from lesions is not entirely clear. Clinically, however, it is important to recognize that aphasia may result from damage to subcortical structures that have important connections to the perisylvian cortical language areas.

Examination of Language

Language assessment can be brief and simple or extensive and detailed, depending on the purposes of examination and the severity of the disorder. Assessment of language should be undertaken early in any examination of mental status, because language deficits can influence performance on parts of the mental status examination, including verbal thought, verbal learning and recall, calculation, verbal abstraction and information, and right-left orientation in response to verbal command.

History

The history of the communication deficit contributes to an understanding of the time course of the disease, its localization, and possibly its cause. The manner in which a patient communicates the history often yields enough information to differentiate aphasia from nonaphasic communication deficits.

The following questions elicit general language complaints, establish the patient's awareness of deficits, and provide clues to differential diagnosis.

1. Do you have difficulty expressing yourself? If so, describe it.
2. Did you recognize your difficulty in speaking, or did others point it out to you?
3. Do you know what you want to say but are unable to find the words? Or do you have trouble organizing your thoughts or recalling facts before you even try to put them into words?
4. Do you ever use a wrong word that is close in meaning to the one you meant (for example, "table" for "chair")?
5. If you are unable to find a word, do you sometimes intentionally substitute a word close in meaning?
6. Do you make errors in grammar, such as leaving out words like "a" or "the" or saying "will" instead of "did"?
7. Do you have trouble understanding what others say to you, even if you hear without difficulty?
8. Is your difficulty with comprehension a problem of remembering what was said or of not understanding it in the first place?
9. If you have difficulty understanding, is it worse in noise or if several people are conversing? Do you have more trouble if something is lengthy or spoken quickly?
10. Do you have trouble understanding what you read? If so, is it because you don't see the words well? Or is it because you don't understand what they mean?
11. Do you look at a letter or word and not know what it means or take a long time to figure it out? Does this happen with objects, pictures, or people or just with letters or words?
12. Has your writing changed? If so, is it just not as neat, or do you have difficulty with spelling, or finding the words, or putting sentences together?

Because intelligence, education, and occupation influence skills and interest in reading and writing, complaints about written language may not be as reliable or as emphasized by the patient as oral expression or comprehension. In addition, many aphasic patients have good attentional and social skills, are acutely attuned to nonverbal cues provided by the clinician and environment, and appreciate the purpose of the neurologic examination. These traits significantly aid the patient's speech comprehension and may mask comprehension deficits that are only detectable through formal testing.

Essential components of formal language examination

All primary language modalities should be evaluated. Tasks should include items difficult enough to detect mild impairment and others simple enough to permit residual skills to be detected when impairment is severe. Because they contribute to localization within the dominant hemisphere, the ability to repeat verbally presented materials and the fluency characteristics* of conversational speech are also important to assess. Finally, because impaired word retrieval nearly always accompanies aphasia, assessment of naming ability is essential.

Observing language test behavior

Interpretation of language performance cannot be based solely on a computation of errors. Some persons make few correct responses in any language modality but are not aphasic, whereas others exhibit behaviors in the process of responding accurately that are clearly indicative of aphasia. The differential diagnosis of communication impairment must rely as much on qualitative behavioral observations as on numerical test scores; many useful behavioral observations can be made during history-taking as well as during formal testing.

The language test

A number of lengthy, comprehensive, standardized examinations of language are available. However, within the context of the neurologic examination, it is more reasonable to use a screening test. Table 4-2 contains a relatively brief language examination that can be administered with ease at the bedside. Guiding principles and purposes are discussed below. They parallel the test given in Table 4-2.

I. Comprehension
  A. *Listening.* For valid examination, hearing loss should be ruled out. It is important to administer verbal comprehension items without giving nonverbal cues. For example, the examiner should avoid vocal inflections that indicate a response should be "yes" or "no" and should inhibit eye or hand movements that might help identify an object or movement that is part of a command.
  1. *Simple commands* are used to determine residual comprehension when impairment is severe. For example, most aphasic patients follow a command to close their eyes. It is also important to include different types of items, because discrepancies across item types sometimes occur; for example, head and whole body

---

*Fluency in this context refers to the degree to which utterances are normal in length, syntax, pauses, intonation, articulation, and amount of information conveyed per number of words. Specific fluency characteristics encountered in aphasia are discussed in the section on disorders within the section on speaking deficits in aphasia.

Table 4-2 Screening Examination of Language Functions

I. Comprehension.
   A. Listening.
      1. Simple commands:
         a. Close your eyes.
         b. Look at the floor.
         c. Make a fist.
         d. Show me your chair (or bed).
         e. Touch your chin.
      2. Yes-no questions (head nod, eye blink, or verbal response acceptable):
         a. Are you standing up?
         b. Is a mother older than her child?
         c. The hat is newer than the coat. Is the coat older?
      3. Right-left commands:
         a. Show me your left hand.
         b. Show me your right ear.
         c. Touch your right ear with your left thumb.
      4. Complex commands:
         a. Before touching your nose, point to the light.
         b. Look at the ceiling after you point to the floor.
         c. Touch your chin and your nose, but first close your eyes.
   B. Reading.
      1. Letter identification: "Point to these letters" (print letters on paper):

         P   W
         M   B

      2. Letter reading: "Read the letters above."
      3. Single words: "Read these and show me where they are" (present printed words to patient, each on a separate card):
         a. Floor.
         b. Chair.
         c. Nose.
         d. Wrist.
         e. Ceiling.
      4. Commands: "Read this and do what it says to do" (present printed sentences to patient, each on a separate card):
         a. Make a fist.
         b. Close your eyes.
         c. Touch your right ear with your left thumb.
         d. Look at the ceiling after you point to the floor.

II. Expression.
   A. Speaking.
      1. Conversational speech (assessed during history).
      2. Narrative: "Tell me about what's happening in this picture" (hand patient a pictured action scene; see Fig. 4-1 for example).
      3. Repetition: "Repeat these words and sentences":
         a. Please sit down.
         b. What time will the bus pick you up?
         c. I ordered a ham sandwich, a glass of milk, and a piece of apple pie.
         d. Catastrophe.
         e. Methodist Episcopal Church.
         f. No ifs, ands, or buts.

Continued

Table 4-2	Screening Examination of Language Functions — cont'd

II. Expression.
    4. Object naming: "Tell me the name of this" (point to each object):
       a. Watch.
       b. Wrist.
       c. Knuckles.
       d. Chair.
       e. Pen (or pencil).
       f. Stomach.
    5. Sentence completion:
       a. You sleep in a _____.
       b. We wash with soap and _____.
       c. The American flag is red, white, and _____.
    6. Automatic speech:
       a. Count from 1 to 10.
       b. Say the days of the week.
    7. Singing (have the patient sing "Happy Birthday" or another familiar song).
    8. Word definitions and proverb explanations: "Tell me what these words and sayings mean":
       a. Island.
       b. Bargain.
       c. Don't cry over spilled milk.
       d. Don't count your chickens before they're hatched.
  B. Writing.
    1. Dictated words: "Write these words" (dictate words one at a time):
       a. Man.
       b. Watch.
       c. Basketball.
    2. Dictated sentences: "Write this sentence" (dictate sentences one at a time):
       a. Please sit down.
       b. Some water is not good to drink.
    3. Spontaneous writing: "Write a sentence or two about something you've done today."
    4. Copying: "Copy these" (present the following, leaving space for the patient to copy:
       a. M S W
       b. + ▲ ◨

movement commands (such as look up, stand up) are often simpler than pointing or commands to move the limbs.

  2. *Yes-no questions* carry a liability of 50% accuracy by guessing alone but eliminate the need for motor responses beyond a simple "yes" or "no," head nod, or even eye blink. Thus, accuracy varies as a function of stimulus complexity and not motor requirements, a desirable characteristic for measures of comprehension.

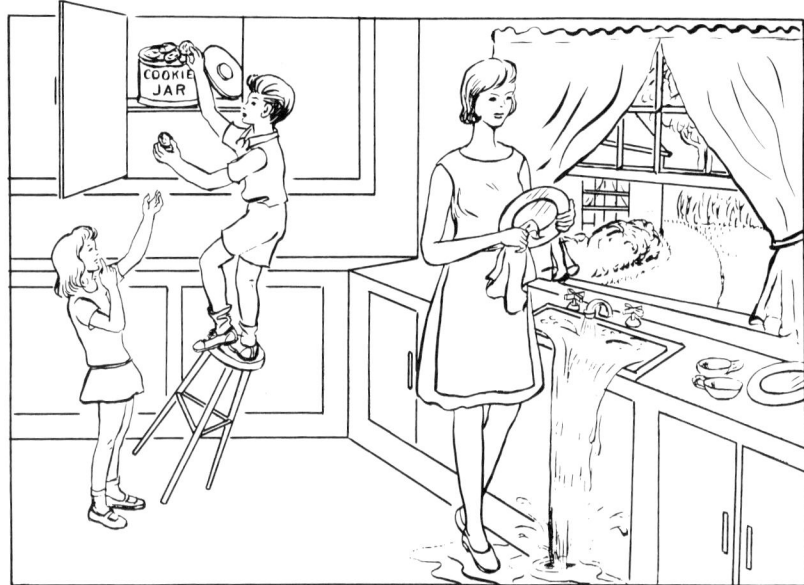

Figure 4-1
Action scene used in narrative portion of screening examination of language functions. *(From Goodglass H, Kaplan E:* The assessment of aphasia and related disorders, *ed 2, Philadelphia, 1983, Lea & Febiger. By permission of the publisher.)*

      3. *Right-left commands,* if there is disproportionate impairment, may reflect dominant parietal or right hemisphere dysfunction.
      4. *Complex commands,* because of their length and grammatical and syntactical complexity, often uncover subtle deficits in comprehension.
  B. *Reading.* Some items should be similar to those used to test verbal comprehension, especially when a discrepancy between listening and reading comprehension is suspected.
      1. *Letter identification* can be used to assess the basic ability to recognize letters. Aphasic errors are more likely to reflect auditory ("p" for "t") than visual ("m" for "w") errors; a consistent tendency toward visual errors is suggestive of left occipital or right hemisphere disease.
      2. *Letter reading* is used to assess recognition and retrieval of letter names. Letter naming is frequently better than picture naming in aphasic patients.
      3. *Single word reading* tasks assess comprehension at a very simple level. Some patients read words aloud inaccurately but

demonstrate accurate comprehension by pointing, whereas others read aloud accurately but fail to demonstrate comprehension.
    4. *Commands* assess reading comprehension at the sentence level. They also permit informal observations of visual field deficits and neglect (that is, when the patient reads aloud, words on the left or right side of the sentence may be consistently omitted).
II. Expression
  A. *Speaking.* Assessment of oral expression is crucial to differential diagnosis and localization, to establishing the functional severity of the communication deficit, and to identifying areas of preserved verbal ability that may be capitalized on during language therapy. For these reasons, a number of abilities should be assessed.
    1. A *conversational speech* sample is especially important for judgments about the fluency of speech. It permits observations of speech rate, articulatory accuracy, prosody, grammatical accuracy and completeness, word retrieval problems, and the amount of information conveyed per number of words. These observations may permit speech to be characterized as *fluent* or *nonfluent,* a categorization that correlates fairly well with postrolandic and prerolandic lesions, respectively. Conversation also reflects relevance, orientation, and organization, behaviors important for differentiating aphasic from some nonaphasic deficits.
    2. *Narrative speech tasks* are especially valuable when a patient gives only brief, unelaborated responses during basic conversational interaction. Showing the patient a pictured scene provides material to talk about and has the added advantage of specifying the content of the conversation. The observations to be made are the same as those made during conversation.
    3. *Repetition* of speech permits several observations. Disproportionately good repetition in contrast to spontaneous speech is associated with dominant hemisphere lesions outside the perisylvian zone. Gradually increasing the length of materials to be repeated is an indirect way of assessing verbal retention span, and repetition of low-content words and phrases (for example, "no ifs, ands, or buts") and complex syllable sequences is useful in detecting apraxia of speech and conduction aphasia.
    4. *Object naming* directly assesses word retrieval; however, it should not be confined to one category (for example, colors, objects, body parts), because relative category preservation or selective impairments sometimes occur. Word retrieval problems are

common to all "types" of aphasia but also occur in patients with confusion, dementia, and right hemisphere injury. However, the nature of the errors can vary among pathologic conditions, and their recognition can aid differential diagnosis.
5. *Sentence completion* is a word retrieval measure that is usually easier than object or picture naming because of the redundant cues provided in the stimulus sentence. For example, many patients, unable to name a picture of a bed, will readily say "bed" to complete the sentence "You sleep in a _____."
6. *Automatic speech* in patients with severe deficits may be fairly well preserved, even for those who are otherwise mute, and the ability to count or say the days of the week in the absence of other speech can be very valuable to diagnosis. For example, preserved counting in the otherwise mute patient rules out anarthria or severe dysarthria, localizes the lesion to the dominant hemisphere, and suggests relative preservation of nondominant hemisphere motor speech functions.
7. *Singing*, like automatic speech, should be assessed in any patient with limited verbal abilities due to aphasia or apraxia of speech. Highly overlearned songs, such as "Happy Birthday," sometimes elicit an adequate tune or even well-articulated lyrics in such patients.
8. Finally, *definition of words* and *explanation of proverbs* are sensitive to the concreteness or bizarreness often seen in demented or confused patients. Aphasic patients often demonstrate appreciation of abstract concepts and rarely give bizarre or irrelevant responses.

B. *Writing.* Writing is usually the most impaired modality in aphasia. In addition to resembling the patient's oral output, writing may reflect spelling and letter formation errors. In aphasia, such errors are typically present regardless of whether the dominant (and often paretic) or the nondominant hand is used.
1. *Dictated words* reduce word retrieval demands and permit the evaluation of written spelling and letter formation ability at a relatively simple level of complexity.
2. *Dictated sentences* are more complex but still do not require word retrieval. Spelling errors, word substitutions, and syntactical errors emerge more readily on these tasks than on dictated words.
3. *Spontaneous writing*, which requires patients to formulate their own expressions, is likely to elicit the full range of language (or cognitively based) errors that may be apparent in their speech, as well as spelling and letter formation errors.

4. *Copying* of letters and basic shapes is useful for assessing motor control and visual-spatial factors that may influence writing. Errors on these basic tasks usually are not attributable to the language deficits associated with aphasia.

The Disorders

With the results of the language examination, the clinician is in a position to answer several questions. Is the patient deficient in verbal comprehension, verbal expression, reading, or writing? Is the patient aphasic? If aphasia is present, does the pattern of deficit provide clues about more precise localization within the dominant hemisphere? Does the aphasia explain all the deficits, or is it embedded within a more diffuse impairment of cognitive function? Are deficiencies in language more consistent with nonaphasic deficits in cognitive, sensory, or motor function? Do nonaphasic deficits suggest a focal lesion outside the perisylvian language zone or diffuse, bilateral, or multifocal involvement?

Aphasia

Aphasia is an *impairment in the interpretation and formulation of language symbols*. In most instances, *impairment is present in all language modalities,* although sometimes to different degrees within and among patients. When aphasia is the only higher level cognitive deficit, and when deficits are present in all language modalities, the lesion includes the *dominant hemisphere* perisylvian area or underlying subcortical structures.

It is important to keep in mind that even with severe aphasia, the individual can be alert, cooperative, and responsive in relevant ways and can exhibit a desire and effort to communicate, however inadequate the result. Although not always cognizant of specific errors, these patients rarely actively deny their deficits and are very often frustrated by them. They also generally follow accepted rules for social interaction and display appropriate affective reactions to people and the environment. When these affective, social, and attentional attributes are abnormal, impairment other than or in addition to aphasia must be suspected.

Listening comprehension deficits

Deficits in listening generally worsen as redundancy and familiarity are decreased and length and complexity are increased. Short-term recall for verbal materials is usually reduced and is reflected in increased errors on lengthy commands, reduced digit span, and omission of information as length increases on sentence repetition tasks. Performance may improve substantially if commands are accompanied by nonverbal cues; this can lead to a perception that comprehension of spoken language is better than it actually is. When verbal comprehension is intact, deficits in other modalities are typically mild.

Reading comprehension deficits

Reading deficits are similar to verbal comprehension problems, although they tend to be more severe. When they are severe, the ability to match spoken to written letters and single words may be impaired. Mild impairments may be detected only in response to complex commands or paragraph-level materials. Most errors in reading aloud are semantic ("table" may be read as "chair," "up" as "down"), although visually based errors may occur. Finally, some aphasic patients read aloud without error but with poor comprehension; others may comprehend better than predicted by errors made during reading aloud.

Speaking deficits

Verbal expression deficits are the most striking feature of aphasia. Word retrieval problems are reflected in many ways, ranging from delays, to stated inability to retrieve a word, to *perseveration,* to *jargon* (calling a fork a "four-armed fire-breaker"), to *semantic paraphasias* ("fork" for "knife"), to *phonemic paraphasias* ("flife" for "knife"), to *neologisms* ("dillion" for "pencil"). Efforts at word retrieval may be accompanied by gestures or descriptions that clearly indicate that the concept is known or recognized. Patients who produce numerous phonemic paraphasias or jargon or neologistic responses may be unaware of errors and are generally more severely impaired than those who only delay or make semantic errors.

The fluency characteristics of speech contribute importantly to distinctions among different types of aphasia, distinctions that may reflect lesion locus within or around the perisylvian area. Conversational or narrative speech can be classified as *fluent* or *nonfluent,* although probably not reliably in more than 40% of patients, with the remainder in a gray area between the two categories.

Patients with fluent aphasic speech ("fluent aphasia") typically produce sentences of average length, with a variety of grammatical constructions, and normal rate and rhythm. Abnormalities consist of pauses for word retrieval and frequent semantic, phonemic, jargon, or neologistic errors, and relatively little specific information is conveyed per number of words uttered. Lesions associated with fluent speech characteristics tend to be temporal or parietal, or both.

Nonfluent aphasic speech ("nonfluent aphasia") is often telegraphic (as in a telegram, articles and prepositions are omitted or grammar is simplified; for example, "go to store" for "I went to the store") or simplified in syntactic complexity, with associated short phrases and sentences. Pauses occur frequently, both for word-finding and articulation efforts, and the prosodic features of speech are abnormal. Patients with nonfluent speech usually have an accompanying apraxia of speech. The associated lesion is usually posterior frontal or frontal-parietal.

Most aphasic patients have difficulty with repetition, and the characteristics of the repetition errors are usually similar to those in spontaneous speech or naming tasks. In addition, errors generally increase with increasing length because of short-term recall deficits for verbal materials.

Writing deficits
Writing is generally the most impaired modality. Errors in vocabulary, semantics, and syntax are usually consistent with those heard in speech. Spelling difficulties are usually apparent, devastatingly so in many cases, rendering recognition of intended words impossible (for example, "lotuck" for "fork").

Clusters of symptoms in aphasia
Typologies for aphasia are abundant, and a detailed discussion of them is beyond the scope of this chapter. The classification of aphasia with eponyms having anatomic implications (for example, Broca's aphasia, Wernicke's aphasia), along with a mixture of terms that imply underlying physiology (for example, conduction aphasia), sensory-motor dichotomies (for example, receptive aphasia, expressive aphasia), and symptom descriptions (for example, anomic aphasia), can be more confusing than helpful to clinical diagnosis and frequently promotes the fixing of a label at the expense of careful examination. In clinical practice, it is more important to identify salient behavior and clusters of language symptoms, because only they permit the diagnosis of aphasia and, occasionally, more precise localization within or around the perisylvian language area. Because the severity and behavioral manifestations of aphasia vary considerably, some appreciation of the variety of symptom clusters that may be encountered is of value. Brief descriptions of the most typical clusters of language symptoms follow.

Some aphasic patients exhibit a cluster of symptoms in which verbal comprehension is clearly superior to expression, speech characteristics are nonfluent, apraxia of speech is nearly always present, and repetition and naming ability are impaired. The associated lesion is perisylvian, most often in the frontal operculum and adjacent frontal lobe and in the parietal operculum. Such patients are often said to have *Broca's aphasia, expressive aphasia,* or *nonfluent aphasia.*

Some patients' verbal comprehension is significantly impaired, their speech characteristics are fluent, and verbal and phonemic paraphasias, jargon, and neologisms may be prominent. Repetition and naming are impaired. The associated lesion is perisylvian, often within the posterosuperior temporal and inferior parietal areas. These patients are often said to have *Wernicke's aphasia, receptive aphasia,* or *fluent aphasia.*

Some patients have fluent speech with verbal and phonemic paraphasias and word-finding delays, but there is a relative sparing of verbal and reading comprehension. However, their repetition is noticeably impaired, and it is the distinction between good comprehension and poor repetition that differentiates them from patients said to have Wernicke's aphasia. The lesion is perisylvian, is typically postrolandic, and often includes the supramarginal gyrus at the end of the sylvian fissure. These patients are sometimes said to have *conduction aphasia*.

Some patients have mild aphasia with relatively preserved comprehension and repetition but with obvious naming and word-retrieval difficulty. The lesion is perisylvian, most commonly temporal or temporoparietal. These individuals are sometimes said to have *anomic aphasia*.

Some individuals have severe and persisting aphasia in all modalities, usually with limited available speech and writing, and nonfluent speech. Repetition may be impossible. The lesion typically has destroyed large portions of the perisylvian language area. The term *global aphasia* is often applied to these cases.

Infrequently, patients who may closely resemble those said to have Broca's or Wernicke's aphasia have relatively preserved repetition. Their lesions are usually at the border of or beyond the perisylvian language area, vascularly in more distal portions of the middle cerebral artery or in the border zone with the anterior or posterior cerebral artery. The term *transcortical motor* or *transcortical sensory aphasia* is sometimes applied in these cases.

Prominent modality deficits

Although rare, significant deficits in only one or two language modalities can occur. Such deficits may coexist with aphasia or may occur in the absence of any true language impairment. Their differentiation from aphasia has important implications for diagnosis, localization, and management.

In *pure word deafness* (also called *auditory verbal agnosia* or *severe auditory imperception*), it may be impossible to recognize the meaning of any spoken message, even though hearing acuity is normal. Although usually accompanied by aphasia, this disturbance differs from the severe auditory comprehension impairment of severe aphasia because speech, reading, and writing are significantly better than verbal comprehension. The lesions producing this deficit are typically bitemporal or dominant temporal, although with sparing of Wernicke's area.

Significant reading impairment without significant language or writing impairment is referred to as *alexia without agraphia*. The mechanism of impairment presumably involves a disconnection between visual areas and the dominant perisylvian language area that must decode the written message. The lesion is typically in the dominant occipital lobe and splenium of the corpus callosum. When significant reading *and* writing impairment occur in the relative absence of aphasia in other modalities, the condition is called *alexia with agraphia*. The lesion usually involves the dominant angular gyrus.

Mutism can result from aphasia, though it rarely persists if aphasia is the only deficit. It may also be the product of severe dysarthria (anarthria) or apraxia of speech. Absence of speech may also occur in *akinetic mutism*. The akinetically mute patient, in contrast to the mute aphasic patient, is typically inert, immobile, and unresponsive, both verbally and nonverbally. The condition is usually associated with general cognitive deficits, and when verbal responses appear, they are markedly delayed, brief or unelaborated, low in volume, and concrete. Such patients may have bifrontal, thalamic, or mesencephalic lesions. Finally, mutism may be *psychogenic* or *hysterical*, a condition often differentiated from neurogenic mutism by the absence of deficits in other modalities, an absence of motor speech signs, preservation of oral vegetative functions, absent or bizarre attempts at speech, and, frequently, bland acceptance of the disability.

Other neurologic deficits affecting language and communication

Patients with *general intellectual impairment* or *dementia* often perform poorly on language examination and may appear genuinely aphasic. This is not surprising, because the diffuse nature of their cognitive deficits logically affects language functions. In this sense, demented patients often display aphasia. The challenge, however, is to determine if the language difficulty is the only impairment or if it is embedded within more diffuse cognitive deficits. Demented patients may handle concrete language tasks quite well. Their grammar, syntax, and speech prosody are nearly always fluent, and their language, when defective, most closely resembles that encountered in aphasia with fluent speech characteristics. It is generally believed that their primary language deficit is in the semantic sphere and that other language components are relatively spared. Unlike patients with focal aphasia, they often display disorientation and poor judgment, and their affect and social interaction may be inappropriate. Demented patients usually have short-term memory deficits that are out of proportion to their other language problems, and their handling of abstract tasks like definitions and proverbs is often literal and concrete to a degree that cannot be explained by word-finding problems.

Patients with the neurologic condition of *confusion* may do poorly on language examination. However, their disorientation, their bizarre, irrelevant, and confabulatory responses, their denial of or obliviousness to their deficits, and their inappropriate affect usually differentiate them from patients with aphasia.

Patients with *right (nondominant) hemisphere lesions* occasionally have difficulty on language tasks, but the misdiagnosis of aphasia usually is not made. They may, however, make naming errors that are visually based and may have great difficulty with reading as a result of neglect or visual field defects. Their writing, in addition to reflecting left neglect, may be poorly organized spatially and contain letter omissions, extra loops on letters, and repeated letter series, errors that reflect visual-perceptual rather than linguistic deficits. Also, many patients with right hemisphere impairment, although not linguistically impaired, have significant communication problems that often reflect a nearly mirror image of aphasic deficits. Among the receptive communication deficits that have been noted are difficulty interpreting implicit and implied meanings (for example, that "Can you tell me the time?" is usually a request, not a yes-no question), difficulty grasping the figurative meaning of metaphors and idiomatic expressions, and difficulty interpreting the moods conveyed by people's voices and body language. Expressively, they may digress in conversation or talk about unimportant components of a situation, have difficulty staying on topic, and have reduced ability to convey information through speech melody, facial expression, and body movements.

Chapter 5

The Cranial Nerves
Except II, III, IV, and VI

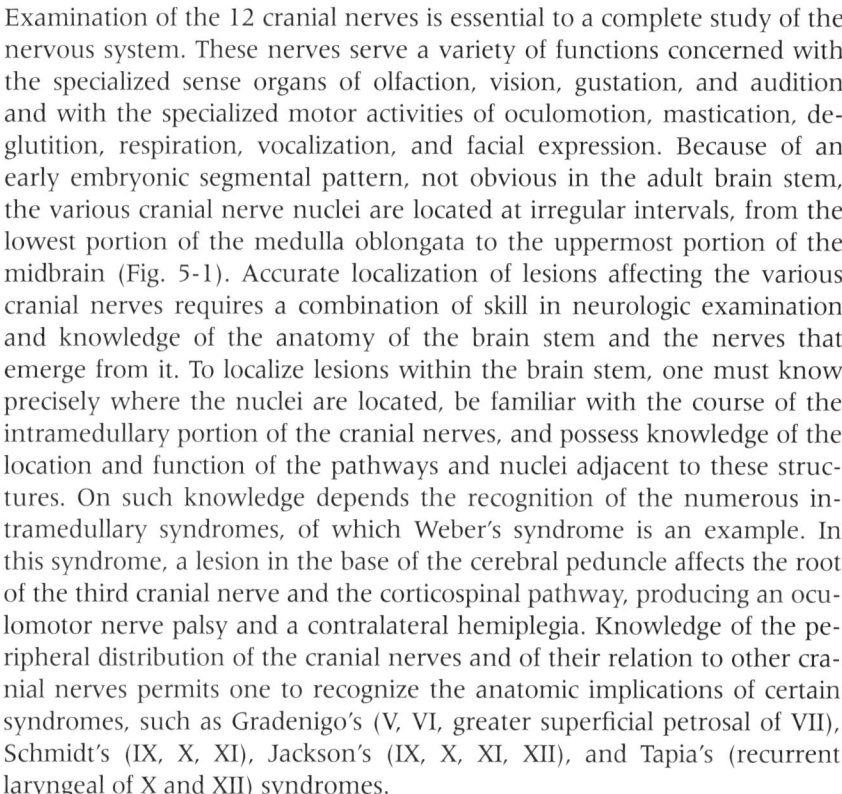

Examination of the 12 cranial nerves is essential to a complete study of the nervous system. These nerves serve a variety of functions concerned with the specialized sense organs of olfaction, vision, gustation, and audition and with the specialized motor activities of oculomotion, mastication, deglutition, respiration, vocalization, and facial expression. Because of an early embryonic segmental pattern, not obvious in the adult brain stem, the various cranial nerve nuclei are located at irregular intervals, from the lowest portion of the medulla oblongata to the uppermost portion of the midbrain (Fig. 5-1). Accurate localization of lesions affecting the various cranial nerves requires a combination of skill in neurologic examination and knowledge of the anatomy of the brain stem and the nerves that emerge from it. To localize lesions within the brain stem, one must know precisely where the nuclei are located, be familiar with the course of the intramedullary portion of the cranial nerves, and possess knowledge of the location and function of the pathways and nuclei adjacent to these structures. On such knowledge depends the recognition of the numerous intramedullary syndromes, of which Weber's syndrome is an example. In this syndrome, a lesion in the base of the cerebral peduncle affects the root of the third cranial nerve and the corticospinal pathway, producing an oculomotor nerve palsy and a contralateral hemiplegia. Knowledge of the peripheral distribution of the cranial nerves and of their relation to other cranial nerves permits one to recognize the anatomic implications of certain syndromes, such as Gradenigo's (V, VI, greater superficial petrosal of VII), Schmidt's (IX, X, XI), Jackson's (IX, X, XI, XII), and Tapia's (recurrent laryngeal of X and XII) syndromes.

CRANIAL NERVE I—OLFACTORY NERVE

Olfactory neurons of the first order consist of bipolar sensory cells, the ciliated distal axons of which pass to the superior part of the nasal

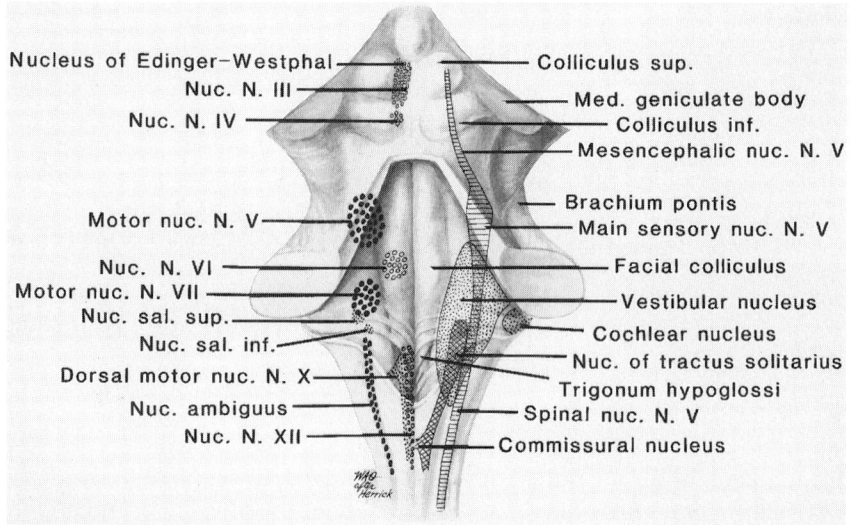

Figure 5-1
Cranial nerve nuclei. *(After Herrick, from Ranson SW, Clark SL: The anatomy of the nervous system: its development and function, Philadelphia, 1947, WB Saunders Co.)*

mucosa and the central axons (unmyelinated) of which are grouped together in small bundles to constitute the olfactory nerve. After passing through the cribriform plate of the ethmoid bone, the central processes reach the olfactory bulb, which lies in contact with the cribriform plate. The neurons of the second order, located in the olfactory bulb, form the olfactory tract and course posteriorly from the bulb along the olfactory groove of the frontal bone to the olfactory trigone and then into the brain and to the hippocampal gyrus of the same side. Further complex connections, including those to the hippocampus, fornix, mamillary bodies, piriform area, septum pellucidum, anterior commissure, amygdaloid nuclei, and habenular nuclei, exist but are not of great clinical significance in olfaction.

Clinical Examination

Odoriferous but nonirritating substances, such as crushed cloves, coffee, wintergreen, and camphor, are used for testing olfactory sensation. The ability to perceive such substances is tested separately in each nostril by having the patient sniff the test substance while the patient or the examiner closes the other nostril. The patient is asked first to state whether an odor is perceived. If the answer is "yes," the patient is asked to identify the smell. Although the patient may be unable to name the test substance, the appreciation of an odor is sufficient to exclude anosmia.

Interpretation

Unilateral brain lesions do not ordinarily cause loss of the sense of smell unless the olfactory tracts are damaged. Intranasal disease is a common cause of impaired olfactory sense and should be excluded before a diagnosis of neurogenic anosmia is made. Lesions of one olfactory tract produce unilateral anosmia. The most common cause of anosmia is trauma. Tumors at the base of the frontal lobe, such as a meningioma arising from the olfactory groove, also can cause anosmia.

Cranial Nerves II, III, IV, and VI

These nerves are discussed in the following chapter on neuro-ophthalmology.

CRANIAL NERVE V—TRIGEMINAL NERVE

Anatomy

The trigeminal nerve is the largest of the cranial nerves; it is sensory to the face and buccal and nasal mucosae and motor to the muscles of mastication.

Most of the cell bodies of the sensory portion of the trigeminal nerve lie in the gasserian ganglion; a few are located in its mesencephalic nucleus. Gasserian ganglion cells are unipolar, giving origin to fibers that bifurcate; the peripheral branches enter one of the three divisions of the nerve. The proximal branches form the sensory root, enter the lateral portion of the pons, and there divide into ascending and descending fibers. The ascending branches pass to the main sensory nucleus (concerned primarily with the sensation of touch) and to the mesencephalic root of the nerve (concerned with proprioception from muscles of mastication and periodontal membranes). The descending branch forms the descending root of the trigeminal nerve and mainly subserves the sensations of pain and temperature. It extends on the same side through the pons and medulla to reach the uppermost segments of the spinal cord, giving off terminals and collaterals to the nucleus of the spinal trigeminal tract en route. From the main sensory nucleus most of the fibers of the second order cross to the opposite side and ascend to the ventral posteromedial nucleus of the thalamus. The exact course of the fibers of the second order originating in the nucleus of the trigeminal tract is controversial, but at least some also end in the ventral posteromedial thalamic nucleus. The cortical representation for facial sensation is in the inferior portion of the postcentral gyrus of the opposite side.

The motor nucleus of the trigeminal nerve lies at the midlevel of the pons, medial and ventral to the main sensory nucleus. The efferent fibers from this nucleus leave the pons and pass underneath the gasserian ganglion to become incorporated in the mandibular nerve.

The three divisions of the trigeminal nerve are the ophthalmic, the maxillary, and the mandibular.

The first division, the ophthalmic nerve, passes into the upper part of the orbit through the superior orbital fissure and is distributed to the conjunctiva, cornea, upper lid, forehead, bridge of the nose, and scalp as far posteriorly as the vertex of the skull. It supplies sensation to the area shown in Figure 10-5.

The second division, the maxillary nerve, leaves the middle fossa through the foramen rotundum and enters the sphenomaxillary fossa. The nerve then goes through the inferior orbital fissure, crosses the floor of the orbit, and emerges through the inferior orbital foramen. The maxillary nerve conducts tactile, pain, and temperature sensation from the skin of the cheek and lateral aspects of the nose, the maxillary teeth and jaw, and the mucosal surfaces of the uvula, hard palate, nasopharynx, and lower part of the nasal cavity (see Fig. 10-5).

The third division, the mandibular nerve, leaves the skull through the foramen ovale. This nerve carries sensory and motor impulses. The sensory distribution is from the skin of the mandibular jaw, pinna of the ear, anterior portion of the external auditory meatus, homolateral side of the tongue, mandibular teeth, gums, floor of the mouth, and buccal surface of the cheek. The motor supply is to the muscles of mastication (temporal, pterygoid, and masseter).

Clinical Examination

The technique of testing pain, thermal, and other sensations in the area supplied by the trigeminal nerve is described in Chapter 10.

The corneal reflex is tested by having the patient look to one side while the cornea is lightly touched with cotton wool that has been twisted into a compact cylinder or drawn out into a point. Sometimes it seems advantageous to moisten the cotton before the test is performed. The cotton should be introduced from a direction other than that of the gaze in order to minimize reflex defensive blinking. The normal response to this stimulus is a prompt, partial or complete closure of the eyelids. The reflexes of each eye are compared, and if a defect seems to exist, the patient is asked whether the sensation is equal on the two sides. (The efferent portion of the reflex is mediated through the facial nerves; see *Facial Nerve*, below.)

After corneal sensation is tested, the wisp of moistened cotton is rolled into a pointed cylinder, the patient is instructed to close the eyes, and the cotton is carefully and gently inserted into the right (or left) nostril. Normally the patient will draw away slightly and wrinkle the nose. Then the other nostril is tested. This test provides an easy way of quantitating sensation by the nasociliary division of each ophthalmic branch of each trigeminal nerve.

The temporal and masseter muscles are examined by having the patient clamp the jaws together while the examiner palpates the muscles and attempts to separate the jaws by applying pressure downward on the chin. Complete absence of contraction or severe degrees of weakness of the temporal and masseter muscles are readily detected, but minor degrees of weakness may be ascertained with difficulty. In unilateral weakness of the pterygoid muscle, the jaw is seen to deviate toward the side of the weakened muscle as it is opened slowly. Furthermore, the partially opened jaw is easily pushed toward the side of the weakened pterygoid muscle.

Tumors in the middle fossa and in the cerebellopontine angle may affect one or more portions of the trigeminal nerve. Such lesions more commonly produce impairment of sensory function than of motor power. Cerebellopontine angle tumors frequently produce a decrease in the corneal reflex on the same side before there is subjective or objective sensory disturbance in the face. A previous injection of alcohol into one or more divisions of the nerve as a treatment for trigeminal neuralgia may account for a defect in function.

CRANIAL NERVE VII—FACIAL NERVE

Anatomy

The seventh cranial nerve is motor to the muscles of facial expression and mediates taste to the anterior two-thirds of the tongue and general sensation to portions of the external ear.

The motor nucleus of the facial nerve lies deep in the pons. From the nucleus the fibers course dorsomedially, looping around the nucleus of the abducens nerve, and then proceed ventrally, laterally, and caudally to emerge from the pons at the pontomedullary junction. Passing into the internal auditory meatus with the eighth cranial nerve, the seventh nerve enters the facial canal of the temporal bone. The canal bends around the anterior boundary of the vestibule of the inner ear, and at this angle lies the geniculate ganglion. Distal to the geniculate ganglion, the facial nerve gives off a small branch to the stapedius muscle and then the chorda tympani, which carries fibers of taste from the anterior two-thirds of the tongue via the lingual nerve (Fig. 5-2). The facial nerve leaves the facial canal through the stylomastoid foramen, passes through the parotid gland, and supplies the muscles of the face, the posterior belly of the digastric, the stylohyoid, the buccinator, and the platysma.

The sensory portion of the facial nerve arises from the geniculate ganglion and consists of peripheral and central branches coming from

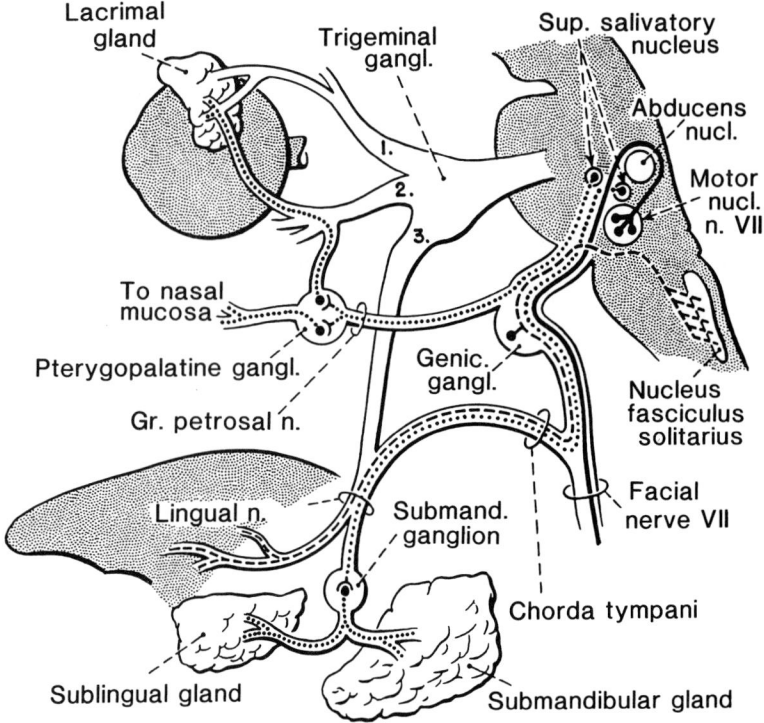

Figure 5-2
Diagram of the components of the facial nerve. *(Modified from Strong OS, Elwyn A: Human neuroanatomy, Baltimore, Williams & Wilkins Co. By permission of the publisher.)*

unipolar cells in the ganglion. The central branches form the intermediate nerve (nerve of Wrisberg) and end in the upper part of the nucleus of the tractus solitarius in the pons. The peripheral branches come from the taste buds of the anterior two-thirds of the tongue. The pathway these taste fibers follow to the brain stem is not clear from present evidence, which suggests that it is variable. In most cases, the taste afferents reach the geniculate ganglion by way of the lingual nerve, the chorda tympani, and a short segment of the facial nerve. A few fibers mediating general somatic sensory impulses from the external ear also have cells of origin in the geniculate ganglion.

The facial nerve also carries parasympathetic fibers (secretory and vasodilator) from the superior salivary nucleus. These fibers leave the facial nerve over the chorda tympani nerve as well as via the greater superficial petrosal nerve, passing to the submaxillary and sphenopalatine ganglia, where they synapse with postganglionic cells whose fibers innervate the maxillary and lacrimal glands and the vessels of the mucous membrane of the palate, nasopharynx, and nasal cavity (see Fig. 5-2).

Clinical Examination

Examination of facial nerve function begins with the initial observation of the patient; during talking and smiling, significant abnormalities, such as slowness of contraction of one corner of the mouth on smiling, may be noted. The motor portion of the nerve innervates muscles that wrinkle the forehead, close the eyes, purse the lips, and retract the buccal angles in a smile or grimace. The patient is instructed to wrinkle the forehead by looking upward and to resist the examiner's attempts to smooth out the forehead by forcefully running his or her fingers down the forehead on both sides. The ability to close the eyelids tightly is tested against the attempts of the examiner to pry them open. The patient is asked to show his or her teeth by retracting the buccal angles, to whistle, and to purse the lips against the pressure of the examiner's fingers. Slight unilateral weakness or slowness of movement may be made more apparent by having the patient quickly alternate between smiling and pursing the lips.

The lower facial musculature can be tested in stuporous or uncooperative patients by observing the wincing reaction occasioned by pressing firmly over the styloid processes just posterior to the angles of the jaw. In infants, the facial movements are observed during crying.

The detection of a lag or droop of one corner of the mouth on smiling is often of sufficient importance that the examiner should specifically attempt to make the patient smile. Some people smile after whistling or in response to a remark from the examiner such as "I wish I could think of some joke to make you smile." Some examiners may resort to a stock joke that experience has proved effective in provoking a smile from the most dour patient.

The platysma can be observed to contract when the patient makes a maximal effort to draw the lower lip and angle of the mouth downward and outward, at the same time tensing the skin over the anterior surface of the neck. The examiner demonstrates the test and instructs the patient to mimic the movements.

There are two types of facial nerve motor weakness, namely, that resulting from involvement of corticobulbar pathways (upper motor neuron) and that from involvement of lower motor neurons. The former is characterized by inability of the patient to retract the corner of the mouth normally while the forehead function remains intact on the same side. There may be moderate weakness of eyelid closing, but this is less pronounced than the weakness at the corner of the mouth. Usually, the palpebral fissure is also widened on the involved side. The primary motor neurons of the brain stem supplying the forehead muscles of each side receive upper motor neuron innervation from both sides of the cortex. A unilateral lesion, therefore, does not impair forehead muscle function. Lesions in the facial nucleus, or facial nerve, cause paralysis of half of the entire face, including the forehead, eyelids, and lips.

As can be seen in Figure 5-2, a lesion of the facial nerve peripheral to its junction with the chorda tympani will not produce impairment of taste on the anterior two-thirds of the tongue.

Taste is examined with the use of sugar, tartaric acid, sodium chloride, quinine, or similar substances. The patient is told to protrude the tongue; a small quantity of the test substance (on wet cotton on an applicator) is gently rubbed on one side of the tongue, and the patient signals identification of the test substance before drawing the tongue into the mouth. Thus, diffusion of the taste to the opposite side or to the posterior third of the tongue, which would obscure the test result, is prevented.

Most cases of facial paralysis of lower motor neuron type have no apparent cause and are therefore best classified as idiopathic facial palsies. The name "Bell's palsy" is also commonly used to describe cases of idiopathic facial palsy. It should be recalled that facial paralysis of the lower motor neuron type is a syndrome that may have many different causes, including infection by herpes zoster, otitis media, meningitis, Lyme disease, syphilis, or leprosy; inflammation, such as that in sarcoidosis or inflammatory polyradiculoneuropathy; and neoplasm, such as acoustic neuroma, cerebellopontine angle meningioma, neurofibroma of the facial nerve, or leptomeningeal carcinomatosis. Several possible causes have been proposed for the idiopathic facial palsies, including an autoimmune-mediated inflammatory focal neuropathy, herpes simplex viral infection of the nerve, and swelling of the nerve induced by exposure to cold air or allergic factors leading to compression by the bony facial canal.

Central types of facial palsy (upper motor neuron) may result from any type of lesion, be it vascular, neoplastic, inflammatory, or other, that involves the portion of the motor cortex that supplies the face or the projections therefrom in the corticobulbar pathways through the internal capsule, cerebral peduncle, or pons.

CRANIAL NERVE VIII—ACOUSTIC NERVE

Anatomy
The acoustic nerve is made up of two divisions: the cochlear, subserving the sense of hearing, and the vestibular, subserving the sense of balance.

Cochlear division
The cochlear division arises from bipolar cells in the spiral ganglion of the cochlea in the petrous portion of the temporal bone. The central fibers enter the cranial cavity through the internal auditory meatus,

ending in the cochlear nuclei of the medulla. Each cochlear nucleus is connected with the cortex of both temporal lobes; therefore, unilateral cortical or subcortical lesions do not produce a unilateral loss of hearing.

Vestibular division
Bipolar cells in the vestibular ganglion within the internal auditory meatus give off peripheral fibers, which end in the neuroepithelium of the vestibular portion of the labyrinth (cristae ampullaris of the semicircular canals and the maculae of the utricle and saccule), and central fibers, which enter the medulla beside those of the cochlear nerve. In the medulla, the fibers terminate in the vestibular nuclei, which have connections through the vestibulospinal tracts for reflex movement of the limbs and the trunk in response to stimulation of the vestibular end organs, through the medial longitudinal fasciculus for control of conjugate eye movements in relation to movements of the head, and with the cerebellum to assist in the control of muscle tone as it relates to postural adjustments.

Projections to the cerebral cortex, especially the posterior portions of the temporal lobes, undoubtedly exist but have not been accurately identified. Lesions of the vestibular nuclei cause severe vertigo and nystagmus that are difficult to differentiate symptomatically from labyrinthine vertigo. Lesions of the medial longitudinal fasciculus cause internuclear ophthalmoplegia but do not cause dysequilibrium.

Clinical Examination
Cochlear division
The sense of hearing may be tested by a number of techniques. The so-called dollar watch is a commonly used test object. In a quiet room, the dollar watch may be heard approximately 40 inches from the normal ear. If the room is less quiet, it may be heard normally at 30 inches or less from the ear. The watch is first held outside the hearing range of one ear while the other ear is closed. The patient is instructed to indicate the first detected sound as the watch is gradually moved nearer to the ear. In recording hearing on the neurologic record, a fraction is used. The numerator represents the number of inches at which the watch can be heard by the patient. The denominator is the distance in number of inches at which the watch can be heard by a normal ear. (Watches differ in size and form, and the examiner must know the normal value for the test object being used.) Thus, 10/10, 20/20, or 40/40 hearing would represent a normal result with different watches or with the same watch under different conditions. A recording of 10/30 would indicate that a watch had been heard 10 inches from the ear and that the same object would have been heard 30 inches from a normal ear. If a watch normally heard at 30 inches was not heard on contact with the ear, the hearing would be recorded as 0/30; if heard only on contact, as c/30.

Another object for testing air conduction is a vibrating tuning fork of medium pitch (C = 256 vibrations per second). These are not accurate quantitative tests of hearing. To measure hearing sense accurately, the electric audiometer is used and an audiogram is made.

In the normal ear, air conduction is greater than bone conduction. The comparison of bone conduction and air conduction is known as the Rinne test. The activated tuning fork is placed against the mastoid bone, and the patient is instructed to indicate when it can no longer be heard. The fork is then placed beside the external auditory meatus and estimation of air conduction is made. The test result is said to be positive, or normal, when the tuning fork is heard about twice as long by air conduction as by bone conduction. An abnormal Rinne test result is a sign of a middle ear defect or of blocking of the external auditory canal. In involvement of the cochlear nerve, air conduction and bone conduction are quantitatively decreased, but the Rinne result is positive (normal).

The base of the vibrating tuning fork is next placed on the vertex of the skull (Weber's test). If hearing is normal, the sound is heard equally in both ears; that is, the sound is not lateralized. In middle ear disease or in blocking of the external auditory canal, the sound is better heard on the affected side (lateralized to the affected side). If the cochlear nerve is involved on one side, the sound is better heard on the opposite, or normal, side.

In the differentiation of labyrinthine and acoustic nerve or brain stem lesions, special auditory studies are often essential and can be most helpful in localizing the site of the vestibular disturbance. These audiologic tests require special equipment and personnel trained in audiology to apply and to interpret the results.

Over the past 50 years, numerous tests of auditory function have been used to try to differentiate eighth nerve lesions from cochlear lesions. Acoustic reflex tests measure the contraction of the stapedius muscle in response to intense acoustic stimuli. They require relatively inexpensive equipment and can be completed in a short time. The true-positive rate for eighth nerve disease is about 85%. The true-positive rate for cochlear involvement is about 85%. Since auditory reflex tests are relatively simple to perform, they provide a good screen for patients.

Brain stem auditory evoked potentials measure the electrophysiologic response of the auditory system to stimuli. Waveforms are generated and measured to determine if the disorder is in the cochlea or more proximal. These evoked potentials are more difficult to perform and require a more expensive apparatus.

Brain stem auditory evoked potentials form the most accurate test and can identify eighth nerve lesions in about 95% of patients. The true-positive rate in patients with cochlear disease is 89%.

Békésy audiometry, the alternate binaural loudness balance test, and the short increment sensitivity index are the three tests previously used to further evaluate acoustic function. These tests are far less accurate and therefore less reliable.

Vestibular division
Caloric and rotational stimuli are used to produce changes in the endolymph current in the semicircular canals and thus test the vestibular apparatus. The performance and interpretation of these tests constitute a complex examination. The student is referred to standard textbooks of otolaryngology, neurology, and neurophysiology for details concerning this type of examination.

Patients thought to have disease of the vestibular system may have vestibular function more simply tested by means of a modified caloric (Bárány) test. After being told to signify the onset of dizziness or nausea, the patient is placed upright with the head tilted 60 degrees backward, and the external auditory canal is irrigated with 100 to 200 mL of cold (19°C to 21°C) water or 5 to 10 mL of very cold (0°C to 10°C) water. The patient is then examined for nystagmus and past pointing with each hand. The time elapsed before the onset of dizziness or nausea is noted.

The normal findings after irrigation of the right ear, with the patient in the position described earlier, are sensation of nausea, horizontal nystagmus with the slow component to the right, past pointing to the left, and falling to the right. With complete interruption of vestibular nerve function, there is no dizziness, nystagmus, past pointing, or falling. With incomplete interruption of nerve function, the usual responses are decreased on the involved side. If the normal response is obtained save for the absence of nystagmus, it is possible that the vestibular connections with the medial longitudinal fasciculus are defective.

Patients with hyperirritability of the vestibular system have increased responses to these tests. The complaint of dizziness may be simply produced or exaggerated by rapidly turning the patient's head from side to side a few times. Nystagmus may appear immediately after this maneuver, and observations should be made for its presence.

A much more accurate and now rather widely practiced method of recording nystagmus is *electronystagmography*. This procedure is based on a voltage difference in the eye, the retina being negative and the cornea positive. This corneal-retinal potential allows the eye to act as a dipole. Electrodes are placed on either side of the eyes in the plane of the eye movement to be recorded. On ocular rotation associated with nystagmus, the electrodes detect a displacement of the corneal-retinal potential as the positive pole at the front of the eye moves closer to one electrode and the negative charge at the back moves toward the other. These changes are registered by electronic instruments and can be analyzed quantitatively and qualitatively.

Electronystagmography allows one to record nystagmus behind closed eyelids or in the dark, hence eliminating the suppressive effect of visual fixation. As a result, the sensitivity with which spontaneous and induced nystagmus can be traced is significantly enhanced, and a permanent objective record is obtained against which to compare later findings.

All patients complaining of vertigo should undergo the test for positional nystagmus (Nylén-Bárány test), especially when the results of otologic and neurologic studies are negative and when no cause for the vertigo has been found. It is specifically helpful in patients who have had head injuries and in whom positional dizziness is the chief complaint.

The patient (in this example, male) is seated on the examining table so that when he reclines, his head will hang over the edge of the table (Fig. 5-3). He should be reassured and be told to keep his eyes open, to relax with his hands in his lap, and not to be alarmed if he becomes dizzy. The examiner then gently turns the patient's head to the left and, fairly rapidly, lowers him to a reclining position with head hanging over the edge of the table. The examiner supports the patient's head with one hand while asking him to look toward the examiner's finger, which is held to the left, so that the patient's eyes are directed laterally and slightly downward. If no nystagmus appears in 15 seconds, the patient is raised to the upright position for 15 seconds with the head in the neutral position. The test is then repeated with the head in the neutral position, in other words, hanging over the end of the table with the eyes

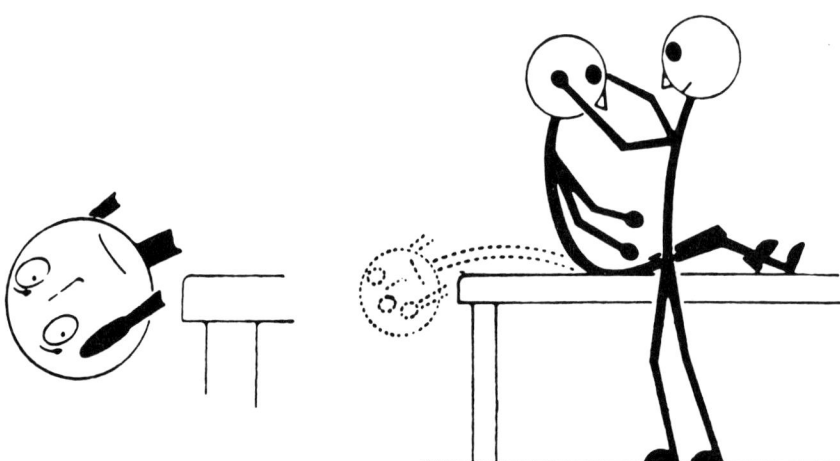

Figure 5-3
Seating of patient on table to test for positional nystagmus. *(From Harrison MS: Benign positional vertigo. In Wolfson RJ, editor: The vestibular system and its diseases, Philadelphia, 1966, University of Pennsylvania Press, pp 404–427. By permission of the publisher.)*

directed upward. Again the patient assumes a sitting position for 15 seconds, and the test is repeated with the head turned to the right. If no nystagmus or vertigo appears within 15 seconds, the patient is returned to the sitting position. Often the patient becomes dizzy momentarily on sitting up, and if his eyes are directed toward the side opposite that toward which his head was turned when he was reclining, brief horizontal nystagmus may be noted.

Various classifications of the results of this test have been proposed. About 90% of the patients in whom nystagmus develops during the test demonstrate rotatory nystagmus toward the lowermost ear while the head is turned to one side or the other. Nystagmus appears on recumbency after a brief (1 to 5 seconds) latent period, rapidly reaches a peak (4 to 8 seconds), and is accompanied by variable but often rather severe vertigo. Thereafter, nystagmus and vertigo decrease rapidly (within a few seconds) and disappear. This type of response usually appears with the head turned to one side only and is easily fatigued; in other words, it is not reproducible more than once or twice unless an hour or more is allowed between tests. Also, it is often referred to as "benign positional nystagmus" because it usually does not reflect significant, identifiable, or progressive vestibular disturbance. However, this response, along with the other types of responses to be described, has been observed occasionally with lesions in any part of the vestibular system; benign positional nystagmus is allegedly caused by derangement of the utriculus toward which the rotatory nystagmus beats.

In the test for positional nystagmus, the occurrence of persistent nystagmus with the patient in the "head hanging" position, with direction changed or fixed, with or without vertigo, and without fatigue on repeated testing is more commonly associated with lesions of the brain stem or cerebellum. This is true also when the nystagmus is vertical in direction. Persistent direction-changing or direction-fixed nystagmus is encountered in only a small percentage (10% to 15%) of patients with positive responses to the test for positional nystagmus. Occasionally, a patient, when tested, shows vigorous nystagmus without complaining of vertigo; this reaction is also apt to be found with lesions of the brain stem rather than with peripheral disturbances.

If hearing loss and vertigo or positional lightheadedness are present, it may be advisable to obtain trispiral tomograms of the petrous bones to rule out otosclerosis.

CRANIAL NERVE IX—GLOSSOPHARYNGEAL NERVE

Anatomy
The glossopharyngeal nerve contains sensory and motor fibers. The visceral sensory fibers mediate taste from the posterior third of the tongue,

information from the carotid body and aortic baroreceptors and chemoreceptors, and general sensation from the tympanic membrane, lining of the tympanic cavity, external auditory meatus, skin at the junction of the ear and mastoid, and mucous membranes of the posterior pharynx, tonsils, and posterior soft palate. These afferents arise from cells in the inferior (petrosal) ganglia and end in the tractus solitarius in the medulla. Through the tractus solitarius, fibers connect with cells in the superior salivary nucleus to complete reflex arcs concerned with salivation. Secretory fibers arise in the inferior salivary nucleus and pass into the middle ear and then through the lesser petrosal nerve to the otic ganglion, from which postganglionic fibers supply the parotid gland. The glossopharyngeal nerve emerges through the jugular foramen. A few somatic sensory fibers mediating sensation from the external ear arise from the superior ganglion and pass into the descending tract of the fifth nerve. Motor fibers arise from a nucleus in the medulla that is rostral to the nucleus ambiguus and pass to the stylopharyngeus muscle (branchial striated muscle).

Clinical Examination
The ninth nerve is tested by touching the posterior wall of the pharynx with a tongue depressor or applicator stick. The normal response is prompt contraction of the pharyngeal muscles, with or without gagging. However, because the posterior pharyngeal wall is also supplied by the tenth cranial nerve, this maneuver does not test the ninth nerve in isolation. The testing of taste sensation on the posterior one-third of the tongue is technically difficult and of little clinical value. Glossopharyngeal neuralgia and its rare association with syncope is an infrequent clinical condition that emphasizes the importance of glossopharyngeal anatomy.

CRANIAL NERVE X—VAGUS NERVE

Anatomy
The vagus nerve has somatic motor fibers that arise from the nucleus ambiguus and autonomic fibers that arise from the dorsal motor nucleus. The motor fibers from the nucleus ambiguus innervate the striated muscles of the pharynx, tongue (palatoglossus), and larynx (except stylopharyngeus and tensor veli palatini). The fibers from the dorsal motor nucleus of the vagus are autonomic and pass via the peripheral parasympathetic ganglia to activate the smooth muscles of the trachea, bronchi, esophagus, and gastrointestinal tract up to the splenic flexure. These general visceral efferents also activate the secretory glands of the pharynx, larynx, lungs, gastrointestinal tract, liver, and pancreas, inhibit the sphincters of the upper gastrointestinal tract, and slow the heart rate.

The sensory, or afferent, fibers from cells in the inferior (nodose) ganglia end in the tractus solitarius of the medulla. They convey visceral sensation from the lower pharynx, larynx, trachea, bronchi, heart, esophagus, and most of the gastrointestinal tract and impulses from stretch receptors in the wall of the aortic arch and chemoreceptors in the aortic bodies. General somatic afferent fibers with cell bodies in the superior (jugular) ganglion mediate sensation from the back of the ear, external auditory canal, part of the tympanic membrane, part of the pharynx and larynx, and part of the dural floor of the posterior cranial fossa via the spinal tract of the fifth nerve.

Clinical Examination
Clinical testing of the vagus nerve is difficult despite its size and many functions. Unilateral paralysis of the motor portion causes ipsilateral paralysis of the muscles of the palate, pharynx, and larynx. Weakness of the vocal cord causes the voice to be hoarse, and weakness of the palate, particularly if bilateral, can cause hypernasal speech. Lesions of the recurrent laryngeal branch of the vagus nerve produce weakness or paralysis of the ipsilateral vocal cord, causing dysphonia. The soft palate is observed as the patient says "ah." Normally, the median raphe rises in the midline and the uvula hangs in the midline. In unilateral weakness, there is deviation to the intact side. Some persons without weakness may have an asymmetrical soft palate. Unilateral impairment of the vagus does not usually affect swallowing. Bilateral lesions can cause dysphagia and regurgitation. The sensory component of the vagus nerve is difficult to assess clinically.

CRANIAL NERVE XI—ACCESSORY NERVE

Anatomy
The accessory nerve consists of a cranial portion and a spinal portion. The cranial accessory nerve emerges from the caudal nucleus ambiguus and joins the vagus nerve to form part of the inferior laryngeal nerve. The spinal portion arises from cells in the ventrolateral anterior horn of the upper five cervical cord segments. The motor fibers unite between dorsal and ventral roots along the upper cervical cord, enter the skull through the foramen magnum, and exit through the jugular foramen. The nerve innervates the sternocleidomastoid and trapezius muscles.

Clinical Examination
The accessory nerve is examined by having the patient turn the head forcibly against the examiner's hand away from the muscle being tested while the sternocleidomastoid muscle is observed and palpated. The function of the trapezius muscle is assessed by having the patient shrug

and retract the shoulders against resistance. Unilateral paralysis of the trapezius results in the inability to elevate and retract the shoulders and difficulty raising the arm above the horizontal. There is depression in the shoulder contour (trapezial ridge), with downward and lateral displacement of the scapula.

CRANIAL NERVE XII—HYPOGLOSSAL NERVE

Anatomy
The hypoglossal nerve supplies the somatic muscles of the tongue. The nucleus is located in the midline medullary tegmentum near the floor of the fourth ventricle. The nerve emerges from the skull via the hypoglossal canal.

Clinical Examination
The patient is asked to protrude the tongue, and the movements are evaluated. Observations should include the position of the tongue, the strength and rapidity of movement, paralysis, atrophy, and abnormal movements. The strength of the tongue can be tested by having the patient push the tongue against each cheek while the examiner pushes against the protruding cheek. Direct palpation may confirm atrophy. An upper motor neuron lesion may cause some contralateral loss of function of the hypoglossal nerve and deviation of the tongue away from the lesion. Bilateral upper motor neuron lesions cause the alternate motion rate of the tongue to be slow. When the hypoglossal nucleus or nerve is involved, the protruded tongue deviates to the side of the lesion and is atrophic.

Chapter 6

Neuro-Ophthalmology
Including Cranial Nerves II, III, IV, and VI

CRANIAL NERVE II (OPTIC NERVE) AND VISUAL PATHWAY

Anatomy

The optic nerve extends from the optic disk to the optic chiasm and is composed of axons originating in the ganglion cells of the retina, which lie near its surface. The terminal organs of sight are the rods and cones. The rods subserve black-and-white vision and the cones color vision. The rods and cones are found in the deepest layers of the retina, separated from the choroid by a layer of pigment cells. Cones alone are found at the fovea, and they predominate over the rods in the rest of the macula. However, elsewhere in the retina the rods are more numerous than the cones. The rods and cones relay impulses to the ganglion cells through the bipolar cells.

The fibers of the ganglion cells converge toward the optic disk, where they emerge from the eye as the optic nerve. The macula, the site of the most highly developed end-organs of sight and likewise of the most acute vision, is located somewhat less than two disk diameters to the temporal side of the optic disk. Fibers from ganglion cells in this region pass, in a special arrangement called the "papillomacular bundle," to the temporal portion of the optic disk. The nerve fibers pierce the sclera through a sievelike modification, the lamina cribrosa. At this transition point, the nerve becomes myelinated. Since there are no rods or cones at the optic disk, a corresponding blind spot in the field of vision is produced.

The optic nerve courses posteriorly through the orbit and enters the cranial cavity through the optic foramen (which also contains the ophthalmic artery) (Fig. 6-1) and joins its fellow of the opposite side to form the optic chiasm. As seen in Figure 6-2, a partial decussation of the fibers from the two sides takes place in the optic chiasm. In this decussation, fibers from the nasal retina, subserving the temporal visual field,

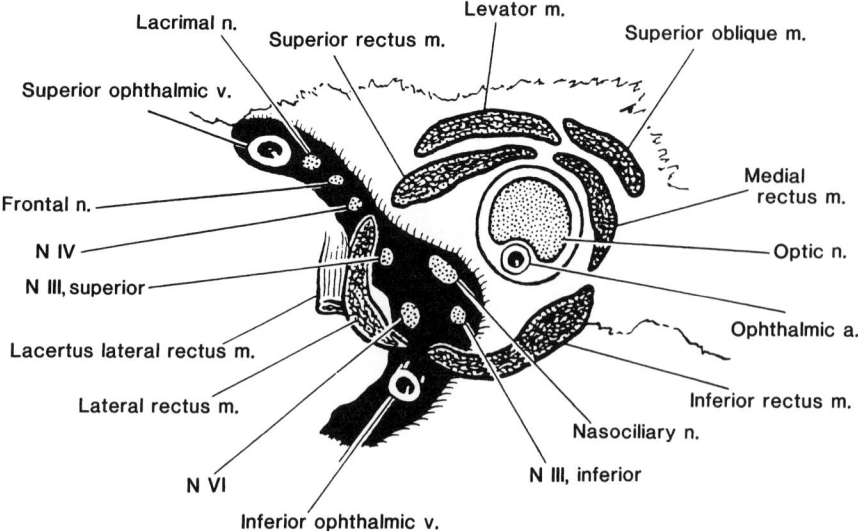

Figure 6-1
Apex of the right orbit showing the relationship of the sites of extraocular muscle attachment (annulus of Zinn) and adjacent structures. *(From Burian HM, Von Noorden GK: Binocular vision and ocular motility: theory and management of strabismus, St Louis, 1974, CV Mosby Co. By permission of the publisher.)*

cross to the opposite side, with the inferior nasal fibers (superior temporal field) looping forward as von Willebrand's knee into the opposite optic nerve before crossing. Fibers from the temporal retina remain uncrossed. The fibers of the optic tract partially encircle the cerebral peduncle and pass to the lateral geniculate body (Fig. 6-3). A few fibers end in the pretectal region of the midbrain and are concerned with pupillary reflexes.

Certain cells of each lateral geniculate body give rise to long axons that form a thick band, the optic radiation. These geniculocalcarine fibers lie close to the outer wall of the lateral ventricle. The fibers first course laterally. The upper fibers soon turn posteriorly, coursing through the parietal lobe, but the lower ones loop forward a variable distance around the inferior horn of the lateral ventricle in the temporal lobe (forming Meyer's loop) before they pass posteriorly and join the upper fibers to pass into the occipital lobe, where they terminate in the primary visual cortex (Brodmann's area 17).

Visual Acuity

The optic nerve is a sensory nerve. Its function is tested by measuring the visual acuity (test chart) and color vision (color plates),

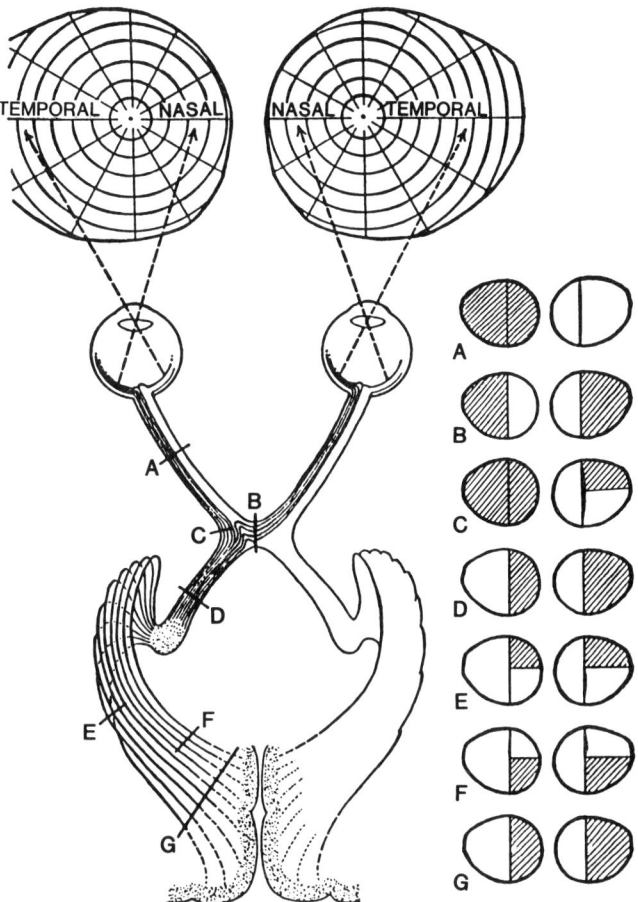

Figure 6-2
Lesions of optic pathways. *(From Homans J: A textbook of surgery, ed 6, Springfield, Illinois, 1945, Charles C Thomas, Publisher. By permission of the publisher.)*

determining the extent of peripheral vision (visual fields), and inspecting the retina and optic nerve head by means of the ophthalmoscope.

Visual acuity of each eye is tested separately for distance and near vision. (In neurologic work, there usually is no reason for the patient not to wear glasses to correct any refractive error that may exist.) The best corrected visual acuity is the acuity of neurologic significance. Any uncorrectable decrease in acuity requires explanation.

Distance vision is determined with the patient wearing distance correction. The Snellen chart (Fig. 6-4) is placed 20 feet from the patient. On the chart, the number beside each line of letters indicates the

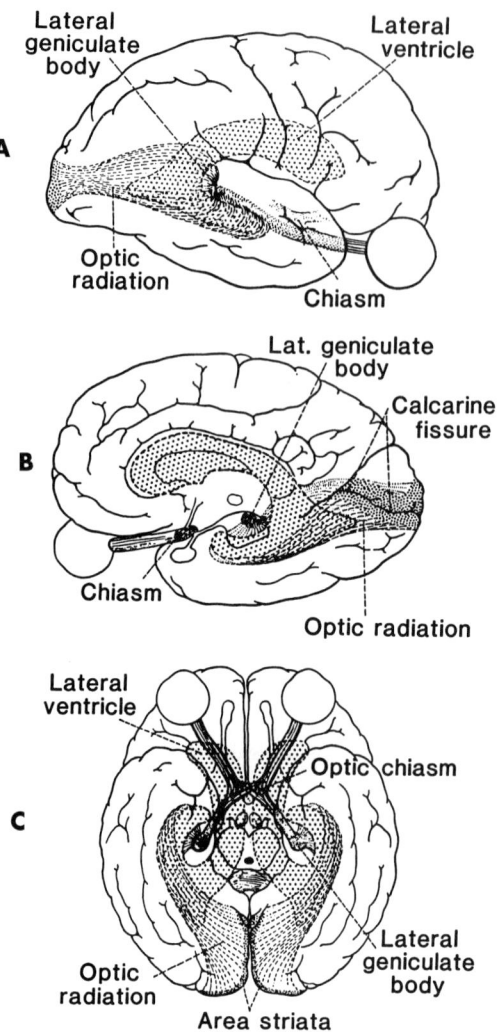

Figure 6-3
The course of the visual pathway within the brain: **A**, viewed from the right side; **B**, in midsagittal section; and **C**, from below. (From Rucker CW: The interpretation of visual fields, ed 3, San Francisco, 1957, American Academy of Ophthalmology and Otolaryngology. By permission of the publisher.)

number of feet at which the letters can be read by a person who has normal vision. Thus, normally, the small letters in the line designated "20" can be read at 20 feet, and normal visual acuity for distance is recorded as "20/20." If distance vision is defective, the smallest letters the patient is able to read may be the larger ones in the line designated "40," in which case the visual acuity is recorded as "20/40," the denominator indicating the distance at which letters of the size read should be discernible to a person with normal vision.

The best acuity that can be attained without a functioning macula is 20/200. An acuity better than this implies macular function.

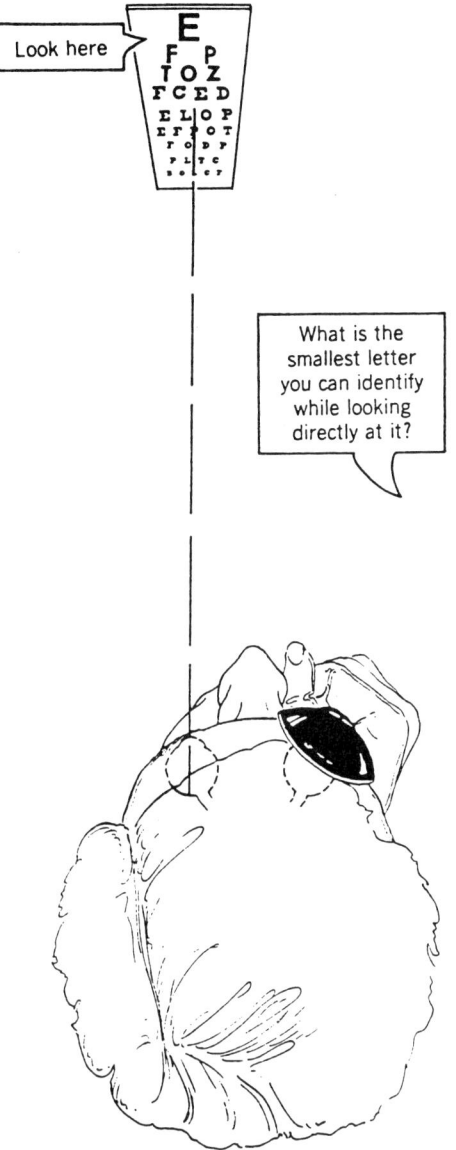

Figure 6-4
Testing the field of vision. *(From Anderson DR: Testing the field of vision, St Louis, 1982, CV Mosby Co. By permission of the publisher.)*

The largest letter on the Snellen chart is the "E," a 20/200 target. A person with 20/200 acuity sees this letter at 20 feet; one with normal acuity sees it at 200 feet. A person who can read it only at 10 feet has 10/200 vision; at 5 feet, 5/200 vision; and so on.

The three middle fingers of one hand, straightened and spread apart, are about the same size and configuration as the "E" and can be used in the clinical setting to obtain an approximate measure of acuity. An acuity of "counts fingers at 5 feet" (CF at 5 feet) is equivalent to 5/200 vision, CF at 1 foot to 1/200 vision.

For patients who cannot respond verbally or for children, the "E" or three fingers can be oriented in different directions and the patient asked to point in the direction of the prongs or digits.

If a patient is unable to count fingers, the ability to see light should be tested. A dark room and a bright light (generally that of an indirect ophthalmoscope) are needed. Light perception vision is designated "LP." Light perception with projection (LP with P) indicates that the patient can tell the direction from which the light is shining.

A patient may have only a small area of seeing field, and the target (letters, an "E," fingers, or light) must be moved around in front of the patient in a search for the seeing field.

Near vision is tested with the patient wearing bifocals or other near correction. Near correction is usually prescribed so that reading material is in focus at 14 inches. Undercorrection increases and overcorrection decreases this distance. Since the ability to accommodate to a near target decreases sharply between the ages of 45 and 65, undercorrection is quite common, and the patient should hold a "near card" ("reading card") where it is in the best focus to approximate the best acuity.

With a good refraction, however, a near card is held 14 inches from the patient, and the line of smallest letters the patient can read is determined. A subject with normal vision can read the line of letters designated "14/14," and the acuity is so recorded. Patients whose glasses are unavailable can have their near vision tested using "universal reading glasses." These are +3.00-diopter (D) glasses purchased without prescription. For the emmetropic patient who has lost all ability to accommodate to near vision with age or drugs, with +3D lenses the near card will be in focus at 0.33 m, or about 14 inches. The vision so obtained is an approximation only and should not be used as a final measure of acuity.

A refractive error can be eliminated by having the patient view the distance letters or the near card through a pinhole. The hole must be a millimeter or so in diameter, large enough to eliminate refraction at its edges. Through a pinhole, the only light entering the eye is that coming directly along its long axis. This light is always in focus at the fovea.

In small children and mentally impaired older children and adults, a rough measure of acuity can be obtained by showing the patient small toys or tiny objects, such as nonpareils. If the patient is alert to these or reaches for them, one can estimate the acuity by noting their size and distance from the patient. Each eye can be tested separately by occluding the fellow eye.

Optokinetic responses can be used to determine the ability to see. Each eye is tested separately. An optokinetic nystagmus drum is rotated in front of the patient. The elicitation of optokinetic nystagmus is an indication that the patient sees the stripes on the drum. An optokinetic nystagmus target with smaller stripes, such as a tape measure, can also be used. A rough estimate of acuity can be made by using optokinetic nystagmus strips with stripes the same width as the bars on the standard "E" card or "E" on the Snellen distance test chart. The "E" is a 20/200 target; that is, it is designed so that a person with normal acuity sees it at 200 feet and a person with 20/200 vision sees it at 20 feet. If, for example, a patient's vision is 20/400, the "E" or optokinetic stripes of the same width are seen at 10 feet.

In the patient who claims not to be able to see, the optokinetic nystagmus drum is helpful, as described earlier. In another useful test, the patient is placed, eyes open, facing a mirror. When the mirror is tilted, the gaze of a seeing patient reflexly follows the image in the mirror, and this eye movement can be seen. Normal visual acuity should double when the distance is halved or when the image is magnified two times, and discrepancies in these expected findings should be assessed. Comments written on cards and shown to the patient sometimes evoke a telltale facial expression. Patients who see but claim they cannot usually manage to negotiate obstacles in the examining room without serious errors.

Color Vision

Defects in color vision, especially for red, are very sensitive indicators of optic nerve disease. Color plates designed to assess this deficiency are the standardized pseudoisochromatic plates, with geometric figures made up of dots of varying hues on a ground of dots of similar hues. Patients with optic nerve disease cannot discern all the figures. (Color plates of another type, the Ishihara plates, are designed specifically to test for inherited red-green color blindness and are not as useful for assessment of the optic nerve.) The Farnsworth 100-hue test requires the ordering of 100 blocks of different shades of the spectrum. It is more sensitive than the use of plates but is time-consuming and is therefore mainly a research tool.

At the bedside, color vision can be assessed with a red object such as a bottle cap. The cap is viewed with each eye separately, and the apparent colors are compared. Viewed with an eye with an abnormal optic nerve, the color appears washed out, browner, or less red. A penlight viewed in the same way appears dimmer to the abnormal eye. In fact, the entire environment may appear darker and less vibrant in hue.

The Field of Vision

The field of vision may be defined as that portion of space in which objects are visible during fixation of gaze in one direction. The normality of the visual field depends on the intactness of the visual pathways from the retina through the optic nerves, chiasm, tracts, and radiations to the visual cortex in the occipital lobes. Since lesions interrupting various parts of the pathway cause specific types of defects in the visual fields, it is possible, from the nature of the defect in the field, to determine the site of the lesion.

There are three major areas of the visual field: the central field, extending 20 degrees from the point of fixation and subserved by the macula and surrounding retina; the midfield, extending from 20 to 40 degrees; and the periphery (Fig. 6-5).

Amsler grid testing

The Amsler grid (Fig. 6-6) is a standardized piece of graph paper marked in the center with a dot for fixation. The patient's near correction lenses are worn, and one eye is occluded. The patient is asked to fix the gaze on the center dot and to note any distortions, irregularities, or missing areas in the graph paper. The procedure is repeated with the second eye. This testing is especially sensitive to defects in the central part of the field. It is used extensively in detecting and following macular lesions and their resultant field defects. These abnormalities can cause apparent bending or distortions in the lines, or positive scotomata (dark spots) near fixation. The Amsler grid also reveals field defects of other causes if they involve the area of the field covered by the grid, that is, the central 20 degrees. Lesions located posterior to the retina (in the optic nerve or beyond) cause negative scotomata. The lines of the grid are simply "missing."

Tangent screen perimetry

This form of testing, which examines the field out to 30 degrees from fixation, is done with the patient wearing distance correction. One eye is occluded. The patient is seated facing a black felt screen marked with black stitching showing a fixation dot, the outlines of the blind spot on each side, and concentric circles at 10, 20, and 30 degrees from fixation (Fig. 6-7). A target, either a small red or white disk of standard size (1 mm, 3 mm, etc.) mounted on a black stick or a projected spot of light, is placed on the screen at different locations or brought in from the periphery. Fixation is monitored by putting the target into the physiologic blind spot and ascertaining that the patient cannot see it.

Goldmann fields and computerized perimetry

The Goldmann perimeter is a bowl-shaped device that uses small targets of light. It works on the same principle as the tangent screen but measures the full extent of the visual field. Computerized devices are similar. They have computer programs designed for various disease processes, such as glaucoma and chiasmal lesions. These concentrate the testing on those areas of the field most likely to be affected by the process under study.

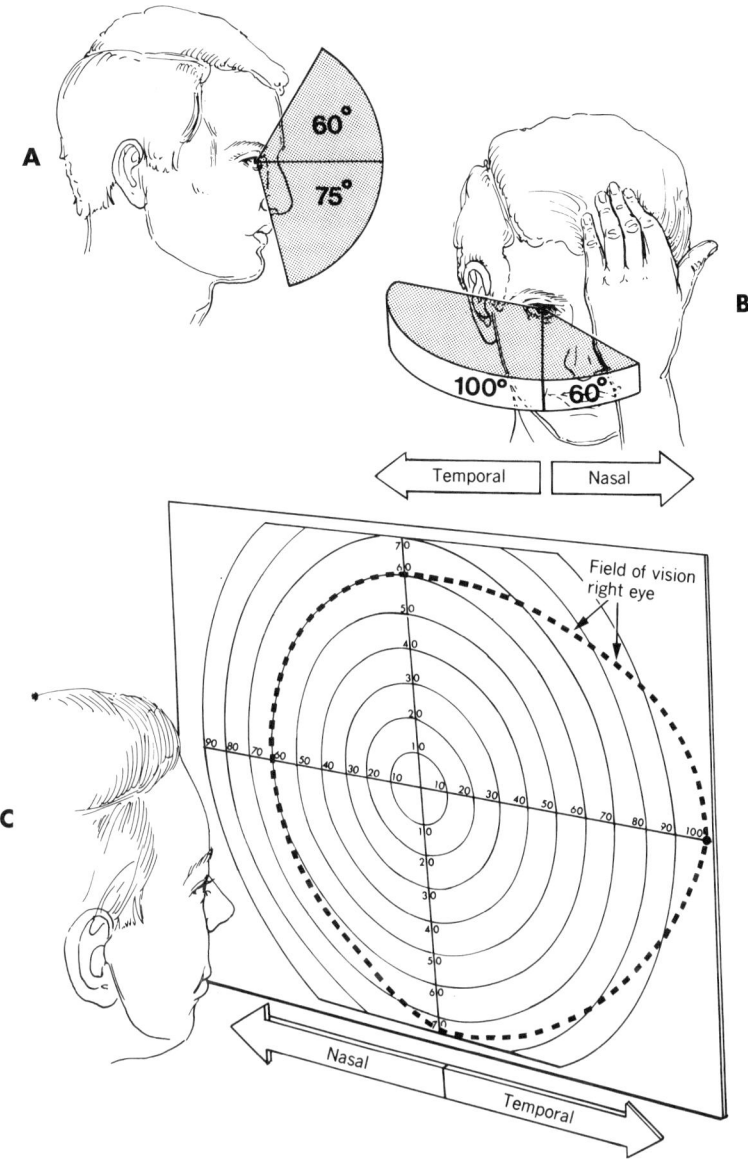

Figure 6-5
The field of vision. *(From Anderson DR: Testing the field of vision, St Louis, 1982, CV Mosby Co. By permission of the publisher.)*

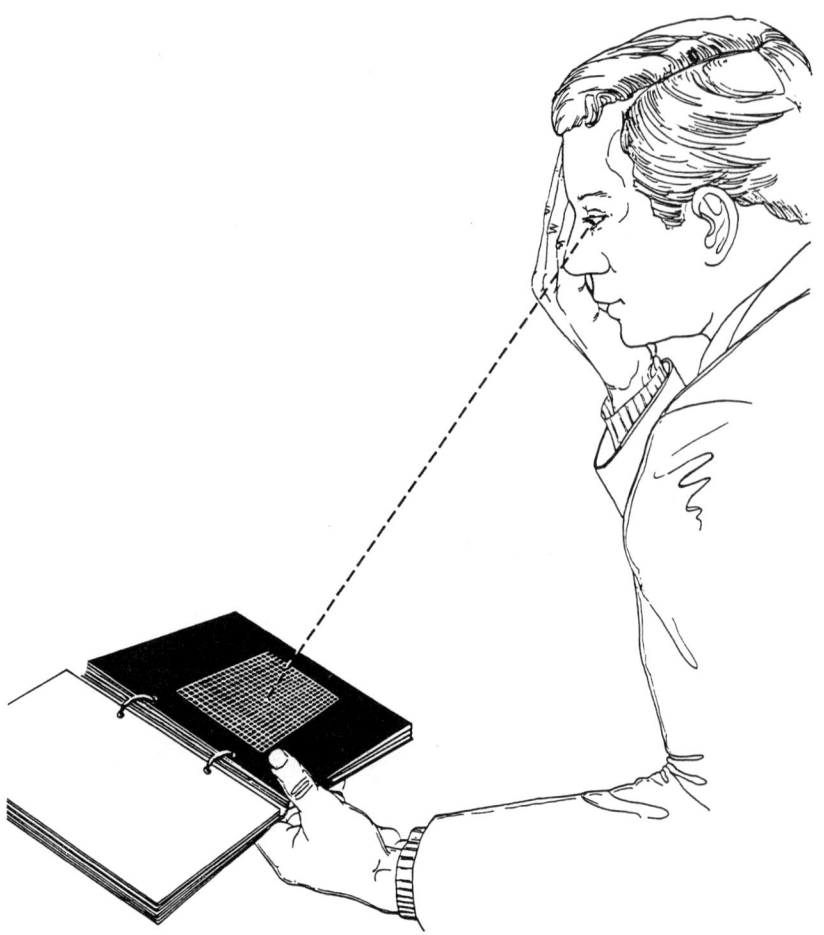

Figure 6-6
Testing the field of vision. *(From Anderson DR: Testing the field of vision, St Louis, 1982, CV Mosby Co. By permission of the publisher.)*

Bedside testing of the visual fields

The commonest methods of bedside testing are the confrontation tests, in which the examiner confronts or faces the patient being tested and compares his or her own visual field with that of the patient. Each eye is tested separately without correction. To examine the patient's right eye, the examiner uses his or her own left eye.

A reliable confrontation test is that of *finger-counting fields,* done by the examiner presenting his or her hands in each of the two hemifields. The patient is asked whether both hands can be seen and whether any differences are noted in clarity or brightness. The examiner's hands are

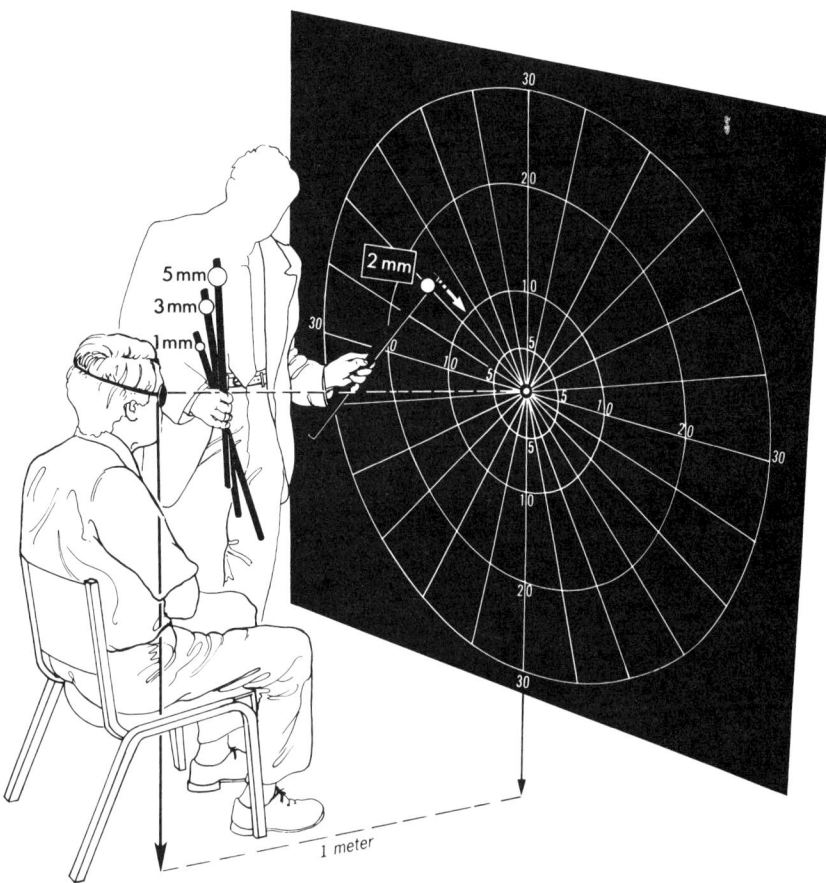

Figure 6-7
Tangent screen testing. *(From Anderson DR: Testing the field of vision, St Louis, 1982, CV Mosby Co. By permission of the publisher.)*

then presented in two quadrants at a time, and again the patient is asked to make comparisons. Finally, one, two, or five fingers are presented in each quadrant, and the patient is asked to report how many fingers are seen. The fingers can be presented for just a moment or for a longer period. When an area of depressed field is discovered, the examiner's hand is moved from the depressed field to the normal field, and the patient is asked to indicate when targets are seen clearly. The parietal lobe syndrome of visual neglect is tested by presenting fingers in the right and left hemifields simultaneously and noting whether the patient is aware of both sets of stimuli at once or whether those on one side are extinguished. Because fingers can be presented very briefly, this method has the advantage of not suffering from inaccuracies due to the distractibility of the patient. Many patients have trouble maintaining fixation and keeping their head and eyes from turning toward the target. It also has the advantage of testing the midfield, an area often abnormal in patients with optic nerve or chiasmal lesions. Moving rather than static fingers can be presented in the quadrants (see the discussion of the Riddoch phenomenon, below).

Another method of confrontation perimetry is referred to as *outline perimetry*. Again, the examiner covers one of the patient's eyes and closes his or her own corresponding eye, and the patient fixes the gaze on the examiner's open eye. The patient is told to tell the examiner when a target the examiner moves slowly into the patient's field of vision is first seen. The target is held to the side of the patient's face outside the field of vision and is moved into the field. The four quadrants of vision, namely, upper and lower nasal and upper and lower temporal, are tested separately for each eye. The target may be the hand, a moving finger, or a small red or white bead. The examiner uses his or her own field of vision as a control by moving the target from outside this field in a line equidistant from the eye of the examiner and the patient. Thus, the patient and the examiner should see the target at approximately the same point.

Some patients with posterior parietal lesions may be able to detect movement in an area of field but not static targets (Riddoch phenomenon). Outline perimetry may therefore appear to be normal when finger counting in each quadrant is not. Optic nerve and chiasmal defects may be densest in the midfield and may be evident on finger counting in the quadrants testing but not on outline perimetry.

The confrontation testing methods described above can be done with a red target such as a bottle top in the quadrants or approaching from the periphery. This increases their sensitivity to field defects caused by optic nerve, chiasm, and temporal lobe lesions. Red appears brown or washed out in comparison with color seen by the fellow eye or in the normal areas of field.

In the examination of uncooperative patients and children, the resourcefulness and patience of the examiner are challenged. In such instances, the examiner may find the observation of optically elicited eye movements of value. An attractive object, such as a small hand puppet or toy, is brought into the periphery of the visual field. If the patient looks in the direction of the object, that portion of the field probably is intact.

Another method occasionally of value in examination of uncooperative patients is to determine whether defensive blinking reactions are elicited by swiftly moving the hand in a threatening manner toward the eyes while being careful to confine the movement to one quadrant or one half of the field of vision.

Recording observations

The visual field obtained on the perimeter or screen is recorded on a chart that represents the field as the patient sees it. The field for the right eye is placed to the right on the chart, its upper portion above, its temporal portion to the right, its nasal portion to the left. The test objective used is recorded by a fraction, the numerator indicating the size of the test object, the denominator the distance at which it was used. For example, 3/330 indicates that a 3-mm bead was used on the arm of the perimeter, which had an arc radius of 330 mm measured from the eye of the subject to the point of fixation.

Thus, a complete left homonymous hemianopsia observed by perimetry and on the tangent screen would be recorded as in Figure 6-8.

The results of confrontation tests may be recorded on circles divided into quadrants, which allow for ready transposition of any defects that may be found. Generally, these records are made by the same rules used for recording data from perimeter and tangent screen. The Department of Neurology at the Mayo Clinic uses an idiosyncratic convention for recording these results, however, and it will be described here to avoid confusion. When the results of confrontation tests are charted, the chart

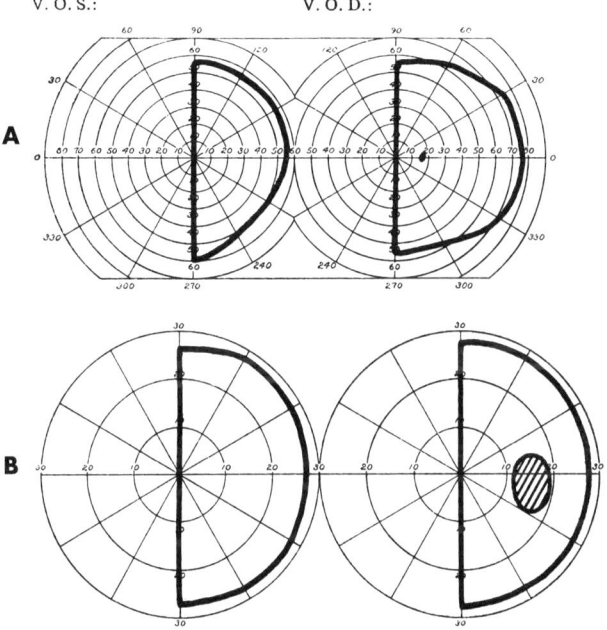

Figure 6-8
Record of complete left homonymous hemianopsia observed **(A)** by perimetry and **(B)** on the tangent screen.

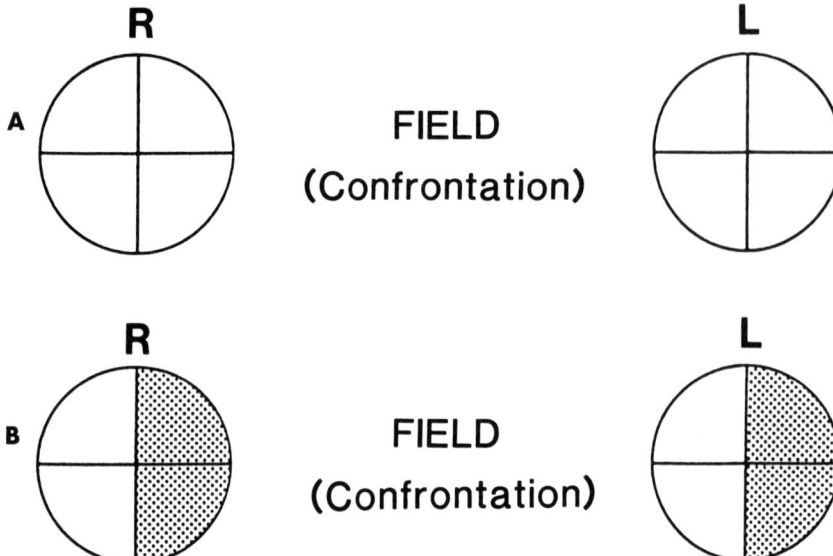

Figure 6-9
Record of the results of confrontation tests. **A**, the blank form. **B**, record of left homonymous hemianopsia.

of the left eye is on the right and the nonseeing areas are shaded. This result is the mirror image of that recorded by general convention. For example, if while confronting the patient the examiner discovers that the patient cannot see in the temporal field of the left eye or the nasal field of the right eye, the left homonymous hemianopsia is indicated by shading the nonseeing areas on the charts, as in Figure 6-9.

Interpretation of Visual Field Defects
In Figure 6-2, the fibers from the inner half of each retina cross in the chiasm, whereas the fibers from the outer half are uncrossed. This illustrates that ordinarily lesions affecting the optic nerve anterior to the chiasm produce unilateral impairment of vision, whereas lesions of the chiasm or those posterior to it produce bilateral visual field defects. The various fields of vision are named according to their proximity to the nose or temple, as shown in the diagram. Loss of vision in half the field of one eye is called "hemianopsia," and loss of vision in corresponding halves of both visual fields is called "homonymous hemianopsia" and is further designated right or left. A lesion at "A" causes total blindness in the left eye. A lesion at "C" causes a "junctional" field defect because it damages the junction between the optic nerve and the chiasm. It involves von Willebrand's knee (see Fig. 6-2) and causes an optic nerve type of defect on the side of the lesion and a superior temporal defect in

the opposite eye. A lesion at "D" causes a right homonymous hemianopsia, and one at "B" produces a bitemporal hemianopsia. Lesions posterior to the chiasm, at "E," "F," and so forth, produce different types of right homonymous defects. If the lesion is in the optic radiations after they have expanded into a sizable anatomic area, partial (quadrantic) homonymous defects may occur. When the lesion is in the optic tract, the field defects are very incongruous, that is, highly dissimilar in the two eyes. Lesions in the optic radiations are more congruous; the more posterior the lesion, the more congruous the fields become. Occipital lesions cause perfectly congruous field defects. This phenomenon occurs because the topological organization of the array of visual fibers becomes more ordered as the fibers course posteriorly.

Scotomata

A scotoma is a defect within the field of vision. The normal blind spot may be considered a physiologic scotoma. Scotomata may be considered positive when the patient sees them as dark spots. *Positive* scotomata are due to changes in the media or the retina. Motile scotomata result from opacities floating in the vitreous. *Negative* scotomata exist as defects in the field of vision and are caused by a lesion at the optic nerve head or posterior to it. Patients are not necessarily aware of their scotomata. Scotomata may be referred to as absolute when perception of light is entirely lost over the defective area and as relative when it is not. Scotomata are further classified by their location in the field of vision. A central scotoma involves the point of fixation and seriously impairs central visual acuity. It is caused by a lesion in the macula. Paracentral scotomata are situated adjacent to the point of fixation. Cecocentral scotomata involve the point of fixation and extend into the normal blind spot and are characteristic of optic nerve lesions. Ring, or annular, scotomata encircle the point of fixation. One cause is Leber's disease. Scintillating scotomata are subjective experiences in which bright colorless or colored lights are observed in the field of vision. They usually occur as a part of migraine and less commonly occur as a seizure involving an occipital lobe.

Retinal lesions

Vascular lesions of the nerve fiber layer of the retina produce wedge-shaped positive scotomata corresponding to the area of vascular supply of the arteriole involved. Because no vessels cross the horizontal raphe, this line is always respected in the visual fields. Branch retinal artery lesions at the disk cause altitudinal defects, positive scotomata coming on like a shade going down or up if they are embolic and progressing somewhat more slowly if they represent local thrombosis. In some cases, a cilioretinal artery, a branch of the ophthalmic artery taking off behind the optic disk, pierces the sclera near the edge of the disk to supply the macula. Occlusion of the artery causes a small central positive scotoma, and, conversely, occlusion of the ophthalmic artery distal to the branching off of a cilioretinal artery results in infarcted retina with macular sparing. A small central field is preserved. Lesions of the choroid (choroiditis, tumor, trauma, choroidal degenerations) or of the deeper layers of the retina (retinal detachments, chorioretinitis) produce visual defects corresponding to the area of interference with the rods and cones, and these defects have an irregular shape approximating their ophthalmoscopic appearance. Choroidal crescents, usually associated with high-grade myopia, are seen around the optic disk when the retina does not meet the edge of the disk and choroidal pigment shows through. They produce a variety of defects in the field of vision corresponding to the site of the associated defective retina.

Optic disk lesions

Compressive and vascular lesions of the optic disk, such as those caused by glaucoma or by hyaline bodies of the disk (disk drusen), characteristically produce arcuate scotomata secondary to wedge-shaped infarcts of the disk. If the lesion is large, the scotoma may break through to the periphery of the visual field. Such arcuate defects usually arise near or at the blind spot, arch either above or below the fixation point, and fan out into the nasal field, where they invariably terminate at the horizontal meridian and may produce a "nasal step." Tilting of the optic disks may cause bitemporal depression of the visual fields, which may be erroneously ascribed to a lesion at the optic chiasm. Inflammatory lesions of the optic disks (papillitis) cause disk swelling, loss of visual acuity, and cecocentral scotomata. These are scotomata involving the fixation area, the blind spot, and the "waist," that part of the field between the two. They result from significant involvement of the maculopapular bundle, that is, the fibers in the disk that arise from the macula and the retinal tissue between the macula and the disk. Common causes are the papillitis of multiple sclerosis and toxic (tobacco, alcohol) amblyopia.

Papilledema

Papilledema is swelling of the optic disk caused by raised intracranial pressure. Blocked axonal transport at the lamina cribrosa causes the axonal swelling seen ophthalmoscopically. Visual function is initially well preserved. The condition is distinguishable from papillitis, which is inflammation and swelling of the disk with associated visual loss. Early signs of papilledema are best seen on direct examination of the disk. These signs are described below. The earliest perimetric evidence of papilledema is enlargement of the blind spot. Later signs include reduction in acuity and peripheral constriction of the fields, beginning nasally. In cases of papilledema, size of the blind spot should be plotted routinely as a baseline and as a means for following the course of the condition.

Retrobulbar optic nerve lesions
When these lesions are caused by inflammatory or metabolic lesions of the nerve, the field loss is like that seen in papillitis. Compressive lesions, on the other hand, with their local ischemic and axonal transport changes, cause cecocentral, diffuse, midfield, or peripheral defects, depending on their exact anatomy and physiology.

Junctional lesions
These lesions occur at the junction between the optic nerve and the chiasm. They affect the ipsilateral optic nerve fibers and in addition involve von Willebrand's knee, fibers from the inferior nasal retina of the opposite eye as they loop forward into the opposite optic nerve after decussating at the chiasm (see Fig. 6-2). When there is an obvious optic nerve lesion on one side, measurement of the superior temporal field of the opposite eye is of considerable importance. A lesion that has spread from the optic nerve back to the junctional area is no longer surgically resectable.

Chiasmal lesions
Bitemporal hemianopsia is the characteristic field defect resulting from chiasmal lesions. Tumors of the pituitary gland and craniopharyngiomas are the commonest lesions involving the chiasm. Aneurysm, dilated third ventricle, trauma, glioma of the chiasm, meningioma, and inflammatory lesions less commonly involve this structure. The earliest perimetric evidence of a chiasmal lesion is depression, especially to red targets, in the temporal midfields or periphery, superiorly if the lesion comes from below the chiasm and inferiorly if the lesion comes from above. Occasionally, fusiform aneurysms of the carotids compress non-decussating fibers and cause binasal field loss.

Neoplasms
Neoplasms, by their tendency to displace neighboring structures, interrupt fibers of the visual pathway by direct pressure and by interference with their nutrient blood supply. Since an early tumor does not usually interrupt all of the fibers, the resulting hemianopsia frequently is incomplete, the defects in the fields are relative, and the blind areas slope gradually into the seeing areas. Moreover, the defects relentlessly enlarge and become more dense from month to month. A progressive defect with sloping margins thus suggests the presence of a neoplasm.

Vascular events
Circulatory disturbances tend to produce infarction in isolated masses of brain tissue. Portions of the visual pathway included in the infarcted areas are likely to be totally interrupted. The corresponding defects in the visual fields tend to occur suddenly and to be blind to large test objects, and the border between the blind and the seeing areas may be sharply demarcated. This is especially true in old infarctions.

Patterns of field loss

Complete homonymous hemianopsia has lateralizing value only. It signifies a loss of function of the visual pathway somewhere behind the chiasm but gives no more information than that. Incomplete homonymous hemianopsia, on the other hand, supplies more specific information. Congruity is exact in lesions of the occipital cortex and less exact in lesions of the temporal and parietal radiations. Further forward, in lesions of the optic tract, congruity is not maintained. In principle, the more posteriorly the lesion is located, the more congruous the field defect between the two eyes.

Macular sparing sometimes occurs in occipital lobe lesions. This is because of a rich anastomotic network between terminal branches of the middle cerebral artery and the posterior cerebral artery.

Lesions of the temporal lobe affect the optic radiations in Meyer's loop (see Fig. 6-3). They produce the characteristic "pie in the sky" homonymous defect, denser superiorly. Parietal lobe lesions involve the superior radiations and cause homonymous defects that are denser below.

Occipital lesions can have an apparent incongruity due to preservation of the monocular temporal crescent. Although most of the field of vision is seen with both eyes, the far temporal fields are seen with the ipsilateral eye only. Consequently, a lateral occipital crescent of cortical tissue on each side receives radiations from one eye only. Since this cortex is a vascular watershed area, insults to the posterior cerebral artery territory often spare it and hence preserve the monocular temporal crescent.

Bilateral homonymous hemianopsia is encountered infrequently. It may be due to a tumor arising in the falx between the occipital lobes or to trauma or infarct in both occipital lobes or in each of the two optic pathways. The latter may occur as a result of obstruction in the basilar artery near the point of division into the two posterior cerebral arteries or as the result of multiple occipital emboli.

Contraction of the field of vision is the commonest defect due to psychogenic causes. In extreme cases, tubular or gun-barrel vision results. The tendency of the fields to remain small rather than to enlarge appropriately when the patient is moved away from the screen is characteristic. Identical fields are occasionally detected in the presence of organic brain disease, particularly in tumor of the occipital lobe. A psychogenic type of field defect does not necessarily eliminate the possibility of a cerebral lesion, and organic and psychogenic defects may be combined.

Although central scotomata are said not to occur in psychogenic disturbances, paracentral or annular scotomata do occur occasionally and can be recognized by their failure to enlarge and to move away from the point of fixation when the patient is placed at a greater distance from the screen. "Spiral" fields rather than concentric oval ones are sometimes obtained on formal testing. Fields are often not reproducible.

Ophthalmoscopy

The neurologist's main interest in ophthalmoscopy lies in examining the optic disk, the retina, and the vessels for evidence of neurologic disease.

The patient is asked to look at a distant object. For examination of the right retina, the examiner holds the ophthalmoscope in the right hand and uses his or her own right eye; this technique is reversed for examination of the left eye. Errors of refraction in the eyes of the patient or examiner can be corrected by the use of lenses in the ophthalmoscope. The neurologist ordinarily begins the examination of the retina by finding the optic disk. The macula and the surrounding retina are then surveyed. The pupil can be dilated with 1% tropicamide (Mydriacyl) for a better view of the retina, but tests of corneal sensitivity and pupillary function should be performed before this is done.

The red-free (green) light on the ophthalmoscope is useful for examining the nerve fiber layer of the retina. When this layer is thinned, the choroid behind it is more prominently visible. Because of its vascularity, it appears blackish with the green light. The red-free light also enhances the visibility of blood vessels, hemorrhages, and vascular lesions.

It is useful to inspect the media by focusing the ophthalmoscope on the cornea, anterior chamber, lens, and vitreous in turn. Clues to non-neurologic reasons for visual loss (for example, corneal scars, cataracts) can often be seen.

The optic disk

Ophthalmoscopically, the optic disk, or papilla, is a yellowish red, plate-like structure, typically flat, with clearly defined margins; the arterioles of the retina diverge from, and the veins converge toward, the disk. It is the center of observation from which the examination of the fundus proceeds. Normally, the disk has sharp borders. In myopic (longer, near-sighted) eyes, choroidal pigment may be visible as a crescent around the disk because the retina does not come fully up to meet its edge. In hyperopic eyes (shorter, farsighted) the disk may appear rather full, and no choroidal crescent is visible. The rim of the disk takes on a pinkish hue because of surface capillaries. In the center of the disk is the "physiologic cup," a central depression, yellower than the rim, in which can be seen a suggestion of the crosshatched appearance of the lamina cribrosa, which is formed by scleral fibers. The cup:disk ratio is a measurement of the diameter of the cup to the diameter of the disk. It is expressed as a decimal value from 0.1 to 1.0. The normal value varies widely, but the ratios are usually equal bilaterally. An increase in this ratio over time or an asymmetry in the ratio between the two eyes may indicate an enlargement of the cup caused by raised intraocular pressure (glaucoma). In this condition, the rim may appear slightly pale and there is a sloping from the central cup up to the rim rather than a distinct edge.

In 80% of normal patients, venous pulsations are visible on the disk. These are best seen by focusing the ophthalmoscope on the veins and watching to see if they go in and out of focus in a pulsatile manner. When present, these pulsations indicate that the intracranial pressure is less than 200 mm Hg. When they are known to have been present and subsequently disappear, the intracranial pressure has increased to a level above 200 mm Hg.

Papilledema and papillitis

Swelling of the optic disk may be due to active inflammation or passive congestion. According to current usage of terms, when the former factor is responsible, the swelling is called "optic neuritis," or "papillitis," and is associated with loss of vision in the form of a cecocentral scotoma. When the inflammatory lesion is in the posterior portion of the optic nerve, the disk is not swollen and the condition is termed "retrobulbar neuritis." Swelling of the disk due to increased intracranial pressure with blockage of axonal transport at the level of the lamina cribrosa is termed "papilledema." In this condition, visual acuity is not affected until secondary optic atrophy ensues and the fields become contracted.

The earliest sign of papilledema is hyperemia of the rim of the disk. Later, the margins of the disk blur slightly, the veins appear full and engorged, and hemorrhages develop in the nerve fiber layer (splinter hemorrhages). The disk becomes elevated, and nerve fiber infarctions (cotton wool spots) appear. Folds may develop in the retina. Protein leaks from the nerve fibers and vessels (waxy exudates). In massive papilledema, large areas of the nerve fiber layer may become infarcted, and these areas then appear dull and boggy because of cotton wool spots and waxy exudates as well as massive hemorrhage. Around the macula, a "macular star" of hard white exudates from leaked protein can be seen.

The findings of papillitis of the disk are similar to those of early papilledema: hyperemia, swelling, protein leakage, and hemorrhages. If the diagnosis of demyelinating disease is suspected, the veins in the periphery of the retina should be examined for perivenous sheathing. This usually has the appearance of sugarcoating on the veins and is due to perivenous collections of extravasated protein and white cells.

Since one examines the retina and disk with monocular vision, the usual power of depth perception is absent. It is, therefore, necessary to measure the elevation (swelling) of the disk above the surrounding retina by the system of lenses of the ophthalmoscope. In measuring the amount of elevation of the optic disk, one should focus on the smallest blood vessel that can be seen on the most elevated portion of the disk and then determine the most plus lens with which the vessel can be seen clearly and note the value of the lens. The same procedure is repeated for a small vessel near the macula. Using this method, the examiner cannot exert his or her own accommodative power and thereby introduce a needless error in measurement. The difference, in diopters, in the lenses required to see clearly the two vessels is a measure of the amount of papilledema. (For example, a +2D lens is required for the vessel on the disk, a −2D lens for the vessel in the macula. The disk is elevated 4D.)

A number of developmental conditions can be confused with papilledema. A common one is the structurally full disk. In the myope, the eyeball is long and the retinal ganglion cell layer does not meet the edge of the disk, so that a dark crescent of choroidal pigment is visible around it, and the edge of the disk is easy to judge. In the hyperope, however, the eyeball is shorter and the retinal ganglion cell layer meets the edge of the disk, so that the margins are indistinct. A search for the features of papilledema discussed above helps differentiate this structurally full disk from papilledema. If a question remains, fluorescein angiography is helpful. A papilledematous disk has neovascularization, and these vessels leak dye. A structurally full disk does not leak.

As a rule, glial veils or excess of glial tissue is not difficult to diagnose; the excess tissue is readily recognizable as a plaque or as shreds extraneous to the normal substance of the disk. Ordinarily, the glial tissue follows along the vessels in the form of a sheath. It may extend beyond the margins of the optic disk.

Hyaline bodies or drusen in the disk substance produce appearances that may simulate one of several pathologic entities. Ophthalmoscopically, drusen appear as shiny or glistening "sago-like" bodies on the surface or in the substance of the optic disk. Within the optic nerve, the hyaline bodies or drusen may be located anywhere on or near the surface of the disk, deep in the substance of the nerve, extending into the physiologic excavation, or at the margins of the nerve head and extending even into the surrounding retina. The number of hyaline bodies present and their location determine the ophthalmoscopic appearance of the disk. Drusen buried in the disk can elevate it. This elevation is mistaken for papilledema when no consideration is given to features of edema other than elevation.

Occasionally, the normal myelin of the retrobulbar optic nerve continues out onto the nerve head and in the nerve fiber layer of the retina. This medullated (myelinated) nerve fiber layer appears pearly white and may obscure disk structures. Its appearance can be confused with that of papilledema, but hyperemia, hemorrhages, and other stigmata of papilledema are lacking.

Anterior ischemic optic neuropathy

The sudden or subacute onset of an altitudinal or segmental visual field loss, that is, a loss in the territory of an artery at the disk, is the mark of anterior ischemic optic neuropathy. Occasionally this clinical entity is due to vasculitis, a hypercoagulable state, or polycythemia, but more often it is idiopathic. On ophthalmoscopy, there are altitudinal or segmental swelling and hyperemia with hemorrhages, signs of infarction of a portion or even all of the disk. The ratio of cup to disk in an unaffected fellow eye may be quite small, a suggestion of an underlying anatomic predisposition to this entity at the level of the lamina cribrosa.

Venous occlusion
This entity, which may be acute or chronic, causes partial visual loss with dilated, dusky veins, disk swelling, and hemorrhage.

Retinal emboli
The most common emboli are Hollenhorst plaques, which are composed of cholesterol crystals. They appear shiny orange-yellow and are often situated at the bifurcation of retinal arterioles. Such a plaque may appear to be wider than the arteriole, because one sees the outer dimension of the column of red blood cells rather than the wall of the arteriole. Pressure on the eye often changes the position of the embolus slightly, and the material may appear to glint or change shade, a characteristic sometimes referred to as a "heliographic reflection." The blood flow in the arteriole is often seemingly unimpeded by these bright orange-yellow plaques. These emboli may move distally, and often they disappear in a few days. The presence of one or more cholesterol retinal emboli indicates that there is or has been an ulcerated atheromatous intimal lesion of the ipsilateral internal carotid artery or the heart.

Another important type of embolus in retinal vessels consists of gray-white material, thought to be formed by blood, platelets, and fibrin. These emboli may be long and may be seen to move through an arteriole, but commonly they are stationary; pressing on the eye does not move the embolus, and there is no heliographic reflection. Blood does not appear to flow past the emboli; there may be infarction of the retina. Special studies show that some of these emboli have a high lipid content. In many instances, the source of the emboli is an atheromatous lesion at the origin of the ipsilateral internal carotid artery.

Particles of calcium are another type of retinal emboli. They are white, generally short, and stationary. Calcium emboli commonly come from heart-valve lesions. Septic emboli, talc, and cornstarch emboli as well as others may be seen in the retina but are less common than those already described.

Optic atrophy
Optic atrophy is associated with decreased visual acuity and a change in color of the optic disk to light pink, white, or gray, depending on its degree. There are six subgroups in the ophthalmoscopic classification of optic atrophy. *Primary* atrophy occurs as a result of a lesion behind the optic nerve head when retrograde degeneration of nerve fibers takes place. The disk is pale. Because it has never been swollen, its margins are sharp. When the lesion is relatively mild, the pallor is mostly evident

temporally where the large papillomacular bundle passes. *Secondary* atrophy occurs in a disk that was once swollen. The disk is pale, the margins are blurred from old protein deposits, and the veins are sheathed with protein deposition as well. *Segmental* atrophy is altitudinal or wedge-shaped, resulting from old anterior ischemic optic neuropathy with a branch retinal artery occlusion. *Cavernous* atrophy occurs in glaucoma when the physiologic cup enlarges and the rim thins, becomes pale, and is finally obliterated. *Consecutive* atrophy occurs with attenuated retinal arterioles or pigmented retinal lesions. It is due to diffuse retinal disease, such as retinitis pigmentosa, diffuse chorioretinitis, or quinine intoxication. *Congenital* atrophy is due to hypoplasia or other developmental abnormality of the disk. The disk is often small, has sharp edges, and may be misshapen.

Signs of optic atrophy may be observed in the nerve fiber layer as well. When retrograde degeneration occurs, the nerve fiber layer thins, diffusely if the process is generalized and segmentally following the arcuate fiber projections if the process is segmental. These changes are best seen if the red-free (green) light on the ophthalmoscope is used. The dark-appearing vascularity of the choroid is prominent in atrophied areas.

CRANIAL NERVES III, IV, AND VI (OCULOMOTOR, TROCHLEAR, AND ABDUCENS NERVES), OCULAR MOTILITY, AND AUTONOMIC FUNCTIONS

The third, fourth, and sixth cranial nerves are discussed together, since they all supply muscles concerned with ocular movement. The third cranial nerve, in addition, innervates the levator of the eyelid, the constrictor of the pupil, and the ciliary muscle, which controls accommodation. Consequently, a discussion of ptosis and pupillary reflexes is appropriate at this point. Convenience dictates that a discussion of the remaining neuro-ophthalmologic tests be included in this section.

Anatomy
Oculomotor nerve

The third nerves, the oculomotor nerves, arise from a paired nucleus situated in the midbrain ventral to the aqueduct of Sylvius at the level of the superior colliculi and the red nuclei. The oculomotor nucleus sends efferent fibers to extraocular muscles (superior rectus, inferior rectus, medial rectus, and inferior oblique). In addition, the Edinger-Westphal nucleus, the visceral subnucleus of the oculomotor nerve, lying superiorly in the nuclear complex, sends parasympathetic fibers to the levator palpebrae superioris, the pupillary constrictor muscle in the iris, and the ciliary body. The neurons innervating each superior rectus muscle lie beside each other. The caudal subnucleus, which supplies both levator palpebrae superioris muscles, is a single midline structure. All the projections from the third nerve nucleus are ipsilateral except those to the superior rectus, which are crossed (the crossing occurring within the nucleus), and those to the levator palpebrae superioris, which are both crossed and uncrossed (again, the crossing occurs within the nucleus itself). The root fibers arising from each side of the oculomotor nucleus pass ventrally through the medial longitudinal fasciculus, the red nucleus, the substantia nigra, and the medial part of the cerebral peduncle and emerge as several rootlets in the interpeduncular fossa. The nerve runs forward between the posterior cerebral and the superior cerebellar arteries (Fig. 6-10). It goes through the basal cistern lateral to the posterior communicating artery and below the uncus, where it runs over the petroclinoid ligament medial to the trochlear nerve and just lateral to the posterior clinoid process. Then, piercing the dura between the anterior and the posterior clinoids, it comes to lie in the lateral wall of the cavernous sinus, where it divides into a small superior and a large inferior branch. Both of these divisions pass forward into the orbit through the superior orbital fissure, the superior division supplying the superior rectus muscle and the levator of the upper lid and the inferior divisions supplying the medial rectus, inferior rectus, and inferior oblique muscles, and, via parasympathetic fibers, the constrictor of the pupil and the ciliary body.

Unilateral nuclear lesions cause bilateral superior rectus and levator palpebrae superioris weakness as well as involvement of other muscles ipsilaterally. They may also cause pupillary dilatation. Such lesions are very rare. Fascicular lesions in the midbrain can involve the medial longitudinal fasciculus, the red nucleus, and the medial portion of the peduncle. Complete paralysis of the oculomotor nerve results in ptosis, dilatation of the pupil with iridoplegia and cycloplegia, and rotation of the eye outward and slightly downward as a result of unopposed action of the lateral rectus (VI) and the superior oblique (IV) muscles, with inability to move the eye upward, inward, or downward.

Common causes of oculomotor nerve palsy are, in the nuclear portion, lacunar infarctions; in the fascicular portion, infarcts, hemorrhages, and tumors; in the subarachnoid portion, posterior communicating artery aneurysms, infarcts of the nerve itself, and pressure from herniation of the uncus; in the cavernous sinus portion, inflammatory and mass lesions and thrombosis of the sinus; and, in the orbit, mass lesions and nerve infarctions. Neuromuscular diseases can also weaken the muscles innervated by the third nerve. More proximal third nerve lesions tend to have quite large pupils because the sympathetics are uninvolved. More anterior lesions (after the sympathetics join the third nerve in the cavernous sinus) display pupils of more moderate size.

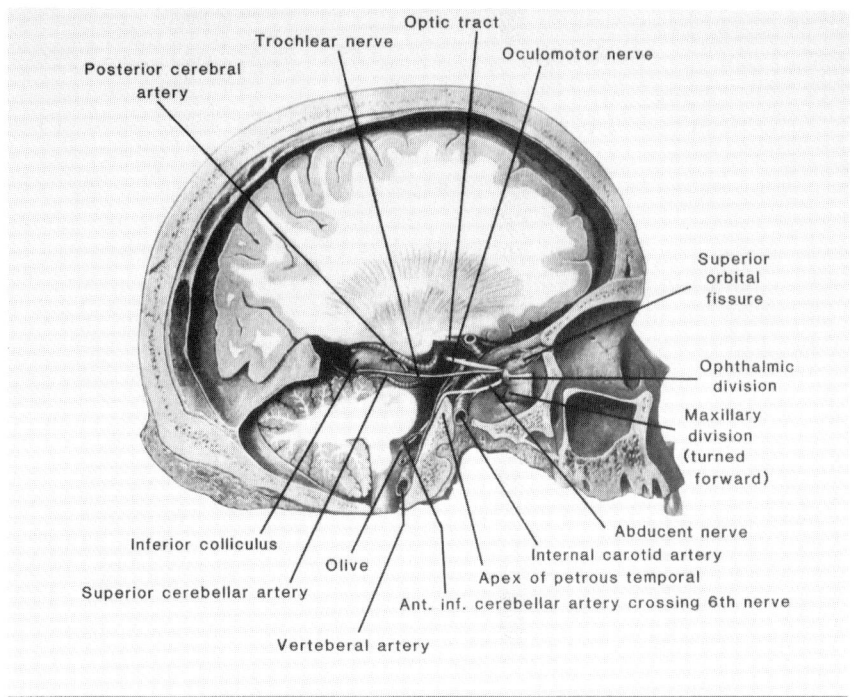

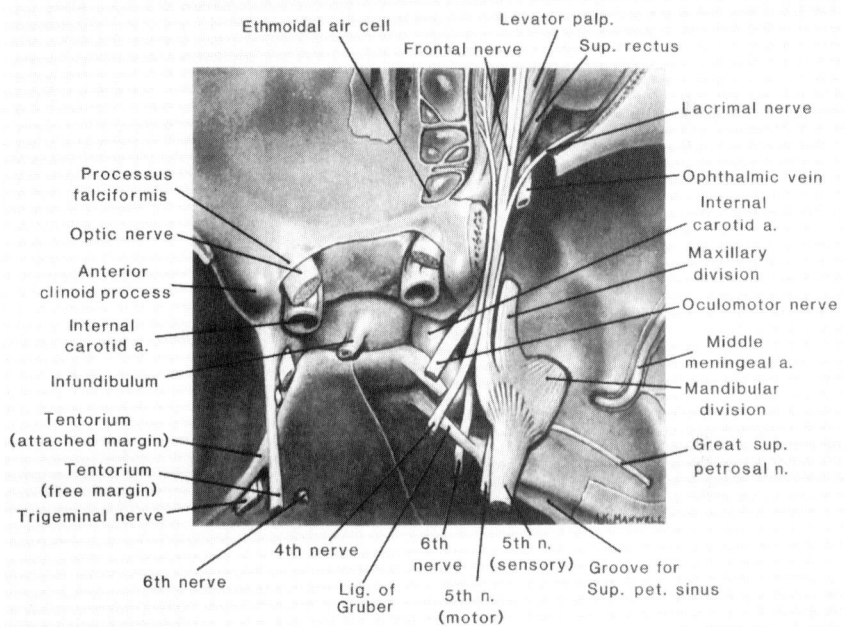

Figure 6-10
The intracranial courses of the third, fourth, and sixth cranial nerves. *Top*, Parasagittal view. *Bottom*, Superior view. Lig. of Gruber: petroclinoid ligament. *(From Warwick R: Eugene Wolff's anatomy of the eye and orbit, ed 7, London, 1976, HK Lewis & Co. By permission of Chapman and Hall.)*

Trochlear nerve

The fourth nerves arise from a paired group of cells in the midbrain at the level of the inferior colliculi near the ventral margin of the central gray substance that surrounds the aqueduct of Sylvius. Axons arise from these nuclei of origin, pass laterally and then dorsally around the central gray substance, and decussate on the dorsal surface of the brain stem at the lower margin of the inferior colliculi within the anterior medullary velum (see Fig. 6-10).

Each trochlear nerve passes forward around the side of the cerebral peduncle, coursing between the two uppermost branches of the basilar artery, the posterior cerebral branch above and the superior cerebellar branch below. Here it takes a long and vulnerable course in the subarachnoid space below the free margin of the tentorium cerebelli. Continuing forward, it pierces the dura in the angle between the free and the attached margins of the tentorium cerebelli to enter the lateral wall of the cavernous sinus. Still continuing forward, it enters the orbit through the wide portion of the superior orbital fissure. It passes over the upper surface of the levator of the lid and enters the belly of the superior oblique muscle. When the trochlear nerve is paralyzed, the eye cannot be turned downward when it is rotated inward.

Common causes of trochlear nerve palsy are, in the nuclear portion, lacunar infarctions; in the subarachnoid portion, entrapment against the tentorium in herniation and trauma; and, in the cavernous sinus and orbit, causes the same as those listed for the oculomotor nerve.

Abducens nerve

The sixth nerves arise from a paired group of cells in the floor of the fourth ventricle near the midline within the lower portion of the pons. Each is capped by the genu of the facial nerve. The abducens nucleus contains two distinct populations of neurons: those that innervate the lateral rectus muscle and those that project via the medial longitudinal fasciculus to the motor neurons of the contralateral medial rectus muscle. Fibers destined for the lateral rectus muscle travel ventrally in the pons through the medial lemniscus and lateral to the corticospinal tract and emerge at the lower margin of the pons. The nerve leaves the pons immediately dorsal to the anterior inferior cerebellar artery and, after an *upward* course of 15 mm through the subarachnoid space anterior to the pons, pierces the dura overlying the basilar portion of the occipital bone (see Fig. 6-10). Under the dura it runs up the back of the petrous portion of the temporal bone and then bends forward at a sharp angle under the petrosphenoidal ligament to pass on through the cavernous sinus. Although all the other nerves traversing the cavernous sinus lie within its lateral wall, the abducens nerve often lies within the sinus itself, surrounded by a separate sheath. The nerve enters the orbit through the superior orbital fissure and then pierces the lateral rectus muscle. The intrapontine portion of the facial nerve loops around the sixth nucleus, so that a lesion, such as an ependymoma or a subependymal glioma of the fourth ventricle, may affect both nerves and produce homolateral paralysis of the lateral rectus and facial muscles. When the abducens nerve is paralyzed, the ipsilateral eye is turned in toward the nose and abduction of the eye is impaired.

Common causes of abducens nerve palsy are, in the nuclear portion, lacunar infarctions; in the fascicular portion, infarctions, hemorrhages, and tumors; in the subarachnoid portion, stretching due to downward herniation and trauma at the petrosphenoidal ligament when the pons is pushed against the clivus and downward in trauma; and, in the cavernous and orbital portions, causes the same as those listed for the other nerves.

Sympathetic innervation to the eye

The sympathetic fibers to the eye form a polysynaptic pathway (Fig. 6-11). The first-order neurons have their cell bodies in the hypothalamus and descend in the lateral brain stem and spinal cord to the corticospinal center of Budge, located in the spinal cord at the C-8, T-1, and T-2 levels. Here the neurons synapse, and second-order neurons leave the spinal cord via the anterior ramus and travel in the thoracic sympathetic trunk. They take a course around the lung and under the subclavian artery and ascend in relation to the carotid artery as it leaves the chest cavity. A second synapse is located at the superior cervical ganglion near the bifurcation of the carotid artery. The third-order sympathetic neurons to the face send axons via the external carotid and its branches to blood vessels, sweat glands, and ciliomotor fibers. The third-order neuron sympathetic supply to the orbit travels via the internal carotid. In the cavernous sinus, the fibers leave the carotid, some traveling with the first diversion of the trigeminal nerve via the long ciliary nerve to the dilator muscle of the pupil. Other fibers travel via the ophthalmic artery to the lacrimal gland, orbital vasomotor targets, and Müller's muscles of the eyelids. The parasympathetic fibers are discussed with the anatomy of the third nerve.

External Examination
The globes

The eyes are inspected for exophthalmos. Myopic globes, because they are longer, may sometimes give the appearance of exophthalmos when they are not abnormal. A history and examination of old photographs will help to clarify this. Exophthalmos is best seen by standing behind the seated patient and observing the eyeballs from above. Comparative measurements between the two eyes can be made with an exophthalmometer, a device with rules and mirrors. The globes are gently retropulsed over closed lids. They normally have a resiliency. Masses behind them can be detected in this way. Also, ocular tension can be

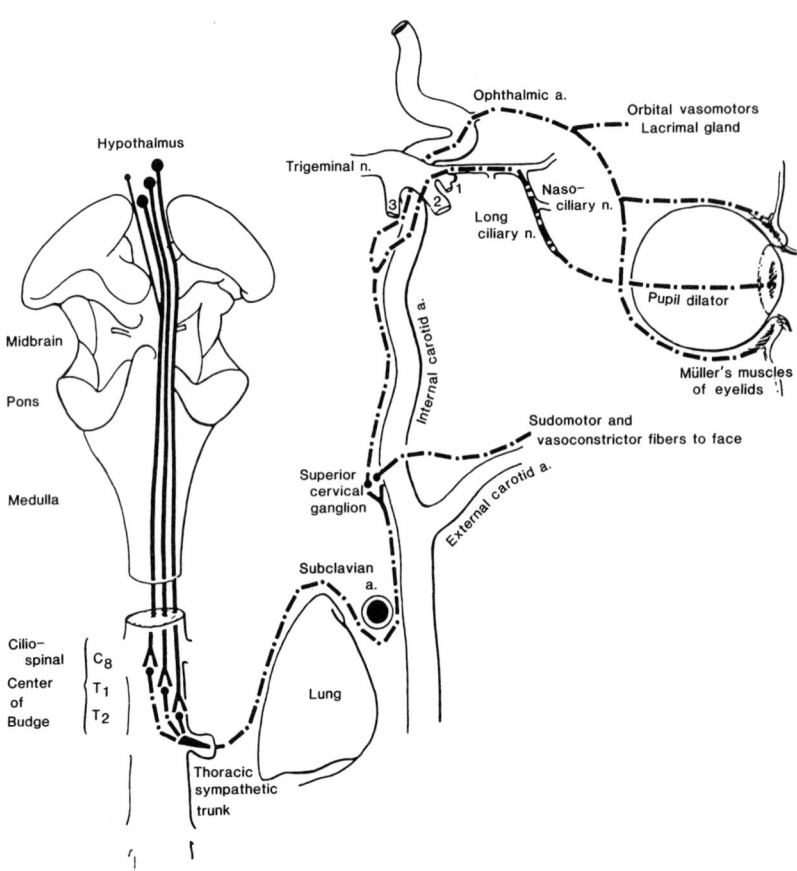

Figure 6-11
Ocular sympathetic pathways. Hypothalamic sympathetic fibers form a polysynaptic system as they descend to the ciliospinal center. This intra-axial tract is functionally considered the first-order neuron. The second-order neuron takes a circuitous course through the posterosuperior aspect of the chest and ascends in the neck in relationship to the carotid system. Third-order neurons originate in the superior cervical ganglion and are distributed to the face with branches of the external carotid artery and to the orbit via the ophthalmic artery and ophthalmic division (1) of the trigeminal nerve. (From Glaser JS: Neuro-Ophthalmology, ed 2, Philadelphia, 1990, JB Lippincott Co. By permission of Lippincott-Raven Publishers.)

approximated in this way. Comparison with a normal eye helps to distinguish a pathologic condition.

The lids

In its normal position, the upper eyelid covers 1 to 2 mm of the iris. The lower lid touches the limbus. The height of the palpebral fissure is measured with a ruler when an abnormality is suspected. The lids are examined for color, heliotrope lids being characteristic of polymyositis-dermatomyositis and red, injected lids of inflammation or venous obstruction. Common positional abnormalities of the lids are ptosis, lid retraction, lid lag, and blepharospasm (affecting muscles other than just those of the lids). Ptosis of 1 to 2 mm and miosis are components of Horner's syndrome, which is discussed later. Senile ptosis results from muscle and connective tissue laxity in the levator muscle. It may be unilateral or bilateral. It is fixed and is often accompanied by compensatory furrowing of the forehead in an effort to raise the lids out of the pupillary axis. The ptosis of an oculomotor nerve palsy may be either partial or complete. It is accompanied by weakness in the extraocular muscles supplied by the nerve and sometimes by pupillary abnormalities. It is discussed in the section on the oculomotor nerve. The ptosis of myasthenia gravis is characteristically variable, although it may seem quite stable. The lids are assessed for fatigability by asking the patient to sustain upgaze (this maneuver simultaneously tests the superior recti). Ptosis will increase if the lids are fatigable. The lids are rested by having the patient close the eyes. After eye opening, the ptosis may lessen for a time.

Cogan's lid twitch is another sign of myasthenia. The patient is asked to look down and then to quickly move the eyes to the primary position. A ptotic lid, given the chance to rest in downgaze, will overshoot on returning to primary gaze, twitching before coming to rest in primary position. Cogan explained this on the basis of easy recoverability and irritability of the muscle.

Lid retraction and stare are hallmarks of hyperthyroidism. As the eyes make following movements into downgaze, the lids can lag behind the globes. This condition is known as "lid lag."

Sometimes ptosis is present on one side and lid retraction on the other, so that one must decide whether ptosis is the primary problem and the contralateral lid retraction is merely compensatory because the person is making an effort to see with the ptotic eye and to elevate the lid or whether the retraction is a separate abnormality. If lifting the ptotic lid eliminates the contralateral retraction, it is merely compensatory. Similarly, if covering the ptotic eye manually eliminates the retraction, again, it is merely compensatory. If, with either of these maneuvers, the retracted lid remains retracted, the lid retraction is primary. Since there is some association between Graves' disease and myasthenia gravis, it is in this combination of conditions that this finding is most likely to be seen.

The orbicularis oculi is innervated by the seventh cranial nerve. To test its strength, the examiner tells the patient to squeeze the eyes shut. This muscle is normally very strong and should not be overcome with this test. The eyes are observed for evidence of squinting and blepharospasm, repeated unwanted contractions of the orbicularis with lid closure and often with contraction of other facial muscles.

Enophthalmos and blepharospasm and squinting narrow the palpebral fissure from below as well as from above. Ptosis changes only the position of the upper lid.

The iris
Both irides are normally the same color. A blue iris on one side suggests the possibility of Horner's syndrome occurring on that side before the age of 2 years. Inspection with an ophthalmoscope shows the normal iris to be opaque to light. Holes indicate atrophy. Capillaries seen on the surface indicate rubeosis, a neovascularization of the iris secondary to anterior segment ischemia. Neurofibromas may occur on the iris. These are elevated, whereas the normal iris freckles are not. The brown inner edge of the iris, the "ruff," may atrophy, particularly in small-fiber neuropathies.

As the pupil is studied, one should look for the Kayser-Fleischer ring of Wilson's disease. This is usually a complete ring of gray-green or golden brown pigmentation near the posterior layer of the cornea. It is approximately 2 to 3 mm wide and is separated from the periphery by a narrow zone of clear cornea. It is best seen, especially when poorly developed, with the slit lamp. It is always bilateral and is made up of fine pigment granules situated in Descemet's membrane.

The ophthalmoscope and slit lamp also allow inspection of the media, cornea, anterior chamber, lens, and vitreous for cells, protein, blood, and pigment. Each of these structures should be focused on with the ophthalmoscope. Early cataracts, for example, can be easily seen. When a patient's vision is less than 20/20, it is important to rule out abnormalities in the media as well as refractive errors before proceeding with further investigations.

The pupil
The size of the pupil is controlled by a sphincter muscle and a layer of dilator fibers that lie on the anterior surface of the pigment layer of the iris. The sphincter, or constrictor, muscle is supplied by parasympathetic fibers of the oculomotor nerve that arise in the Edinger-Westphal nucleus and synapse in the ciliary ganglion. The dilator muscle is supplied by sympathetic fibers (Fig. 6-12). Most individuals have pupils equal in size, although some have "simple anisocoria," normal pupils that differ slightly in size.

The size of the pupil is influenced by many factors, chief of which is the intensity of light falling on the retina. The afferent pathway for constriction of the pupil by a light stimulus is from the retina via the optic nerves, chiasm, optic tracts, and the brachium of the superior colliculus to the pretectal region, where there is a synapse. From there a second-order neuron continues the pathway to the Edinger-Westphal nucleus, from which the efferent pathways arise. The normal pupil contracts promptly when light is shone on the ipsilateral retina, the direct light

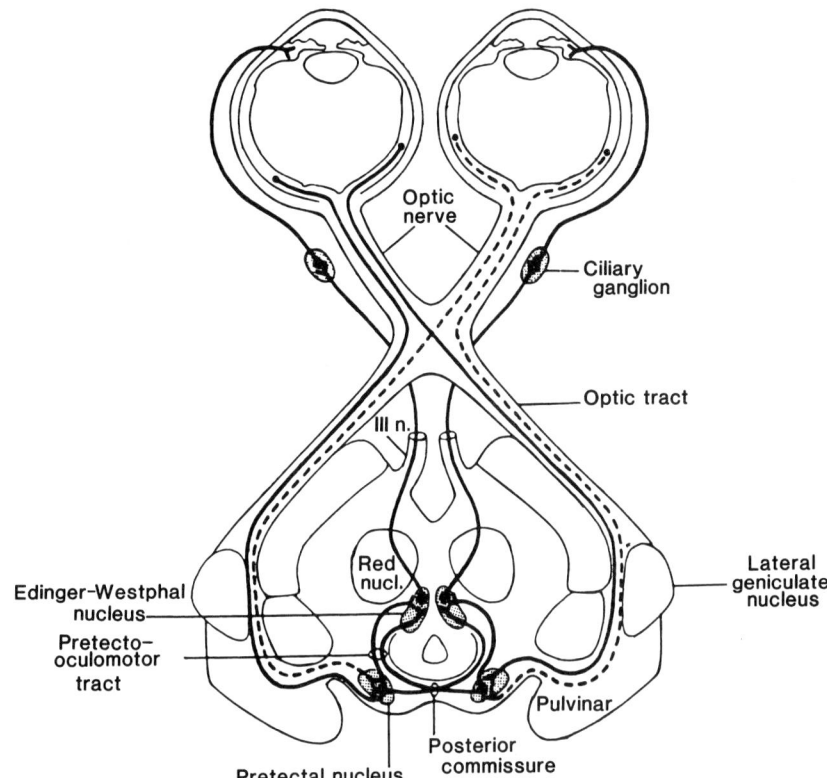

Figure 6-12
The pathway of the pupillary reaction to light. *(From Walsh FB, Hoyt WF: Clinical neuro-ophthalmology, ed 3, Baltimore, 1969, Williams & Wilkins Co. By permission of the publisher.)*

reflex. As a result of semidecussation of fibers, both in the optic chiasm and in the pretectal region, the contralateral as well as the ipsilateral pupil responds; this is known as the "crossed light reflex," or "consensual light reflex."

The pupils also constrict under the stimulus of accommodation and convergence. The pathways for these reflexes are ill-defined at present.

The pupil may respond to a painful stimulus directed toward a neighboring or a distant portion of the body. The pain reflexes are as follows:

1. The ciliospinal reflex, which consists of a dilatation of the pupil on painful stimulation of the skin of the neck on the ipsilateral side.
2. The oculosensory reflex, which consists either of constriction of the pupil or of dilatation followed by constriction in response to painful stimulation of the eye or its adnexa.

Forceful closing of the eye, closing the eyes in sleep, and upward deviation of the eyeballs are followed by constriction of the pupils. This is known as the "orbicularis reflex."

The variation in the size of the pupils in response to various pharmacologic preparations may be designated as the "drug reflexes." These consist of (1) dilatation either on stimulation of the sympathetic division of the autonomic nervous system or with paralysis of the parasympathetic division and (2) constriction either with paralysis of the sympathetic elements or on stimulation of the parasympathetic pathways. Atropine, homatropine, and scopolamine act as mydriatics by a depressing or paralyzing action on structures innervated by postganglionic cholinergic nerves. Epinephrine, ephedrine, amphetamine, and cocaine dilate the pupil by stimulating structures innervated by postganglionic adrenergic nerves. Pilocarpine, acetylcholine, and muscarine constrict the pupil by stimulating structures innervated by postganglionic cholinergic nerves, and physostigmine and neostigmine do so by inhibiting the action of cholinesterase. Hippus is the alternating widening and constricting that is the normal result of changes in the balance between sympathetic and parasympathetic innervation.

The pupillary light response should be tested with a bright light. The source is held below the eyes, out of the line of vision, and the patient is told to focus in the distance to avoid the artifact of constriction of the pupil to accommodation. The most common cause of sluggish pupils is a weak light.

An amaurotic pupil shows absolutely no reaction to light. It is the pupil of a blind eye whose retina or optic nerve has been completely destroyed. The eye is often referred to as "NLP," no light perception. There is no consensual light response in the fellow eye. The direct response in the fellow eye is normal, and the consensual response in the blind eye is intact.

With impaired function of a very large area of retina, or of the optic nerve, a unilateral afferent pupillary defect or Marcus Gunn pupil may be found. When a light is shone into the eye on the side of the afferent pathway defect, both pupils may appear to constrict sluggishly. When the eye on the normal side is stimulated, both pupils constrict normally. The swinging flashlight test is done to better evaluate this subtle and sometimes barely perceptible difference. The flashlight is directed back and forth, first into one eye and then across the nose into the other eye. Normally, the first pupillary movement elicited in each eye is constriction. If an eye has an afferent defect, however, the first movement when the light is swung to that eye is dilation of the pupil, because the brain perceives less light via the damaged pathway. This observation of the first pupillary movement is an invaluable test for detecting optic nerve damage. It has now been standardized by use of a series of gray filters of different densities. These are placed in succession in front of the good eye until the dilation response disappears.

Interruption of the sympathetic nerve supply (Horner's syndrome) to the iris and eyelids results in a small pupil and narrowing of the palpebral fissure, the latter being due to a slight ptosis of the upper lid and slight elevation of the lower lid. The enophthalmos sometimes said to accompany these changes is only apparent and is seldom confirmed by the exophthalmometer. The anisocoria is greater in dim light, because the affected pupil fails to dilate. The pupil reacts promptly to light and on convergence, and it usually fails to dilate on instillation of a 10% solution of cocaine. If the lesion is in the third-order neuron, the pupil should also fail to dilate with a 1% solution of hydroxyamphetamine hydrobromide (Paredrine). Occasionally, there is a disturbance in sweating of the face on the affected side, indicating that the lesion is proximal to the bifurcation of the carotid. The reason is that the fibers for autonomic function on the face travel via the external carotid, whereas those destined for the eye go via the internal carotid. This syndrome was described by Horner in 1869. The site of the interruption of the sympathetic fibers may be in the brain stem, the cervical portions of the spinal cord, the anterior roots of C-8, T-1, T-2, or T-3, the cervical sympathetic trunk, or any portions of the postganglionic pathway. The interruption may be due to adenomatous goiter, trauma, or a lesion within the cavernous sinus. Horner's syndrome may also be the result of injury to the brachial plexus or of certain lesions in the thorax, such as Pancoast's tumor.

The myotonic pupillary reaction (tonic pupil) described by Saenger and by Strasburger in 1902, and sometimes referred to as "Adie's pupil," may lead the unwary into diagnostic difficulties. The patient is generally a young woman with a large pupil and a complaint of trouble focusing or blurring of vision. The reaction to light is absent if tested in the customary manner, although the size of the pupil changes slowly on prolonged exposure to a bright light or if the patient remains in the dark for a considerable time. The reaction on convergence is slowed, sometimes requiring 5 seconds or more for completion, and the widening of the pupil on gaze into the distance is prolonged over a similar period. This slow dilation of the pupil is the most useful diagnostic feature. The tonic pupil reacts promptly to the usual mydriatic and miotic drugs and is abnormally sensitive to a 2.5% solution of mecholyl instilled into the conjunctival sac. This solution will not affect a normal pupil but will constrict a myotonic pupil. Slit lamp examination shows irregular segmental contractions of the iris. The lesion is commonly associated with absence of or a decrease in the activity of muscle stretch reflexes.

Of the abnormal pupillary reactions, that described by D. Argyll Robertson in 1869 has elicited perhaps the greatest interest. According to his description, the retina is quite sensitive to light, and the pupils are small; the pupils react promptly on accommodation for near objects but do not contract on exposure to bright light, and they constrict still further under physostigmine salicylate but dilate slowly and only partially with atropine. The site of the lesion responsible for Argyll Robertson's pupils is not known. Adie pointed out that if Argyll Robertson's original definition is adhered to, this pupillary disturbance is an almost infallible sign of syphilis. Large pupils that react on convergence but not to light may be indicative of syphilis, but they occur also in many other diseases, including tumor of the brain, meningitis, and chronic alcoholism.

In light-near dissociation, reaction of the pupil in the seeing eye to light is less strong than the reaction to near. (The examiner must beware. The commonest cause of this phenomenon is weak batteries in the ophthalmoscope, and the next most common is doing the test in a brightly lighted room.) Causes include syphilis, diabetes, tectal lesions, myotonic dystrophy, familial amyloidosis, aberrant regeneration of the third nerve, and Adie's pupil. The lesion may be, at least in some cases, in the periaqueductal gray matter.

Aberrant regeneration of the third nerve is a misdirection-in-regeneration syndrome after mechanical trauma to the nerve. The fibers grow back along each other's pathways. This lesion is discussed more fully below. The pupil can remain dilated and fixed, can return to normal, or can develop pseudo–Argyll Robertson features, with poor response to light and modest response on convergence but also with reaction on adduction due to innervation from fibers originally destined for the medial rectus.

After head injuries, a dilated and fixed or sluggish pupil may be observed on the side of the cranial trauma. Called "Hutchinson's pupil," it is caused by a herniation of the hippocampal gyrus through the tentorium, with resultant pressure on the third nerve of the same side.

The convergence reflex is observed by watching the pupil as gaze is shifted from a distant object to a near object. It is best to encourage an optimum response by making the near target interesting and easy to see. The examiner's finger does not meet these criteria. It should be remembered that a person who has normal distance vision but has lost the ability to accommodate is not able to focus at a distance closer than 1 m. A near target is not seen clearly. This patient can be tested wearing bifocals. The patient with poor vision is asked to look at his or her own finger. Proprioception assists in obtaining a good response.

Ocular Movements

Limitation of rotation of the eyeballs may be due to paresis of the third, fourth, or sixth cranial nerves, to interruption of the prenuclear connections, or to disturbance within the extraocular muscles themselves, as in myasthenia gravis, exophthalmic goiter, or Duane's retraction syndrome. Tumor or inflammation within the orbit also may restrict movements of the globe. The limitation of ocular rotations associated with cavernous sinus thrombosis is caused by involvement of the third, fourth, and sixth nerves in the sinus rather than by swelling in the orbit.

Range of motion of the eyes and alignment of the visual axes

Ductions are the rotations of each eye alone when only that eye is viewing. Versions are the rotations of both eyes with both eyes viewing. These must be tested separately, because imbalances between the two eyes may affect the way they move in concert with each other.

Examination and recording of ocular movements

Ocular rotations are tested by having the patient turn the eyes in the cardinal directions of gaze and by having the eyes converge on a near point. Paralysis or weakness of a single or several ocular muscles or of conjugate movements (movements of both eyes in the same direction) and the presence or absence of nystagmus on conjugate deviation are observed.

Direct observation in a good light is usually adequate for examination of the function of the external muscles. Most persons can rotate their eyes readily until the outer margin of the cornea reaches the outer canthus and can rotate them medially until the inner margin of the cornea is buried under the caruncle. The limits of upward and downward rotation vary greatly in normal individuals, but differences between the two eyes are readily recognized and are more important in the diagnosis of paralysis of single ocular muscles.

The muscles that turn the eyeball are yoked in pairs (Fig. 6-13); the medial and lateral recti turn the eye in and out, the superior and inferior

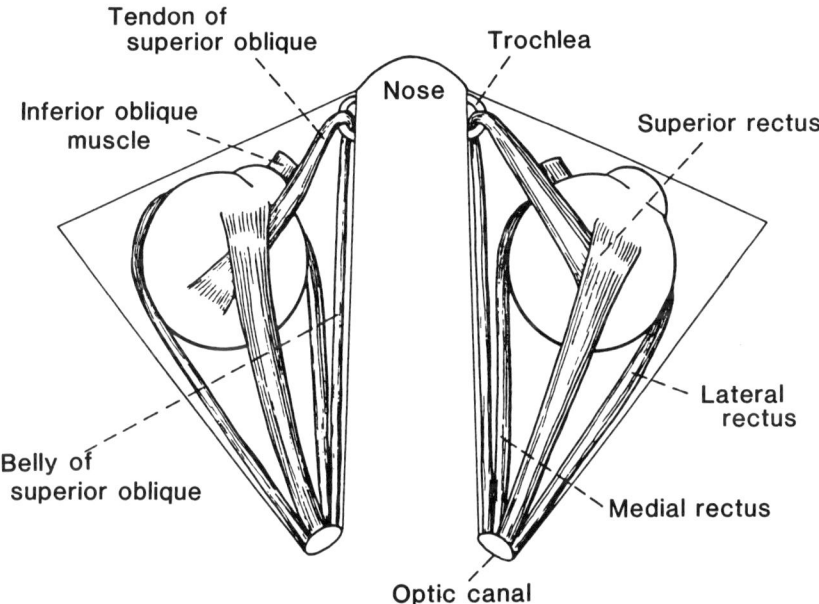

Figure 6-13
Rucker's "schematic representation of extraocular muscles" as portrayed in Baker AB: *Clinical Neurology. (By permission of Lippincott-Raven Publishers.)*

recti turn the eye up and down when it is looking out, and the inferior and superior obliques turn the eye up and down when it is looking in. The medial and lateral rectus muscles turn the globe in the direction indicated by their names. When the eye is turned out, the oblique muscles are more effective in producing a torsion of the eye than in elevation or depression. However, when the eye is turned in toward the nose, the obliques become efficient elevators and depressors, and the superior and inferior recti produce torsion. From the primary position, with the gaze straight ahead, rotation up and down is participated in by several muscles. The function of individual muscles is tested most readily by observing them in the field of their greatest efficiency. Consequently, the patient is first asked to look to one side and then to the other to test the lateral and medial recti. Then, while looking to one side, the patient is told to look up and down. In this position, the out-turning eye is elevated and depressed by the superior and inferior recti muscles and the in-turning eye by the inferior and superior oblique muscles. Then the patient is asked to look to the opposite side, and the procedure is repeated, testing the opposite pair of muscles. It should be remembered that although the recti act in the directions indicated by their names, the obliques do not, the superior oblique rotating the eye downward, the inferior oblique rotating it upward.

The following chart used for recording observations of ocular rotation also serves as a guide for positioning the eyes to separate the actions of the individual muscles in testing their strength:

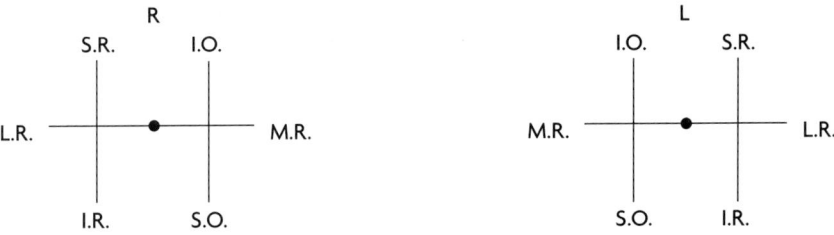

The observations are made while confronting the patient, so that the chart for the left eye is to the right and vice versa. The dot on the center line indicates the primary position of gaze with the patient looking straight ahead. The initials near the end of each line are those of the individual eye muscles primarily concerned with rotation of the eye in the direction of the line away from the primary position. For example, upward rotation of the right eyeball after the gaze has been directed toward the left is chiefly performed by the inferior oblique muscle. Weakness or normality of that muscle can be indicated by inscribing the appropriate symbol above the vertical line to the right on the chart for the right eye.

Since there may be an imbalance in ocular muscle pull, each eye must be tested individually for power of rotation. A cover is placed over one eye of the patient, and the patient is told to look at the examiner's target with the other eye while the target is moved to the right, left, up, and down. It may be found that, although there is one full rotation of one eye or the other when the two eyes are fixing on the object, each eye has full power of rotation when fixing by itself.

Strabismus

Strabismus is a misalignment of the visual axes. It shows itself either as a phoria, which is a latent deviation held in check by fusional vergence mechanisms, or as a tropia, which is a manifest deviation not held in check by fusion. Strabismus may be either paralytic or nonparalytic. A paralytic strabismus is caused by actual weakness of one or more of the muscles controlling gaze. It is very often noncomitant, that is, varying with the direction of gaze. A nonparalytic strabismus is caused not by any muscle weakness per se but by an imbalance in the way the two eyes act together. Very often, the strabismus does not change in different positions of gaze with either eye fixating. It is therefore comitant.

Because they are latent deviations suppressed by fusion, phorias are detected by the alternate cover test. They are detected when binocular vision is not allowed. The patient is asked to look at a distant target. An occluder is quickly moved from one eye to the other, and any movements made by the eyes to take up fixation are noted. The test is done with the eyes in different cardinal positions of gaze. This is most readily accomplished by having the patient maintain fixation on a distant target and turning the head so that the eyes are in right gaze, left gaze, and so forth.

An esophoria is a deviation medially under the cover with the eye moving outward to take up fixation when the cover is switched to the opposite eye. An exophoria is a deviation laterally with a medial movement to take up fixation. A hyperphoria is a tendency for vertical misalignment. It is always named by the higher eye no matter where the disease is located. (Tropias can also be detected with this test. See later discussion.)

Common nonparalytic phorias include the squints that are suppressible by fusion. Many people have a tendency to be walleyed (exophoria) or cross-eyed (esophoria) when fusion is broken by covering one eye. Occasionally there is a tendency to a vertical deviation (hyperphoria), which, as with the tropias, is always named by the higher eye. Many nonparalytic esophorias and exophorias have larger deviations either in upgaze or in downgaze. They are called "V" pattern and "A" pattern, respectively.

An example of paralytic phoria is a very early sixth nerve palsy. The eye under cover turns in because of subtle lateral rectus weakness. This sort of phoria is worse (the deviation is greater) in the direction of gaze of the weak muscle. The earliest sign of herniation downward may be very subtle bilateral sixth nerve palsies manifested by the turning in of each eye under the cover. The patient is still able to overcome these by the drive for fusion.

Patients with phorias do not complain of double vision unless or until their phorias break down into tropias, manifest deviations unsuppressible by fusion. Nonparalytic phorias can break down with age, fatigue, drug effects, alcohol intoxication, and head injury. They then become nonparalytic tropias, and their assessment will be discussed below. Paralytic phorias often also break down, and the muscle weakness becomes greater with the progress of disease. They become paralytic tropias.

A tropia is a misalignment of the visual axis when both eyes are viewing. When it is acquired, it produces diplopia. A congenital tropia results in visual suppression amblyopia or anomalous retinal correspondence, and no diplopia results. It is detected by the cover-uncover test, which is done with the eyes in the different cardinal positions of gaze. For each position in turn, each eye is covered and uncovered. If a tropia is present when the fixing eye is covered, the other eye turns to take up the target. When the cover is removed, the eye that was underneath turns to take up the target (if it is the preferred eye for fixation) or else no movement occurs (if neither eye is preferred). When the nonfixing eye is covered, no movement of the other eye is seen. The deviation of the sound eye under cover (the "secondary" deviation) is greater than that of the paretic eye under cover (the "primary" deviation).

Walleyed and cross-eyed patients who fix with one eye or with each eye alternately have nonparalytic tropia. The extraocular movements of each eye are full, but the eyes are out of alignment. Paralytic tropias include weakness in any muscle or combination of muscles that causes diplopia.

The Bielschowsky head tilt test is used in addition to the tests described above to analyze a vertical deviation. The side of the hypertropia and whether it is greater in right or left gaze and in up or down gaze are determined. Then, the deviation is measured with the head tilted to the left and the right (Bielschowsky's head tilt test). When the head is tilted, the vertical eye muscles are no longer driven in their usual yoked pairs. The reason is that the otoliths cause compensatory cyclorotation by coinnervation of the ipsilateral (to the side of the tilt) superior oblique and superior rectus muscles, which produces intorsion and coinnervation of the contralateral inferior oblique and inferior rectus muscles, in turn producing extorsion. With a left superior oblique palsy, the left hyperdeviation becomes more marked on leftward head tilt and less marked on rightward tilt. The result of this test is positive in most cases of superior oblique palsy but not in cases of palsy of a vertical rectus muscle.

Acute paralytic strabismus shows greater deviation in the direction of gaze of the paralytic muscle; that is, the strabismus is noncomitant. With time, however, comitancy spreads so that the deviation becomes equal in all directions of gaze.

Maddox rod testing

A red glass or a red glass with prisms molded into it (Maddox rod) is placed before the right eye. It breaks fusion. The patient is asked to look at a small white light in the distance. The right eye sees a red dot (with the red glass) or a red line (with the Maddox rod), and the left eye sees the white light. The head is turned so that the eyes are in the nine different cardinal positions of gaze, and the separations between the images are charted. The position in which the separation of the two images is greatest is determined (Fig. 6-14). The following rules should be applied to detect the paretic extraocular muscle.

1. The distance between the true image ("good" eye) and the false image (eye with paretic muscle) increases in the direction of action of the paretic muscle. Example: An object is moved to the patient's left, and diplopia is noted. As the object is moved farther and farther to the patient's left, the images move farther and farther apart. Either the right medial rectus or the left lateral rectus muscle is weak.
2. The more peripherally seen image is the false image (image seen by the eye having the paretic muscle). Example (continued from rule 1): The patient is told to watch the object carefully and to note whether the outside (to the patient's left) or the inside image disappears as the examiner's hand is placed over the right eye. The patient notes that the inside image (true image) disappears. Therefore, the peripheral image (false image) is being seen by the left eye, and the left lateral rectus muscle is the defective muscle.
3. If in the paresis of a vertical rotator the distance between the true image and the false image is greater in the abducted (outwardly rotated) position of the affected eye, a rectus muscle is involved, but if it is greater in the adducted (inwardly rotated) position of the affected eye, an oblique muscle is involved. Example: The patient complains of diplopia on looking up. Application of rule 2 shows that the left eye is involved. The object is now moved so that the patient must look up and to the right (left eye adducted) and then upward to the left (left eye abducted). The distance between the images is greater in the abducted position. Therefore, the superior rectus is the defective muscle.

Another useful test for evaluating diplopia is the Lancaster red-green test. The patient wears glasses with red glass in front of one eye and green in front of the other. The patient can see only red objects with one eye and only green with the other. Fusion is broken. With a red and a green flashlight, one held by the examiner and the other by the patient,

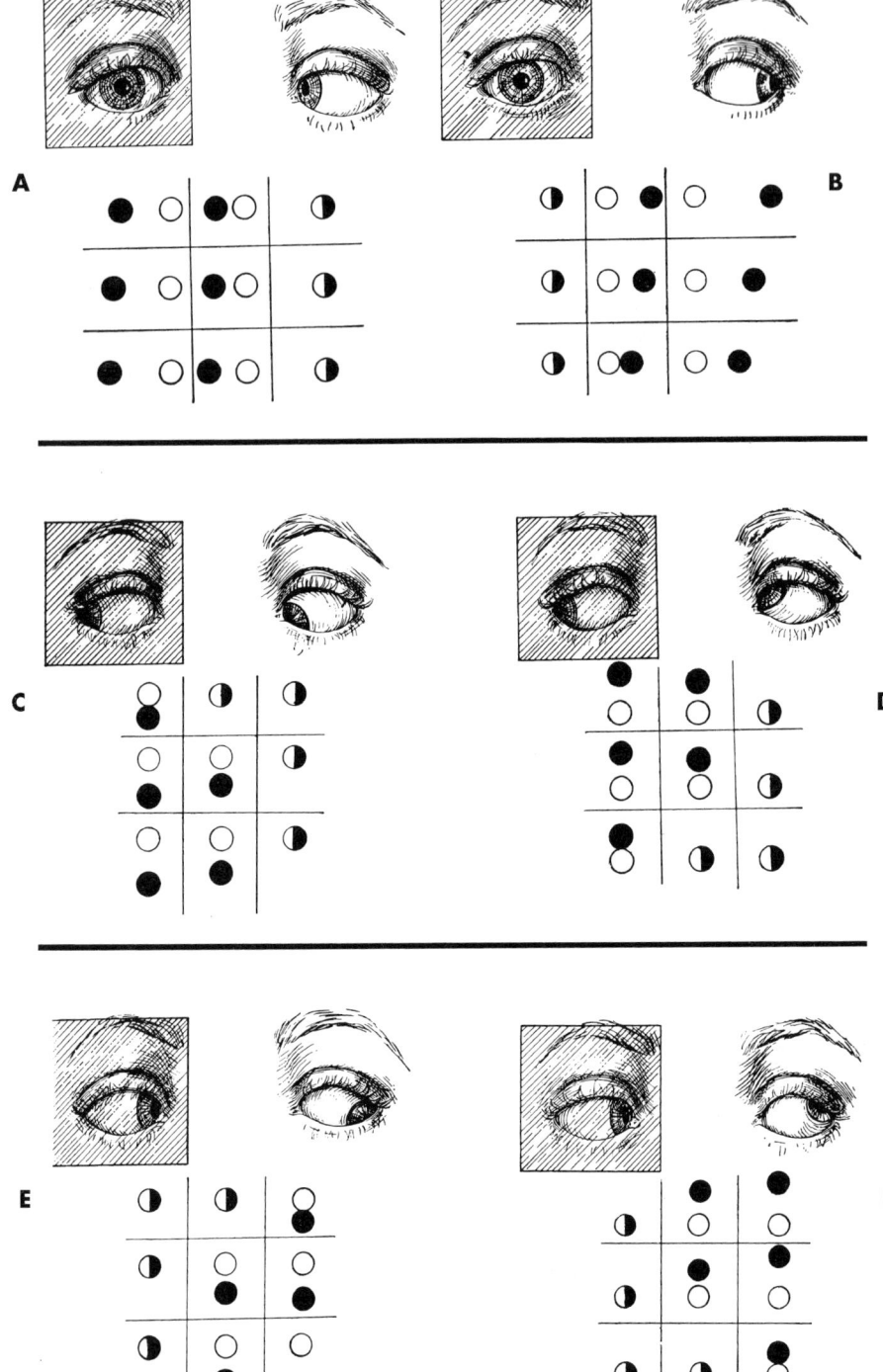

Figure 6-14
The red glass test. The findings are shown for paralysis of individual extraocular muscles of the right eye. In each case, the red glass is placed over the right eye. The charts below each case are displayed as the subject indicates to the examiner the position of the red *(filled circle)* and white *(open circle)* images in the nine cardinal positions of gaze. **A**, Paralysis of the right lateral rectus muscle. The right eye cannot abduct beyond the primary position. The uncrossed diplopia increases on looking into the patient's right field of gaze. **B**, Paralysis of the right medial rectus muscle. The right eye cannot adduct beyond the primary position. The crossed diplopia increases on looking into the patient's left field of gaze. **C**, Paralysis of the right inferior rectus. The right eye cannot be depressed in the abducted position. The separation of the images is greatest on looking down and to the right, with the red image localized lower. **D**, Paralysis of the right superior rectus. The right eye cannot be elevated in the abducted position. The separation of the images is greatest on looking up and to the right, with the red image localized higher. **E**, Paralysis of the right superior oblique. The right eye cannot be depressed in the adducted position. The separation of the images is greatest on looking down and to the left, with the red image localized lower. **F**, Paralysis of the right inferior oblique. The right eye cannot be elevated in the adducted position. The separation of the images is greatest on looking up and to the left, with the red image localized higher. *(From Cogan DG: Neurology of the ocular muscles, ed 2, Springfield, Ill, 1956, Charles C Thomas, Publisher. By permission of the publisher.)*

---

the fixation points of the two eyes in various fields of gaze can be plotted on a screen.

The patient's head should be observed for any turns, tilts, or thrusts used to compensate for abnormalities in motility.

Ocular motility is controlled on three different levels in the brain. The lowest level is mediated entirely via the brain stem. The patient is asked to look at a distant target, and the head is moved while fixation is constant. With head movements, the semicircular canals are stimulated and input is sent from the vestibular nucleus to the gaze centers in the pons (for horizontal gaze) and the midbrain (for vertical gaze) and thence to the third, fourth, and sixth nerve nuclei and, in the case of horizontal gaze, from the sixth nerve nucleus to the third via the medial longitudinal fasciculus. With each movement of the head, compensatory movements of the eyes are made, and gaze remains fixed on the target. In a comatose patient, the semicircular canals are stimulated by head movements, and this maneuver is the basis of the "doll's eye" test. Intact reflex eye movements indicate intact brain stem connections. (The original "doll's eyes" were fixed, like the eyes painted on doll faces, indicating a brain stem lesion. This has resulted in some confusion about how to report results. Specifying whether the pathways are intact eliminates this confusion.) This same system can be tested with a stronger stimulus—

cold or warm water in the auditory canal (ice-water calorics). The head is elevated 30 degrees. Cold water drives the eyes tonically toward the stimulus, with quick phases of nystagmus away from it. Warm water does the opposite. Cold water in both ears drives the eyes down, and warm water drives them up, with corrective quick phases in the opposite direction.

The next higher level of gaze control is that of following movements. The patient is asked to pursue a target. The pathway involves vision, visual cortex, and frontal eye fields and requires a relatively small amount of cortical input. The highest level involves eye movements to abstract verbal commands to look right, left, up, or down. It involves auditory processing and frontal eye fields and implies intact high-level functioning. The second and third levels involve "supranuclear" or "prenuclear" control of gaze, that is, control before the final common pathway of the brain stem nuclei. These higher level movements are particularly impaired in progressive supranuclear palsy and in other degenerative disorders as well.

Ocular skew is a vertical tropia not explainable by any muscle or nerve abnormality. It may be either comitant or noncomitant. It is caused by a prenuclear abnormality, usually a lesion in the midbrain.

Fixation and gaze-holding mechanisms

The eyes should be examined while the patient, with eyes in the primary position, is fixing on a distant target. The eyes should be still and steady. Ocular motor neurons fire at a steady rate during fixation. Extraneous eye movements may be observed. Square-wave jerks are composed of a tiny conjugate saccade (rapid eye movement) off the target, with a pause in this position and then a saccade back to the target. Eye-movement recordings demonstrate a pattern of square waves, hence the name. They are a mark of vestibulocerebellar abnormality and are seen in various diseases, including cerebellar disorders and progressive supranuclear palsy.

Another abnormality of gaze-holding is ocular flutter. This consists of small-amplitude back-to-back horizontal saccades, that is, saccades without any interval between them. The eyes appear to be rapidly quivering back and forth. Oscillopsia consists of the same back-to-back saccades, this time occurring in all directions of gaze. Both of these abnormal movements reflect disorders in the pause cells of the raphe; those controlling horizontal gaze are in the pons, and those for vertical gaze are in the midbrain.

Ordinarily, burst cells in the brain stem would fire all the time, projecting onto the nuclei of the third, fourth, and sixth cranial nerves, were they not inhibited by pause cells in the raphe. When a saccade is about to begin, the pause cells are inhibited, and the burst cells fire, projecting onto the cranial nerve nuclei. Lesions in or impinging on the raphe, such as encephalitis, autoimmune disorders, and tumors near the dorsal brain stem, cause flutter and oscillopsia. Flutter occurs when the disorder is limited to the pons, oscillopsia when it extends to the midbrain.

The eyes are also examined in primary gaze and eccentric gaze. Sometimes there is a gaze preference toward a particular direction. The left frontal eye fields send projections to the right (contralateral) gaze center in the pons to drive the right sixth nerve nucleus (right lateral rectus muscle) and, via the medial longitudinal fasciculus, the left third nerve nucleus (left medial rectus). The eyes turn right. Persistent irritative activity in a frontal eye field drives the eyes to the opposite side. An ablative frontal lesion allows the eyes to deviate toward the lesion, forced there by the unopposed contralateral frontal eye field. Very often, these changes are transient, occurring in the early period after the development of a lesion. Later, forced eye closure by the patient causes the eyes to deviate toward the side of the lesion, whereas no deviation is seen with the eyes open. Bilateral frontal or frontoparietal lesions may cause an acquired apraxia of the gaze that limits voluntary eye movements.

Abnormalities of gaze may also be seen in stupor and coma. Some patients have "ping-pong gaze," with the eyes first deviating right and then deviating left. Other patients have roving eye movements. Both of these abnormalities probably represent abnormal patterns of frontoparietal neural firing, with one side overtaking the other repeatedly. Cortical gaze abnormalities can often be overcome by strong vestibular stimulation (head movements and calorics), because brain stem connections exist between the vestibular nuclei and gaze centers in the pons and midbrain. This can be useful in patients in stupor and coma, since it is possible to demonstrate that local brain stem connections are intact.

Gaze palsies can also occur on the basis of disease in the brain stem itself. A lesion in the sixth nerve nucleus causes a gaze palsy because the nucleus contains two populations of neurons, those that turn the eye outward and those that, projecting via the medial longitudinal fasciculus to the contralateral medial rectus subnucleus of the third nerve, bring the contralateral eye inward. The eyes cannot turn in the direction of the lesion. A lesion in the gaze center in the pons (in the paramedian pontine reticular formation) also causes an ipsilateral gaze palsy. If the lesion extends to the ipsilateral medial longitudinal fasciculus, an ipsilateral gaze palsy and a contralateral internuclear ophthalmoplegia are present. Therefore, the only horizontal eye movement is abduction of the contralateral eye. This is "Fisher's one-and-a-half syndrome." An internuclear ophthalmoplegia is caused by a lesion in the medial longitudinal fasciculus. This tract runs from the sixth nerve nucleus immediately across to the contralateral raphe area and then up to the medial rectus subnucleus of the third nerve. A lesion located here may interrupt adduction completely or cause it to be slowed. This can be tested by asking the patient to make saccades back and forth between two targets. Slow adduction can be seen by the observer. Convergence can be preserved if the lesion is more dorsally located.

Gaze difficulties can also occur with midbrain lesions. Supranuclear lesions impair upgaze and can drive the eyes down (setting-sun sign). The eyes may bob downward and drift back up (ocular bobbing).

The vestibular system

The peripheral vestibular apparatus consists of the semicircular canals, which detect angular acceleration, and the otoliths, which are sensitive to linear acceleration and gravity. The incoming nerve synapses at Scarpa's ganglion, and then axons project to the vestibular nuclei and the cerebellum. Projections go from the vestibular nuclei up to all three ocular motor nuclei. There is a precise relationship between each of the semicircular canals and eye movements in the plane of that canal. The vestibular organs are paired for a push-pull action. The vestibular commissure connects the two vestibular nuclei. The purpose of the vestibular system is to keep gaze on the target during rapid and brief head movements.

Nystagmus

Nystagmus is a repetitive to-and-fro movement of the eyes. It may be either smooth and sinusoidal (pendular nystagmus) or an alteration of a slow drift and a quick corrective saccade back (jerk nystagmus). Reliable diagnosis can rarely be made on the basis of the waveform alone. The entire clinical picture must be considered.

Nystagmus may arise through stimulation of the peripheral vestibular apparatus. For clinical diagnostic purposes, otologists study the eye movements after turning the patient in a Bárány chair and after irrigating the outer ear canal with warm or cold water.

Rotation of the head produces a nystagmus in the plane of rotation, regardless of the position of the head. It is due to inertia of the fluid within the semicircular canals. At the beginning of turning, there is a lag of the endolymph; when turning stops suddenly, the momentum of the endolymph tends to keep it moving. The eyes are drawn in the direction of flow of the endolymph. This represents the slow phase of the nystagmus. The quick phase is in the opposite direction. Because the direction of flow of the endolymph relative to the canals is reversed when turning is suddenly stopped, the direction of the nystagmus is reversed then, too.

Clinically, only the nystagmus persisting after the turning has ceased is studied. Its slow component is in the direction of turning; its quick component is in the opposite direction. Its amplitude is increased on looking in the direction of the quick phase and diminished on looking in the direction of the slow phase. Change of gaze, although it alters the intensity of the nystagmus, does not alter the direction of its quick and slow components. The vestibulo-ocular reflex is normally suppressible by fixation. The patient sits in a swivel chair and holds a target fixed in relation to patient and chair. The chair is turned. The eyes normally stay on the target. There is no nystagmus. This suppression can fail to occur in vestibular and brain stem and cortical disease.

Caloric stimulation of the vestibule also brings about a pronounced nystagmus. Flushing the ear canal with cold water causes a rhythmic movement of the eyes with the quick component to the opposite side; warm water produces a rhythmic movement with the quick component to the same side.

In the presence of a labyrinthine fistula, pressure within the semicircular canals can be modified by a rubber bulb inserted in the ear canal. An increase of pressure causes a nystagmus with its quick component to the same side; a decrease of pressure causes a nystagmus with its quick component to the opposite side.

Destruction of one vestibule or of one vestibular nerve causes an extreme depressive defect; deviation of the head and eyes and the slow phase of the nystagmus are toward the side of the lesion, the quick phase of the nystagmus being to the opposite side. As in rotational and caloric nystagmus, turning the eyes toward the quick phase increases its amplitude, but change of gaze does not alter the direction of the quick and slow components. In this respect it differs from the central nervous system types. A distressing vertigo accompanies this disorder, and both the nystagmus and the vertigo persist for from one to several weeks. Nystagmus of vestibular type is also present during the episodes of vertigo in Meniere's disease and postural vertigo and in these instances is of a mixed vertical and rotatory type.

In the diagnosis of postural vertigo, we have frequently obtained help by the simple maneuver of having the patient sit on the end of the examining table, then laying him or her back quickly with the head turned toward one shoulder, and repeating this procedure with the head toward the other shoulder (Nylén's maneuver). Often when the patient falls back with the head in one specific position, a latent period of 1 or 2 seconds is followed by true vertigo and mixed rotary and vertical nystagmus of several seconds' duration. It sometimes aids the patient to know that one can arise and lie down without becoming dizzy if movements are made slowly and the head is kept turned toward the side that does not cause vertigo.

When impairment of the vestibular nerves is bilateral and equal on the two sides, either partial or complete, even in the acute phase there is no nystagmus or vertigo. Instead, the patient reports that the environment seems unstable during head movement. This is oscillopsia due to poor functioning of the vestibulo-ocular reflex.

Nystagmus originating in the vestibular nucleus is jerk-type rotatory and linear, not positional, and is associated with vertigo. Central vestibular nystagmus is often downbeat and worse looking down and out. The lesion causing it is generally in the posterior fossa near the craniocervical junction. The pathogenesis has not been settled. There may be unopposed action from the anterior semicircular canals because the posterior canals may be injured as their projections cross in the floor of the fourth ventricle. The lesion may also be in the cerebellum. Another form of central vestibular nystagmus is upbeat nystagmus. The lesion can be in the anterior vermis of the cerebellum and other locations. Excitatory connections from the anterior semicircular canals to the brachium conjunctivum may be disturbed. Side-beat nystagmus originates close to the vestibular nuclei in the medulla.

Gaze-evoked nystagmus is brought on by the eye assuming an eccentric position in the orbit. The eyes drift off the target and make a saccade back on. Gaze-evoked nystagmus along with impaired smooth pursuit (see later discussion) is often caused by cerebellar diseases. In an internuclear ophthalmoplegia, there is horizontal gaze-evoked nystagmus in the abducting eye. Drugs and fatigue also cause gaze-evoked nystagmus. In these cases, the nystagmus is horizontal in lateral gaze and vertical in vertical gaze.

Congenital nystagmus is irregular, conjugate, and horizontal, even in upgaze. It is accentuated by fixation and anxiety and diminished by convergence. It has a null point, a direction of gaze in which its amplitude is minimized. It may be pendular or jerky in type. The cause is unknown. Latent nystagmus appears when one eye is covered. It is seen in both eyes. Manifest latent nystagmus is present with both eyes seeing and accentuated when one eye is covered. It is associated with upward deviation of the covered eye and with strabismus. As with latent nystagmus, the cause is unknown.

Pendular nystagmus may be acquired. It may be horizontal, vertical, or a combination and is either conjugate or disconjugate. It is associated with upbeat nystagmus and can be seen with palatal myoclonus. The disease is in the dentatorubro-olivary connections.

Seesaw nystagmus is alternating elevation and intorsion of one eye with depression and extorsion of the other. The lesion is in the midbrain.

Convergence-retraction nystagmus consists of quick eye movements that converge or retract the eye. It probably actually consists of opposing saccades and is not a true nystagmus. It indicates dorsal mesencephalic disease.

Periodic alternating nystagmus beats in one direction, stops, and then beats in the other. It has a 4-minute (approximately) cycle. Lesions in the vestibular commissure and pathways to the caudal brain stem and cerebellum cause it.

Saccades

Saccades are rapid eye movements. They are seen in foveate animals and redirect the eyes after a following movement. An invariant relationship obtains between the peak velocity and the size of the movement, larger saccades being faster. Because of elevated threshold for light detection and visual masking, one does not see during saccades. A burst of phasic activity drives the eyes to the new position, and a tonic level of innervation keeps them there. The pause cells, which normally inhibit the burst cells, are turned off; the burst cells supply a phasic burst, and the tonic cells keep the eyes on target.

Saccades are tested by asking the patient to look first at one target and then at another. The eyes should be quite accurate, although they sometimes undershoot or overshoot slightly and a corrective saccade is required. Significant overshooting indicates dysmetria, a sign of cerebellar system disease. In myasthenia gravis, saccades may appear to be too fast. These are large, fast saccades that stopped in flight because of fatigue. Slow saccades are caused by drugs, central nervous system disorders, and fatigue. Patients with ocular motor apraxia cannot initiate saccades. In Parkinson's disease, saccades are hypometric and akinetic. Saccades may be inappropriate, as in square-wave jerks and ocular flutter and opsoclonus, discussed above. Saccades can also be evaluated with the optokinetic nystagmus drum. This is a cylinder with vertical stripes that is rotated along horizontal and then vertical axes in front of the patient. The eyes normally make a following movement, and a corrective saccade ensues.

Smooth pursuit

Smooth pursuit allows vision to remain clear during movements of the head and eyes. The stimulus is an object at the edge of the fovea—a proprioceptive stimulus, such as the person's own finger or the imagination. The cerebellum and both cerebral hemispheres are important in its physiology. It is tested by asking the patient to follow a slowly moving target. At slow speeds, pursuit should be smooth, the eyes keeping up with the target. Pursuit has too low a gain and the eyes lag behind in instances of weakness, medication, age, or cerebellar disease. Too high a gain causes the eye to go ahead of the target and produces ocular instability and pendular oscillations. A diseased hemisphere causes an imbalance in pursuit tone and a deviation of the eyes.

Vergence

Vergence movements are slow movements bringing both eyes onto a near target. They are stimulated by disparity in the locations at which the images fall on the retina and by blur. Blur induces the near triad of vergence movement, change in the shape of the lens to a more spherical form, and pupillary constriction. Vergence movements are tested by bringing an interesting target from far to near. In patients with poor vision, vergence movements can be stimulated by proprioception. The patient's finger is brought from far to near, and the patient is told to imagine that he or she is looking at it. Abnormalities in accommodative convergence synkinesis cause strabismus. Convergence may be insufficient. Convergence abnormalities may also be acquired. These are often associated with abnormalities of vertical gaze and are seen in Parkinson's disease and progressive supranuclear palsy. With pineal tumors, there can appear to be too much convergence. Actually, the patients are unable to converge at all and are making adducting saccades.

The physiology of convergence movements has not been worked out. Important areas are the midbrain, the third nerve nuclei, the cerebellum, and the hemispheres.

Chapter 7

Motor Function. Part I: Central Integration

The various signs of neurologic normality or abnormality are basically the examining physician's interpretations of the muscular activity of the patient, be it facial expression, gait, dressing or undressing, verbal responses, or performance of the formal part of the examination. Reflex responses and acknowledgment of sensory stimuli are further examples of the physician's dependence on muscular activity in assessing neural function. Even the mental status examination depends ultimately on the interpretation of muscular activity of the patient.

Motor dysfunction may result from involvement of muscle, neuromuscular junction, peripheral nerve, or central nervous system. Although damage to almost any portion of the central nervous system may result in a disturbance of muscular performance, certain portions of the nervous system are concerned primarily with muscular activity; these are the pyramidal and extrapyramidal systems and the lower motor neurons in the brain stem and the spinal cord. The cerebellum also is included among the components of the central nervous system involved with motor function.

The terms "pyramidal" and "extrapyramidal" are used to denote major descending neural systems concerned primarily with motor activation through their total effect on the lower motor neurons. The output of these two systems is influenced by all other neural activity.

The *pyramidal* system can be defined as consisting of neurons whose fibers are contained within the medullary pyramids. It is the only nonrelay corticospinal pathway. Actually, the minority of its fibers arise from neurons in the rolandic cortex (area 4) and only 3% to 4% are of Betz cell origin. Most of its fibers originate from adjacent frontal (area 6) and parietal (areas 1, 2, 3, 5, and 7) cortices. The total effect of most fibers is facilitory, but some are inhibitory. They descend through the internal capsule, basis pedunculi, and medullary pyramids, and the majority decussate in the caudal portion of the medulla to become the lateral corticospinal tracts of the spinal cord. Unilateral "pure" lesions of the medullary pyramid result in flaccidity rather than spasticity, with a Babinski sign, absent abdominal reflexes, impairment of manual dexterity, and less prominent and less persistent weakness of the leg. However, because the "pyramidal" tract at the level of the pyramids is not usually affected in clinical isolation, the classic upper motor neuron constellation is weakness, spasticity, hyperreflexia, and a Babinski sign. These clinical findings represent damage to a combination of the direct motor pathway projecting from cerebral cortex and the multisynaptic modifying motor pathways traveling in association with it.

The *extrapyramidal system* in its broadest sense includes all other descending neural pathways acting on the lower motor neuron. Like the pyramidal system, it also contains fibers originating in cortical areas 4, 5, and 6, and, in addition, in area 8; but unlike the pyramidal system, it acts through one or more internuncial neurons in the basal ganglia, the nuclei of the brain stem (red nucleus, vestibular nuclei, reticular nuclei), and the cerebellum. Most of these components are inhibitory in total effect (a notable exception being the cerebellum), and the usual consequence of extrapyramidal dysfunction is now thought to be spasticity or rigidity.

The foregoing separation of motor systems is entirely arbitrary and is based on a peculiarity of descriptive anatomy: the medullary pyramid. A lesion duplicating pyramidal transection is difficult to achieve at higher or lower levels in the nervous system. Most lesions occurring naturally are likely to spare some pyramidal fibers and to involve associated extrapyramidal fibers. The spasticity associated with most lesions affecting the pyramidal system but missing in "pure" pyramidal lesions can be explained by damage to inhibitory fibers in association with the pyramidal tract. The selective changes in flexor and extensor strength can also be explained on this basis. In an upper motor neuron lesion, the "antigravity" muscles are more likely to be spared. The upper motor neuron innervation in humans is distributed in such a way that the extensors of the lower limbs and the flexors of the upper limbs are relatively spared and exhibit greater resting tone.

The *gamma loop* is an important functional concept in the maintenance of muscle tone. Skeletal muscles contain fusiform structures (muscle spindles) consisting of several specialized muscle fibers of two types, that is, the nuclear bag and the nuclear chain fibers, each supplied by afferent and efferent nerve endings (Fig. 7-1). The nuclear bag fibers have striated contractile elements at each pole and a passive, encapsulated clear structure—the nuclear bag—at the center. An annulospiral nerve ending winds around the nuclear bag and is sensitive to its elongation. The poles of these fibers are supplied by small motor fibers—the gamma efferents.

The muscle stretch reflex is a monosynaptic arc with annulospiral fibers having excitatory synapses on alpha motor neurons, which

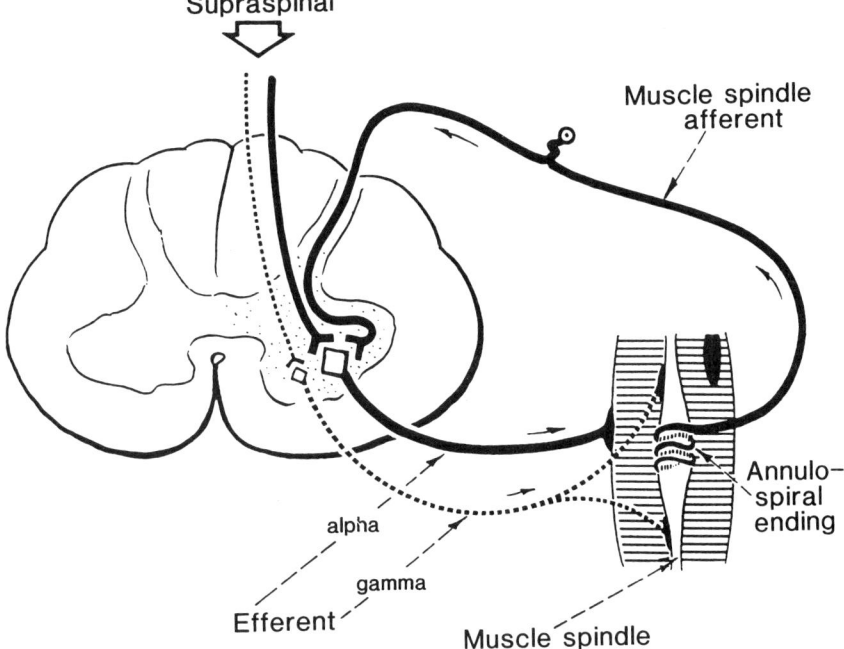

Figure 7-1
An intrafusal nuclear bag muscle fiber with its spindle afferent and gamma efferent nerves is graphically illustrated and labeled *muscle spindle*. It is surrounded by an extrafusal muscle fiber with its alpha efferent nerve. Descending or supraspinal pathways that influence gamma and efferent neurons may have either an excitatory or an inhibitory effect. *(From Thomas JE: Muscle tone, spasticity, rigidity. J Nerv Ment Dis 132:505–514, 1961. By permission of Williams & Wilkins.)*

innervate *extrafusal* muscle fibers of the parent muscle. Their contraction results in passive shortening of the spindles and the nuclear bags and decreases the firing of the annulospiral fibers.

Gamma efferent firing causes contraction of *intrafusal* fibers and passive lengthening of the nuclear bags, increasing their sensitivity to further stretching (hyperreflexia). The converse is also true. The level of activity of this system is set by descending (supraspinal) facilitory and inhibitory influences of both tonic and phasic character. The suprasegmental influences on tone are now thought to be most influential at the presynaptic output of the IA afferents. Many disorders of central nervous system motor function (spasticity, rigidity, ataxia, tremor) created by different lesions can now be understood in terms of imbalances in this system.

Stretch receptors of higher threshold are found in the muscle tendons (Golgi), which, through a polysynaptic arc, inhibit the alpha motor neurons of the parent muscle and facilitate its antagonists.

MUSCLE TONE

All movement, whether reflex or voluntary, normal or abnormal, is the result of total neural activity derived from many sources, acting upon primary motor neurons (the final common pathway) and, in turn, being further influenced by the physiologic status of the peripheral nerve, neuromuscular junction, and muscle fiber. Muscle tone is one of the recognizable end-results of this complex of multiple sources of neural energy.

Electromyography has enabled the physiologist to learn much about the nature of neuromuscular contraction and is providing the clinician with useful information on the nature and differentiation of neuromuscular disorders. Needle electrodes placed within muscle tissue detect action potentials whenever neighboring fibers contract. We now know that complete relaxation does exist when the skeleton is fully supported and there is no need for the maintenance of posture. As a rule, however, postural reflexes involving some muscle groups are constantly active and bring about various degrees of contraction of the antigravity muscles. *Long latency stretch reflexes* are the basis for reflex postural positioning and enable the body to remain in the upright position without conscious effort. These stretch reflexes, especially when elicited by postural changes, are modified by impulses reaching anterior horn cells from the vestibular system, visual centers, and proprioceptive receptors in the neck. Changes in posture are most modified by the extrapyramidal system. These "righting reflexes" thus modify the stretch reflexes and result in a degree of chronic contraction of certain muscles, compensating for the effects of gravity. Thus, the tone of any group of muscles depends on its location, the position of the person, and the ability to relax muscles voluntarily. The determination of tone is a matter of personal experience and is difficult to evaluate quantitatively.

Symptoms and Signs of Disturbances of Muscle Tone

Variations from normal muscle tone result in increased tone (hypertonicity) or decreased tone (hypotonicity) and may be subclassified as follows.

Spasticity

Spasticity is the result of loss of suprasegmental influence on the tonic contraction of muscle. It usually involves opposing muscle groups to differing degrees, so that the limb tends to assume a posture resulting from this imbalance and to retain this posture when passively displaced. With upper motor neuron lesions in humans, the flexors of the upper extremity and the extensors of the lower extremity exhibit this increase in tone. With rapid passive displacement, resistance of the muscle increases and then relaxes (clasp-knife phenomenon), the muscle relaxation being the result of inhibitory impulses from the tendon receptors of Golgi. Thus, in spasticity, resistance varies with both the speed and the direction (that is, flexors versus extensors) of passive motion. When severe, it may lead to permanent contractures.

Rigidity

Rigidity is a form of increased muscle tonus in which steady contraction of flexors and extensors leads to increased resistance to passive movement, which, as a rule, varies to a lesser extent with the speed in either direction of the movement. In rigidity, the tendon reflexes are normal, and the condition is not accompanied by abnormal plantar responses unless there is concomitant involvement of the pyramidal system. In parkinsonism, the rigidity is often termed *cogwheel*, because when the extremity is passively moved, rhythmic interruptions in the resistance are detected.

Hypotonicity

Hypotonicity is a loss of normal tone in which the muscle feels soft and flabby and offers less than normal resistance to passive movement. It is usually the result of damage to the proprioceptive or motor innervation of the muscle. A less marked hypotonicity may be seen with lesions affecting regions with a facilitory influence on the gamma efferent system, such as the cerebellum. Muscular disuse also may result in hypotonia.

Patients seldom complain directly of increased or decreased tone but generally refer to the associated disorder of motility. In rigidity and spasticity, spontaneous complaints usually refer to the dragging of a foot or to slowness of movement. Occasionally, a patient speaks of stiffness, heaviness, weakness, or even "numbness" when referring to increased tone in an extremity. Either rigidity or spasticity may lead to pain, especially in the axial and girdle muscles.

Examination of Muscle Tone

In hypertonia, particularly spasticity, the extremities at rest tend to assume a fixed posture. This posture may be one of overextension or, more often, of increased flexion. The muscle bellies tend to stand out more prominently. Palpation demonstrates increased firmness and increased resistance to lateral displacement of the affected muscles. In hypotonia, the extremities tend to assume a position dictated by gravity.

Associated arm movements in walking may be diminished in both hypotonia and hypertonia. The normal slight degree of forearm flexion is aggravated in both spasticity and rigidity, whereas it is usually lost in hypotonia.

Resistance to passive movement

Adequate evaluation of muscle tone requires that the patient be as relaxed as possible. Instructions include allowing the extremities to "go loose, relax as if asleep" or "go floppy like a dishrag" so that the physician can move them freely. If this fails, the patient may respond to such suggestions as "Let me do the work. Don't try to help." Diverting the patient's attention may be useful. The examiner then moves each extremity through its range at each joint. Normally, a mild, even resistance to movement is noted through the entire range. Hypertonicity may be mild or so extreme that passive movement is prevented. Mild degrees of rigidity of the wrist may be enhanced as the patient performs repetitive movements with the opposite hand. Hypotonia is recognized by increased ease of passive movements, and when the extremity is "shaken," flailing of the distal portion takes place. In severe hypotonia, the joints may be passively hyperextended.

The tone of the neck muscles may be tested by passively moving the head or by the head-dropping test. In the latter, the patient lies relaxed in a supine position. The examiner lifts the patient's head off the examining table with one hand and allows it to drop unexpectedly, catching the head with the other hand. Normally, the head drops heavily, almost like a dead weight, whereas with rigidity the head drops slowly.

Pendulousness

When an extremity is displaced passively so that it swings freely, there is a regular precise pendular motion that diminishes in a steady, even manner. This pendulousness may be increased or decreased in range and duration, and in addition it may be irregular instead of in a straight line. It is important to observe the number of oscillations, the regularity of the diminution of the swinging, the pattern described by the movement, and the comparison of the two sides. Pendulousness is largely a function of muscle tone, and again the patient should be encouraged to relax.

Upper extremities are tested by moving the standing patient's shoulders back and forth through an arc with the trunk as a pivot point. One shoulder is pulled forward as the other is pushed backward and vice versa. The resultant to-and-fro swinging of the upper extremities is observed by the examiner. A different test for the same purpose can be performed with the patient standing. The examiner places his or her hands on the patient's hips and briskly flips the patient's upper extremities away from the body. The speed, range, regularity, and pattern of movement may be seen, heard, and felt by the examiner as the arms swing away from the body and return.

The lower extremities are examined with the patient sitting on the edge of a table with the legs hanging freely over the edge. The examiner lifts the legs (extending them at the knees) and allows them to drop, observing the duration, regularity, and pattern of swinging. Pendulousness of the legs also may be observed if the examiner briskly flips the patient's legs forward or backward to start free-swinging.

With hypotonia, the pendulousness is increased, the swinging being freer; the pattern described is irregularly zigzag. With rigidity of extrapyramidal origin, the duration of swinging is greatly reduced and the pattern is regular. In spasticity, the duration is normal or slightly diminished. However, the forward swing is jerky, irregular, and brisk, whereas the backward swing is slower and of diminished range. The pattern is irregular and not in a straight line.

In the supine position, the knee and hip can be quickly passively flexed without the patient's awareness. The heel in normal tone remains in contact or is only slightly raised off the surface of the examining table. In hypertonicity, however, the heel becomes prominently elevated off the examining surface.

Postural fixation

The normal extremity maintains a desired posture for a reasonable time without the need for voluntary correcting movements. This postural fixation is impaired with disorders of muscle tone as well as with weakness, loss of joint position sense, and vestibular dysfunction. It is examined by means of deviation tests. The patient extends the arms horizontally in front of the body with the fingers spread, the wrists extended, and the eyes closed. The hypotonic or weak arm tends to drop. If the outstretched arms are tapped sharply by the examiner, the hypotonic arm may oscillate several times before returning to the original position. The *rebound phenomenon* is of complex origin but is due in part to hypotonia and in part to a loss of synergistic control by the opposing muscle groups; the normal outstretched arm returns promptly without oscillation when depressed slightly, whereas the affected arm overshoots its original position and may oscillate several times before stopping. This abnormality is most commonly seen in disorders of the cerebellar control circuits. With vestibular dysfunction, there may be slow rotation to one side of the upper part of the trunk and horizontal displacement of the outstretched fingers. The test also brings out a variety of movement disorders, including chorea, athetosis, pseudoathetosis, myoclonus, asterixis, and tremors (see the section on involuntary movements).

COORDINATION

The cerebellum receives information about limb position and the degree of muscle contraction from proprioceptive endings in muscle spindles, tendons, and joints via the spinocerebellar pathways and the inferior and superior cerebellar peduncles. Vestibular as well as touch, visual, and auditory information also reaches the cerebellum. Furthermore, the cerebellum receives impulses, via the brachium pontis, that are concerned with voluntary activity and that originate in the cerebral cortex. Cerebellar efferents return to the cortex via connections in the brain stem nuclei (rubral, vestibular, olivary, and reticular) and the thalamus. Other cerebellar efferents reach the spinal cord via connections in the same brain stem nuclei. Through these circuits, the cerebellum coordinates posture, equilibrium, and voluntary movement. Its control of voluntary movement at the spinal level is chiefly through phasic facilitory influences. The basal portion of the cerebellum is concerned with the maintenance of equilibrium, the anterior portion with the coordination of postural activities and gait, and the lateral portions with the coordination of ipsilateral skilled voluntary movements.

Disturbances of movement simulating cerebellar incoordination may be caused by lesions of muscles, of peripheral nerves, of posterior columns, and of the frontal and postcentral cerebral cortex. Paralysis of an extremity prevents carrying out tests for coordination.

Testing of Coordination

In the course of taking the history and before formal testing, the examiner should observe the patient during normal activity, such as undressing, picking up objects, and buttoning clothing. Incoordination consists of errors in rate, range, direction, and force. The movement may start slowly; the range of motion and the force applied may be excessive. Different components of the movement are called into play at the wrong time. Attempts to compensate result in sudden corrective movements, thus giving an irregular, jerky pattern often overreaching the mark.

Nose-finger-nose test

The examiner illustrates while instructing the patient in this test. The patient touches the tip of the index finger alternately to his or her nose and to the tip of the examiner's finger, repeating the sequence several times. The examiner moves his or her own finger about during the test. The two sides are tested separately. The patient should have to extend the arm fully in this test, since terminal tremors may appear only with maximal extension.

Knee pat (pronation-supination) test

In the sitting position, the patient is instructed to pat the knee alternately with the palm and dorsum of one hand and then with the other, slowly and gradually increasing the rate of patting to a maximum. Abnormalities in rate, rhythm, and precision may be observed. The test is particularly useful in detecting cerebellar dysfunction, in which the rate is slow and irregularities in rhythm and amplitude are prominent. An abnormality of rhythm or amplitude is recorded in the space designated for this test, and observations concerning the rate are recorded on the chart under "alternate motion rate."

This test cannot be carried out easily with the patient in the supine position. However, the same information can be obtained by having the supine patient extend the arms without supporting the elbows on the bed and pat the palm of one hand alternately with the palm and dorsum of the other.

Toe-finger test
The patient, while supine, touches the examiner's finger with the great toe and holds it there until the examiner moves the finger to a new position. After the patient has done so, the examiner quickly moves the finger to another position, a foot or two away, the patient pursuing the examiner's finger with the toe. The test usually begins with the examiner holding the finger several feet above the patient's hip. It is well to inform the patient to bend the knee in the performance of the test.

Finger-nose test
The test is started from a position of full extension at the elbow with the upper part of the arm in the horizontal plane. It is performed initially with the eyes open and then with the eyes closed. The patient is instructed to touch the index finger to the nose and return to the starting position, repeating the sequence at varying rates. The examiner may stop the test at any time and place the patient's upper arm in another horizontal starting position.

The test is easily performed in a supine position, but it is important that the patient not be allowed to support the elbow on the bed.

Heel-knee test
This test is best performed in the supine position. The patient lifts the lower extremity being tested and places the heel on the opposite knee while keeping the ankle dorsiflexed. After touching the knee, the patient slides the heel downward over the shin and dorsum of the foot toward the great toe. The patient should be encouraged to do this in one smooth motion and not too slowly. Some examiners ask the patient to slide the heel back up the shin, giving them an opportunity for longer observation.

ALTERNATE MOTION RATE

Although a decrease in the speed with which the fingers can be wiggled or the foot patted can result from many causes, experience has shown this test to be of particular value to the neurologist. Often the history, although inconclusive, suggests that an organic disease of the central nervous system may be present. At times in such cases, the most careful examination fails to disclose any abnormality in motor function or tone, coordination, or sensation; and the finding of a persistent decrease in alternate motion rate, for instance, the speed of finger wiggle in one hand, is the only observation of significance.

In these tests, one also observes the amplitude, rhythm, and precision of movement, and if abnormalities are noted, they must be recorded. A perceptible decrease in alternate motion rate may be evident in diseases giving rise to spasticity and rigidity before one can detect an abnormality in tone by passive movement, posture, or pendulousness. The decrease in alternate motion rate and the irregularity of its rhythm, precision, and amplitude may be manifestations of cerebellar disease, in which instance it is designated *dysdiadochokinesia*. Furthermore, alternate motion rate may be slowed by local conditions, such as arthritis of the fingers, and by a variety of disorders, organic and functional, affecting the higher integrative functions of the brain. Its greatest value, however, lies in the fact that in parkinsonism and other so-called extrapyramidal disorders as well as in pyramidal disorders, it may be one of the earliest manifestations. Often, however, the *amplitude* rather than the rate is reduced in parkinsonism, particularly when the test is prolonged for more than a few seconds.

Tongue Wiggle

The patient is asked to wiggle the tongue rapidly from side to side, and the examiner illustrates the test. Occasionally a patient has difficulty in this unpracticed maneuver and yet can rapidly protrude and retract the tongue. Either or both methods may be used at the discretion of the examiner. The commonest causes for a decrease in tongue wiggle other than local weakness, such as that associated with myasthenia gravis or bulbar palsy, are the rigidity of parkinsonism and the spasticity resulting from bilateral corticobulbar deficit in pseudobulbar palsy.

Finger Wiggle

The patient is asked to wiggle the fingers up and down, as if playing a piano or using a typewriter, while the examiner demonstrates the test. It is advisable to have the test performed while the upper extremity is held loosely and incompletely outstretched. It is preferable to test each hand separately. At the time of this test, it is well to ask about the handedness of the patient, since a failure to wiggle the fingers of the nondominant hand as rapidly as those of the dominant hand is of less significance. A refinement of the test is to have the patient tap the interphalangeal joint of the thumb with the tip of the index finger of the same hand. The number of taps in 10 seconds may be counted and recorded.

Foot Pat
While sitting with feet resting comfortably and flat on the floor, the patient is instructed to pat the floor as rapidly as possible with the ball of the foot while keeping the heel in place. Depending on leg length, the patient may have to move forward on the couch or chair for proper placement of the feet. The test can be quantitated by counting the pats in 10 seconds. In the supine position, the test is carried out by having the patient pat the foot against the palm of the examiner.

ABNORMAL INVOLUNTARY MOVEMENTS

Abnormal involuntary movements (hyperkinesias) often challenge not only the novice physician but also the seasoned clinician. The unusual appearance of certain dyskinetic movements may make classification difficult and even raise a question of a psychogenic basis. Skill in recognizing and classifying abnormal involuntary movements is one of pattern recognition and requires experience in the clinic. As one develops this expertise, however, certain definitions and guidelines help in the proper diagnosis of dyskinetic movements.

Before defining the different types of abnormal involuntary movements, one must decide what differentiates normal from abnormal. A broad spectrum of human motor behavior is considered "normal." This includes movements or activities that are essentially involuntary, such as blinking or arm swinging while walking. In addition, most or all persons display mannerisms, especially when engrossed in a sedentary activity or when anxious, such as rubbing an earlobe while reading, foot tapping when nervous, or nail-biting. On the other hand, movements defined as "abnormal" meet the following criteria:

1. A general consensus that the movements, or the degree of the movements, are outside the limits of normal human motor behavior.
2. Interference of the movements with goal-directed motor tasks or with social relationships.
3. An inability to completely inhibit the movements when necessary and appropriate.

Abnormal movements can be subdivided into two categories: (1) those occurring as a response to an uncontrollable urge or sensation, and (2) those initiated completely outside conscious awareness. Various inappropriate motor behaviors are also seen in major psychiatric disorders (for example, schizophrenia and obsessive-compulsive disorders); abnormal motor behavior due to major psychiatric disease is not considered further in this discussion.

Abnormal Movements Provoked by an Uncontrollable Urge
Tics

Tics are simple or complex stereotyped motor behaviors that occur in response to an irresistible urge. They are typically under partial voluntary control, and the individual may be able to voluntarily suppress the movement for a short time. Voluntary suppression, however, escalates the urge, often resulting in an explosion of movement. Tics can be "simple," such as eye blinking, shoulder shrugs, grimacing, grunting, and sniffing. On the other hand, tics may be quite complex, such as vocalizations (echolalia, coprolalia), jumping, kicking, squatting, or compulsive touching. If the patient displays only a simple tic, it may be quite difficult to be certain whether it is a manifestation of some other movement disorder or truly a tic. Simple involuntary movements can sometimes be identified as a tic based on the company they keep; that is, they may be associated with complex tics, which are easily distinguishable from true chorea or dystonia. With more severe disease, the ability to suppress the tic may be quite difficult or impossible. By definition, a chronic tic disorder starting in youth that includes vocalizations may be classified as Gilles de la Tourette's syndrome. Transient and nondisabling tics are not infrequent during adolescence and hence are not necessarily a cause for alarm (or treatment).

Chronic tic disorders are thought to have an organic basis and not to simply reflect psychologic factors. Supporting evidence is as follows:

1. Tics may be displayed during sleep.
2. Familial occurrence suggests autosomal dominant inheritance with variable penetrance.
3. Cortical premovement electrical potentials are absent. They can be recorded just before a *voluntary movement* but are not found in association with spontaneous tics. However, if the patient is asked to voluntarily imitate the tic, the premovement potential is seen.

Akathisia

The term "akathisia" implies a subjective feeling, defined as a sense of inner restlessness, that may be associated with adventitious movements. The sensation of inner restlessness tends to elicit movements that help relieve the inner tension. These movements in response to akathisia are most commonly seen in "tardive" syndromes associated with the prolonged use of a dopamine antagonist drug. Drugs of this type, including neuroleptic medications used to treat psychosis, as well as metoclopramide or other antiemetics, may also induce a variety of other "tardive" syndromes, which are further discussed below. Akathisia is also frequently experienced by patients with Parkinson's disease, although they typically do not move in response to the akathisia.

Restless legs syndrome

Patients with this condition complain of an inability to get comfortable when sedentary. They feel as if they have to move and especially to move their lower extremities. This is particularly a problem at night when these persons cannot get comfortable in bed. They may repetitively rise from bed and pace the floor. They may also display stereotyped movements as a response to this sensation. Typically, this condition is not confused with other movement disorders, since patients focus on the uncomfortable sensation in their lower extremities, and it is easy to identify this as the cause of the movements.

Individuals with restless legs syndrome also frequently display "periodic movements of sleep," which are elicited outside conscious awareness. Often, these periodic movements of sleep are characterized by dorsiflexion of the foot, associated with knee and hip flexion, recurring at definite intervals (for example, every 20 to 40 seconds). In some, these may intrude into wakefulness.

Abnormal Movements Initiated Outside Conscious Awareness
Tremor

Tremor, the most common type of involuntary movement, is defined as a rhythmic (periodic) movement of a body part. The fixed recurring interval between movements differentiates tremor from certain other repetitive movements, such as repetitive (phasic) dystonia. Tremor of a limb is typically subdivided into four categories: rest, postural, action, and terminal.

Rest tremor occurs when the limb is in a position of repose. It may be seen in the hands when in the lap or during walking with the arms at the sides.

A *postural tremor* can be observed when a limb is maintained against gravity. Upper limb postural tremor should be assessed both with the arms extended in front of the body and with the elbows flexed and the hands held in front of the face. This elbow-flexed position often brings out the most severe forms of postural tremors.

An *action tremor* occurs with movement. In the upper limbs, it can be assessed during finger-nose maneuvers.

Terminal tremor is the component of tremor seen as the moving limb nears the target. The term "intention tremor" has been used interchangeably with "terminal tremor" but is misleading, and we prefer not to use it.

The most common clinical conditions characterized by prominent tremor are described below.

Physiologic tremor occurs as a transient state in normal persons who are under emotional stress or extremely fatigued or is induced by sympathomimetic medications.

Toxic tremor occurs in toxic-metabolic derangements, sometimes in conjunction with encephalopathy. Disorders such as uremia, thyrotoxicosis, and alcohol or drug withdrawal may be precipitants.

Parkinsonian tremor occurs with other manifestations of parkinsonism and is characterized by tremor when the limb or other body part is at rest. The tremor may persist with sustained posture but usually attenuates with action. It may involve the jaw but spares the head and voice.

Essential tremor, by definition, is unassociated with any other neurologic abnormalities, such as cerebellar or extrapyramidal signs. It involves the limbs, head, and voice in various combinations. This tremor is typically absent in the resting position but develops with sustained postures and action. The hand tremor often becomes exacerbated with action as the target is approached (terminal tremor). An essential voice tremor may be apparent during normal conversation or may be appreciated only when the patient is asked to hold a musical note ("ahhh. . ."). A family history is prominent in approximately half the cases.

The severe tremor that occurs with lesions of the superior cerebellar peduncle (cerebellar dentatorubrothalamic pathway) goes by a variety of names that either connote the presumed anatomic substrate *(cerebellar outflow tremor, rubral tremor)* or emphasize the severity *(wing-beating tremor, severe postural tremor)*. The term "wing-beating" refers to the appearance when the arms are held in front of the trunk with the elbows flexed, reminiscent of a bird flapping its wings. The term "rubral tremor" refers to the red nucleus, previously thought to be the anatomic source of this type of tremor. This tremor is typical of that seen in multiple sclerosis or Wilson's disease. It also occurs in the aftermath of certain brain injuries. It is characterized by a wide tremor amplitude that is prominent with sustained postures or action. The tremor involves proximal portions of limbs, accounting for the wide tremor excursions. If present at rest, it is usually less pronounced. It is often so disabling that patients have difficulty feeding themselves. Although most obvious in the upper limbs in most patients, the tremor also frequently involves the trunk and head and sometimes involves the lower limbs. This type of tremor is seen in association with other neurologic deficits and typically other cerebellar signs.

Orthostatic tremor ("shaky legs syndrome") is a unique but less common tremor disorder. In this condition, tremor is typically absent in the sitting and supine positions, but a lower limb and truncal tremor develops when the person stands. The tremor may either persist or attenuate with walking. In some persons, the tremor may be difficult to see because of the characteristic very high frequency (for example, 16 to 18 Hz); in such patients, postural unsteadiness may be the primary manifestation. The tremulousness can usually be easily appreciated, however, by manual palpation of the thigh while the patient is standing.

Dystonia

Dystonia is characterized by an abnormal posture of one or more parts of the body and involves co-contraction of agonist and antagonist muscles. Although torsion is often present, the dystonic movement can also involve flexion-extension or lateral deviation. The sustained, *tonic* deviation of a body part is usually easy to identify as dystonic. However, dystonic movements may also be *phasic,* occasionally making proper identification more difficult. These phasic movements can be rapid and repetitive; however, they can be differentiated from other movement disorders by several features, including a tendency to be sustained at peak, stereotyped characteristics, and association with more characteristic tonic dystonic movements.

Repetitive phasic dystonic movements can be differentiated from true tremor by a varying interval between the phasic movements (see below). On the other hand, tremor frequently coexists with dystonia.

Dystonia may involve only one isolated segment of the body (focal), contiguous regions (segmental), or major portions of the body (generalized). An example of focal dystonia is spasmodic torticollis (cervical dystonia), with the neck involuntarily rotated or bent to one side. Segmental dystonia could be a combination of spasmodic torticollis with dystonic jaw opening. Primary focal and segmental dystonias are typical of those that begin later in life, well into adulthood. Dystonias that begin in childhood often become generalized and are more likely to be familial.

Dystonia is frequently associated with other forms of adventitious movements. For example, tremor is a frequent accompaniment and in this context is called "dystonic tremor." Dystonia in combination with lightning-like jerks may be referred to as "myoclonic dystonia." Dystonia and chorea frequently occur together and are then termed "choreodystonia" or "choreoathetosis." The term "athetosis" implies slow, writhing dystonic posturing of the distal limbs, especially fingers, hand, and wrist. Myoclonus and chorea are discussed below.

Certain involuntary movements under a variety of names are, in fact, forms of dystonia. Included are blepharospasm (involuntary eye closure), oculogyric crises induced by dopamine antagonist medications, and numerous focal dystonias provoked during specific tasks, such as "writer's cramp" and "musician's cramp" syndromes. The "cramping" of Parkinson's disease is also a type of dystonia. Although the term "cramp" is used to denote some of these syndromes, it is somewhat of a misnomer; as discussed below, true cramps reflect peripheral neuromuscular disorders.

Many types of dystonia are due to pathologic conditions within the basal ganglia, but origins in other cerebral regions have also been documented.

Chorea

Chorea, an involuntary rapid and flowing movement of one or more body parts that is not stereotyped, is manifested as a *random* event. Constantly changing movements may be observed in different parts of the body at irregular intervals. These choreiform movements may be subtle, such as unnecessary arching of an eyebrow or twitching of a corner of the mouth. The person may appear very restless but deny feeling that way. At times, the movements may seem to be modified by the patient to give an appearance of voluntary activity, as if the individual were "covering up" to avoid embarrassment. The randomness and lack of stereotypy distinguish chorea from most other abnormal involuntary movements. Patients with chorea typically cannot keep the involved body part in one position for very long (motor impersistence); this may be shown by an inability to sustain a firm grip on the examiner's fingers ("milkmaid's grip") or to maintain tongue protrusion for more than a few seconds ("tongue darting").

Chorea may be elicited by medications; for example, levodopa therapy can provoke "dyskinesias" in patients with Parkinson's disease. It may also be inherited, as in families with Huntington's disease, or acquired, as in autoimmune disorders (for example, Sydenham's chorea linked to rheumatic fever). The pathologic source is in the basal ganglia.

Ballismus

Ballismus may be considered a subtype of chorea. It is manifested by wild, flailing, sometimes violent movements. These movements are of greater amplitude and tend to involve more proximal muscles than simple choreiform movements. This disorder is typically associated with a lesion of the subthalamic nucleus. In most cases, the ballistic movements are confined to one side of the body, hence the term "hemiballismus."

Myoclonus

Myoclonus is characterized by an involuntary lightning-like jerk of an area of the body. The movements are simple and never complex; that is, a single myoclonic jerk is characterized by displacement of one or more body parts in one direction only. Myoclonus may be subtle, appearing as a sudden flick of the fingers, foot, or other limited area of the body. Myoclonus may also be violent, such as a large jerk of the trunk that causes the person to lurch to the side.

Myoclonus may be spontaneous, or it may be induced by visual, tactile, or auditory stimuli (stimulus-sensitive myoclonus). Myoclonus elicited by use of the involved limb is called "action myoclonus." It may occur as a single jerk or be repetitive.

Myoclonus differs from fasciculations because some part of the body is actually displaced by the former and only a limited segment of muscle is affected by the latter. Myoclonus is also distinguished by its origin within the central nervous system; fasciculations originate in the peripheral nervous system.

Unlike phasic dystonia, myoclonic jerks are not sustained at the peak of movement. Sometimes it is difficult to differentiate phasic dystonia from myoclonic dystonia, but special electrophysiologic studies may allow this distinction to be made.

Myoclonus can originate from any level of the central nervous system, including cortex, basal ganglia, brain stem, and spinal cord. In some cases, myoclonus occurs in conjunction with epilepsy (myoclonic epilepsy) and can be considered a fragment of a seizure. Myoclonus may be one sign of central nervous system electrophysiologic instability in patients with toxic-metabolic encephalopathy. Myoclonus also frequently occurs in the aftermath of cardiorespiratory arrest (postanoxic myoclonus).

In certain clinical situations, such as myoclonus of spinal cord origin, myoclonus may be repetitive with a periodic pattern. If truly periodic, it could be argued that such movements represent tremor rather than myoclonus.

Hiccup (singultus) is actually a form of myoclonus that is produced by a sudden contraction of the diaphragm in association with adduction of the vocal cords. Its cause ranges from lesions of the upper gastrointestinal tract, diaphragm, or mediastinum to disease within the brain stem. It may also develop in toxic-metabolic conditions such as uremia.

Palatal myoclonus is characterized by rhythmic contractions of the soft palate, sometimes in association with other components of the branchial musculature. Some argue that these contractions might be better termed "palatal tremor," since they have a regular frequency like true tremor and are not as lightning-like as typical myoclonus. The term "palatal myoclonus," however, is entrenched in the medical nomenclature.

Asterixis

First described in relation to hepatic failure, asterixis has an appearance similar to myoclonus. It can be seen in affected persons when they hold their arms in front of them with the wrists fully extended, like a policeman stopping traffic. Asterixis is characterized by an inability to maintain this position against gravity, with a resultant slow and irregular flapping of the wrists. These movements result from sudden relaxation of the muscles held against gravity, with intermittent pauses in the muscle tone. Thus, asterixis might be considered a form of "negative myoclonus." Although usually seen in the clinical context of toxic-metabolic encephalopathies, it can also be a manifestation of structural lesions of the cerebral hemispheres.

Tardive dyskinesias

Chronic use of drugs that block dopamine receptors can induce a variety of involuntary movements that may persist indefinitely, long after the offending medication has been stopped. Included are the neuroleptic agents used to treat psychosis as well as some antiemetic drugs. The term "tardive dyskinesias" is used in two ways. First, it connotes the typical orobuccolingual movements that are the hallmark of this class of disorders. Second, it is a general term encompassing all the various types of movements that can occur as "tardive" syndromes (that is, related to chronic use of dopamine antagonist drugs).

Classic tardive dyskinesia that is manifested as orobuccolingual movements is characterized by to-and-fro motions of the mouth and tongue that continue in a repetitive, stereotyped pattern. Typically, opening and closing mouth movements with pursing of the lips are intermixed with intermittent protrusion of the tongue. Sometimes, stereotyped rocking movements of the trunk, adventitious movements of the respiratory musculature, and other repetitive movements accompany the orobuccolingual dyskinesias. The repetitive, stereotyped nature of these movements differentiates them from chorea (although chorea may also occasionally occur as a tardive syndrome).

The other types of movement syndromes that can be seen in tardive disorders include dystonias, movements secondary to akathisia, and, rarely, tics, as well as chorea. Given the wide spectrum of adventitious movements that can be induced by dopamine antagonist drugs, a careful medication history is important in any evaluation of a new patient with a movement disorder.

Spasms

"Spasm" is a general descriptive term applied to a hypercontractile state of muscle associated with reduced mobility across an involved joint or joints. It can be applied to a variety of involuntary muscle contraction states of both central and peripheral origin. In its most elementary form, it occurs as an involuntary reaction to local painful conditions, such as an injury to the spinal vertebrae; spasm developing in this circumstance may contribute to the pain. The term "spasm" is also frequently applied to hypercontractile states originating in muscle, neuromuscular junction, nerve, or spinal reflex arc.

Cramps are painful spasms of muscle that may develop consequent to primary disorders of muscle (for example, metabolic myopathies, such as glycogen storage diseases), of neuromuscular junction (for example, anticholinesterase poisoning), or of motor neuron (for example, amyotrophic lateral sclerosis). They tend to be provoked by a strong voluntary contraction of an already shortened susceptible muscle and are relieved by stretching that muscle. In otherwise normal persons, they may be precipitated by electrolyte disturbances or muscular fatigue with depletion of muscle energy reserves.

Tetany refers to a state of neuromuscular hyperexcitability and repetitive motor neuron firing due to reduced concentrations of ionized extracellular calcium or to metabolic alkalosis. Characteristic of tetany in the upper extremities is carpopedal spasm, manifested by involuntary flexion of the wrists and metacarpophalangeal joints with approximation of the extended digits. Brisk contraction of the ipsilateral facial muscles in response to tapping over the facial nerve in the region of the parotid gland is also seen in tetany (Chvostek's sign).

Spasms may also be seen in disorders that block or attenuate the effects of the inhibitory neurotransmitters (γ-aminobutyric acid, glycine) that modulate spinal and brain stem reflex arc activity. They may occur in certain toxic reactions, such as strychnine poisoning and specific infectious processes (tetanus). In these cases, spasms of the jaw (trismus), face (risus sardonicus), and trunk (opisthotonus) may be striking. Spasms due to loss of spinal inhibitory neurotransmitter function may also occur in the autoimmune disorder *stiff-man syndrome*. In this condition, the truncal muscles and often the proximal lower extremity muscles are in a hypercontractile state sufficient to result in a rigid back with hyperlordosis.

Hemifacial spasm is characterized by paroxysms of rapid, irregular twitching of the facial musculature on one side. It results from an irritative lesion pressing on the facial nerve, most often a pulsating blood vessel. Associated with hemifacial spasm is the phenomenon of synkinesis on the ipsilateral side. Synkinesis can be seen when voluntary contraction of a muscle or a group of muscles elicits abnormal co-contraction of adjoining muscles. For example, in hemifacial spasm, synkinesis may be manifested by inappropriate hemicontraction of the perioral muscles when the eyes are voluntarily closed. Presumably, synkinesis results from regeneration within a damaged nerve, with misdirection of the newly sprouting nerve fibers.

GAIT AND STATION

Gait

Although the act of walking is largely automatic and is taken for granted as a relatively simple process, gait is a highly complex activity. When performed normally, walking requires the proper integration of a number of neural mechanisms involving all levels of the nervous system. Most of these same mechanisms are operative in the maintenance of posture and station. The peripheral nerves must obviously be intact to carry proprioceptive information to the spinal cord and higher centers and to transmit motor impulses to the muscles involved. The muscle stretch reflexes, as well as more complex postural reactions, are mediated by spinal cord centers. In animals, integrative mechanisms capable of producing simple alternating movements of the extremities reside within the spinal cord. Such spinally mediated stepping has not been demonstrated in primates. In humans, the spinal pathways concerned with gait are largely controlled and activated by descending impulses arising from the upper brain stem region and influenced by labyrinthine, visual, and proprioceptive inputs. Postural, righting, and more complex reflexes are further influenced by the cerebellum and basal ganglia as well as voluntary control. Thus, the accurate observation of gait enables the experienced examiner to learn a great deal about the functioning of the peripheral and central nervous systems.

As a rule, a patient's description of the difficulty experienced in walking rarely approaches the value of actually observing the impairment. Nevertheless, it is well to listen attentively to the patient's story about gait dysfunction. If the patient is examined at a time following recovery from the disturbance, the deductions of the examiner must be based on an understanding of the description. Although few patients display sufficient confidence in their dramatic abilities to imitate the past impairment, encouraging them to act out the derangement of gait they previously experienced may prove diagnostically helpful.

Valuable observations of gait may be made as the patient enters the examining room and during movements about the room, such as getting on and off the examining table and going to and from the dressing area. Such observations give rise to impressions that will be confirmed or discarded later by more formal testing of the gait. It is well to have the patient walk fully clothed as one of the initial steps in the neurologic examination. A hallway can be used for more room in which to maneuver. Watch intently as the patient walks. A person does not walk with the legs alone. The attitude of the trunk, arms, and even the face may be altered if the gait is abnormal. Witness the writhing body of torsion dystonia, the unswinging arms of Parkinson's disease, and the smiling indifference of hysteria. After disrobing, the patient should walk in the examining room, where deformities of the spinal column or extremities and their influence on gait may be observed. Watch for any unsteadiness as the patient turns, which can be evidence of a mild ataxia. In addition to walking in the usual manner, the patient may be asked to walk backward and sideways. This change in direction may exaggerate or suppress abnormalities noted in the course of ordinary walking. Ask the patient to walk on his or her heels and then toes. This maneuver not only tests the strength of the dorsiflexors of the foot and of the calf muscles, respectively, but also sometimes reveals an ataxia not otherwise apparent. Balancing and hopping on each foot separately may reveal muscular weakness or minimal ataxia or spasticity of one lower extremity. Elderly or infirm patients should usually omit this test, since a misstep might result in injury. Ataxia not apparent during the foregoing tests may be shown by having the patient walk tandem, that is, by placing the heel of the advancing foot directly in front of the toe of the weight-bearing foot, as though measuring the room. Finally, it is well to listen to the patient's gait. With practice, one can detect irregularities in the rhythm and force with which the feet are brought down or slight shuffling that might escape ordinary observation.

Normal gait
The patient with no gait disturbance walks with a sense of freedom because movements are almost automatic and the walker is practically unaware of making them. In doing so, the weight is alternately shifted from one extremity to the other, allowing the extremity freed of weight to be moved forward with certainty and ease. As this movement takes place, the pelvis is held more or less at a right angle to the weight-bearing extremity. At the same time, the opposite upper extremity moves forward; that is, the arm "swings." This movement is slight in the shoulder and increases distally. The posture of the trunk varies with each individual but, in general, is more or less erect. There is wide individual variation in gait. Some gaits are so distinctive that persons can be recognized at a distance or by the sound of their footsteps. Some gait characteristics tend to run in families. The history of a change in gait may be noteworthy even if the patient's walking is within the limits of normal on examination.

Hemiplegic gait
Most "upper motor neuron" lesions produce an increase in muscular tone and give rise to a "spastic" gait. When this is unilateral, as in a hemiparesis, the affected lower limb is moved forward with difficulty caused by the lack of freedom of movement in all the joints and the characteristic distribution of weakness. As a result, the toe of the affected extremity tends to be forced downward. This necessitates an abduction and a circumduction of the limb to move it forward. In doing so, the toe of the shoe is dragged and may be noticeably worn on the toe and outer aspect. The involved upper limb is held to the patient's side in a flexed posture, and normal arm swing is reduced or lost.

Spastic gait
When both lower extremities are spastic, the gait may be scissorlike, as in congenital spastic paraplegia. The lower extremities are moved forward in a stiff, jerky manner, often accompanied by extreme compensatory movements of the trunk and upper extremities.

Ataxic gait
An ataxic gait is characterized by clumsiness and uncertainty. It may result, for example, from loss of position sense in the lower extremities, such as that occurring in tabes dorsalis. The patient plants the feet too widely apart and in taking a step lifts the advancing leg abruptly and too high. The foot is then brought down solidly in a slapping or stamping

manner. The steps are not spaced evenly, and there is a tendency to sway or totter. An attempt is made to guide the uncertain steps by watching the floor. If asked to close the eyes while walking, the patient has increased difficulty and may fall.

The gait of a person with a disturbance of the vestibular apparatus may be "drunken" and reeling, usually with deviations to one side more than the other. If the condition is severe and accompanied by vertigo, the patient may have so little control of movements that walking becomes hazardous.

Cerebellar disease may produce a gait characterized by apparent looseness of the extremities. Movement of the advancing limb starts slowly; then with unexpected vigor it may be flung erratically forward or sideways. The patient may sense the error and attempt to correct it. Overcompensation follows and adds to the difficulties. Stopping the movement is equally uncoordinated, with the result that the patient stamps the foot to the floor, similar to a person with tabes.

The cause of an ataxic gait cannot regularly be discovered from observation of the gait alone. It is usually wiser to be content to recognize ataxia and to interpret its significance after other portions of the neurologic examination have been completed.

Mixed spastic ataxic gait

A combination of spasticity and ataxia in the lower extremities gives rise to a characteristic gait best described as "jiggling" or "bobbing." The ataxia can be of spinal or cerebellar type, and either the spasticity or the ataxia can predominate. In addition to the stiffness and uncertainty that are readily noted, the weight-bearing extremity displays dancing or bouncing movements of small amplitude that are rapidly repeated. This results in a quick, irregular, up-and-down movement of the whole body. This type of gait is seen most commonly in patients with multiple sclerosis.

Steppage gait

The patient who has a drop foot tends to lift the affected extremity higher than the normal one to avoid dragging or stubbing the toe. When drop foot is bilateral, the gait may resemble that of a high-stepping horse. Steppage gait usually occurs in conditions that affect the lower motor neurons serving the foot dorsiflexors, such as peripheral neuropathy, peroneal palsy, L-5 radiculopathy, motor neuron disease, and poliomyelitis.

Waddling gait

In muscular dystrophy, weakness of the trunk and pelvic girdle muscles results in a swaybacked and potbellied posture and a waddling gait. The waddle results from an inability to maintain the pelvis at a proper angle to the weight-bearing extremity, with a slump of the pelvis toward the non-weight-bearing side. This, in turn, produces an exaggerated compensatory sway of the trunk toward the weight-bearing side. In addition to muscular dystrophy, other conditions producing weakness of the muscles that stabilize the hip girdle can cause a waddling gait. These conditions include other myopathies and progressive spinal muscular atrophy. Congenital dislocation of the hips also can cause a waddling gait.

Parkinsonian gait

In Parkinson's disease and parkinsonian syndromes, the gait and posture are so constantly affected that a stereotyped picture is produced. In a moderately advanced stage of the illness, the head and shoulders are stooped forward, the forearms are partly flexed, the wrists are slightly extended, and the fingers are flexed at the metacarpophalangeal joints and extended at the interphalangeal joints. The characteristic "pill-rolling" tremor of Parkinson's disease may be present while the patient walks. As the patient starts to walk, the movements of the lower extremities may be quite slow to the point that the patient's feet appear to stick to the floor. The patient may lean or tend to fall forward while walking (propulsion), so that the steps are hurried. The result is a shuffling of the feet, which may increase in rapidity until the patient is almost running, the so-called festinating gait. Similarly, a deviation of the center of gravity to the sides or backward can produce lateropulsion or retropulsion, respectively. A tendency to retropulsion contributes to the difficulty in arising from chairs, especially low ones, that is common in Parkinson's disease and parkinsonian syndromes. The parkinsonian patient often moves en bloc when making about-face turns; movement is slow, with many small steps, while the upper body is held relatively motionless. In less advanced stages of the illness, examination of the gait may reveal only a slight forward stoop and a loss of associated swinging of the affected arm or arms during walking.

Dystonic and choreic gaits

Dystonia can seriously affect the gait, often in bizarre and unusual ways, so that hysteria is suspected. Gait disturbances can be the first and, for a time, the only manifestation of dystonia. In dystonia musculorum deformans and in symptomatic dystonia, there can be involuntary contraction with sustained inversion and plantar flexion of one foot, flexion of the hip, or abnormal postures of the upper limb or spine. Initially, the examination when the patient is supine or seated may be unrevealing, and the involuntary movements appear only during attempts to walk.

In patients with chorea, the brief, quick movements impart an irregular jerkiness to the gait accompanied by purposeless brief movements of the upper limbs, head, neck, and face. When the choreiform movements are severe, walking can be lurching and dangerous, and when they are mild, it can have a dancing or lilting quality.

Apraxia of gait

This term is used to describe gait impairment without demonstrable sensory loss, weakness, or cerebellar deficit. The impairment is seen in patients with widespread cerebral disease, especially that affecting the frontal lobes. The patient has difficulty arising and standing and initiating steps. Like someone with Parkinson's disease, the patient may be bent forward and take hesitating, short, shuffling steps. Unlike the characteristics of Parkinson's disease, upper limb movements are normal, tremor is absent, and there is no true rigidity, although gegenhalten is frequently present. Despite the difficulty walking, when seated the patient initially can perform complex coordinated movements with the lower extremities. Later, movements when sitting and supine are also affected.

Normal pressure hydrocephalus gait

Normal pressure hydrocephalus is characterized by the triad of gait disturbance, slowness of thinking, and incontinence of urine more often than stool. Gait disturbance, usually the first symptom, has no specific characteristics. The patient may have difficulty arising, usually has a slightly widened base, takes small steps, is unsteady, and often has a tendency to fall backward. Gegenhalten may be present. There are characteristics of a parkinsonian gait and some elements of apraxia. The difficulty with mentation and sphincter control and imaging evidence of hydrocephalus help to confirm the diagnosis.

Hysterical gait

Although a gait disorder may seem bizarre, it does not follow that it must be the result of a conversion disorder. However, when gait is disturbed in conversion hysteria, the disturbance is likely to be bizarre, even fantastic. Wildly weaving, bobbing, lurching movements of the body can appear to put the patient in imminent danger of falling. Another patient may proceed by painfully slow, hesitant steps, with long balancing on one foot before putting the other to the floor. Another with a purportedly weak leg might drag the toe of a strangely inverted or everted foot noisily along the floor. Variations are too numerous to allow a complete listing. In general, a hysterical gait is characterized by inconsistency. The person who balances too long on one foot is indulging in gymnastics that would be impossible without good muscle strength and coordination. The "weak" leg is found to have no sign of muscle atrophy, and the muscle stretch reflexes are normal. The patient who seems about to pitch over with every step can cross and uncross the legs, lie down and sit up without difficulty, and, in general, manage the lower extremities rather well while on the examining table. This incongruity, within the gait itself and between the gait and results of other neurologic tests, helps in deciding whether a gait is hysterical. The term "astasia-abasia" refers to a condition in which patients are unable to stand or walk because of hysterical conversion disorder.

Limping gait

A limping gait may be produced by various conditions, such as shortening of one lower extremity and deformity of a foot. A common cause for limping can be the pain experienced when weight is borne on one lower extremity (antalgic gait). The patient puts the affected extremity down gingerly and takes a short step to remove the weight from the painful limb as soon as possible. At the same time, the good limb is brought forward rapidly and lands more vigorously than usual.

Although patients with vascular claudication and pseudoclaudication both experience lower limb discomfort and need to stop walking after a certain distance, the patient with pseudoclaudication from lumbar spinal stenosis can have the same symptoms (pain or numbness or weakness in the lower limbs) from simply standing in an erect position for a certain length of time. The patient with pseudoclaudication can gain relief by flexing at the waist, and many patients with lumbar spinal stenosis are noted to stand and walk flexed at the waist to help avoid or delay the onset of lower limb symptoms.

Finally, the patient with a painful sensory neuropathy may appear to be walking on hot coals. Quick, uncomfortable steps are taken, and sometimes the patient walks on the sides of the feet to limit discomfort.

Station

Station, the patient's manner and posture in standing, is conveniently evaluated during testing of the patient's gait. The patient is asked to stand with feet together, head erect, and eyes open. Some examiners prefer to have the patient extend the arms. The patient can be given gentle pushes to see if there is any tendency to fall forward, to the sides, or backward. After assuming a stable standing position, the patient is asked to close the eyes. Any tendency to sway or fall is noted. The degrees of steadiness shown with eyes open and with eyes closed are compared and recorded.

The result of the Romberg sign is said to be positive when unsteadiness is increased by closure of the eyes. Characteristically, it is present in diseases such as tabes dorsalis, subacute combined degeneration, and polyneuritis in which there is a loss of proprioceptive sensation from the lower extremities. As a matter of fact, the average person does not stand as steadily with the eyes closed as with them open, and the unsteadiness of station associated with cerebellar disease or with loss of vestibular function can be aggravated perceptibly by closing the eyes. Hence, when the Romberg test result is positive, careful neurologic examination of the various systems concerned with balance is required before a decision can be made about the lesion responsible for it.

The Romberg sign result can be falsely positive in a patient with hysteria, who might sway dramatically at the waist instead of the ankles and maintain stance despite wild gyrations. If stance is broken, the eyes are sometimes kept closed. The "abnormalities" can sometimes be minimized by instructing the patient not to sway or by asking that a second task, such as finger-to-nose testing or tongue wiggle, be performed simultaneously.

Some examiners prefer that the foregoing tests be performed with the patient fully clothed or at least wearing shoes; others prefer to have the shoes removed. In doubtful cases, it is best to observe the patient under both conditions.

Chapter 8

Motor Function. Part II: Specific Study of Muscle

Even in this day of computerized measurements of force and electrical activity, no machine has been devised that even begins to replace the careful clinical examination. Mastery of the clinical examination of muscle is a prerequisite to assessment of the entire motor system and to intelligent use of the important aids of electromyography and biopsy. The basic methods of inspection, palpation, and percussion used in physical diagnosis are also used for the examination of muscles. These methods, along with training and experience in the testing of muscle strength, form the basis for clinical study of neuromuscular disorders.

DISORDERS OF MUSCLE SIZE

The size of muscles varies greatly with the age, gender, body build, occupation, state of nutrition, and training of the individual. Consequently, considerable experience with many patients is required before the physician gains confidence in concluding that a particular muscle is unusually small or large or of unusual configuration.

Atrophy

Atrophy, as applied to muscles, refers to a loss of bulk: the muscle was once larger and is now smaller. By history, comparison with other muscles, or repeated observation, atrophy can usually be differentiated from congenital absence of a muscle or failure of muscular development.

To determine whether atrophy is present, the examiner assesses the bulk of the muscle by inspection and palpation and compares the muscle with neighboring muscles, with the same muscle on the opposite side of the body, and with general muscular development. A change in contour or configuration of muscle frequently corroborates muscle atrophy. Minor differences in the circumference of extremities are an unreliable means of determining atrophy, since asymmetrical development, for example, of the calves, is not uncommon. Comparative measurements are often of value, however, in determining progression of atrophy. Atrophy resulting from disease of the lower motor neuron or of the muscle itself is almost always associated with significant weakness of the muscle. In an elderly or inactive person, skeletal muscles may appear small, yet they may retain the ability to contract forcefully.

Hypertrophy

Hypertrophy describes an increase in the size of muscle. It is also identified by inspection, palpation, and comparison with other muscles. A muscle of normal size appears hypertrophic in the midst of atrophic neighboring muscles. For example, it is often difficult in progressive muscular dystrophy to decide whether the calves are hypertrophic or only appear so in contrast to the atrophic muscles of the thigh.

INTRINSIC MUSCLE MOVEMENTS

Fasciculations

Fasciculations are the twitches observed in resting muscle that result from the spontaneous firing of one or more motor units. They can be seen, palpated, and, at times, heard with a stethoscope. Fasciculations are best differentiated from other muscle movements by examining the patient supine or prone with the muscles at rest. Fasciculations differ from other spontaneous movements by their random recurrence. They occur as single, isolated twitches rather than as runs of rapid twitches. Fasciculations usually do not produce joint movements except for small movements of fingers or toes. A brief twitch of a muscle that produces joint movement is more likely to be due to chorea.

There is considerable variability in the ease with which fasciculations can be seen. In some cases, fasciculations are obvious because of their number and large size. They are difficult to observe in deep-lying muscles and in obese persons. Often, they are harder to find in women and young children than in men. It is well to search for them diligently in a well-lighted room. Usually, they can be seen best with oblique lighting. Sometimes it is helpful to moisten the skin over the muscle and to look for the flickerings in reflected light. At times, deep fasciculations can be palpated when they cannot be seen. Light percussion of a muscle may activate fasciculations. Administration of neostigmine to a susceptible person may activate dense fasciculations; the muscles may appear to be alive with twitches from head to toe.

Contraction fasciculations are rhythmic twitches of motor units observed during weak contraction of muscle. They are seen most frequently in patients who have an old or continuing involvement of the nerve supply to skeletal muscle that results in enlargement of its motor units. For example, contraction fasciculations are common as a result of poliomyelitis, amyotrophic lateral sclerosis, or chronic compression of a nerve root. Contraction fasciculations are differentiated from spontaneous fasciculations by their rhythmic recurrence and disappearance on relaxation of the muscle.

Shivering, the result of cold, may give rise to rapid twitches of muscle, and for that reason the patient being observed for fasciculations must be kept comfortably warm to avoid confusion.

Tremor may produce intrinsic muscle movements that resemble fasciculations. Particularly in tremor of the tongue, confusion may arise. Since tremor of the tongue is almost always of the action type and seen when the tongue is protruded, it is well to observe the tongue for fasciculation through partially opened lips while it lies at rest in the mouth. The tremor of thyrotoxicosis, with or without myopathy, produces intrinsic muscular movements that superficially resemble fasciculations.

Fasciculations vary in size with variations in the size and distribution of muscle fibers and in the number of muscle fibers that contract simultaneously. In muscles containing long fibers, hypertrophic fibers, or motor units with widespread muscle fibers, the contractions may be inches in length. In the tongue, the twitches are much smaller, since the units are smaller.

Fasciculations derive their connotation of malignancy from their association with amyotrophic lateral sclerosis, in which they are regularly seen. However, it must be remembered that they can occur in normal individuals and as a result of any disease that produces degeneration or irritation of the lower motor neuron. Consequently, they may be present in a number of disorders of the peripheral nerve, in radiculopathies, in poliomyelitis, and in intrinsic diseases of the spinal cord, such as syringomyelia and intramedullary tumor.

Furthermore, fasciculations are a normal phenomenon occasionally seen in persons who have no neurologic or muscular disease, in which case they may be referred to as *benign fasciculations.* Frequently such patients are physicians, whose knowledge of the potential prognostic significance of fasciculations engenders the anxiety that leads them to consult the neurologist. It is extremely rare for a patient who has amyotrophic lateral sclerosis to seek medical attention because of fasciculations alone. Although roughly one-half of such patients are aware of their fasciculations, they almost always seek medical advice because of dysfunction resulting from weakness or spasticity and not because of twitches in their muscles.

Fasciculations that have been present for several months and are unassociated with other evidence of denervation determined clinically and electromyographically are benign. Benign fasciculations are quite common but often not recognized. They occur most commonly in muscles that have been stressed without adequate training and may be increased for several hours after exercise. Minimal exercise may strikingly accentuate fasciculations in deconditioned muscles.

Cramps

Cramps are normal phenomena whose frequency is increased in some neurologic diseases. They are most commonly identified on the history but occasionally occur during the examination of the muscle. Although typically painful and transient contractions of a whole muscle or groups of muscles, cramps can be painless and limited to a segment of muscles. They occur most often in muscles being used frequently and actively, such as the calf and intrinsic foot muscles. They may be brought on by vigorous contraction of a muscle in a shortened position and can be relieved by stretching and rubbing the involved muscle. The occurrence of cramps during the muscle examination should be noted.

Myokymia

Myokymia is a condition in which there are spontaneous brief tetanic contractions of one or more motor units. Usually, adjacent motor units contract alternately and intermittently, producing a continual undulation, or rippling, of the surface of the muscle. The movements are slower and more prolonged than those produced by the brief single twitches of fasciculation. Although in rare instances myokymia in the limbs results from radiation damage, local decompression of peripheral nerve, or a metabolic disease, it is most commonly a benign form of muscle twitching in overstressed muscles. (See also the discussion of fasciculation and myokymia in the "Electromyography" section of Chapter 15.)

Facial myokymia is an unusual type of unilateral facial spasm characterized by continuous, fine, rhythmic, undulating movements of an area of the face. The surface of the skin moves like the surface of a bag containing worms. Myokymia limited to the eyelids is almost always benign. More widespread facial myokymia may result from multiple sclerosis, brain stem tumors, or demyelinating cranial neuropathies.

Fibrillation

The term "fibrillation" is used to refer to the spontaneous, independent contractions of individual muscle fibers. The contractions are minute and cannot be seen through the intact skin. Electromyographic evidence of them is found regularly in denervated muscle beginning 10 to 21 days after the muscle has been deprived of its nerve supply. They may persist as long as the fibers remain viable. Fibrillations have been detected in partially denervated muscle for as long as 20 years.

RESPONSE TO PERCUSSION

Normal

Normal muscle contracts in response to sharp percussion. The excitability of the muscle judged in this way roughly parallels the excitability to stretch. However, in complete absence of the stretch reflex, the muscle may remain excitable to percussion. Consequently, in the study of stretch reflexes, direct percussion of the muscle being tested should be avoided.

Only the fibers that have been percussed directly contract. Therefore, if the small tip of the percussion hammer is used, a narrow band of fibers is seen to contract, producing a brief longitudinal depression in the muscle.

Myotonic Reaction

Myotonia is characterized by the persistence of a strong contraction of muscle after stimulation has ceased, whether the contraction be initiated voluntarily, mechanically, or electrically.

In suspected myotonia, the patient is instructed to grasp the examiner's hand or fingers strongly. After the grasp has been maintained for 5 seconds or so, the patient is told to release the grasp quickly. A persistence of contraction while the patient is obviously trying to comply with the examiner's request is one manifestation of myotonic reaction.

Percussion myotonia

Myotonia detected by the method just described can be verified readily by eliciting a prolonged contraction in response to sharp percussion. In different patients, myotonia may be more readily elicited in some muscles than in others, and tests should be done in more than one area. The finger extensors are particularly sensitive for the demonstration of myotonia. A quick tap on the normal extensor digitorum communis muscle results in a rapid, brief extension of one or more fingers. If myotonia is present, the finger or fingers remain extended for several seconds. The thenar eminence may also readily demonstrate myotonia when it is struck sharply with the smaller tip of the percussion hammer. This causes a quick contraction, producing opposition of the thumb that persists for several seconds before gradual relaxation begins.

Figure 8-1
Percussion myotonia.

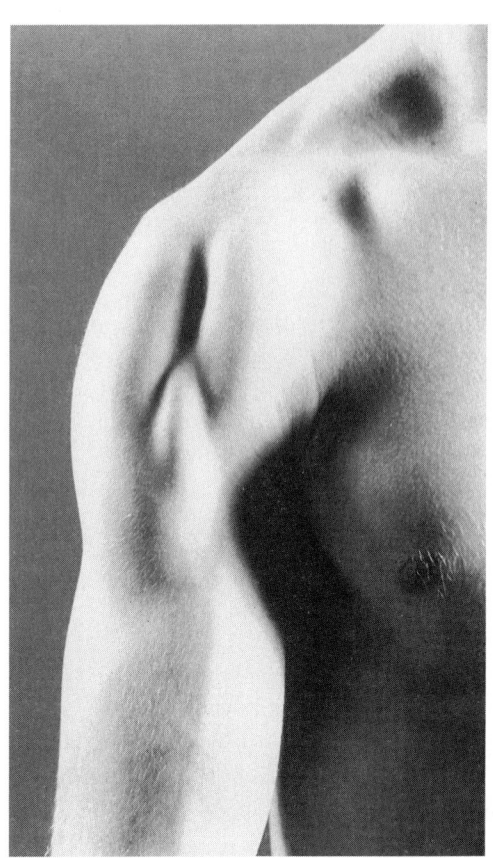

Other exposed muscles, such as the tongue and the deltoid, may be similarly used to elicit percussion myotonia (Fig. 8-1). In these muscles, the portion of muscle struck contracts, producing a depression in the muscle that persists for several seconds.

Myoedema
Occasionally in normal persons and frequently in myxedema and in debilitative states, the localized portion of the muscle percussed forms a hillock that persists for several seconds (Fig. 8-2). The formation of the hillock is referred to as "myoedema." The response differs from that of myotonia in that it is not accompanied by electrical activity of the muscle. Also, the raised hillock of myoedema is in contrast to the persistent focal depression observed in percussion myotonia.

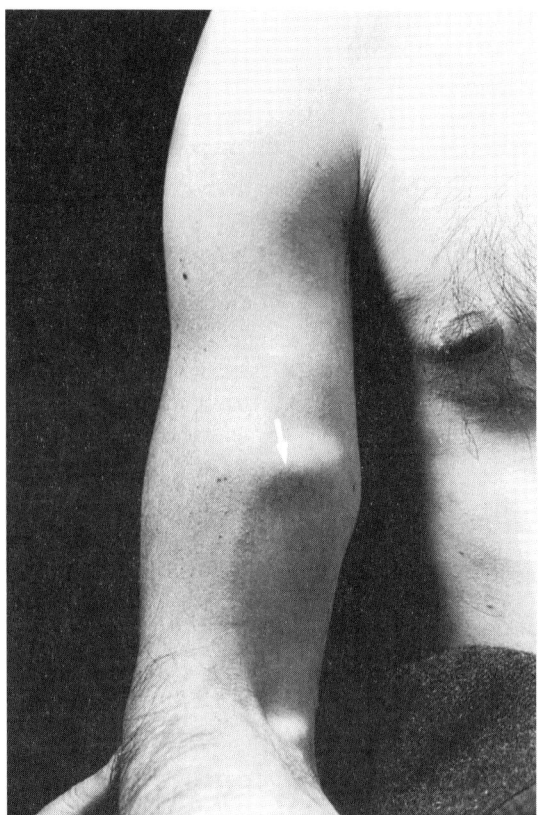

Figure 8-2
Myoedema.

PALPATION OF MUSCLE

Tenderness

Tenderness of muscle is determined by squeezing. However, since muscle is covered by skin and subcutaneous tissue, one should try to exclude tenderness of these structures before concluding that the muscle is tender. This is done by lightly touching and pressing the skin and by squeezing a fold of the skin overlying the muscle. Comparing pressure of the skin against bone with pressure over a muscle, such as the anterior tibial, is helpful in testing for tenderness of muscle. Furthermore, tenderness of a specific muscle often can be demonstrated when the muscle is brought into action, as in testing the strength of the muscle.

Consistency

The consistency of muscles varies considerably in normal healthy persons. The limits of these variations cannot be described concisely. They are best learned by repeated observation and testing of patients whose muscles are normal. Disease of the muscle or of the nervous system may result in striking alterations in the consistency of muscles. Muscular dystrophy, polymyositis, and Volkmann's contracture may produce an increased consistency ranging from rubberiness to woodiness. Sometimes the muscle is diffusely affected; sometimes the increased consistency is patchy, so that fibrous longitudinal bands can be palpated.

Acute denervation produces an atony that is recognized by flabbiness to palpation. Chronic denervation may produce self-perpetuating electrical discharges in muscle that result in a firm muscle consistency and sometimes hypertrophy from continuous muscle contraction. Electromyographic testing readily identifies these characteristic, complex, repetitive potentials.

Conditions such as meningitis and herniated intervertebral disk may cause irritation of spinal nerve roots. This, in turn, may result in protective muscle spasm. Lesions of the central nervous system may give rise to spasticity or rigidity that augments the consistency of muscle.

Contracture

If a muscle is maintained for weeks or months in a shortened condition, a contracture usually develops as a result of changes in the fibrous constituents of the muscle. Such a muscle cannot be stretched to normal limits without the application of considerable pressure and the production of pain. In women who regularly wear high-heeled shoes, a shortening of the gastrocnemius and soleus muscles not infrequently develops, and tightening of the heel cord may be sufficient to prevent them from extending the ankles as fully as needed in walking on the heels.

Contractures of muscles are detected on passive motion of joints. The tendon of the affected muscle is seen to tighten passively, limiting the range of movement of the joint being tested. If limitation of movement is encountered, careful observation usually enables the examiner to differentiate limitation due to fibrous-tissue changes about the joint or to spasm of muscle from true contracture of muscles. In uncertain cases, spasm can be readily differentiated from contracture by electromyographic testing. Of course, spasm, contracture of muscles, and structural fixation of joints may all occur simultaneously, limiting motion of joints. Contractures are most often found in the extensors of the back, the adductors and internal rotators of the shoulder, the extensors or flexors and the adductors of the hip, the flexors and pronators of the forearm, and the other flexor muscles of the extremities.

To detect contracture, the examiner must move each joint passively through its full range of motion. In addition, the toe-touching test in full sitting position is valuable in detecting contractures in the extensors of the back, hips, and hamstrings. The patient is instructed to try to touch the toes without bending the knees while sitting upright with the knees fully extended.

A distinction should be made between how clinicians and how physiologists use the term "contracture." The clinician uses the term to denote any state of fixed shortening of skeletal muscle that is not produced by nerve impulses. Usually, the shortening is caused by changes in the fibrous and elastic supporting tissues of the muscle. To the physiologist, the term classically has a more precise meaning and denotes a prolonged reversible shortening of muscle fibers caused by action of the contractile mechanism of the fibers without the occurrence of the action potentials associated with the usual tetanic contraction. When the shortening becomes irreversible, it is known as "rigor." Contractures in the physiologic sense can be produced experimentally by acids, alkalis, acetylcholine, veratrine, and other substances. The "myoedema" produced by mechanical stimulation of a muscle is a physiologic contracture.

MUSCLE STRENGTH

The testing and grading of the strength of individual muscles are among the most difficult segments of neurologic examination to master. They cannot be learned without experience in testing a wide variety of patients who are weak or strong. The student who is armed with determination to learn, has a reasonable knowledge of anatomy repeatedly replenished by reference to texts and atlases, and has access to a variety of patients can gain reasonable proficiency in testing muscular strength within months.

The effort is most rewarding. Without confidence in testing strength, one may fail to detect some diseases if they are minimal in degree. Furthermore, without confidence in detecting muscular weakness, one cannot pinpoint neurologic lesions capable of being localized precisely and cannot understand or properly treat obvious disturbances in gait or function. Even important clues to the psychogenic nature of an illness may be recognized by the examiner proficient in muscle strength testing. And lastly, the determination of progression or regression of a disease often depends on reliable methods of testing and grading strength.

Symptoms

Little experience with patients is needed before one becomes impressed by how often they complain of weakness and how infrequently actual weakness is found. The language of such patients is filled with the words "tiredness," "fatigue," "weakness," and "exhaustion." Often the patient insists that he or she is "too tired to move" or "more tired in the morning" after sleep than at any other time. On judicious questioning, however, it is found that although experiencing a sense of utter exhaustion while lying in bed, the patient is able to arise, bathe, dress, eat, and drive an automobile or even run to catch the morning train.

On the other hand, the patient who has neuromuscular weakness usually describes disturbances in function that result from inability to contract and to sustain the contraction of muscles with normal vigor. This person's complaints are more specific. Although no sense of illness may be experienced in the lying or sitting position, when the patient begins to move or act, deficiency in performance is encountered. There may be difficulty in lifting the head from the pillow and trouble rolling over in bed. The patient may find it impossible to arise from a low chair without pushing up with the hands. Perhaps the knees cannot be crossed without assistance of the hands in flexing the thigh. On walking, the patient may describe a tendency for the ankles to turn or the feet to flop if the evertors or dorsiflexors are weak. Often, ascending and descending stairs and squatting and arising are difficult, and the leg cannot be lifted over the edge of the bathtub.

Weakness of the upper extremities gives rise to complaints of inability to turn doorknobs, to lift heavy objects, or, in the case of a woman, to hold the arms overhead for the period required in preparing her hair.

Weakness of the neck muscles most often produces complaints of inability to lift the head off the pillow or of a tendency for it to fall forward.

The complaints referable to weakness of muscles supplied by the cranial nerves are similarly specific. Drooping of the eyelids and diplopia are produced by extraocular weakness. Weakness of the lips is proclaimed by inability to enunciate clearly, whistle, blow up a balloon, or suck through a straw or, when unilateral, by drooling on the weakened side. With weakness of the orbicularis oculi, the patient may be unable to keep soap out of the eyes during washing of the face or the eyelids may remain partly open during sleep. Often a change in facies or inability to smile properly is described. Tiring of the jaws and inability to bite hard are complaints indicative of weak jaw muscles. Dysphagia, dysarthria, nasal speech, and regurgitation are the usual complaints resulting from weakness of the tongue, palate, and pharynx. When weaknesses of both the tongue and the buccinator muscles exist together, as is so often the case in myasthenia gravis, even the most fastidious person may admit that food lodges between the teeth and the cheeks and must be dislodged by the fingers.

Of course, many other complaints are indicative of muscular weakness, varying with the activities and occupations pursued by the patient and the degree, number, and location of muscles involved. The foregoing complaints are typical and indicative of the type of complaint produced by actual weakness of muscles.

Perhaps the greatest confusion in the reporting of symptoms arises from the tendency of many patients to attribute erroneously to weakness the deficiencies in function that result from spasticity, rigidity, or even pain and stiffness. The examiner must be alert to this misuse of words. As a rule, it is the responsibility of the examiner to determine by muscle testing whether weakness is present when a patient believes that he or she is weak or describes deficits in function that could result from weakness. For instance, the differentiation of a nonspecific febrile illness from acute poliomyelitis often depends on the detection of a minimal degree of muscular weakness.

Grading and Recording of Muscle Strength

Various methods of grading muscle strength are in use. Undoubtedly, all have merit, and yet many are unsuited for the purposes of neurology. Under these circumstances, it is important to define criteria for the designation of specific grades of weakness so that the limits of each grade are recognized by all. Otherwise, the records of one examiner are meaningless to the next in determining whether the weakness is worsening, improving, or stationary.

Throughout the years, we have found that two types of grading are of practical value. One type is for the novice, and the other, more specific type is gradually used as experience is acquired. In both types, "0" represents normality, "−4" records complete paralysis, and "−1" represents the slightest degree of loss of strength that one is able to detect. For the novice, "−2" is used to designate moderate weakness (±50%) and "−3" to indicate severe degrees of weakness (±75%). To indicate the slightest detectable contraction, usually a perceptible twitch, the symbol "−3, 4" is of value.

With experience, the examiner finds it desirable to record more accurately weakness of moderate to considerable degree, which the novice does well to record with reasonable accuracy as "−2" or "−3." This has entailed the introduction of an additional symbol, "g," meaning gravity, which can be used in recording the strength of several muscles. The symbol "g" is qualified by the insertion before it of a plus or minus sign. Thus "−g" as applied to the quadriceps (or any other muscle in which the effect of gravity is useful in grading) represents inability of the quadriceps to extend the knee completely against gravity. The symbol "+g" is used to indicate ability barely to accomplish this movement. With introduction of the symbol "g" and the qualifying use of the preceding plus or minus sign, the symbol "−3" must be more specifically defined as ability to move through the full range against gravity plus pressure made by the examiner. Naturally, these more specific designations must be avoided in recording the strength of muscles, such as the brachioradialis, whose function cannot be isolated. They are also valueless as applied to smaller muscles, such as those of the hands or feet. Seldom are they applied to muscles other than the flexors and extensors of the neck, deltoids, triceps, flexors of the forearm, and flexors and extensors of the wrist and, in the lower extremities, to flexors and abductors of the thigh, extensors and flexors of the knee, and dorsiflexors of the ankle.

Not infrequently, there is doubt as to the normality or the complete absence of contraction. In such cases, our indecisiveness can be expressed conveniently and clearly by placing a question mark after the symbol that most nearly describes our opinion.

An outline defining the various degrees of weakness and comparing the symbols used in the rough and the more precise methods is given in Table 8-1.

Normal Strength

Normal strength may be defined as the degree of strength of a muscle or muscle group that is contracted with maximal vigor in the test situation by a fully cooperative and healthy person. Thus, the definition implies experience on the part of the examiner and cooperation on the part of the patient.

Table 8-1 Grading of Muscle Strength and Weakness

Experienced Examiner	Novice Examiner
0 = Normal	Normal = 0
0, −1 = Questionable weakness	Questionable weakness = 0, −1
−1 = Slightest detectable weakness	
−1, 2 = Slight but not slightest weakness; loss of strength considerably less than 50%	Slight weakness (25%) = −1
−2 = Moderate weakness; 50% strength	
−2, 3 = Between grades above and below (−2 and −3, respectively)	Moderate weakness (50%) = −2
−3 = Severe weakness but capable of moving extremity against gravity and appreciable resistance made by examiner	Severe weakness (75%) = −3
+g = Severe weakness; ability barely to move extremity through full range against gravity alone	
−g = Severe weakness; inability to move extremity through full range against gravity	
−3, 4 = Very severe weakness (minimal detectable contraction)	Very severe weakness (minimal detectable contraction) = −3, 4
−4 = Complete paralysis	Complete paralysis = −4

As is often the case in neurology, confidence in testing is attained by doing. For this reason, we require the novice in neurology to test and record the strength of a number of muscles in every instance in which a complete neurologic examination is indicated. It is required that this portion of the examination be completed even though there is no reason to believe that abnormalities will be detected. This procedure ensures experience in the testing of strength when weakness does not exist. Thus, the examiner has an opportunity to learn the limits of normality against which comparisons can be made and becomes capable of detecting the slighter but significant degrees of abnormality. Only through extensive experience with normal individuals can an examiner become able to recognize and accurately grade weakness in patients ranging from well-muscled male weight lifters to frail elderly women. In each case, the grading of strength must be in comparison with that in similar healthy individuals.

In the precise estimation of muscle strength, it is necessary that the patient be able to cooperate fully. Consequently, in the examination of comatose and disturbed patients and in infants and young children, these tests cannot be performed as reliably. However, rough estimates of strength can usually be based on observations of performance. Does the patient move the extremities voluntarily? Is spontaneous movement or withdrawal from an unpleasant stimulus vigorous or weak? Is it of the same degree on both sides? Is there an asymmetry of the face on the display of emotion, as in the crying of an infant? In the comatose patient, is there any resistance to gravity when a lifted extremity is dropped?

Of course, deformity and pain induced by muscle contraction can prevent full cooperation of the patient. Often, even if pain is present, the patient can be urged to make a maximal contraction if the pressure used by the examiner is applied gingerly and the patient is made to understand that only a brief strong contraction is required.

General Survey of Motor Function

These performance tests are not intended as substitutes for specific tests of muscle strength except in very young children or in patients who cannot cooperate sufficiently for reliable specific testing. Perhaps they are of greatest value in determining whether a disease characterized by muscular weakness, such as polymyositis, is progressing or abating.

Of course, failure to perform normally the maneuvers required in the "General Survey of Motor Function" (Table 8-2) is not necessarily the result of weakness. Deformity, contracture, pain, involuntary movements, spasticity, rigidity, ataxia, and, at times, psychiatric disorders, such as conversion hysteria, interfere seriously with function in persons with normal strength.

Table 8-2	General Survey of Motor Function	
R		L
Arise from chair, arms folded		
	Walk on toes	
	Walk on heels	
	Hopping	
Squat fully and arise		
	Lift foot to step	
	Step up on step	
	Abduct arms to horizontal	
	Reach fully overhead	
	Winging of scapulae	
	(Supine)	
Lift head off table		
	Flex thigh lifting extended lower extremity	
Hands on occiput, arise to sitting position		
	(Prone)	
Fully extend neck		
Lift head and shoulders off table, hands on buttocks		

Testing Muscle Strength

Although there are variations in the techniques of examiners expert in performing tests of muscle strength, all make use of fundamental anatomic knowledge about location, origin, and insertion of muscles and an understanding of muscle actions. Armed with anatomic knowledge and experience, the clinician attains unrivaled superiority in testing strength. It is safe to say that no machine has been devised to substitute for the examiner in positioning the patients, directing pressure, applying resistance, detecting substitution, and, finally, in determining whether the patient is making a full effort.

Two methods of testing are used. The first, and usually the preferred, method requires that the patient resist pressure initiated by the examiner. The other method allows the patient to initiate contraction, which is resisted by the examiner. At first, there may seem to be little difference between the two methods, but experience shows that, as a rule, patients more easily comprehend what is wanted of them and cooperate better if they are instructed to hold against pressure initiated by the examiner attempting to overpower the muscle being tested. However, the second method, in which the patient initiates movement that is resisted by the examiner, is particularly advantageous in the testing of very weak muscles. In any event, both methods are used frequently and often as a means of checking the result obtained by the one first applied.

Proper positioning of the patient is important in conducting and evaluating tests of muscle strength. In general, that posture affording the greatest stability of the body is best. Consequently, the supine and prone positions are made use of, but the sitting position is preferred in testing most of the muscles attached to the scapulae. In fact, the sitting position is entirely satisfactory for testing strength of the extremities if the muscles of the trunk and pelvis are not appreciably weak. Proper positioning, of course, is necessary when it is desirable to use or eliminate the force of gravity in the testing and grading of the strength of very weak muscles.

Positioning is of greatest importance in separating the actions of one or more muscles that participate in the production of the same movement. For example, the gluteus maximus and hamstrings combine to extend the hip while the knee is extended, but the hamstring action may be eliminated by flexion of the knee. Consequently, in the prone position while the knee is fully flexed, extension of the hip (lifting the knee from the table) becomes a function of the gluteus maximus. The strength of the hamstrings can best be tested by the patient's resisting an attempt by the examiner to extend the semiflexed knee.

As a result of differences in leverage in various segments of the arc of action, there are apparent variations in the strength of muscle corresponding to the segment of the arc in which it is acting. For example, when the elbow is fully flexed, the triceps is at a mechanical disadvantage and extension of the arm is much weaker than it is when the elbow is extended to midposition or beyond. Consequently, if weakness of the triceps is minimal, as it often is when a lesion such as a protruded cervical intervertebral disk involves only the seventh cervical root, the examiner may fail to detect weakness unless, in addition to the usual test of triceps strength, the patient is told to push against the examiner in an effort to extend the fully flexed elbow. In this instance, as well as others, comparison of the strength on the two sides may be of great value in the detection of minimal weakness.

Although proper positioning tends to separate the actions of muscles that combine to produce the same movement, one must be alert to recognize substitution. Consequently, while testing for strength of a specific muscle, the examiner should observe and palpate the muscle and its tendon and similarly scrutinize neighboring muscles that can substitute for its action. Also, one should watch carefully for lack of fixation of the scapula and pelvis while testing muscles that act on the shoulder or hip joints. It may be necessary to stabilize the scapula or pelvis manually to test the strength of the deltoid or iliopsoas. For example, the novice may mistake weakness of the serratus anterior or trapezius for weakness of the deltoid. In such cases, pressure toward adduction on the abducted arm may be weakly resisted by the patient. However, careful observation will show that the shoulder joint is not being adducted but rather that the scapula is being rotated.

It is important to avoid jerkiness in tests of muscle strength. The patient is instructed to resist pressure initiated by the examiner, and it is necessary that the examiner avoid abrupt application of pressure. It should be initiated gingerly and gradually increased to a maximum. Furthermore, the patient should be made to understand that he or she is to continue resisting pressure made by the examiner until the test is completed. The examiner varies pressure during the test and observes whether the patient continues to resist with maximal effort as the joint affected is allowed to move. Cooperative patients, whether strong or weak, maintain a smooth resistance to pressure and continue to press smoothly against the examiner as pressure is slackened and the joint is allowed to move. This is referred to as "follow-through."

Hysterical Motor Dysfunction ("Weakness")
Behavior of a patient during the test of muscle strength is one of the most reliable indices available to the clinician of the patient's ability to comprehend the examiner's instructions and to withstand pain and of the determination to cooperate. Furthermore, hysterical behavior is manifest as often, if not more often, during tests of muscle strength as it is during examination of sensation or the fields of vision.

The patient who manifests a hysterical type of motor dysfunction (weakness) on request to perform a specific motion, such as extension of the ankle, may respond with the opposite motion and flex the ankle instead of extending it. On being urged, the patient is likely to produce several irregular, briefly sustained contractions. Against pressure created by the examiner, the patient makes a series of poorly sustained contractions of varying strength that often are found to become stronger with encouragement and urging by the examiner. Finally, after much urging, a strong contraction is produced for a second or two, after which abrupt and complete relaxation occurs ("giving way"). Furthermore, although understanding that steadily maximal counterpressure is to be maintained against the pressure made by the examiner, the patient fails to pursue the examiner's hand as it is allowed to retreat in the direction of action. This phenomenon is referred to as "lack of follow-through."

The behavior on muscle testing is in marked contrast to the behavior of the usual cooperative patient, whether weak or strong. Such patients promptly contract maximally the muscle being tested and maintain the maximal contraction steadily and smoothly against varying degrees of pressure without "giving way" and by "following through" as the pressure is decreased.

Experience has shown that the type of dysfunction described as hysterical weakness is usually a reflection of a functional psychiatric disorder, provided that the patient thoroughly comprehends what is wanted, the test is unproductive of pain that results in "giving way," proprioceptive sensation is intact, and cerebral disease resulting in a conceptual type of motor dysfunction (apraxia) is absent.

Scheme Employed in Examining Muscles

It is helpful to follow some sort of routine or sequential scheme in examining the individual muscles of the extremities. This helps the examiner to maintain orientation and facilitates localization of a lesion. For example, a plan based on the anatomy of the brachial plexus and peripheral nerves may prove useful. The muscles of the shoulder girdle and arm are tested in the approximate order in which the nerves of supply originate from the components of the brachial plexus, beginning proximally and proceeding distally. At levels in this sequence where more than one major nerve arises, the muscles are tested in the order in which their nerves originate, beginning with the upper or lateral component of the plexus and proceeding across the plexus to the lower or medial component. The muscles supplied by the radial, median, and ulnar nerves are examined in the following sequence: first those supplied by the radial nerve in the order in which the branches arise, proceeding distally, then those supplied by the median nerve in the same manner, and finally those supplied by the ulnar nerve, again in the same order. With certain deviations from this strict anatomic sequence, this scheme lends itself readily to a clinically convenient and logical procedure for examination.

It is scarcely feasible, and it is unnecessary in clinical work, to test every muscle separately. In the following outline, most of the muscles are tested and in as specific a manner as is reasonably possible, but attention is focused on certain key muscles particularly helpful in clinical evaluation. The muscles omitted are, for the most part, those that are relatively feeble and poorly accessible for individual examination and whose action and nerve supply are duplicated by more powerful and accessible muscles.

Outline of Anatomic Information Required for Tests of Strength of Specific Muscles

In the following descriptions of the tests, the name of each muscle is followed in parentheses by the corresponding peripheral nerve and spinal segmental supply. There is considerable variability in segmental supply, particularly to certain muscles, as given by different authorities. Furthermore, there is some anatomic variation both in the plexuses and in the peripheral nerves. The segments listed cannot, therefore, be regarded as absolute. The principal and usual supply is underlined. The action sections list only the principal and important secondary or accessory functions—those particularly useful in testing and those that may cause confusion by substituting for the activity of other muscles. In the description of the test itself, the position and movement given first refer to the patient unless otherwise clearly stated. In some instances, the movement is adequately indicated by the action of the muscle and, hence, is omitted here. The term "resistance," unless otherwise specifically stated, refers to the pressure applied by the examiner, and this is in the direction opposite to that of the movement. For brevity and uniformity in description of the tests, the method of testing in which the patient initiates action against the resistance of the examiner is given except when the other method is distinctly more applicable. However, *this concession to uniformity and brevity of description is not meant to imply a preference for the method of testing in which the patient initiates action.* The location of the belly of the muscle and its tendon is often given to stress the importance of observation and palpation in identifying the function of that particular muscle. Only those participating muscles are listed that have a definite action in the movement being tested and that may substitute at least in part for the muscle being discussed.

Trapezius (Figs. 8-3 and 8-4)
Spinal accessory N

Action:

- Elevation, retraction (adduction), and rotation (lateral angle upward) of scapula, providing fixation of scapula during many movements of arm.

Test:

- Elevation (shrugging) of shoulder against resistance tests upper portion, which is readily visible.
- Bracing shoulder (backward movement and adduction of scapula) tests chiefly middle portion.
- Abduction of arm against resistance intensifies winging of scapula.

In isolated trapezius palsy with the shoulder girdle at rest, the scapula is displaced downward and laterally and is rotated so that the superior angle is farther from the spine than the inferior angle. The lateral displacement is due in part to the unopposed action of the serratus anterior. The vertebral border, particularly at the inferior angle, is flared. These changes are accentuated when the arm is abducted from the side against resistance. On flexion (forward elevation) of the arm, however, the flaring of the inferior angle virtually disappears. These features are important in distinguishing trapezius palsy from serratus anterior palsy, which produces an equally characteristic winging of the scapula but in which movement of the arm in these two planes has the opposite effect. Atrophy of the trapezius is evident chiefly in the upper portion.

Participating muscles:

- Elevation — Levator scapulae (cervical Ns 3 and 4 and dorsal scapular N, C 3 4 5).
- Retraction — Rhomboids.
- Upward rotation — Serratus anterior.

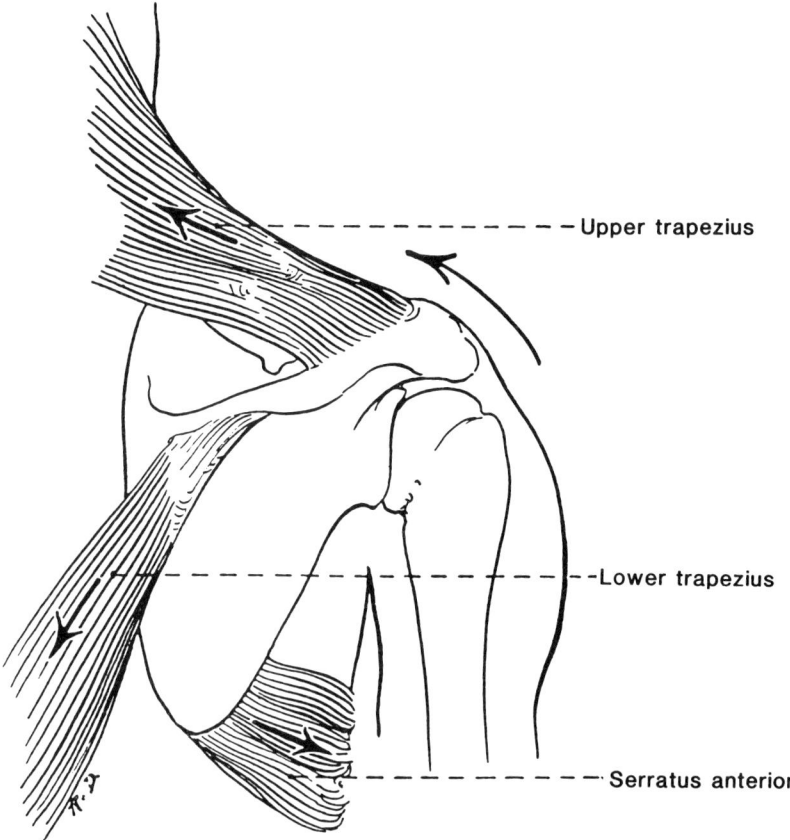

Figure 8-3
Upward rotators of the scapula. *(Redrawn from Hollinshead WH, Jenkins DB: Functional anatomy of the limbs and back, ed 5, Philadelphia, 1981, WB Saunders Co. By permission of Mayo Foundation.)*

Rhomboids (See Fig. 8-4)
Dorsal scapular N from anterior ramus, C 4 5

Action:

- Retraction (adduction) of scapula and elevation of its vertebral border.

Test:

- Hand on hip, arm held backward and medially. Examiner attempts to force elbow laterally and forward, observing and palpating muscle bellies medial to scapula.

Participating muscles:

- Trapezius; levator scapulae — elevation of medial border of scapula.

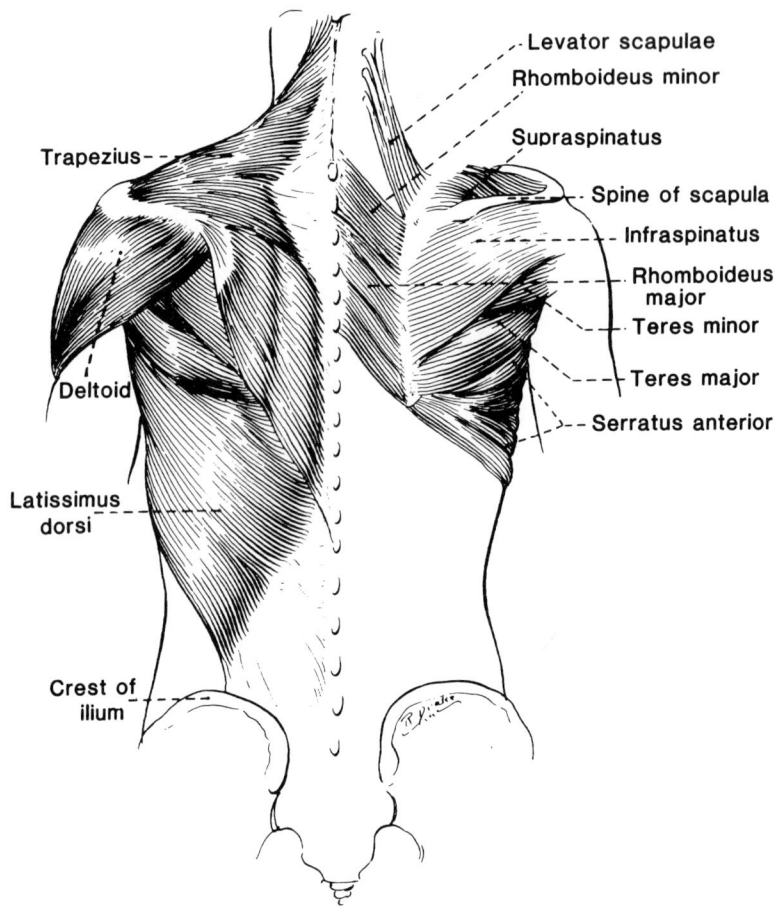

Figure 8-4
Musculature of the shoulder from behind. *(From Hollinshead WH, Jenkins DB: Functional anatomy of the limbs and back, ed 5, Philadelphia, 1981, WB Saunders Co. By permission of Mayo Foundation.)*

Serratus Anterior (See Fig. 8-3)
Long thoracic N from anterior rami, C 5 6 7

Action:

- Protraction (lateral and forward movement) of scapula, keeping it closely applied to thorax.
- Assistance in upward rotation of scapula.

Test:

- Forward thrust of outstretched arm against wall or against resistance by examiner.

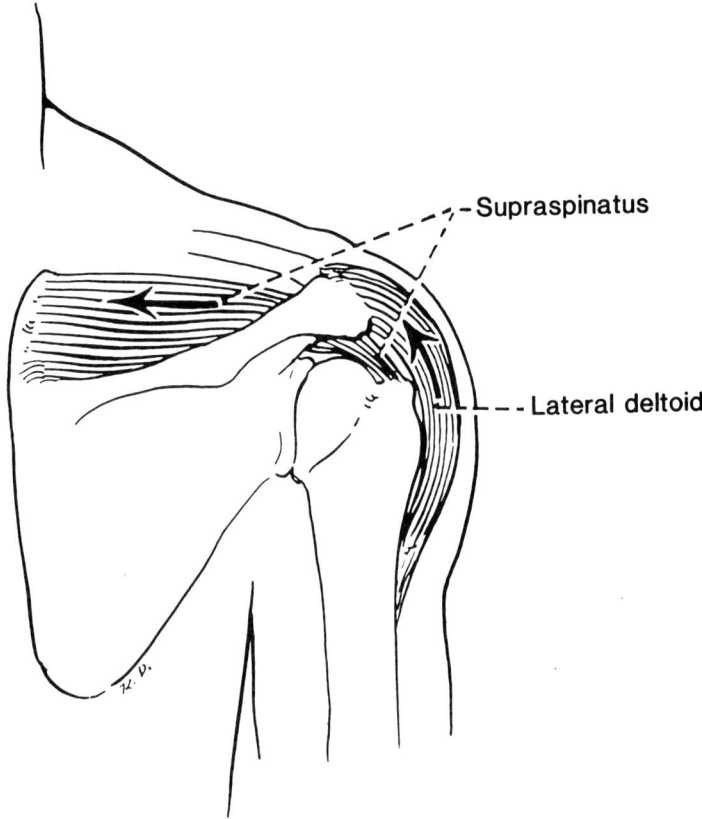

Figure 8-5
Abductors of the humerus. *(From Hollinshead WH, Jenkins DB: Functional anatomy of the limbs and back, ed 5, Philadelphia, 1981, WB Saunders Co. By permission of Mayo Foundation.)*

Isolated palsy results in comparatively little change in the appearance of the shoulder girdle at rest. There is, however, slight winging of the inferior angle of the scapula and a slight shift medially toward the spine. When the outstretched arm is thrust forward, the entire scapula, particularly its inferior angle, shifts backward away from the thorax, producing the characteristic wing effect. Abduction of the arm laterally, however, produces comparatively little winging, demonstrating again an important difference from the manifestations of paralysis of the trapezius.

Supraspinatus (Fig. 8-5)
Suprascapular N from upper trunk of brachial plexus, C 5 6

Action:

- Initiation of abduction of arm from side of body.

Test:

- Above action against resistance.

Atrophy may be detected just above the spine of the scapula, but the trapezius overlies the supraspinatus and atrophy of either muscle will produce a depression in this area. Scapular fixation is important in this test.

Participating muscle:

- Deltoid.

Infraspinatus (Fig. 8-6)
Suprascapular N from upper trunk of brachial plexus, C $\underline{5}$ 6

Action:

- Lateral (external) rotation of arm at shoulder.

Test:

- Elbow at side and flexed 90 degrees. Patient resists examiner's attempt to push the hand medially toward the abdomen.

The muscle is palpable, and atrophy may be visible below the spine of the scapula.

Participating muscles:

- Teres minor (axillary N); deltoid—posterior fibers.

Pectoralis Major (Fig. 8-7)
Clavicular portion (lateral pectoral N from lateral cord of plexus, C 5 $\underline{6}$ 7)
Sternal portion (medial pectoral N from medial cord of plexus, lateral pectoral N, C 6 $\underline{7}$ $\underline{8}$ T $\underline{1}$)

Action:

- Adduction and medial rotation of arm.
- Clavicular portion—assistance in flexion of arm.

Test:

- Arm in front of body. Patient resists attempt by examiner to force it laterally.
- The two portions of the muscle are visible and palpable.

Latissimus Dorsi (Fig. 8-8)
Thoracodorsal N from posterior cord of plexus, C 6 $\underline{7}$ 8

Action:

- Adduction, extension, and medial rotation of arm.

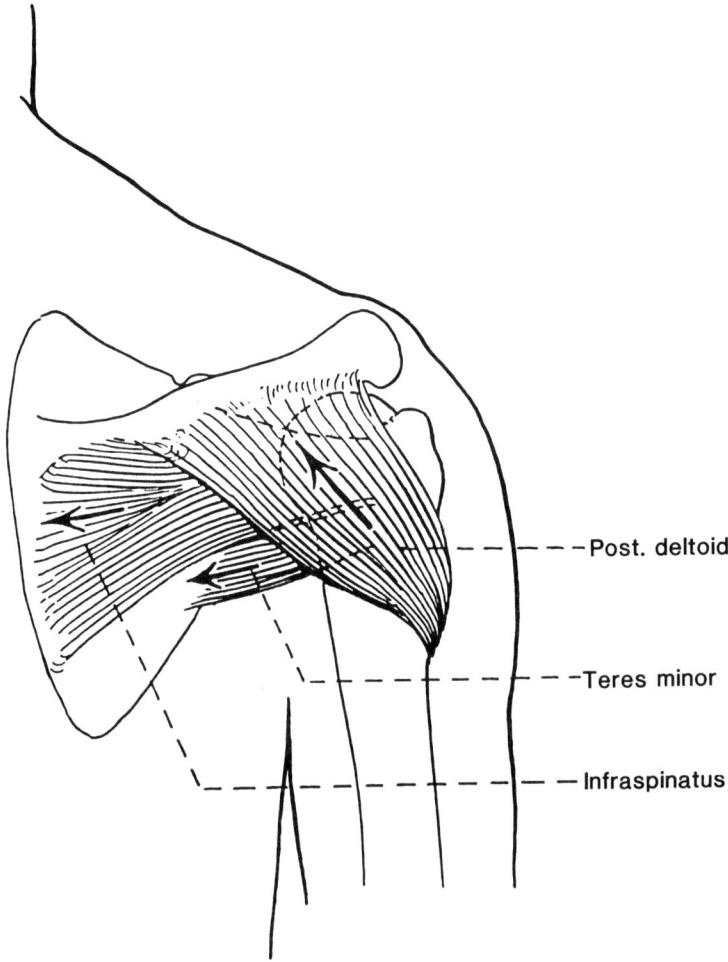

Figure 8-6
The chief external rotators of the humerus. *(From Hollinshead WH, Jenkins DB: Functional anatomy of the limbs and back, ed 5, Philadelphia, 1981, WB Saunders Co. By permission of Mayo Foundation.)*

Test:

- Arm in abduction to horizontal position. Downward and backward movement against resistance applied under elbow.

The muscle should be observed and palpated in and below the posterior axillary fold. When the patient coughs, a brisk contraction of the normal latissimus dorsi can be felt at the inferior angle of the scapula.

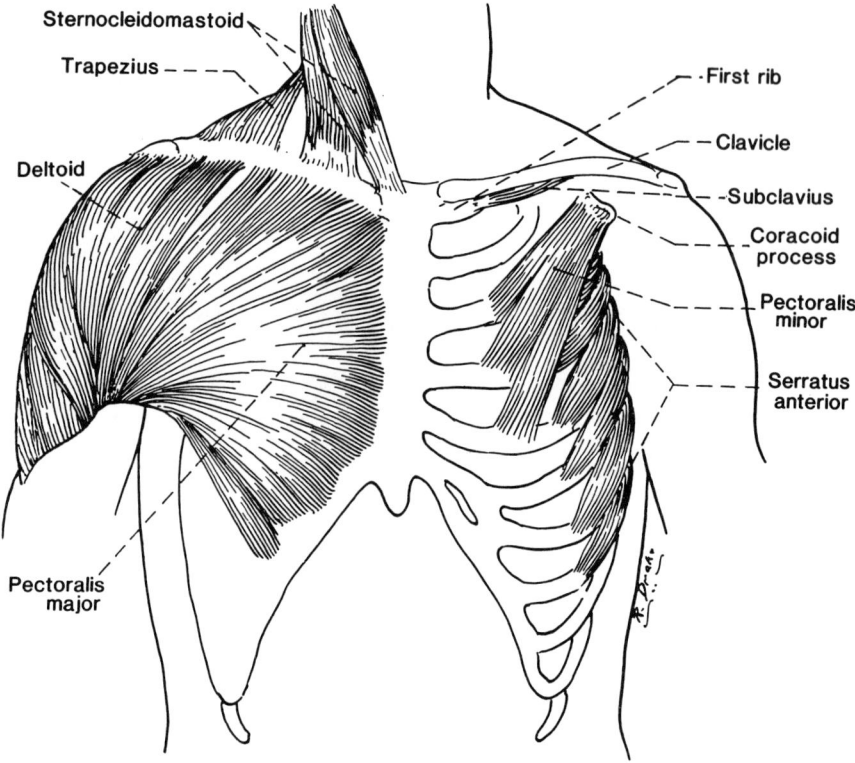

Figure 8-7
Muscles of the pectoral region. *(Redrawn from Hollinshead WH, Jenkins DB: Functional anatomy of the limbs and back, ed 5, Philadelphia, 1981, WB Saunders Co. By permission of Mayo Foundation.)*

Teres Major (See Fig. 8-8 A)
Lower subscapular N from posterior cord plexus, C 5 6 7

Action/Test:

- Same as for latissimus dorsi.

The muscle is visible and palpable at the lower lateral border of the scapula.

Deltoid (See Fig. 8-5 through 8-7 and 8-8 C)
Axillary N from posterior cord of plexus, C 5̲ 6̲

Action:

- Abduction of arm.
- Flexion (forward movement) and medial rotation of arm — anterior fibers.

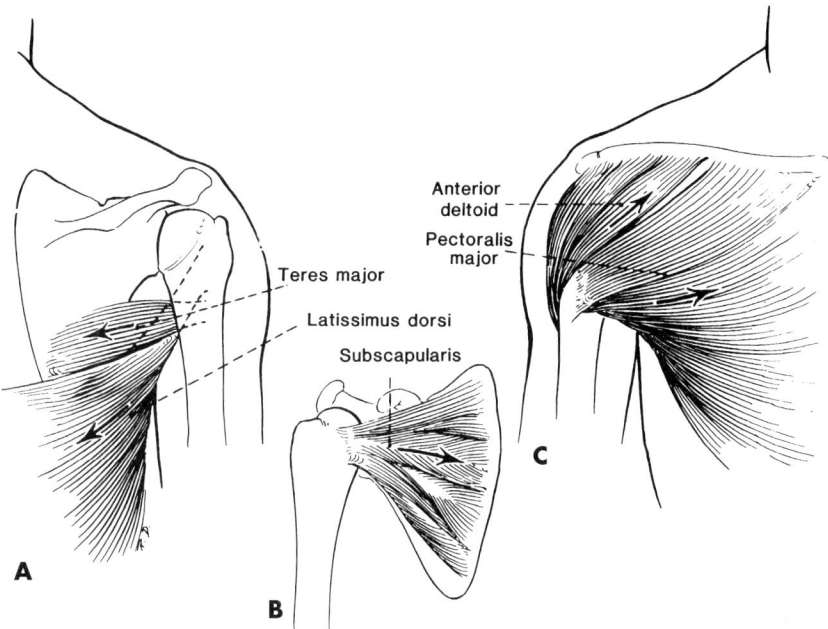

Figure 8-8
The chief internal rotators of the humerus. A, Posterior view. B and C, Anterior views. *(From Hollinshead WH, Jenkins DB: Functional anatomy of the limbs and back, ed 5, Philadelphia, 1981, WB Saunders Co. By permission of Mayo Foundation.)*

- Extension (backward movement) and lateral rotation of arm — posterior fibers.

Test:

- Arm in abduction almost to horizontal. Patient resists effort of examiner to depress elbow.

Paralysis of the deltoid leads to conspicuous atrophy and serious disability, since the other muscles that participate in abduction of the arm (the supraspinatus, trapezius, and serratus anterior — the last two by rotating the scapula) cannot compensate for lack of function of the deltoid.

- Flexion and extension of the arm against resistance.

Participating muscles:

- Abduction — see above.
- Flexion — Pectoralis major — clavicular portion; biceps.
- Extension — Latissimus dorsi; teres major.

Subscapularis (See Fig. 8-8 B)
Upper and lower subscapular Ns from posterior cord of plexus, C 5̲ 6̲ 7

Action:

- Medial (internal) rotation of arm at shoulder.

Test:

- Elbow at side and flexed 90 degrees. Patient resists examiner's attempt to pull the hand laterally.

Since this muscle is not accessible to observation or palpation, it is necessary to gauge the activity of other muscles that produce this movement. The pectoralis major is the most powerful medial rotator of the arm; hence, paralysis of the subscapularis alone results in relatively little weakness of this movement.

Participating muscles:

- Pectoralis major; deltoid—anterior fibers; teres major; latissimus dorsi.

Biceps; Brachialis (Fig. 8-9)
Musculocutaneous N from lateral cord of plexus, C 5̲ 6̲

Action:

- Biceps—Flexion and supination of forearm. Assistance in flexion of arm at shoulder.
- Brachialis—Flexion of forearm at elbow.

Test:

- Flexion of forearm against resistance. Forearm should be in supination to decrease participation of brachioradialis.

• • •

The next group of muscles examined is that supplied by the radial nerve, which is formed as the major branch of the posterior cord of the brachial plexus.

Triceps (Fig. 8-10)
Radial N, which is continuation of posterior cord of plexus, C 6 7̲ 8

Action:

- Extension of forearm at elbow.

Test:

- Forearm in flexion to varying degree. Patient resists effort of examiner to flex forearm further. Slight weakness more easily detected when test is begun with forearm almost completely flexed.

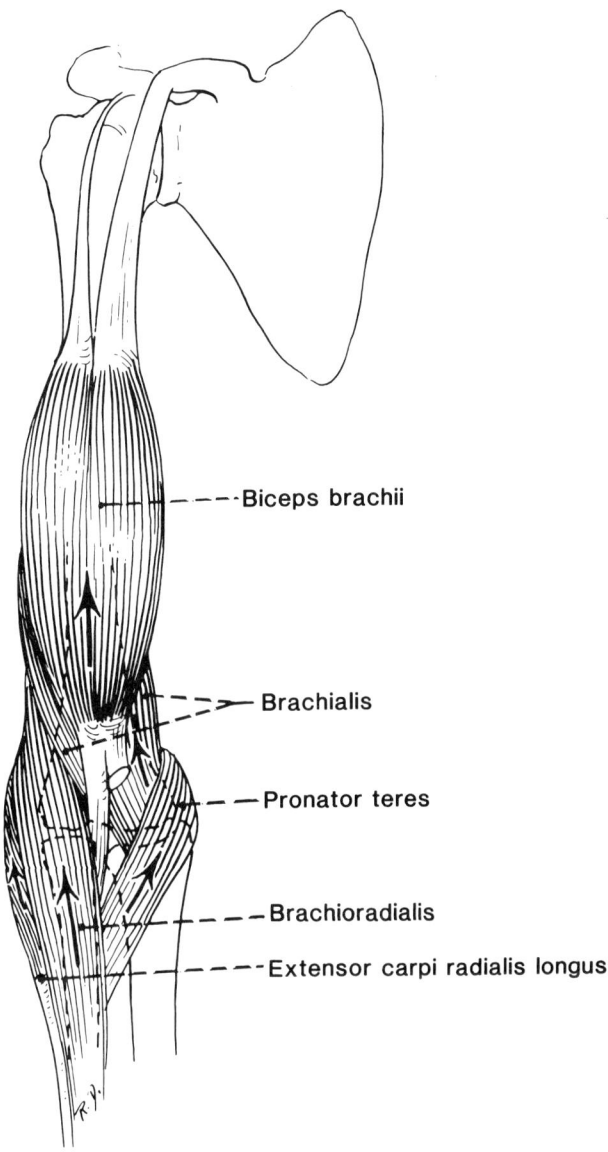

Figure 8-9
The flexors of the elbow. *(From Hollinshead WH, Jenkins DB: Functional anatomy of the limbs and back, ed 5, Philadelphia, 1981, WB Saunders Co. By permission of Mayo Foundation.)*

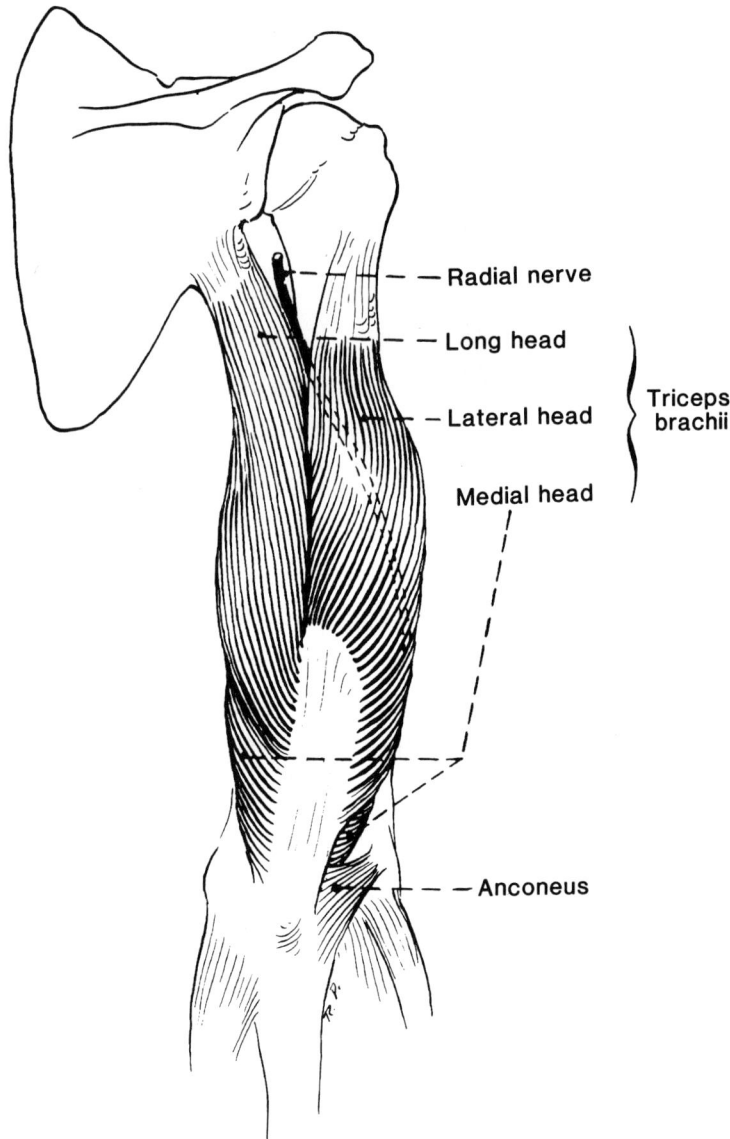

Figure 8-10
Muscles of the extensor (posterior) surface of the right arm. *(From Hollinshead WH, Jenkins DB: Functional anatomy of the limbs and back, ed 5, Philadelphia, 1981, WB Saunders Co. By permission of Mayo Foundation.)*

Brachioradialis (Fig. 8-11)
Radial N, C 5 6

Action:

- Flexion of forearm at elbow.

Test:

- Flexion of forearm against resistance with forearm midway between pronation and supination.

The belly of the muscle stands out prominently on the upper surface of the forearm, tending to bridge the angle between the forearm and the arm.

Participating muscles:

- Biceps; brachialis.

Supinator (See Fig. 8-11)
Posterior interosseous N from radial N, C 5 6

Action:

- Supination of forearm.

Test:

- Forearm in full extension and supination. Patient attempts to maintain supination while examiner attempts to pronate forearm and palpates biceps.

Resistance to pronation by the intact supinator can usually be felt before there is appreciable contraction of the biceps.

Extensor Carpi Radialis Longus (Fig. 8-12)
Radial N, C 6 7

Action:

- Extension (dorsiflexion) and radial abduction of hand at wrist.

Test:

- Forearm in almost complete pronation. Dorsiflexion of wrist against resistance applied to dorsum of hand downward and toward ulnar side.

The tendon is palpable just above its insertion into the base of the second metacarpal bone. The fingers and thumb should be relaxed and somewhat flexed to minimize participation of the extensors of the digits.

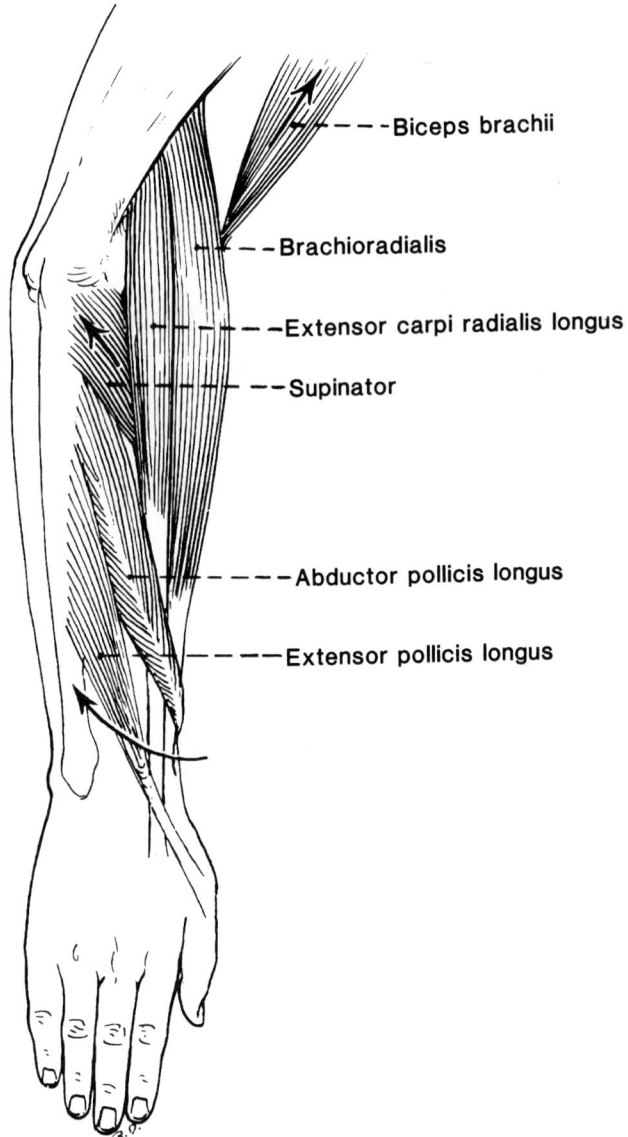

Figure 8-11
The chief supinators of the forearm. *(Redrawn from Hollinshead WH, Jenkins DB: Functional anatomy of the limbs and back, ed 5, Philadelphia, 1981, WB Saunders Co. By permission of Mayo Foundation.)*

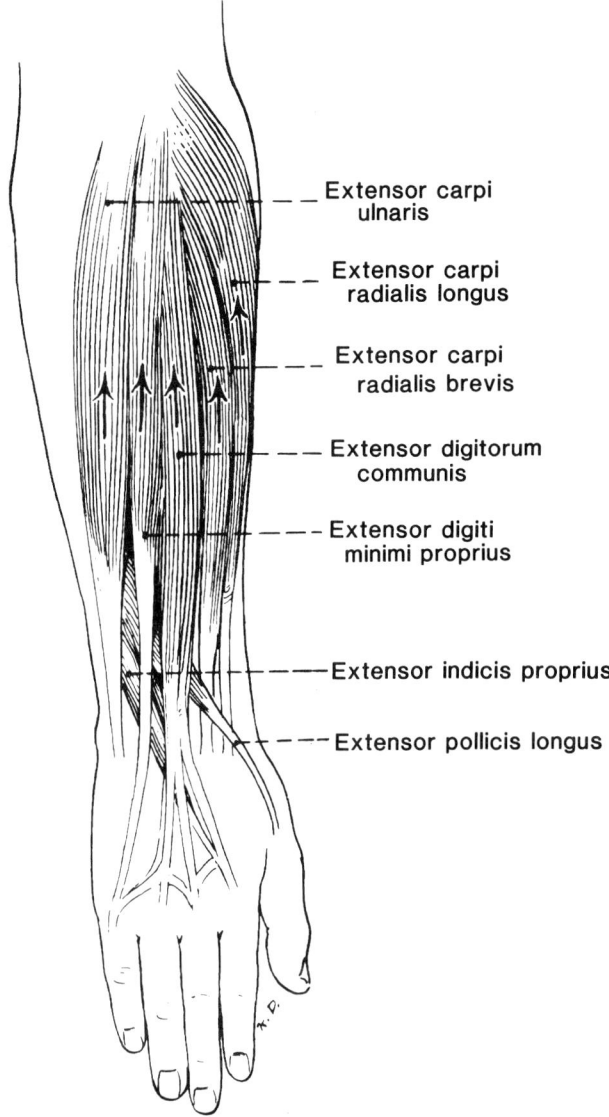

Figure 8-12
The chief extensors of the wrist. *(From Hollinshead WH, Jenkins DB: Functional anatomy of the limbs and back, ed 5, Philadelphia, 1981, WB Saunders Co. By permission of Mayo Foundation.)*

Extensor Carpi Radialis Brevis (See Fig. 8-12)
Posterior interosseous N from radial N, C 6 7

Action:

- Extension (dorsiflexion) of hand at wrist.

Test:

- Forearm in complete pronation. Dorsiflexion of wrist against resistance applied to dorsum of hand straight downward.

The tendon is palpable just proximal to the base of the third metacarpal bone. The fingers and thumb should be relaxed and somewhat flexed to minimize participation of the extensors of the digits.

Extensor Carpi Ulnaris (See Fig. 8-12)
Posterior interosseous N from radial N, C 7 8

Action:

- Extension (dorsiflexion) and ulnar deviation of hand at wrist.

Test:

- Forearm in pronation. Dorsiflexion and ulnar deviation of wrist against resistance applied to dorsum of hand downward and toward radial side.

The tendon is palpable just below or above the distal end of the ulna. The fingers should be relaxed and somewhat flexed to minimize participation of the extensors of the digits.

Extensor Digitorum Communis (See Fig. 8-12)
Posterior interosseous N from radial N, C 7 8

Action:

- Extension of fingers, principally at metacarpophalangeal joints.
- Assistance in extension (dorsiflexion) of wrist.

Test:

- Forearm in pronation. Wrist stabilized in straight position. Extension of fingers at metacarpophalangeal joints against resistance applied to proximal phalanges.

The distal portions of the fingers may be somewhat relaxed and in slight flexion. The tendons are visible and palpable over the dorsum of the hand.

Extension at the interphalangeal joints is a function primarily of the interossei (ulnar nerve) and lumbricals (median and ulnar nerves).

The extensor digiti quinti and extensor indicis (posterior interosseous nerve, C 7 **8**), proper extensors of the little and index fingers, respectively, can be tested individually while the other fingers are in flexion to minimize the action of the common extensor. In a thin person's hand, the tendons can usually be identified.

Abductor Pollicis Longus (See Fig. 8-11)
Posterior interosseous N from radial N, C $\underline{7}$ 8

Action:
- Radial abduction of thumb (in same plane as that of palm, in contradistinction to palmar abduction, which is movement perpendicular to plane of palm).
- Assistance in radial abduction and flexion of hand at wrist.

Test:
- Hand on edge (forearm midway between pronation and supination).
- Radial abduction of thumb against resistance applied to metacarpal.

The tendon is palpable just above its insertion into the base of the metacarpal bone and forms the anterior (volar) boundary of the "anatomic snuffbox."

Participating muscle:
- Extensor pollicis brevis.

Extensor Pollicis Brevis
Posterior interosseous N from radial N, C $\underline{7}$ 8

Action:
- Extension of proximal phalanx of thumb.
- Assistance in radial abduction and extension of metacarpal of thumb.

Test:
- Hand on edge. Wrist and particularly metacarpal of thumb stabilized by examiner. Extension of proximal phalanx against resistance applied to that phalanx while distal phalanx is in flexion to minimize action of extensor pollicis longus.

At the wrist, the tendon lies just posterior (dorsal) to the tendon of the abductor pollicis longus.

Participating muscle:
- Extensor pollicis longus.

Extensor Pollicis Longus (See Fig. 8-12)
Posterior interosseous N from radial N, C 7 8

Action:

- Extension of all parts of thumb but specifically extension of distal phalanx.
- Assistance in adduction of thumb.

Test:

- Hand on edge. Wrist, metacarpal, and proximal phalanx of thumb stabilized by examiner with thumb close to palm at its radial border. Extension of distal phalanx against resistance.

If the patient is permitted to flex the wrist or abduct the thumb away from the palm, some extension of the phalanges results simply from lengthening of the path of the extensor tendon. At the wrist, the tendon forms the posterior (dorsal) boundary of the "anatomic snuffbox."

The characteristic result of radial nerve palsy is wristdrop. Extension of the fingers at the interphalangeal joints is still possible by virtue of the action of the interossei and lumbricals, but extension of the thumb is lost.

• • •

The next group of muscles examined is that supplied by the median nerve, which is formed by the union of its lateral root, from the lateral cord of the brachial plexus, and its medial root, from the medial cord of the plexus. Then the muscles supplied by the ulnar nerve (arising from the medial cord of the brachial plexus) are tested. However, for convenience in order of examination, some of the muscles in the ulnar group are tested with the median group.

Pronator Teres (Fig. 8-13)
Median N, C 6 7

Action:

- Pronation of forearm.

Test:

- Elbow at side of trunk, forearm in flexion to right angle, and arm in lateral rotation at shoulder to eliminate effect of gravity, which, in most positions, favors pronation. Pronation of forearm against resistance, starting from a position of moderate supination.

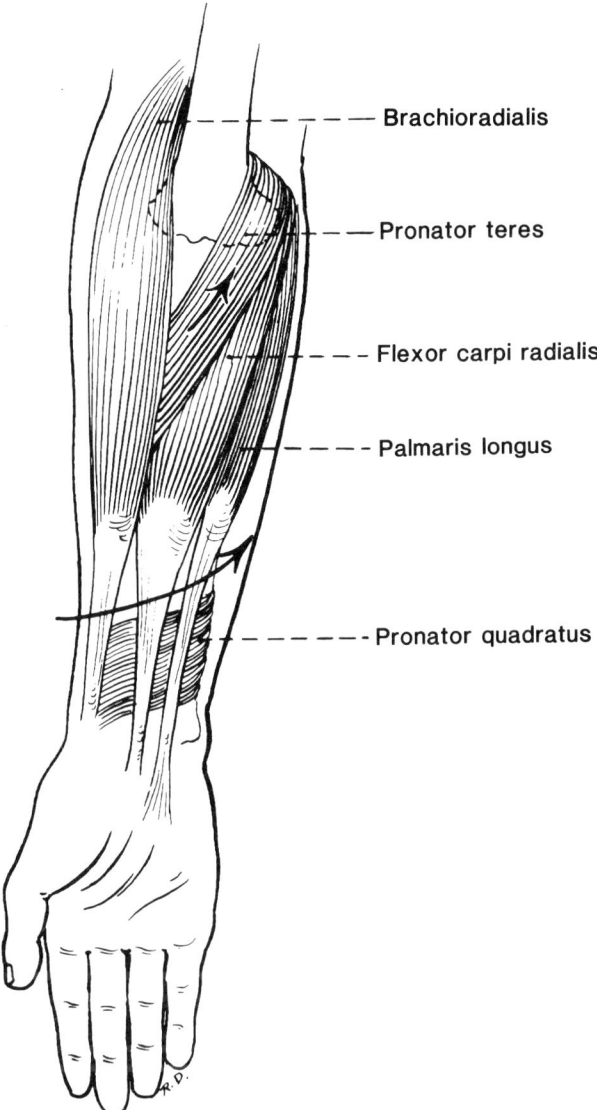

Figure 8-13
Pronators of the forearm. *(From Hollinshead WH, Jenkins DB: Functional anatomy of the limbs and back, ed 5, Philadelphia, 1981, WB Saunders Co. By permission of Mayo Foundation.)*

Participating muscle:

- Pronator quadratus (anterior interosseous branch of median N, C 7 <u>8</u> T 1)

Flexor Carpi Radialis (Fig. 8-13 and 8-14)
Median N, C <u>6</u> <u>7</u>

Action:

- Flexion (palmar flexion) of hand at wrist.
- Assistance in radial abduction of hand.

Test:

- Flexion of hand against resistance applied to palm.
- Fingers should be relaxed to minimize participation of their flexors.

The tendon is the more lateral (radial) of the two conspicuous tendons on the volar aspect of the wrist.

In complete median nerve palsy, flexion of the wrist is considerably weakened but can still be performed by the flexor carpi ulnaris (ulnar nerve) assisted to some extent by the abductor pollicis longus (radial nerve). In this event, ulnar deviation of the hand usually accompanies flexion.

Palmaris Longus (See Fig. 8-13 and 8-14)
Median N, C 7 <u>8</u> T 1

Action:

- Flexion of hand at wrist.

Test:

- Same as that for flexor carpi radialis.

The tendon is palpable at the ulnar side of the tendon of the flexor carpi radialis.

Flexor Carpi Ulnaris (See Fig. 8-14)
Ulnar N, C 7 <u>8</u> T 1

Action:

- Flexion and ulnar deviation of hand at wrist.
- Fixation of pisiform bone during contraction of abductor digiti quinti.

Test:

- Flexion and ulnar deviation of hand against resistance applied to ulnar side of palm in direction of extension and radial abduction. Fingers should be relaxed.

The tendon is palpable proximal to the pisiform bone.

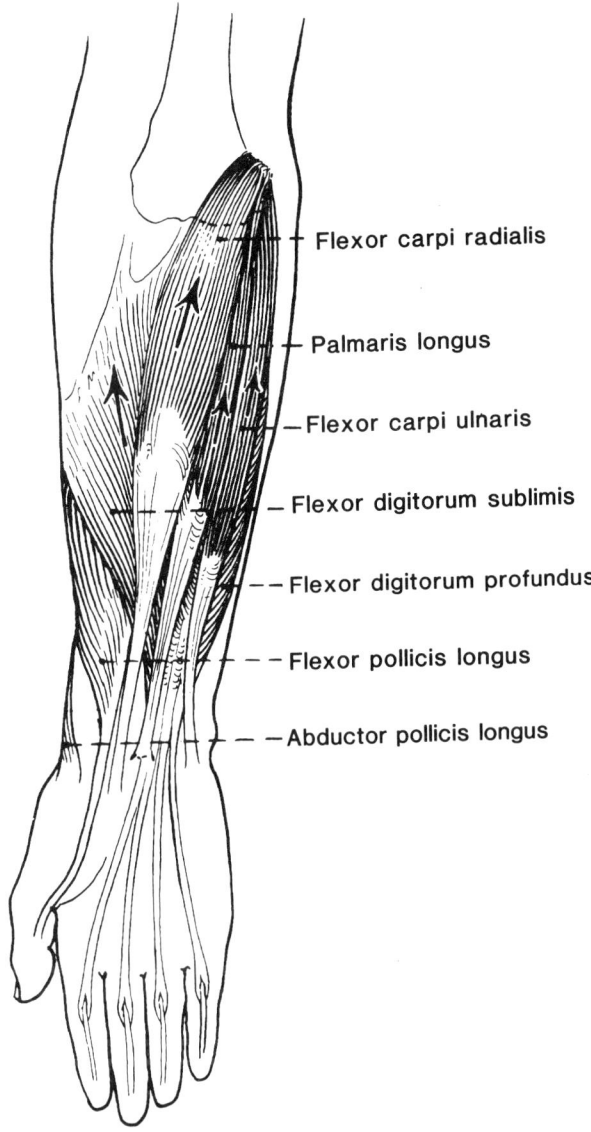

Figure 8-14
The chief flexors of the wrist. *(From Hollinshead WH, Jenkins DB: Functional anatomy of the limbs and back, ed 5, Philadelphia, 1981, WB Saunders Co. By permission of Mayo Foundation.)*

Flexor Digitorum Sublimis (See Fig. 8-14)
Median N, C 7 <u>8</u>

Action:

- Flexion of middle phalanges of fingers at first interphalangeal joints primarily; flexion of proximal phalanges at metacarpophalangeal joints secondarily.
- Assistance in flexion of hand at wrist.

Test:

- Wrist in neutral position, proximal phalanges stabilized. Flexion of middle phalanx of each finger against resistance applied to that phalanx, with distal phalanx relaxed.

Flexor Digitorum Profundus (See Fig. 8-14)
Radial portion—usually to digits II and III (median N and its anterior interosseous branch, C 7 <u>8</u> T 1)
Ulnar portion—usually to digits IV and V (ulnar N, C 7 <u>8</u> T <u>1</u>)

Action:

- Flexion of distal phalanges of fingers specifically; flexion of other phalanges secondarily.
- Assistance in flexion of hand at wrist.

Test:

- Flexion of distal phalanges against resistance with proximal and middle phalanges stabilized in extension.
- With middle and distal phalanges folded over edge of examiner's hand, patient resists attempt by examiner to extend distal phalanges.

Flexor Pollicis Longus (See Fig. 8-14)
Anterior interosseous branch of median N, C 7 <u>8</u> T <u>1</u>

Action:

- Flexion of thumb, particularly distal phalanx.
- Assistance in ulnar adduction of thumb.

Test:

- Flexion of distal phalanx against resistance with thumb in position of palmar adduction and with stabilization of metacarpal and proximal phalanx.

Abductor Pollicis Brevis (Fig. 8-15)
Median N, C <u>8</u> T <u>1</u>

Action:

- Palmar abduction of thumb (perpendicular to plane of palm).
- Assistance in opposition and in flexion of proximal phalanx of thumb.

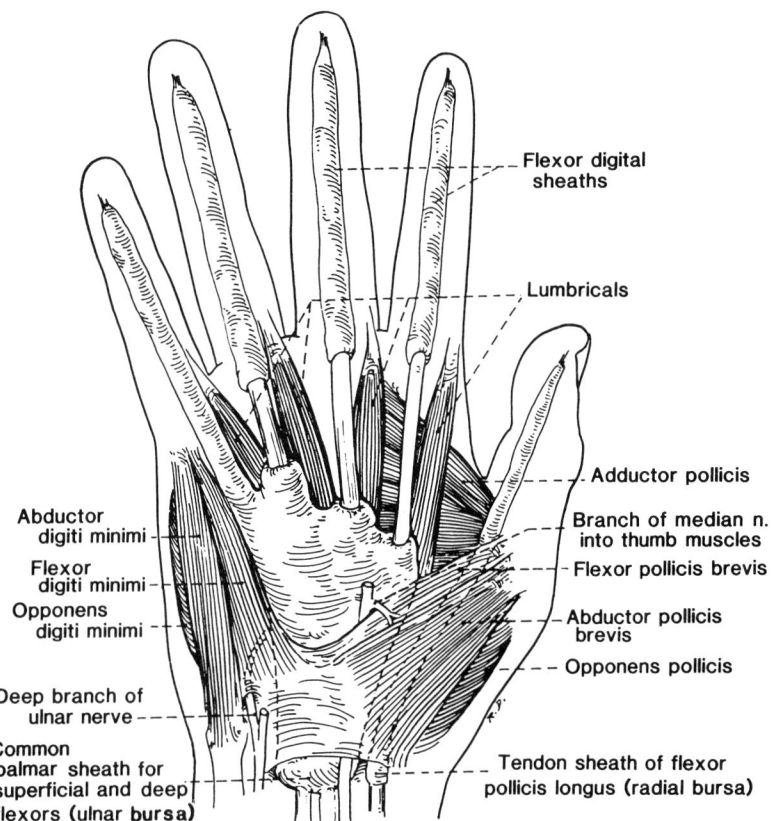

Figure 8-15
Short muscles of the thumb and little finger. *(Redrawn from Hollinshead WH, Jenkins DB: Functional anatomy of the limbs and back, ed 5, Philadelphia, 1981, WB Saunders Co. By permission of Mayo Foundation.)*

Test:

- Palmar abduction of thumb against resistance applied at metacarpophalangeal joint.

The muscle is readily visible and palpable in the thenar eminence.

Participating muscle:

- Flexor pollicis brevis (superficial head).

Opponens Pollicis (See Fig. 8-15)
Median N, C 8 T 1

Action:

- Movement of first metacarpal across palm, rotating it into opposition.

Test:

- Thumb in opposition. Examiner attempts to rotate and draw thumb back to its usual position.

Participating muscles:

- Abductor pollicis brevis; flexor pollicis brevis.

Flexor Pollicis Brevis (See Fig. 8-15)
Superficial head (median N, C 8 T 1); deep head (ulnar N, C 8 T 1)

Action:

- Flexion of proximal phalanx of thumb.
- Assistance in opposition, ulnar adduction (entire muscle), and palmar abduction (superficial head) of thumb.

Test:

- Thumb in position of palmar adduction with stabilization of metacarpal.
- Flexion of proximal phalanx against resistance applied to that phalanx while distal phalanx is as relaxed as possible.

Participating muscles:

- Flexor pollicis longus; abductor pollicis brevis; adductor pollicis.

Severe median nerve palsy produces the "simian" hand, wherein the thumb tends to lie in the same plane as the palm, with the volar surface facing more anteriorly than normal. Atrophy of the muscles of the thenar eminence is usually conspicuous.

Three muscles supplied, at least in part, by the ulnar nerve have already been described: flexor carpi ulnaris, flexor digitorum profundus, and flexor pollicis brevis. The remaining muscles supplied by this nerve follow.

Hypothenar Muscles
Ulnar N, C 8 T 1

Action:

- Abductor digiti quinti and flexor digiti quinti—abduction and flexion (proximal phalanx) of little finger.
- Opponens digiti quinti—opposition of little finger toward thumb.
- All three muscles—palmar elevation of head of fifth metacarpal, helping to cup palm.

Test:

- Action usually tested is abduction of little finger (against resistance).

The abductor digiti quinti is readily observed and palpated at the ulnar border of the palm. Opposition of the thumb and little finger can be tested together by gauging the force required to separate the tips of the two digits when opposed or by attempting to withdraw a piece of paper clasped between the tips of the digits.

Interossei (Fig. 8-16 and 8-17)
Ulnar N, C 8 T 1

Action:

- Dorsal—abduction of index, middle, and ring fingers from middle line of middle finger (double action on middle finger—both radial and ulnar abduction, radial abduction of index finger, ulnar abduction of ring finger).
- First dorsal—adduction (especially palmar adduction) of thumb.
- Palmar—adduction of index, ring, and little fingers toward middle finger.
- Both sets—flexion at the metacarpophalangeal joints and simultaneous extension at the interphalangeal joints.

Test:

- Abduction and adduction of individual fingers against resistance with fingers extended. Adduction can be tested by retention of a slip of paper between fingers, and between thumb and index finger, as examiner attempts to withdraw it.
- Ability of patient to flex proximal phalanges and simultaneously extend distal phalanges.
- Extension of middle phalanges of fingers against resistance while examiner stabilizes proximal phalanges in hyperextension.

The long extensors of the fingers (radial nerve) and the lumbrical muscles (median and ulnar nerves) assist in extension of the middle and distal phalanges. The first dorsal interosseous is readily observed and palpated in the space between the index finger and the thumb.

Adductor Pollicis (See Fig. 8-15)
Ulnar N, C 8 T 1

Action:

- Adduction of thumb in both ulnar and palmar directions (in plane of palm and perpendicular to palm, respectively).
- Assistance in flexion of proximal phalanx.

Test:

- Adduction in each plane against resistance.

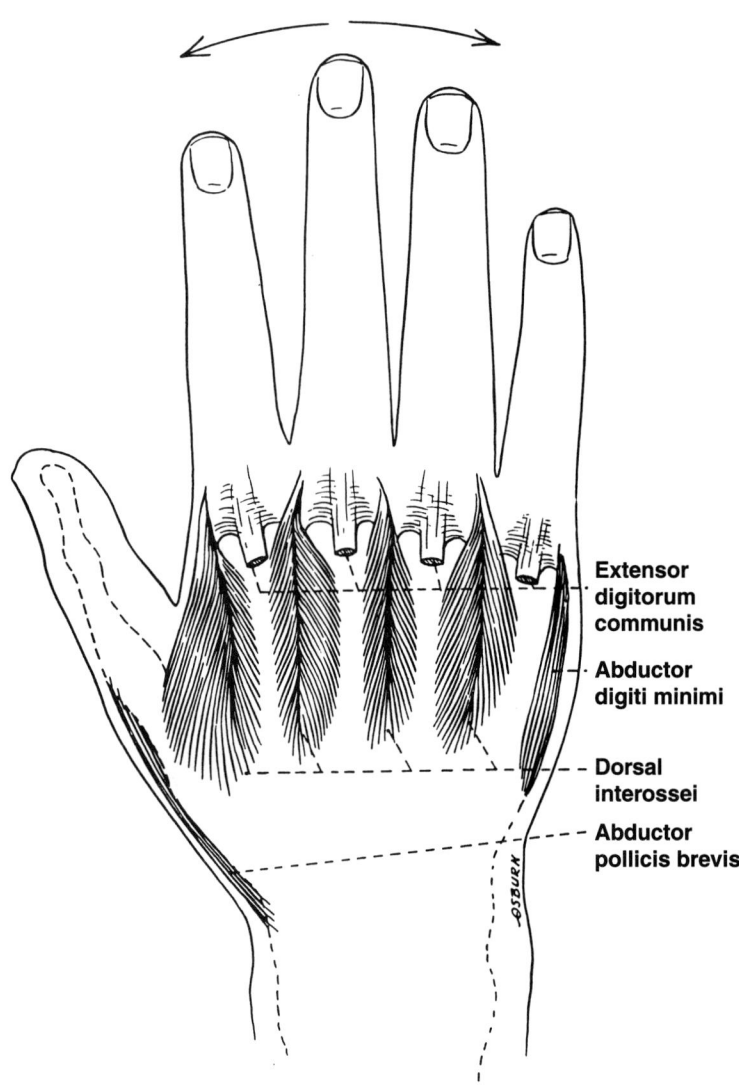

Figure 8-16
Dorsal view of the chief abductors of the digits. *(Redrawn from Hollinshead WH, Jenkins DB: Functional anatomy of the limbs and back, ed 5, Philadelphia, 1981, WB Saunders Co. By permission of Mayo Foundation.)*

- Retention of slip of paper between thumb and radial border of hand and between thumb and palm, without flexion of distal phalanx.

It is often possible to palpate the edge of the adductor pollicis just volar to the proximal part of the first dorsal interosseous.

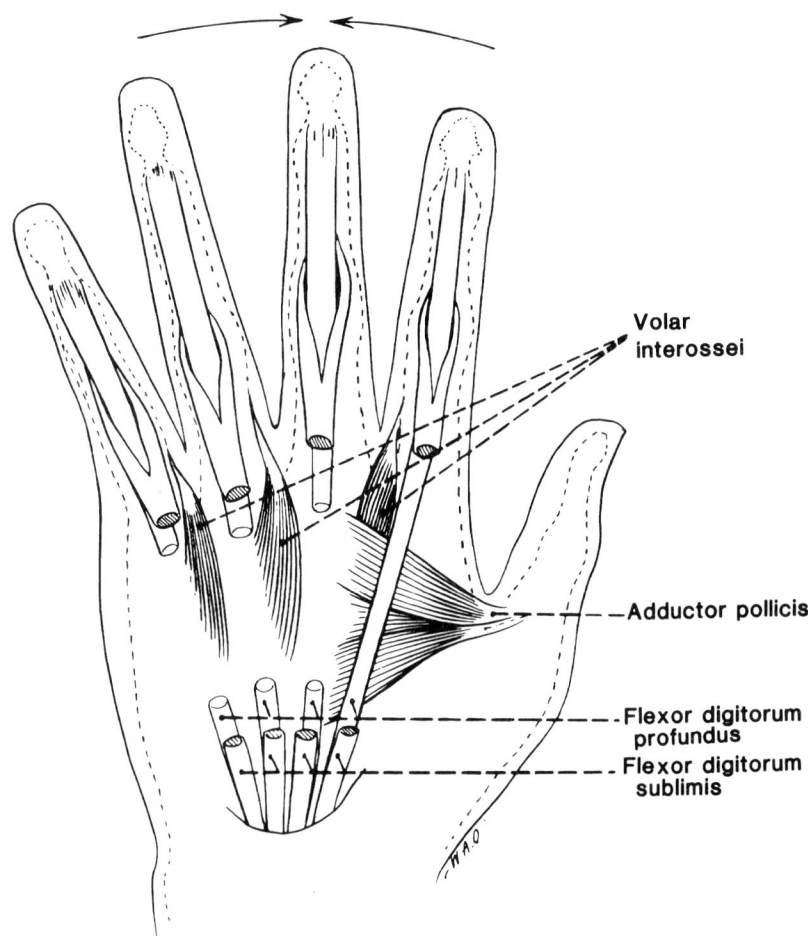

Figure 8-17
The chief adductors of the digits. *(From Hollinshead WH, Jenkins DB: Functional anatomy of the limbs and back, ed 5, Philadelphia, 1981, WB Saunders Co. By permission of Mayo Foundation.)*

Participating muscles:

- Ulnar adduction—first dorsal interosseous; flexor pollicis longus; extensor pollicis longus; flexor pollicis brevis.
- Palmar adduction—first dorsal interosseous particularly; extensor pollicis longus.

In severe ulnar nerve palsy, atrophy is evident between the thumb and index finger, between the extensor tendons on the dorsum of the hand, and in the hypothenar eminence. The little finger is separated

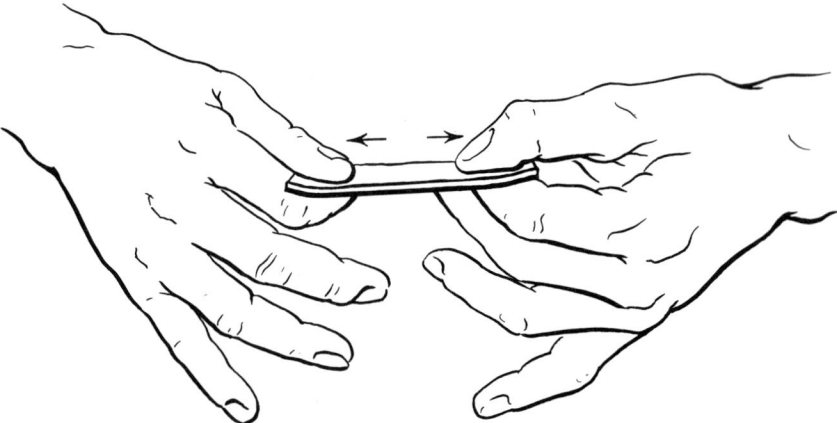

Figure 8-18
Froment's sign of ulnar palsy. Positive in the left hand, as indicated by flexion of the terminal phalanx of the thumb.

from the ring finger and cannot be brought into contact with it. The little and ring fingers, especially, are hyperextended at the metacarpophalangeal joints and flexed at the interphalangeal joints. The index and middle fingers are much less affected because of the intact lumbricals of these fingers (supplied by the median nerve). The true "claw-hand" (main en griffe) is found only in combined median and ulnar nerve palsy. Attempt at adduction of the thumb is usually accompanied by flexion of the distal phalanx, indicating activity of the flexor pollicis longus (median nerve) in an effort to compensate for paralysis of the adductor. Froment's sign of ulnar palsy is an application of this phenomenon (Fig. 8-18). The patient grasps a piece of cardboard firmly with the thumb and index finger of each hand and pulls vigorously. If flexion of the distal phalanx of the thumb occurs, the test result is positive and indicative of ulnar palsy.

Localization of lesions of the brachial plexus (Fig. 8-19) is based on the pattern of muscular weakness (and the distribution of sensory impairment).

Damage to the most proximal elements of the plexus (anterior primary rami) is manifested by weakness or paralysis of one or more of the muscles deriving nerve supply from the rami, such as the rhomboids and the serratus anterior, as well as by segmental distribution of muscular weakness (and sensory deficit) in the more distal portions of the upper extremity. Injury to the anterior ramus T 1 produces Horner's syndrome.

Lesions involving the most distal parts of the plexus spare some of the muscles of the shoulder girdle, and the pattern of muscular

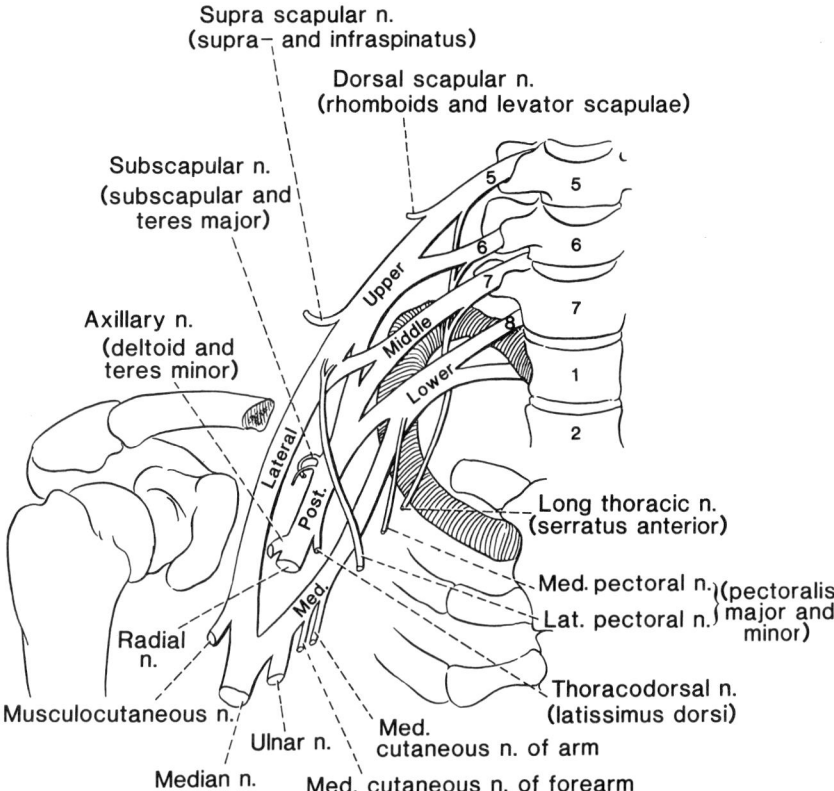

Figure 8-19
The brachial plexus. The muscles supplied by the various nerves are in parentheses.

weakness (and sensory impairment) is more like that due to peripheral nerve injuries.

Lesions affecting the upper portion of the plexus, such as the upper trunk, impair the function of muscles supplied by segments C 5 and 6 (syndrome of Duchenne-Erb), such as the supraspinatus, infraspinatus, deltoid, biceps, brachialis, brachioradialis, and supinator. The arm tends to hang limply at the side, medially rotated and pronated.

Injuries of the lower elements of the plexus, such as the lower trunk, C 8, and T 1 (syndrome of Klumpke), produce disability chiefly of the intrinsic muscles of the hand and flexors of the digits.

These examples illustrate the general principles of localization of lesions on the basis of examination of muscular strength.

• • •

The muscles of the neck and trunk may be examined in groups in most instances.

Flexors of Neck
Cervical Ns, C 1-6

Test:

- Sitting or supine. Flexion of neck, with chin on chest, against resistance applied to forehead.

Extensors of Neck
Cervical Ns, C 1-T 1

Test:

- Sitting or prone. Extension of neck against resistance applied to occiput.

Diaphragm
Phrenic Ns, C 3 4 5

Action:

- Abdominal respiration (inspiration), as distinguished from thoracic respiration (inspiration), which is produced principally by the intercostal muscles.

Test:

- Observation of patient for protrusion of upper portion of abdomen during deep inspiration when thoracic cage is splinted.
- Ability of patient to sniff.
- Litten's sign—successive retraction of lower intercostal spaces during inspiration.
- Fluoroscopic observation of diaphragmatic movements.
- Weakness of the diaphragm should be suspected in diseases of the spinal cord when the deltoid or biceps is paralyzed, for these muscles are supplied by neurons situated very near those innervating the diaphragm.

Intercostal Muscles
Intercostal Ns, T 1-11

Action:

- Expansion of thorax anteroposteriorly and transversely, producing thoracic inspiration.

Test:

- Observation and palpation of expansion of thoracic cage during deep inspiration while maintaining pressure against thorax.
- Observation for asymmetry of movement of thorax, particularly during deep inspiration.

- Other more general tests of function of the respiratory muscles are:
  - Observation of patient for rapid shallow respiration, flaring of alae nasi, and use of accessory muscles of respiration.
  - Ability of patient to repeat three or four numbers without pausing for breath.
  - Ability of patient to hold the breath for 15 seconds.

Anterior Abdominal Muscles
Upper (T 6-<u>9</u>); Lower (T <u>10</u>-L <u>1</u>)

Test:

- Supine—Flexion of neck against resistance applied to forehead by examiner.

Contraction of the abdominal muscles can be observed and palpated. Upward movement of the umbilicus is associated with weakness of the lower abdominal muscles (Beevor's sign).

- Supine—Hands on occiput. Flexion of trunk by anterior abdominal muscles followed by flexion of pelvis on thighs by hip flexors (chiefly iliopsoas) to reach sitting position. Examiner holds legs down.

Completion of this test excludes significant weakness of either the abdominal muscles or the flexors of the hips. Weak abdominal muscles, in the presence of strong hip flexors, result in hyperextension of the lumbar spine during attempts to elevate the legs or rise to a sitting position.

Extensors of Back
Test:

- Prone with hands clasped over buttocks. Elevation of head and shoulders off table while examiner holds legs down.

The gluteal and hamstring muscles fix the pelvis on the thigh.

The movements of the lower extremities are not as complex as those of the upper extremities. Hence, the examination is somewhat simpler. Since the muscles of the pelvic girdle and thigh do not lend themselves as well to a sequence of examination based on the anatomy of the lumbosacral plexus (Fig. 8-20) as the muscles of the upper extremities, the order is determined largely by clinical convenience, with some consideration to segmental innervation.

Many of the muscles are so powerful that when little or no weakness is present, they can be tested profitably by certain maneuvers performed by the patient while upright. Observation of the patient's gait will reveal weakness of certain muscles, and atrophy may be visible:

Iliopsoas—Difficulty in bringing affected leg forward.
Abductors of thigh (chiefly gluteus medius and gluteus

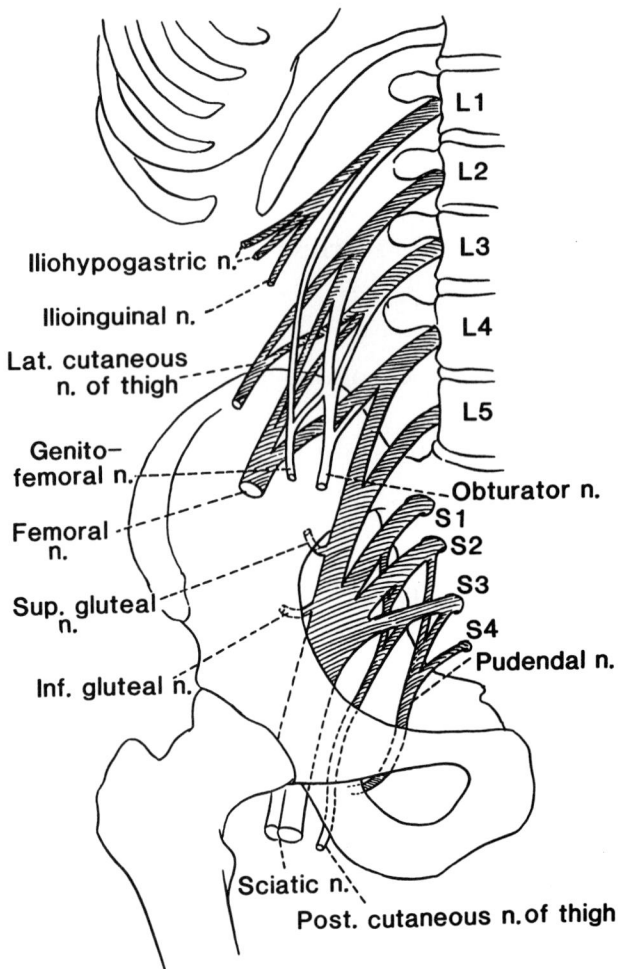

Figure 8-20
The lumbosacral plexus.

minimus)—Sagging of opposite side of pelvis and lateral displacement of pelvis to affected side when weight is on that leg.

Quadriceps—Keeping knee locked when weight is placed on affected leg.

Tibialis anterior and extensors of toes—Various degrees of "steppage gait" and footdrop.

Gastrocnemius and soleus—Limp produced by difficulty in raising heel from floor.

Certain maneuvers by the patient will make muscular weakness more apparent. The principal muscles involved are given:

Stepping up on a step:
  Raising leg up to step—Iliopsoas.
  Raising body—Gluteus maximus and quadriceps.
Squatting and rising—Quadriceps particularly.
Walking on heels—Tibialis anterior and extensors of toes.
Walking on toes—Gastrocnemius and soleus.

When there is little or no weakness, it is feasible to conduct the more detailed examination of the muscles of the lower extremities with the patient in the sitting posture throughout. However, the action of certain muscles is somewhat different in the sitting posture than in the supine or prone position. In particular, some of the lateral rotators of the thigh function also as abductors. Furthermore, the sitting posture interferes seriously with observation and palpation of some muscles—particularly the gluteus maximus and, to a lesser extent, the hamstrings. The muscles mentioned are therefore more accurately tested in the prone position.

In some instances, it is convenient and advantageous to test the corresponding muscles of the two sides simultaneously for comparison. Examples are the adductors and abductors of the thighs and the extensors (dorsiflexors) and flexors (plantar flexors) of the feet and toes.

Iliopsoas (Fig. 8-21)

Psoas major (lumbar plexus [see Fig. 8-20], L 2 3 4); iliacus (femoral N, L 2 3 4)

Action:

- Flexion of thigh at hip.

Test:

- Sitting—Flexion of thigh, raising knee against resistance by examiner.
- Supine—Raising extended leg off table and maintaining it against downward pressure by examiner applied just above knee.

Participating muscles:

- Rectus femoris and sartorius (both—femoral N, L 2 3 4); tensor fasciae latae (superior gluteal N, L 4 5).

Adductor Magnus, Longus, Brevis (See Fig. 8-21)

Obturator N, L 2 3 4; part of adductor magnus is supplied by sciatic N, L 5, and functions with hamstrings

Action:

- Principally adduction of thigh.

Test:

- Sitting or supine—Holding knees together while examiner attempts to separate them.

The legs can also be tested separately and the muscles palpated.

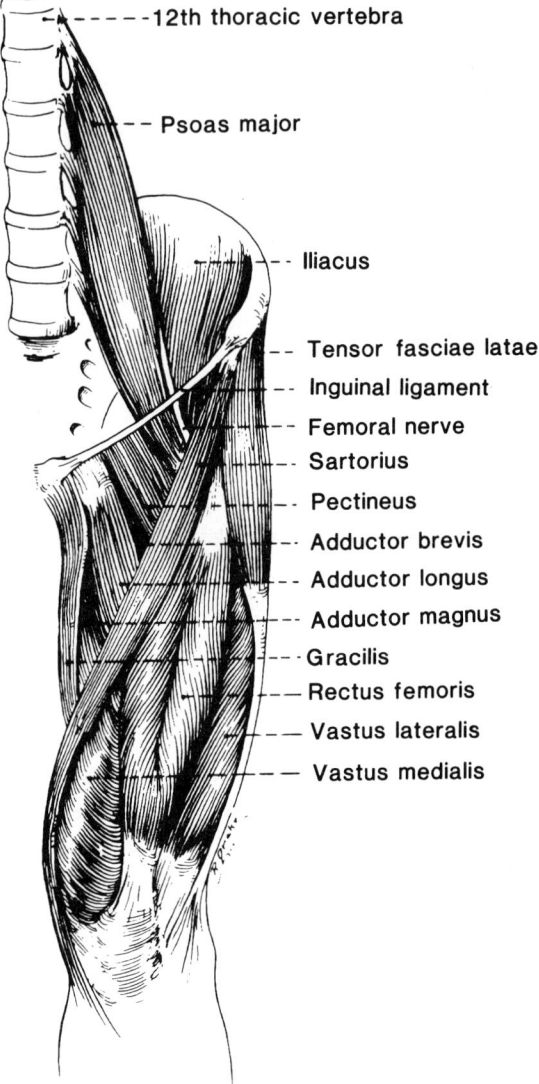

Figure 8-21
The more superficial muscles of the anterior aspect of the thigh. *(From Hollinshead WH, Jenkins DB: Functional anatomy of the limbs and back, ed 5, Philadelphia, 1981, WB Saunders Co. By permission of Mayo Foundation.)*

Participating muscles:

- Gluteus maximus; gracilis (obturator N, L 2 <u>3</u> <u>4</u>)

Abductors of Thigh (Fig. 8-22)
Superior gluteal N, L 4 <u>5</u> S 1
Gluteus medius and gluteus minimus principally
Tensor fasciae latae to a lesser extent

Action:

- Abduction and medial rotation of thigh.
- Tensor fasciae latae assists in flexion of thigh at hip.

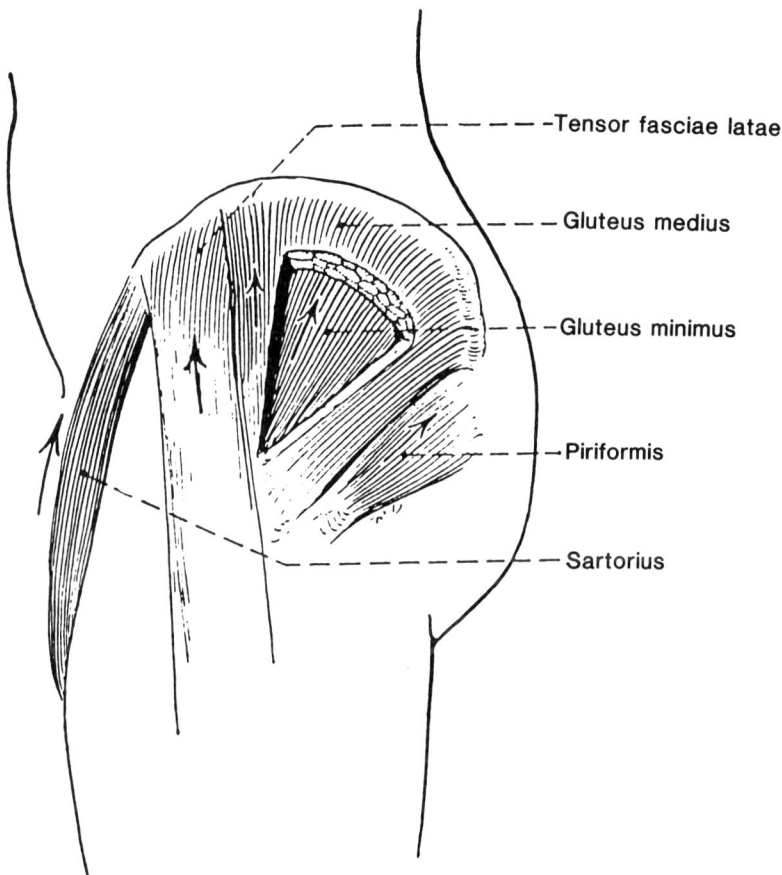

Figure 8-22
The abductors of the thigh. *(From Hollinshead WH, Jenkins DB: Functional anatomy of the limbs and back, ed 5, Philadelphia, 1981, WB Saunders Co. By permission of Mayo Foundation.)*

Test:

- Sitting—Separation of knees against resistance by examiner.

In this position, the gluteus maximus and some of the other lateral rotators of the thigh function as abductors, hence diminishing the accuracy of the test.

- Supine—Same test as for abductors, above. More exact.
- Lying on opposite side—Abduction of hip (upward movement) while examiner presses downward on lower leg and stabilizes pelvis.

The tensor fasciae latae and to a lesser extent the gluteus medius can be palpated.

Medial Rotators of Thigh (See Fig. 8-22)
Same as abductors.
Superior gluteal N, L 4 $\underline{5}$ S 1

Test:

- Sitting or prone—Knee flexed to 90 degrees. Medial rotation of thigh against resistance applied by examiner at knee and ankle in attempt to rotate thigh laterally.

Lateral Rotators of Thigh (Fig. 8-23)
(L $\underline{4}$ $\underline{5}$ S $\underline{1}$ 2)
Gluteus maximus (inferior gluteal N, L 5 S $\underline{1}$ 2) chiefly
Obturator internus and gemellus superior (N to obturator internus, L 5 S $\underline{1}$ 2)
Quadratus femoris and gemellus inferior (N to quadratus femoris, L 4 $\underline{5}$ S $\underline{1}$)

Test:

- Sitting or prone—Knee flexed to 90 degrees. Lateral rotation of thigh against attempt by examiner to rotate thigh medially.

The gluteus maximus is the muscle principally tested and can be observed and palpated in the prone position.

Gluteus Maximus (See Fig. 8-23)
Inferior gluteal N, L 5 S $\underline{1}$ 2

Action:

- Extension of thigh at hip.
- Lateral rotation of thigh.
- Assistance in adduction of thigh.

Test:

- Sitting or supine—Starting with thigh slightly raised, extension

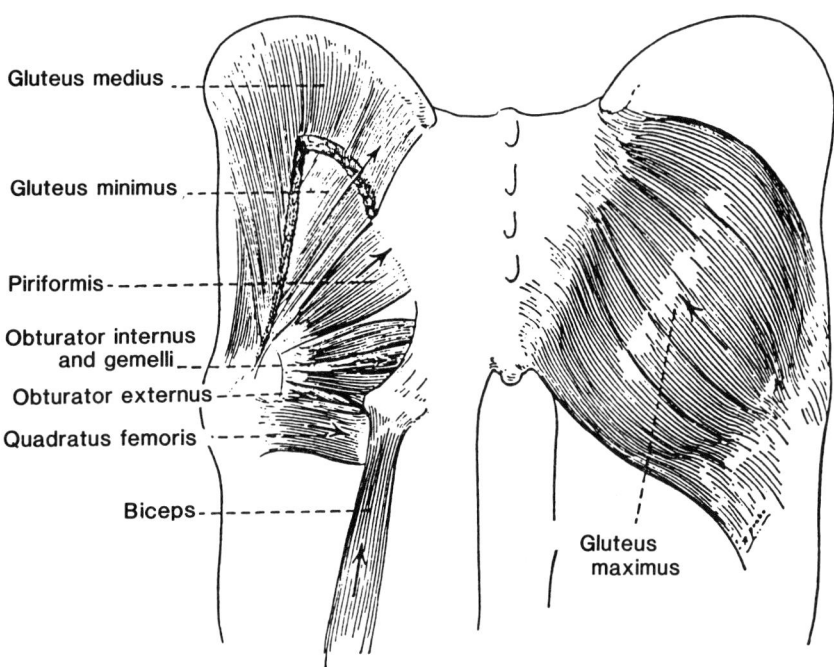

Figure 8-23
The posteriorly placed external rotators of the thigh. *(From Hollinshead WH, Jenkins DB: Functional anatomy of the limbs and back, ed 5, Philadelphia, 1981, WB Saunders Co. By permission of Mayo Foundation.)*

(downward movement) of thigh against resistance by examiner applied under distal part of thigh.

This is a rather crude test, and the muscle cannot be observed or readily palpated.

- Prone—Knee well flexed to minimize participation of hamstrings. Extension of thigh, raising knee from table against downward pressure by examiner applied to distal part of thigh.

The muscle is accessible to observation and palpation in this position.

Quadriceps Femoris (Fig. 8-24)
Femoral N, L 2 3 4

Action:

- Extension of leg at knee.
- Rectus femoris assists in flexion of thigh at hip.

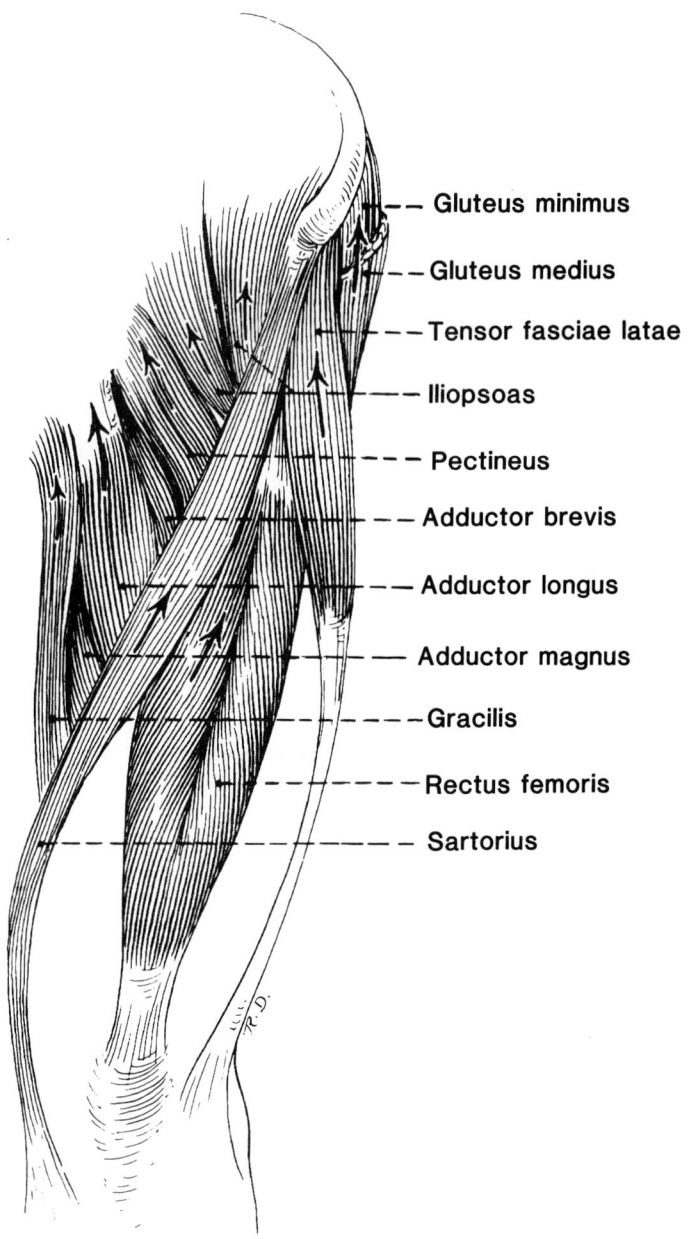

Figure 8-24
Flexors of the thigh. *(From Hollinshead WH, Jenkins DB: Functional anatomy of the limbs and back, ed 5, Philadelphia, 1981, WB Saunders Co. By permission of Mayo Foundation.)*

Test:

- Sitting or supine—Lower leg in moderate extension.
- Maintenance of extension against effort of examiner to flex leg at knee.
- Atrophy is easily noted.

Hamstrings (Fig. 8-25)
Sciatic N, L 4 <u>5</u> S <u>1</u> 2
Biceps femoris—external hamstring (L 5 S <u>1</u> 2)
Semitendinosus   ⎫ internal hamstrings
Semimembranosus   ⎭   (L4 <u>5</u> S<u>1</u> 2)

Action:

- Flexion of leg at knee.
- All but short head of biceps femoris assist in extension of thigh at hip.

Test:

- Sitting—Flexion of lower leg against resistance.
- Prone—Knee partly flexed. Further flexion against resistance. Observation and palpation of the muscles and tendons are important for proper interpretation.

Anterior Tibial (Fig. 8-26 through 8-28)
Deep peroneal N, L <u>4</u>, 5, S1

Action:

- Dorsiflexion and inversion (particularly in dorsiflexed position) of foot.

Test:

- Dorsiflexion of foot against resistance applied to dorsum of foot downward and toward eversion.

The belly of the muscle just lateral to the shin and the tendon medially on the dorsal aspect of the ankle should be observed and palpated to be certain that dorsiflexion is not being accomplished by the extensor digitorum longus without anterior tibial contraction. Atrophy is conspicuous.

Participating muscles:

- Dorsiflexion—Extensor hallucis longus; extensor digitorum longus.
- Inversion—Tibialis posterior.

Extensor Hallucis Longus (See Fig. 8-27)
Deep peroneal N, L <u>5</u> S 1

Action:

- Extension of great toe and dorsiflexion of foot.

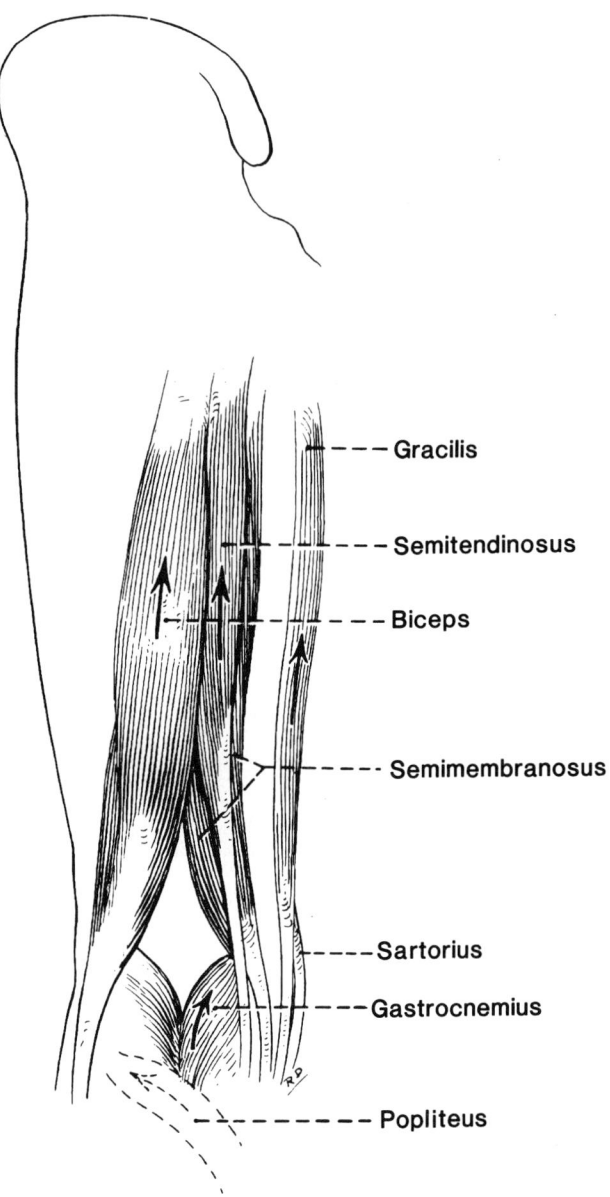

Figure 8-25
Flexors of the knee. *(From Hollinshead WH, Jenkins DB: Functional anatomy of the limbs and back, ed 5, Philadelphia, 1981, WB Saunders Co. By permission of Mayo Foundation.)*

Test:

- Extension of great toe against resistance while foot is stabilized in neutral position.

The tendon is palpable between the tendons of the tibialis anterior and the extensor digitorum longus.

Extensor Digitorum Longus (See Fig. 8-26 and 8-27)
Deep peroneal N, L 4 $\underline{5}$ S 1

Action:

- Extension of lateral four toes and dorsiflexion of foot.

Test:

- Extension of the lateral four toes and dorsiflexion of the foot against resistance.

The tendons are visible and palpable on the dorsal aspect of the ankle and foot lateral to the tendon of the extensor hallucis longus.

Extensor Digitorum Brevis (See Fig. 8-26)
Deep peroneal N, L 4 $\underline{5}$ S 1

Action:

- Assists in extension of all toes except little toe.

Test:

- Observe and palpate belly of muscle on lateral aspect of dorsum of foot during toe extension.

Peroneus Longus, Brevis (See Fig. 8-28)
Superficial peroneal N, L $\underline{5}$ S 1

Action:

- Eversion of foot.
- Assistance in plantar flexion of foot.

Test:

- Foot in plantar flexion. Eversion against resistance applied by examiner to lateral border of foot.

The tendons are palpable just above and behind the external malleolus. Atrophy may be visible over the anterolateral aspect of the lower extremity.

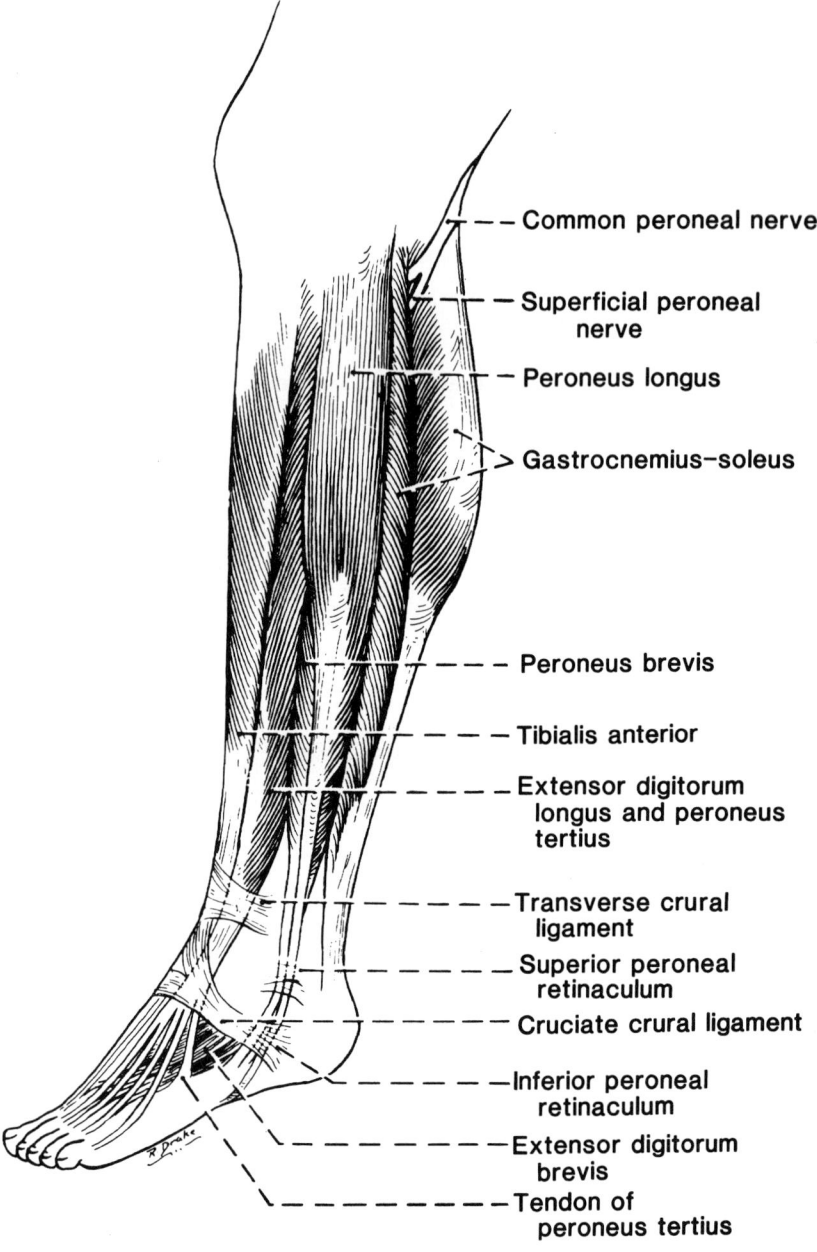

Figure 8-26
The lateral muscles of the leg. *(From Hollinshead WH, Jenkins DB: Functional anatomy of the limbs and back, ed 5, Philadelphia, 1981, WB Saunders Co. By permission of Mayo Foundation.)*

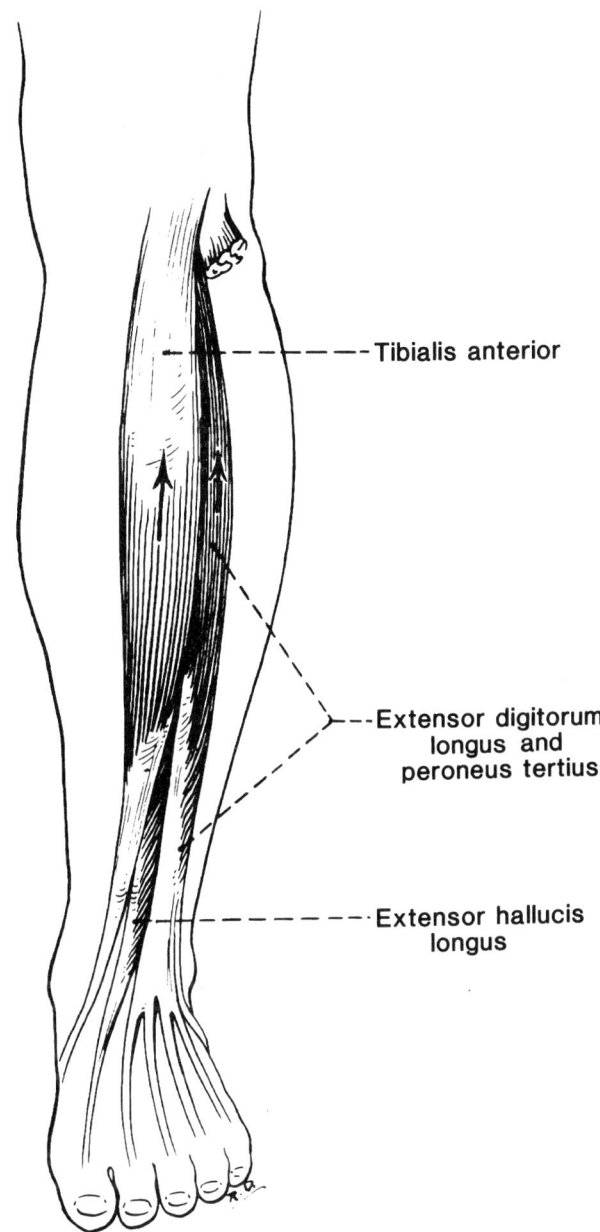

Figure 8-27
The dorsiflexors of the foot. *(From Hollinshead WH, Jenkins DB: Functional anatomy of the limbs and back, ed 5, Philadelphia, 1981, WB Saunders Co. By permission of Mayo Foundation.)*

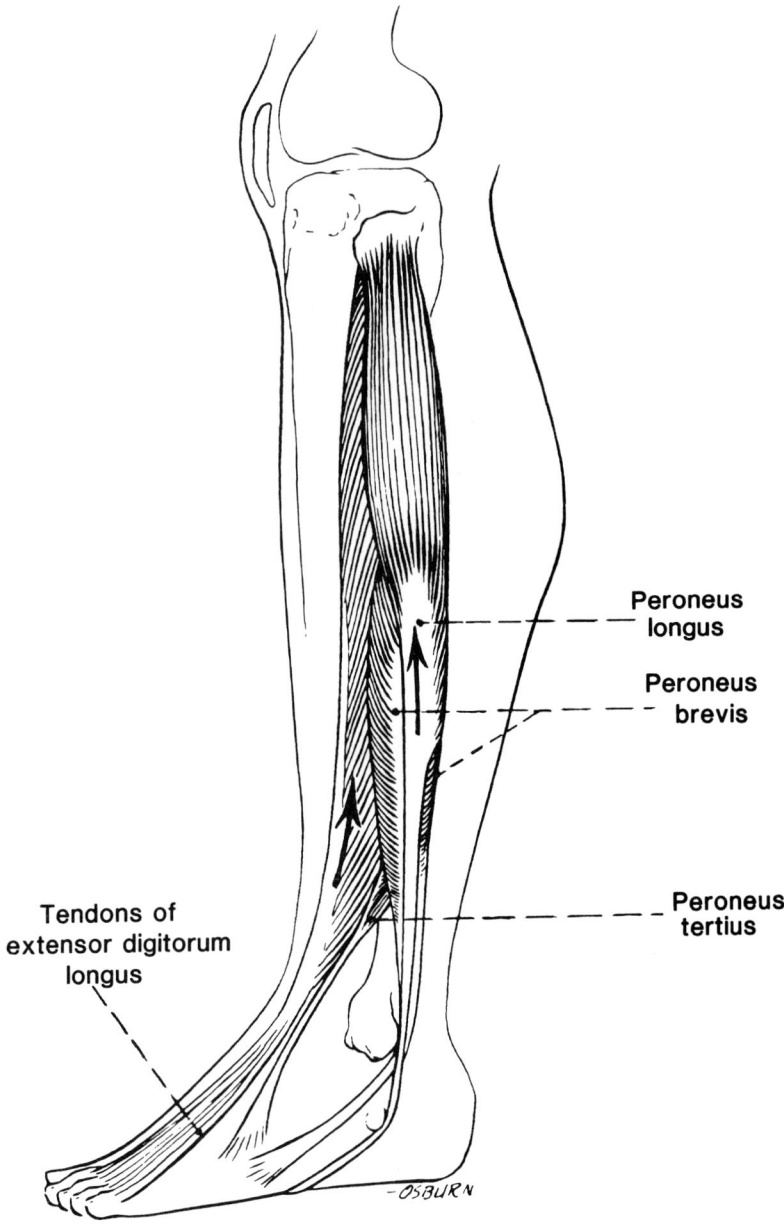

Figure 8-28
Evertors of the foot. *(From Hollinshead WH, Jenkins DB: Functional anatomy of the limbs and back, ed 5, Philadelphia, 1981, WB Saunders Co. By permission of Mayo Foundation.)*

Gastrocnemius; Soleus (Fig. 8-29)
Tibial N, L 5 S <u>1</u> <u>2</u>

Action:

- Plantar flexion of foot.

The gastrocnemius also flexes the knee and cannot act effectively in plantar flexion of the foot when the knee is well flexed.

Test:

- Knee extended to test both muscles. Knee flexed to test principally soleus.
- Plantar flexion of foot against resistance.

The muscles and tendon should be observed and palpated. Atrophy is readily visible. The gastrocnemius and soleus are very strong muscles, and leverage in testing favors the patient rather than the examiner. For this reason, slight weakness is difficult to detect by resisting flexion of the ankle or by pressing against the flexed foot in the direction of extension. Consequently, it is advisable to test the strength of these muscles against the weight of the patient's body. Have the patient stand on one foot and flex the foot so as to lift the body directly and fully upward. Sometimes it is necessary for the examiner to hold the patient steady as this test is performed.

Participating muscles:

- Long flexors of toes; tibialis posterior and peroneus longus and brevis (particularly near extreme plantar flexion).

Posterior Tibial (Fig. 8-30)
Posterior tibial N, L <u>5</u> S 1

Action:

- Inversion of foot.
- Assistance in plantar flexion of foot.

Test:

- Foot in complete plantar flexion. Inversion against resistance applied to medial border of foot and directed toward eversion and slightly toward dorsiflexion.

This maneuver virtually eliminates participation of the tibialis anterior in inversion. The toes should be relaxed to prevent participation of the long flexors of the toes.

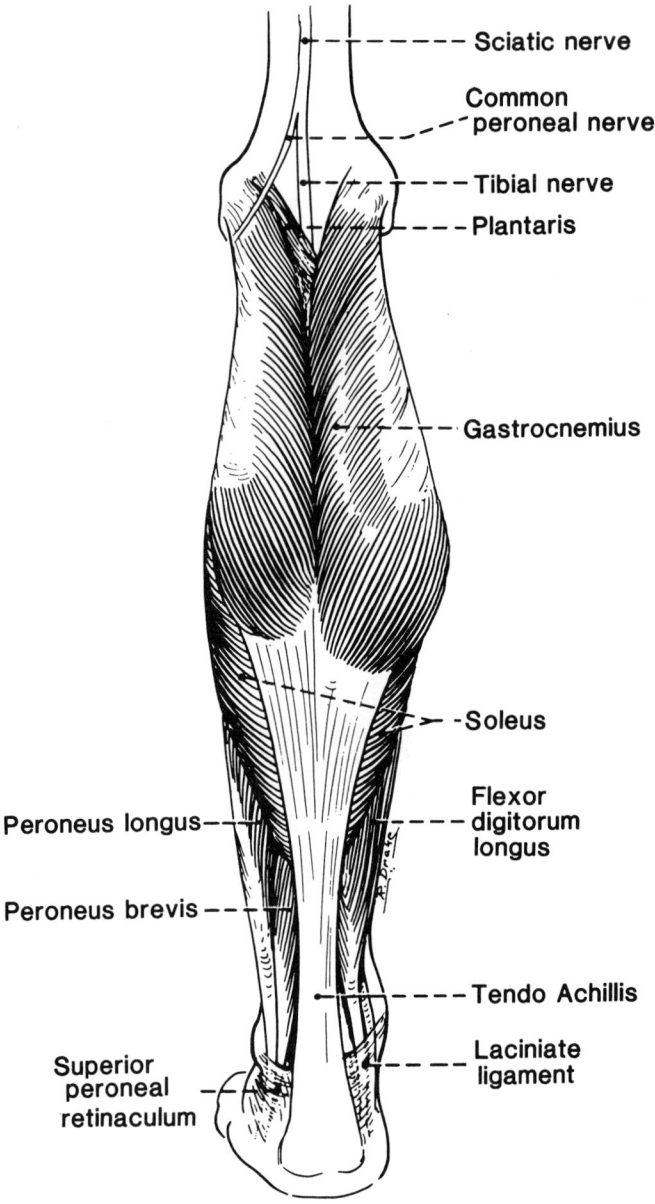

Figure 8-29
The musculature of the calf of the leg, first layer. *(From Hollinshead WH, Jenkins DB: Functional anatomy of the limbs and back, ed 5, Philadelphia, 1981, WB Saunders Co. By permission of Mayo Foundation.)*

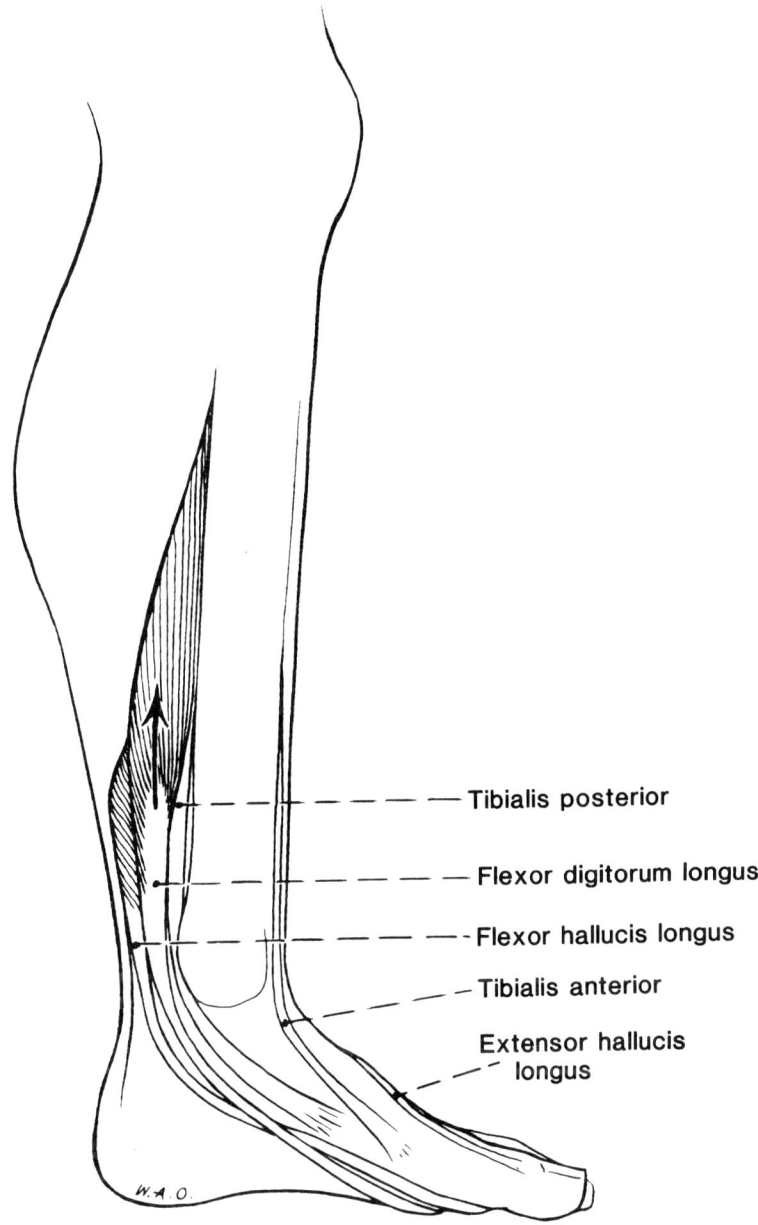

Figure 8-30
Invertors of the foot. *(From Hollinshead WH, Jenkins DB: Functional anatomy of the limbs and back, ed 5, Philadelphia, 1981, WB Saunders Co. By permission of Mayo Foundation.)*

Long Flexors of Toes
Posterior tibial N, L 5 S 1
Flexor digitorum longus
Flexor hallucis longus

Action:

- Plantar flexion of toes, especially at distal interphalangeal joints.
- Assistance in plantar flexion and inversion of foot.

Test:

- Foot stabilized in neutral position. Plantar flexion of toes against resistance applied to distal phalanges.
- Weakness of the long toe flexors results in inability to curl the tips of the toes under the foot against resistance. (See intrinsic foot muscle testing, which follows.)

Intrinsic Muscles of Foot
Virtually all except extensor digitorum brevis (medial and lateral plantar Ns from posterior tibial N, L 5 S 1 2)

Action:

- Comparable to that of intrinsic muscles of hand, with flexion of the proximal phalanges while extending the distal phalanges.

Test:

- Foot stabilized in neutral position. Plantar flexion of the toes against resistance applied to the distal phalanges. (Same maneuver as that in test of long toe flexors.)

If the tibial innervated foot muscles are weak, the examiner easily dorsiflexes the toes at the metatarsophalangeal joint while the distal phalanges remain curled under by the action of the long toe flexors. This sign is an important early manifestation of a peripheral neuropathy or of S 1-2 root lesions. When intrinsic foot muscle weakness is severe, this position becomes a permanent deformity of high arches and "hammer toes," with the toes curled and cocked up on the dorsum of the foot. This position results from the combined action of the long toe extensors and long toe flexors without the opposing action of the intrinsic foot muscles.

Chapter 9

Reflexes

Reflexes provide valuable information about the integrity of the nervous system. Changes in reflex activity may appear before other signs of neurologic dysfunction, and when changes are present, they are distinct between central and peripheral disorders. In addition, the assessment of reflex activity is largely independent of an individual's participation, so that reflexes may be particularly helpful in evaluating patients whose consciousness is altered or whose cooperation is suboptimal or even misleading, such as hostile patients or those with conversion disorders.

Reflexes may be defined as involuntary motor responses to sensory stimuli. They depend on intact afferent and efferent peripheral pathways to transmit an incoming stimulus and effect a response. They are centrally integrated through monosynaptic or polysynaptic connections and modulated or influenced by descending central motor activity. For convenience, reflexes are classified as muscle-stretch, superficial, and pathologic reflexes.

Both muscle-stretch and superficial reflexes are simple segmental reflexes that are present in normal subjects. In both types of reflexes, the afferent impulses are conducted to the spinal cord or brain stem by sensory fibers in the peripheral nerve and sensory (dorsal) root. After passing across one or more synapses within the central nervous system, the impulses act on the anterior horn cells of the spinal cord. Activation of these cells usually results in impulses that emerge from the same segments as those in which the afferent impulses entered. The final common pathway includes the anterior horn cells and their axons, which traverse the motor root and peripheral nerve to reach the effector organ. Stimulation of receptors within the muscles as a result of muscle stretch elicits the muscle-stretch reflexes. Touching, scratching, pricking, and pinching, on the other hand, are the stimuli initiating the superficial reflexes.

Pathologic reflexes are also evoked by muscle-stretch or superficial stimuli, but they differ in two respects from the simple segmental reflexes. First, pathologic reflexes cannot be elicited in normal subjects. Second, despite being segmental, they are often more complex than the simple segmental reflexes and reflect a disturbance in the balance of impulses influencing the final common pathway from many sources and at varying levels within the central nervous system.

MUSCLE-STRETCH REFLEXES

Muscle-stretch reflexes result from a sudden stretch of the muscle. They are sometimes referred to as "tendon," "periosteal," "deep," or "myotatic" reflexes, but the term "muscle-stretch reflex" is preferred, since it is more meaningful physiologically. For example, the designation "radial periosteal reflex" not only lacks the precise meaning of its synonym, "brachioradialis stretch reflex," but also gives an erroneous idea of the anatomy and physiology of the reflex.

Neither the complete absence nor the maximal hyperactivity of muscle-stretch reflexes in itself can be regarded as evidence of abnormality. From time to time, persons are examined who are areflexic and yet seem to be in perfect health. Similarly, persons with maximal hyperactivity of reflexes, including sustained clonus, have been studied thoroughly without detection of organic disease to account for the hyperactivity. The clinical significance of deviations in the activity of muscle-stretch reflexes from the usual or the normal may depend on comparison with other muscle-stretch reflexes—for example, upper compared with lower extremity or comparison of corresponding areas on opposite sides. Finally, the activity of the stretch reflexes must be correlated with the other observations on the neurologic examination before it can be considered to be indicative of disease.

Significant loss or reduction of muscle-stretch reflexes, either segmentally or diffusely, is most often a result of disorders affecting a component of the reflex arc, that is, the peripheral afferent and efferent pathways or their segmental connections in the central nervous system. If such lesions affecting any of these components of the reflex arc are absent, the activity of the muscle-stretch reflexes indicates the balance between inhibitory and excitatory impulses reaching the lower motor neurons from various cerebral and brain stem centers. Lesions of the upper motor neurons produce a loss of the facilitory or inhibitory effects on the final common pathway, and the net result is facilitation of the muscle-stretch reflex. However, interference with projections from the cerebellum and some areas of the brain stem, which are normally facilitating, may result in some decrease in activity of the muscle-stretch reflexes.

Technique of Elicitation

Variations in the technique of eliciting the muscle-stretch reflexes are numerous, but all reliable methods seem to depend on four factors. First, the patient must be completely relaxed. Second, the optimal amount of tension in the muscle is produced by passive manipulation and positioning of the extremity. Third, an adequate stretch stimulus must be applied. Fourth, proper reinforcement should be achieved if reflexes are not obtained by methods that take the first three factors into consideration.

The first two factors, namely, adequate relaxation and the proper degree of tension, depend to a large extent on proper positioning of the patient and the extremity. An appropriate examining table may facilitate positioning. The patient can then sit comfortably with both the upper and the lower extremities in a naturally supported and relaxed position. With the patient's forearms resting on the thighs and feet resting on the step of the examining table, only minor changes in position are necessary to produce the proper amount of tension in the muscle for elicitation of the muscle-stretch reflexes.

Securing relaxation

As a rule, relaxation is greater if the patient is not in pain or fearful of pain being produced by the tests; the position should be comfortable. The examiner can remind the patient to "relax," "not help me," or "let me do the work" to reduce apprehension and achieve relaxation. The extremity is also gently manipulated into a fully supported position, maintenance of which requires no effort by the patient. At times, the ingenuity of the examiner may be severely taxed. Engaging the patient in conversation as a distraction from the test or asking the patient to look elsewhere or think of something else often helps.

Obtaining the proper degree of muscle stretch or tension

After complete relaxation has been achieved, the proper amount of tension within the muscle must be obtained by passive positioning, since the reflex may not be elicited from a muscle that is stretched too much or too little. Although the examiner depends largely on experience, the proper degree of tension is usually obtained when the extremity is placed in a position in which the muscle is approximately midway between its greatest and shortest lengths.

For example, with the patient in the sitting position with forearms and hands resting on the thighs, the proper amount of tension is present for eliciting reflexes of the biceps, triceps, and brachioradialis muscles. The examiner may find it helpful in obtaining the biceps reflex to increase the tension in the biceps muscle by pulling the patient's forearm forward on the thigh, thereby passively extending the elbow slightly, in addition to the tension applied by placing the thumb over the tendon and depressing it. To increase the tension of the triceps muscle in this position, the examiner may find it advantageous to slide the forearm backward or have the patient place hands on hips, movements that increase the flexion of the elbow.

Application of the stretch stimulus

If reflexes are hyperactive, a very light stretch stimulus, such as that produced by tapping the tendon with the tip of a finger, may be adequate to induce the reflex. If the reflexes are decreased and difficult to elicit, however, the maximally rapid stretch of the maximal number of fibers may be required to elicit the reflex. Such a stimulus is not conveniently delivered by a small, lightweight reflex hammer. A longer, well-balanced hammer with adequate weight in its head has many advantages, particularly when the percussing tips are made of rubber that is soft enough to cause no discomfort to the examiner even when the thumb or finger is struck an intense blow.

The technique of indirect percussion of tendons to produce the stretch stimulus in the desired muscle has many advantages. With this method, the tip of the examiner's finger or thumb is placed over the tendon of the muscle to be tested and is struck sharply with the reflex hammer. First of all, palpation of the tendon enables the examiner to determine whether the muscle is completely relaxed and under the desirable amount of tension. In fact, if the tension is not quite sufficient, it can be augmented, often sufficiently, by firm pressure against the tendon. Furthermore, palpation of the tendon enables the examiner to make certain that any reflex action taking place is or is not in the muscle being tested. This may be an important matter. For example, the novice may overlook the absence of the triceps reflex in lesions of the seventh cervical nerve root, usually when the biceps reflex is more active than usual. When the stimulus is applied to the triceps tendon, sudden short extension of the elbow occurs, and this results in sudden lengthening of the biceps muscle and a consequent reflex contraction of the biceps. The examiner notices the reflex action at the elbow but may erroneously conclude that it occurred in the triceps muscle (paradoxical triceps reflex). This example illustrates why it is important to make certain where reflex action is occurring by palpation of tendons and direct observation of the muscle response.

Reinforcement of reflexes

If muscle-stretch reflexes are not obtained after appropriate positioning and with the proper tension in the muscle, an attempt should be made to reinforce the reflex. The most easily applied method of reinforcement is to have the patient contract muscles other than the one being tested. The reflexes of the lower extremities may be reinforced by strong, sustained efforts to pull the hands apart while they are coupled together by means of flexed fingers (Jendrassik's maneuver). The reflexes of the upper extremities may be reinforced by biting the teeth together, squeezing the knees together, making a tight fist with the hand on the other side, and so forth.

A more effective means of reinforcement is to have the patient make a very slight voluntary contraction in the muscle being tested, but this is not feasible in most patients because of their tendency to contract too vigorously. Some patients can obtain the desired degree of contraction if they are instructed simply to think hard about making the movement that is produced by contraction of the muscle being tested. The hoped-for result is a voluntary contraction sufficient to tighten the muscle but insufficient to produce movement of the joint. When a muscle is contracted too strongly, the reflex is abolished; if the muscle is contracted very slightly, the reflex is exaggerated. Incidentally, certain tense people exhibit hyperreflexia as a result of their inability to relax.

The need to reinforce reflexes commonly occurs in patients with suspected peripheral neuropathy or Adie's syndrome; in these situations, depressed reflexes usually remain depressed. In some normal persons, particularly muscular men, reflexes (especially biceps and quadriceps reflexes) may be difficult to elicit in the usual way. With reinforcement, however, they usually improve or normalize. Thus, in most situations in which reflexes increase to a normal or near-normal level of activity with reinforcement, a pathologic process is not found.

Interpretation and Grading of Reflexes

Semiquantitation of a muscle-stretch reflex requires an estimate of the minimal stimulus needed to activate the reflex and an assessment of three components of the reflex contraction. The three components are (1) the speed of contraction and relaxation, (2) the force of contraction, and (3) the degree or range of shortening—in short, the amplitude of the response. Generally, a considerable degree of parallelism exists among the three components, with the force of contraction and the degree of shortening related more to the number of fibers activated than to the speed of contraction. The clinician, in estimating the threshold of reflexes, usually finds it advantageous to determine the lightest percussion that induces the reflex. Then, by observing the response to sharper and stronger blows, the examiner can better estimate the activity of the reflexes on the basis of multiple observations.

The reflex response should be compared on the two sides and graded. Although there are several methods of grading reflexes, we record them on a scale from "−4" to "+4," with "0" being normal. Complete absence is indicated by "−4," pathologic hyperreflexia with clonus by "+4," and intermediate degrees of activity by appropriate numbers preceded by plus or minus signs. A reflex obtained with reinforcement is indicated by encircling the recorded number and sign, for example, ⊖4. This scale for recording reflexes provides a broad range of expression and with experience is quite reproducible.

Reflexes are valuable in supporting disorders that affect regions of the central or peripheral nervous system. Although some central disorders can be associated with hypoactive reflexes (for example, acute spinal cord injuries and diseases of the cerebellum and its components), they are more commonly the result of peripheral disorders. In disorders of the final common pathway, muscle-stretch reflexes are often diminished in proportion to the loss of muscle strength. In contrast, diseases affecting the large sensory neurons or dorsal root are much more prone to reduce or eliminate muscle-stretch reflexes. In a single limb, the segmental pattern may help localize the process. For example, reduction in the triceps and brachioradialis reflexes with a normal biceps reflex supports a radial nerve lesion. If the biceps and brachioradialis reflexes were normal with a hypoactive triceps, a C-7 root lesion would be more probable. Hyperactive muscle-stretch reflexes, on the other hand, are most commonly due to upper motor neuron lesions within the central nervous system. In some situations in which both upper and lower motor neuron involvement occur within the same segment, for example, in amyotrophic lateral sclerosis, the muscle stretch reflex may have a very low threshold for the eliciting of a response but the amplitude or magnitude of the response is reduced.

In addition to the advantages already mentioned of eliciting reflexes by percussion of the examiner's finger, this method is the best available for estimating and comparing the speed of contraction and relaxation of the muscle that has been stimulated reflexly. By no other method is one so likely to recognize *Woltman's sign of myxedema*. Recognition depends on observing the marked slowing of relaxation, particularly easy to detect in the biceps, quadriceps, and gastrocnemius-soleus reflexes. This sign is invaluable as a clinical test for confirming the diagnosis in suspected myxedema; or, as often happens in practice, the recognition of slow relaxation of reflexes may initiate the suspicion of myxedema in the first place.

Specific Muscle-Stretch Reflexes

Although muscle-stretch reflexes can be obtained from almost all accessible muscles, seldom is the elicitation of any except those listed below of significant value.

Jaw reflex

(Synonyms: masseter and temporalis muscle reflex. Cranial N V; mandibular branch of trigeminal.) With the patient's jaw relaxed and about half opened, the examiner gently presses downward on the chin with the index finger and then carefully percusses that finger. Because the reflex is normally difficult to elicit, if it is readily obtained without reinforcement, it is almost always increased beyond the normal degree of activity.

Biceps reflex

(C 5 6; musculocutaneous N.) With the patient in the sitting position, the examiner places the relaxed pronated forearm on the thigh. The amount of tension in the biceps muscle is adjusted by passively positioning the forearm so that different degrees of flexion and extension of the elbow are obtained. The thumb is placed over the tendon and pressed as necessary to secure optimal stretch of the muscle before it is percussed.

When the patient is supine, the upper extremity position is adjusted so that the arm is supported by the mattress and the forearm and hand are resting on the abdomen. Tension is applied to the tendon, and percussion is performed in the same manner as in the sitting position.

Brachioradialis reflex
(Synonym: radial periosteal reflex. C 5 6; radial N.) The positioning of the patient is similar to that for obtaining the biceps reflex except that the forearm should be only midway between pronation and supination. The examiner percusses the tendon over the distal portion of the radius while palpating the muscle and observing for contraction.

Triceps reflex
(C 6 7 8; radial N.) The patient positioning is generally similar to that for the biceps reflex. The very short tendon of the triceps brachii makes it difficult not to percuss some of the muscle fibers directly. Local contraction of directly percussed muscle fibers should be ignored. In normal subjects, the triceps reflex is usually more difficult to obtain than the biceps reflex. Sometimes, the reflex contraction can be more easily detected if the patient's hand is on the hip and the examiner is standing behind the patient.

If the patient is supine, the examiner draws the opposite limb across the chest and abdomen while maintaining the arm in partial flexion at the elbow. The tendon is percussed while the examiner holds the limb, usually at the hand or wrist.

Quadriceps (femoris) reflex
(Synonym: knee jerk. L 2 3 4; femoral N.) In the sitting position, the feet may be allowed to rest on the step of the examining table and positioned for optimal relaxation and tendon stretch. Some examiners prefer to have the feet dangling over the edge of the examining table. The tendon is percussed directly while the examiner observes and feels the muscle contraction. If the patient is large or obese, the examiner may find it helpful instead to place a finger on the patellar tendon to determine the optimal percussion site.

When the patient is supine, the examiner places a hand or forearm under the patient's knees, passively flexing them 20 degrees or so. If an assistant performs this duty, the examiner has the left hand free for placing a finger directly on the tendon. Otherwise, pillows may be placed under the knees to obtain the desired support and position. Sometimes relaxation is best secured by instructing the patient to allow the heel to drag along the sheet while the examiner passively flexes the knee and hip by lifting the knee from the bed.

Adductor reflex

(L 2 3 4; obturator N.) With the patient in the supine position, the legs are separated approximately 30 degrees. The stimulus can be applied to the dorsum of the examiner's finger held against the medial side of the thigh just above the knee. The response is adduction of the leg. Since the magnitude of this response may be difficult to see, especially in large or obese patients, it is often better to use a slightly different technique. In the same position, the leg is allowed to flex at the knee and then is gently rotated externally. The tendinous insertion of the adductor longus is palpated in the middle to upper medial portion of the thigh, and the stimulus is applied again to the dorsum of the examiner's finger while the response is observed and felt.

Although not routinely elicited, the adductor reflex is particularly useful in differentiating a femoral neuropathy from a lumbar plexopathy or radiculopathy when the quadriceps reflex is reduced or absent.

Gastrocnemius-soleus reflex

(Synonyms: ankle jerk, Achilles reflex, triceps surae reflex. L 5; S 1 2; tibial N.) In the sitting position, the feet may be placed on the step of the examining table. In this position, the ankle can be dorsiflexed sufficiently to obtain optimal stretch of the muscles to be tested. If preferred, the foot may be grasped and passively dorsiflexed by the examiner to produce the proper stretch of the muscle while the tendon is struck with the reflex hammer. It is important that the degree of stretch or tension be similar on the two sides. At times, relaxation is difficult to secure without having the patient assume a kneeling position, with the feet and ankles extended unsupported over the front edge of a chair.

In the supine position, relaxation is best secured if the hip is partially flexed and externally rotated and the knee partially flexed. The tendon can be directly stimulated with the reflex hammer in this position. Alternatively, the limbs can be left extended and the tendon indirectly stimulated. To do this, the examiner grasps the forefoot and slightly dorsiflexes the foot before percussing the plantar surface of the forefoot. This maneuver is particularly useful in less cooperative or unresponsive individuals.

Internal hamstring reflex

(Synonyms: semimembranosus and semitendinosus reflexes. L 4 5, S 1 2; sciatic N.) Hamstring reflexes can be elicited, often with difficulty, in a sitting position with the patient's feet resting on the step of the examining table. It is important that the examiner correctly identify the tendon before applying tension to avoid misinterpreting the location of the response.

When the patient is supine, the knee is placed in various degrees of flexion to secure relaxation and the proper amount of stretch. In this position, the muscles can be both observed and palpated during contraction.

External hamstring reflex
(Synonym: biceps femoris reflex. L 5; S $\underline{1}$ 2; sciatic N.) The technique is the same as that described for the internal hamstring reflex, above.

Hoffmann's reflex
(C 7 $\underline{8}$; T $\underline{1}$; median N.) This reflex has been considered by some to be a pathologic reflex, but we agree with Wartenberg and many others that it is simply a finger-flexor stretch reflex elicited in an unusual way. The modification most often used by us is as follows: While the middle phalanx of the middle finger is supported, the distal phalanx is suddenly snapped into flexion and immediately released. After release, the distal phalanx rebounds, resulting in a sudden stretch of that portion of the flexor digitorum profundus muscle that supplies the middle finger and hence evoking the stretch reflex. This is a relatively small stimulus; consequently, the response—flexion of the fingers and thumb—is generally not obtained unless the reflex is hyperactive. The Hoffmann reflex, like other overactive stretch reflexes, has no pathologic significance by itself. For example, it occurs bilaterally in some tense individuals. However, it may be valuable when present unilaterally, particularly if other muscle-stretch reflexes are somewhat more active on the same side.

Rossolimo's reflex
(L $\underline{5}$; S $\underline{1}$ 2; tibial N.) This reflex, too, is simply a muscle-stretch reflex obtained by tapping the plantar surfaces of the toes with a reflex hammer. In a modified method of elicitation, a very quick, short stretch of the toe flexors is produced by briskly brushing them in the direction of extension with a slapping motion of hands or fingers.

Clonus
When muscle-stretch reflexes are accentuated or hyperactive, they may occur repetitively if the examiner simply maintains constant tension on the tendon or muscle being tested. This is clonus, and it may occur in practically any muscle, but routinely it is tested only at the ankle in the gastrocnemius and soleus muscles. The patient is asked to relax the lower extremity being examined while the examiner sharply dorsiflexes the foot and maintains dorsiflexion. Some neurologists consider sustained clonus to indicate organic disease of the central nervous system, but we cannot agree, particularly if it is an isolated finding. Clonus has the same significance as hyperactivity of muscle-stretch reflexes. In most instances, however, sustained clonus and marked exaggeration of muscle-stretch reflexes are associated with organic disease of the central nervous system, but exceptions occasionally are seen.

SUPERFICIAL REFLEXES

Superficial reflexes are those in which the cornea, skin, or mucous membrane is stimulated to produce reflex motor responses. Various stimuli are used in obtaining superficial reflexes. A light touch with a wisp of cotton suffices to elicit the corneal reflex. The pharyngeal reflex is elicited with a touch of a tongue blade or applicator stick, and the superficial abdominal reflexes are usually elicited by a stroke of a blunt stick or pin. A scratch or a pinprick elicits the anal reflex.

Specific Superficial Reflexes
Corneal reflex
(Cranial Ns V, VII.) The cornea is touched lightly with a wisp of cotton. The normal response is a prompt closure of both eyelids. Clean cotton wool twisted into a tight cone (moistening may help obtain the desired shape) is placed on the cornea, the approach to the cornea being made from outside the temporal field of vision and gingerly to prevent reflex defensive blinking. The patient is directed to look upward or away from the side being tested.

If the reflex is decreased on one side, the patient is asked whether any significant difference in sensation is noticed. If the reflex is absent or reduced on one side because of weakness of the orbicularis oculi (the facial nerve), the integrity of the sensory portion of the reflex arc may be judged from the presence of the blink in the opposite eye.

Loss of corneal reflex and sensation is often an early sign of cerebello-pontine-angle tumor.

Pharyngeal reflex
(Cranial Ns IX, X.) The pharynx is touched with tongue blade or applicator stick, producing an involuntary contraction of the pharyngeal muscles (gagging). The pharyngeal reflex may be absent in apparently healthy people. The reflex is absent in lower motor neuron lesions involving the medulla or increased in upper motor neuron lesions above this area.

Superficial abdominal reflexes
(Epigastric [T 6-9], midabdominal [T 9-11], hypogastric [T 11-L 1].) These reflexes usually cannot be elicited if the abdomen is obese, distended, or overly flaccid or if the patient is unable to relax. Their greatest value is based on the frequency with which they are lost during the early stages of multiple sclerosis and their unilateral reduction in unilateral corticospinal deficits and in spinal cord tumors.

Proper relaxation seems best obtained when the patient lies supine with knees comfortably drawn up and supported, arms hanging loosely at the sides, and eyes closed. Sometimes a few deep breaths while the examiner massages the abdomen seem to help.

As a rule, first attempts to obtain the reflexes are made with something blunt, such as an applicator stick, handle of reflex hammer, or key. The strokes are made horizontally on the anterior surface of the abdomen at two levels on both sides. The strokes should be directed toward the umbilicus; at least, they should not be made in a line directed away from the umbilicus. If the latter direction is used, movement of the umbilicus toward the area stimulated may result from traction on the skin, and this movement may be mistaken for an active contraction of the abdominal musculature in the region stimulated. The normal response to the stimulus is a brief, brisk movement of the umbilicus toward the locus of the stimulus. When the reflex is not obtained with blunt instruments, a pin may be used. The novice must be on guard, however, not to injure the patient or produce bleeding by use of the pin.

Cremasteric reflex
(L 1 2.) With the patient supine and thighs abducted slightly, the inner aspect of the thigh is stimulated as in obtaining superficial abdominal reflexes. Reflex contraction of the cremasteric muscle with elevation of the testicle is observed. The reflex is lost in corticospinal tract lesions and in lesions involving the lumbar segments of the spinal cord.

Anal reflex
(S 2 3 4.) The tip of the finger, covered with glove or finger cot, is inserted into the anal ring, and contraction of the anal ring is felt as the skin about the anus and the perineum is scratched or pricked with a pin; or the contraction simply may be observed without palpation. The anal reflex is lost in lesions involving the sacral segments of the spinal cord and cauda equina.

This is a test specifically of the external or voluntary anal sphincter. In the presence of a flaccid paralysis of the external anal sphincter, the normal tonus of the internal sphincter is felt to give way on insertion of the finger. As the finger is withdrawn, the anus remains open or patulous. Apparently, this reaction of the internal sphincter is normal, but it appears to be abnormal, since it can be observed only under the abnormal conditions of paralysis of the external anal sphincter. It does not indicate a loss of the internal anal sphincter function.

Bulbocavernosus reflex
(S 3 4.) The examiner flicks or pinches the foreskin of the penis or pricks foreskin or glans with a pin to evoke a reflex contraction in the bulbocavernosus muscle at the base of the penis. The contraction may be observed, but it is, as a rule, more easily palpated.

Plantar reflex
(L 5; S 1 2.) The plantar reflex is the normal flexion of the toes that results from stimulation of the sole, as is done in attempts to elicit the sign of Babinski.

PATHOLOGIC REFLEXES

The pathologic reflexes are those whose presence signifies an organic interference with function of the nervous system. For instance, the sign of Babinski and related pathologic reflexes result from a failure in function of the corticospinal motor system. Usually, a lesion exists in area 4 or at some point along the corticospinal tract between the motor cortex and the lowest lumbar segment of the spinal cord to account for this pathologic reflex, but that need not be so. The Babinski and confirmatory signs may be strongly positive in severe hypoglycemia, only to disappear within minutes after the intravenous administration of glucose. Thus, a functional defect may exist without demonstrable histologic evidence to account for pathologic reflexes.

In the past, a great deal of discussion centered on the technique of elicitation, the exact nature and significance of the response, the relative virtue, and even the priority of discovery of the numerous reflexes elicited from the foot and leg for the detection of upper motor neuron lesions. This, along with the multiplicity of proper names that have become attached to the reflexes, has made for an endless amount of confusion. We believe it is clearer and simpler to consider these reflexes from a broad physiologic point of view.

The central nervous system is organized not in terms of anatomic segments but according to movement patterns. One of the first of these movement patterns to be described was the defensive reflex withdrawal of an extremity from a painful stimulus. This well-recognized reflex is commonly designated "the flexion reflex" by physiologists. It involves flexion of the hip, knee, ankle (dorsiflexion), and toes in higher vertebrates; and to this, in the chimpanzee and man, is added extension of the great toe. The physiologist looks on the Babinski sign as simply part of the primitive flexion reflex.

The neurons in the motor cortex area (area 4), through their projections (pyramidal or corticospinal pathways), maintain a suppressor action on the flexion reflex. Consequently, when this upper motor neuron is intact, the flexion reflex cannot be elicited by any of the stimuli used in clinical neurology for eliciting reflexes. However, when function of the upper motor neuron fails, its suppressing effect on the flexion reflex is withdrawn and the flexion reflex becomes facilitated or released. When sufficiently facilitated, the reflex is elicited by a variety of stimuli, including the superficial and muscle-stretch stimuli used in the methods of Babinski, Chaddock, Stransky, Oppenheim, and others for obtaining their respective reflexes. In fact, in extreme cases of upper motor neuron deficit, the complete flexion reflex may be exhibited spontaneously and continuously; the patient lies in bed, the hip and knee flexed and the ankle and great toe dorsiflexed.

In other cases of severe upper motor neuron deficit, almost any unpleasant stimulus, such as scratching, pinching, or pricking, evokes the flexion reflex, even though it be applied as high as the thigh, far from the usual reflexogenous zone.

Although we have made a case for the pathologic significance of the reflexes under discussion, at times equivocal reflex responses are obtained. Sometimes even responses that are indistinguishable from the Babinski and confirmatory reflexes are observed; yet after long study and observation, serious neurologic disease is not found. On the other hand, the response, when obtained, is not to be taken lightly, since it frequently signifies central nervous system disease.

Specific Pathologic Reflexes
Babinski's reflex
The method of Babinski is probably the most sensitive and reliable method for eliciting the flexion reflex. Occasionally the reflex may be obtained by the method of Chaddock, even when stimulation of the sole fails to evoke it.

The sign of Babinski consists of extension of the great toe, usually associated with fanning (abduction and slight flexion) of the other toes. Abduction of the great toe may also be seen.

The patient must be relaxed; consequently, it is well to use conversation as a distraction. The initial stimulus should produce neither pain nor tickle. The tip of the finger or the knuckle of the thumb should be pressed against the sole on the lateral side of the heel, from whence it is carried forward toward the little toe and, when the ball of the foot is reached, across it toward the base of the great toe. This often fails to elicit the reflex, and it is necessary gradually to increase the stimulus. The next stimulus to be applied may be sharper. The thumb or fingernail, a key, or the end of the handle of the reflex hammer may be used. However, finally, if an abnormal reflex or a normal plantar reflex has not been obtained by the foregoing types of stimuli, before the examiner concludes that the reflex is absent, a sharp and unpleasant stimulus should be applied. Some of us break a tongue blade to obtain a sharp point with which to apply the stimulus. Often, a painful stimulus, applied with gradually increasing force to the sole at the heel, elicits the reflex without the necessity of extending the stimulus the full length of the foot.

Chaddock's reflex
Stimulus similar to that used in the method of Babinski is applied along the lateral aspect of the foot below the external malleolus.

Oppenheim's reflex
The reflex is elicited in response to a firm, somewhat painful, application of the knuckles of the examiner's index and middle fingers astride the shin, beginning just below the knee and carrying the stimulus rather slowly downward to the ankle.

Stransky's reflex

The little toe is slowly but maximally abducted, and after the maximal abduction has been maintained for 1 or 2 seconds, it is suddenly released. Dorsiflexion of the great toe may occur while the little toe is being held abducted, or it may take place just after release of abduction. The so-called Gonda reflex is similar and is elicited in response to traction and simultaneous flexion of the third or fourth toe, which is released suddenly after a few seconds. Although we consider the Babinski and Chaddock signs to be the most valuable, the other confirmatory signs are often useful, particularly when the patient is very sensitive and when attempts to elicit the sign of Babinski result in defensive movements of flexion and extension that render the test worthless.

Sucking reflex

(Synonyms: lip or snout reflex. Cranial Ns V, VII.) This is a valuable reflex because it is associated with bilateral supranuclear deficit above the level of the facial nucleus in the pons. It is frequently observed in amyotrophic lateral sclerosis, diffuse encephalopathies, and pseudobulbar palsy.

The patient is instructed to relax the jaw sufficiently to part the lips a fraction of an inch. It often helps in securing relaxation to tell the patient to breathe through the mouth. The reflex is elicited by sweeping the end of a tongue blade briskly and lightly over the lips from just lateral to the corner of the mouth to about the center. A brisk, bilateral reflex contraction of the lips is the response evoked. The same reflex action may be elicited by scraping the hard palate with a tongue blade or an applicator stick or by applying other stimuli to the lips, including light percussion with a reflex hammer either directly or through an intervening tongue blade. These "release" reflexes are normally present in the newborn infant and disappear with maturation of the central nervous system.

Chewing reflex

This reflex is an abnormal response obtained by placing a tongue blade in the patient's mouth. When the reflex is well developed, the jaws may bite down, making removal of the tongue blade difficult. This has been called the "bulldog" response. This reflex implies bilateral cerebral upper motor neuron lesions.

Grasp reflex

The examiner grasps the patient's hand and with a finger strokes the patient's palm. The reflex is positive when the patient grasps the examiner's hand or finger. The patient may not release the grasp even on request. This reflex may be present in patients with diffuse bifrontal disease or may be present unilaterally (opposite the side of a frontal lesion).

Chapter 10

The Sensory Examination

If all patients were alert, intelligent, observant, objective, cooperative, and not suggestible, an accurate sensory examination would pose few difficulties. All of these attributes are seldom encountered in any one individual, and thus sensory testing may be one of the most difficult and time-consuming parts of the neurologic examination. Many neurologic problems do not involve the sensory system to any significant degree, and in these the sensory status may be quite quickly established. In other instances, however, the sensory findings may be vital both to the diagnosis and to the handling of the case. A reliable technique for the sensory examination is then of the greatest practical importance.

It should be recognized at the outset that the bedside evaluation of sensation is, at best, a crude procedure, not only because the testing stimuli themselves are ill-controlled but also because both the patient and the examiner introduce intangible human variables.

Much more refined techniques for testing sensation have been developed for research purposes, but from the practical point of view in dealing with patients, the techniques to be described herein are appropriate for identifying significant disturbances in a patient's sensory appreciation.

TYPES OF SENSATION

The physiology of sensation is an exceedingly complex and constantly expanding field of study. No attempt is made herein to explore this aspect of sensation. The aim in this chapter is to suggest a method of sensory examination for the purposes of diagnosis and treatment. The fact that we are still woefully ignorant about how sensory stimuli are really perceived and interpreted is a matter only for acknowledgment. Its amplification must be sought elsewhere.

Depending on the special interest of the investigator, sensation may be classified in many different ways. The neurologist, in searching for the location and cause of neurologic disease, finds it convenient to consider sensation under two main headings: superficial and deep. Each of these main groups includes different modalities, which are discussed separately.

The modalities of sensation, such as the perception of touch, pain, and position sense, are dependent on stimuli that are transmitted from the periphery to the cerebrum along nerve fibers. These fibers are constantly grouping, regrouping, and changing their relationships to one another. The neurologist must become familiar with the longitudinal and lateral relationships of the various groups in nerves, plexuses, roots, and tracts and relate them not only to each other but also to the motor pathways. Then, if the neurologist establishes which of these modalities are impaired and which remain normal, a fairly accurate localization of a neurologic lesion is usually possible.

Superficial Sensation
Included under "superficial sensation" is the perception of light touch, pain, and temperature. Some would consider two-point and traced-figure discrimination here, but it seems more convenient to discuss them later with some of the more complex varieties of sensation.

Deep Sensation
"Deep sensation" includes perception of joint and vibratory sense and pain from the deep-lying somatic structures, such as muscle, ligaments, fascia, and bone.

Cortical Function in Sensation
The role of the cortex in sensory appreciation is discriminative. Destruction of the parietal cortex does not produce loss of any modality of sensation except as a transitory phenomenon. The basic sensations of pain, temperature, vibration, and touch are recognizable as such, but the ability to make fine sensory distinctions is impaired over the contralateral side of the body—facial sensation being least affected.

However, patients with an extensive parietal cortical lesion are unable to identify objects by touch *(astereognosis)*, to identify figures traced on the skin, and to appreciate the direction and degree of passive movements of their joints. Their ability to distinguish between different weights is impaired *(baragnosis)*, and various textures are not recognizable by touch alone.

Thalamic Function in Sensation
In human beings, the thalamus is the main sensory nucleus of the nervous system—a synapsing area of major importance as the nerve impulses proceed to the cortex. The fact that ipsilateral cortical ablation does not prevent the appreciation of painful, thermal, or tactile stimuli does not permit the conclusion that such sensation therefore reaches consciousness at the thalamic level. Conduction across the midline to the opposite cortex has not yet been adequately excluded.

In each thalamus, the sensory fibers of the medial lemniscus (predominantly from the dorsal funiculus) and the more laterally situated spinothalamic and trigeminothalamic tracts are received into the lateral and medial parts of the nucleus ventralis posterior. These fibers, with minor and variable exceptions, are from the opposite side of the body. Within the nucleus there is topical localization, so that, for all modalities of sensation, the body is represented with the head areas medially and the sacral areas most laterally situated. Sensory projections from the thalamus to the cortex are mainly to the posterior central and adjacent gyri.

Certain lesions in the neighborhood of the posterior ventral nuclei of the thalamus and its projection systems may be associated with a peculiar sensory distortion known as "thalamic pain." There is no general agreement on the exact location of these lesions, but it has been suggested that the loss of descending inhibitory fibers to the spinal cord may play a part. Another suggestion is that the destruction of certain lateral thalamic structures may remove an inhibitory effect on the affective activity of midline nuclei.

If such a lesion is present, single stimuli of mild or moderate intensity (with pin or temperature flask, for example) may go unperceived, but more vigorous or repetitive stimulation seems to burst explosively over a sensory threshold, to the patient's considerable distress. Light stroking of the skin may also provoke a very unpleasant sensation *(hyperpathia)*. Sensory distortions of this sort also may be found with partial lesions of peripheral nerves. One additional feature characteristic of spontaneous thalamic pain is the degree to which it may be intensified by an unpleasant emotional disturbance. The pleasure of a happy experience also may be magnified and may cause peculiar "feelings" on the affected side of the body.

GENERAL METHODS OF EXAMINATION

An important preface to each part of the sensory examination is a simple explanation of one's purpose and an actual demonstration of the stimulus to be used and of the responses desired. Above all, the patient should not be tested to the point of fatigue; in cases in which the sensory examination must be painstaking and prolonged, it is often desirable to intersperse less taxing portions of the examination between portions of the sensory testing.

All sensory testing should be carried out in a random, unpredictable order designed to diffuse the patient's attention from any one part of the body and to prevent the anticipation of any particular stimulus. After the preliminary demonstration of each stimulus, it is well to have the patient close the eyes and relax for the ensuing examination. At various times throughout this examination, the patient should be asked to indicate, with a finger, the exact site of stimulation. This practice not only sharpens the patient's attention during a relatively monotonous procedure but also may reveal an unsuspected defect in the ability to localize stimuli *(topagnosis)*.

The sensory examination is most accurately performed when it is carried out purposefully with the clinical history constantly in mind. Only when the history gives no reason to suspect sensory involvement of any kind should one's examination take the form of an anatomic survey of the patient from head to toe. This procedure of excluding, rather than seeking, a sensory deficit can usually be carried out quickly with pin and cotton for superficial sensation and with tuning fork and joint movement for deep sensation.

It should be pointed out here, however, that a specific complaint of sensory disturbance is not the only reason for considering sensory involvement. Take, for example, a patient who has weakness, atrophy, and fasciculations in the muscles of the upper extremities and in whom amyotrophic lateral sclerosis or progressive muscular atrophy might reasonably be suspected. Despite the absence of any sensory complaints in such a patient, during the sensory examination it is particularly important to test those upper extremities and the adjacent shoulder regions with pin and hot and cold probes for impairment in the appreciation of pain and temperature. A deficit of this sort, with normal perception of touch sensation, would suggest syringomyelia rather than one of the aforementioned muscular atrophies.

SPECIFIC METHODS OF EXAMINATION

Figure 10-1 illustrates the most important of the aids required for an adequate sensory examination. The metal disks (glass flasks also may be used) are freshly filled with hot and cold water just before the temperature sense is tested. The long-fibered cotton may be used both for the corneal reflex and for the testing of light touch. Pins should be *sharp* so that with minimal pressure the quick bright response of superficial pain can be elicited. The tuning fork in the illustration is made of a magnesium alloy and vibrates 128 times per second. Many experienced examiners have their own favorite forks of various designs, but the most important thing is to become familiar with the characteristics of one's own instrument.

In general, responses to the sensory examination should be elicited by single choices. Sensitivity can then be increased by varying the intensity of a stimulus. Thus, for joint position sense, the choice should be up or down; for temperature, hot or cold; and for superficial pain, sharp or dull. When the tuning fork is applied, the patient should be asked, "Is it vibrating or just touching?" If the patient answers incorrectly, the stimulus should be increased until correct responses are consistently obtained or the maximum intensity is reached.

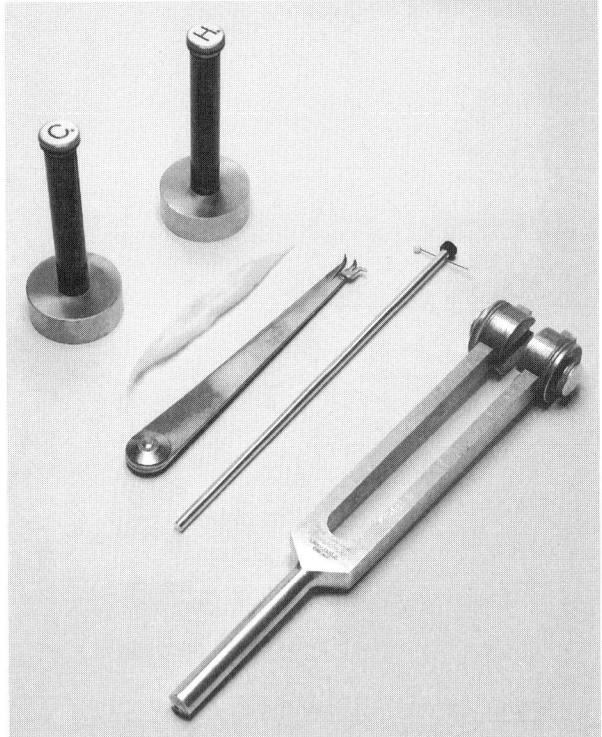

Figure 10-1
Important aids in sensory examination.

Tests for Superficial Sensation
Light touch

Although there is still some disagreement about the specificity of various sensory receptors, it is generally agreed that in the peripheral nerves, the impulses conveying light touch travel predominantly in large myelinated fibers. The cell bodies of these fibers are located in the dorsal root ganglia of the spinal cord and homologous ganglia of the cranial nerves. The central branches of these unipolar cells enter the spinal cord through the posterior root and, as they ascend through the cord, are concentrated mainly in the dorsal fasciculi of the same side and in the opposite ventral spinothalamic tracts (Fig. 10-2). Because of this double distribution, the sensation of touch is often preserved when other modalities are profoundly affected by lesions involving the spinal cord.

Light touch may be investigated with the opposite unpointed end of the cotton used in testing the corneal reflex. Hence, the testing of light touch conveniently follows corneal testing in the examination, and the sequence of proceeding from the head downward becomes a natural

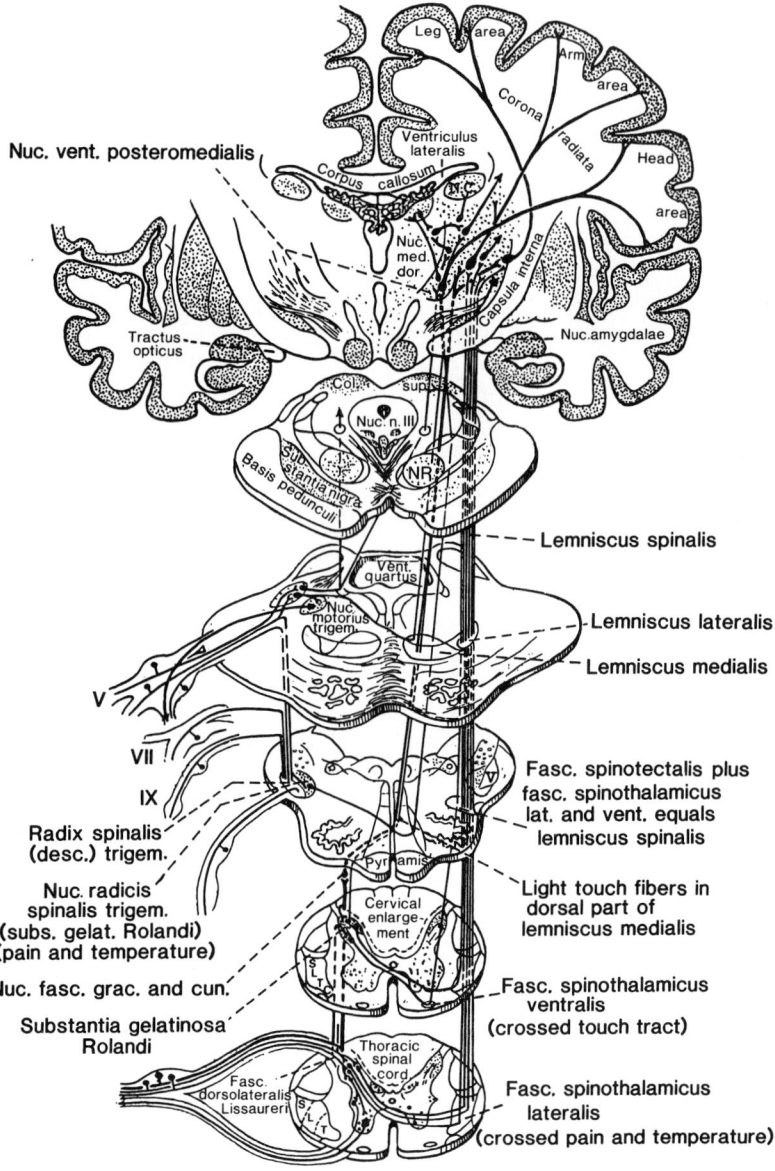

Figure 10-2
Pain, temperature, and light touch conduction. *(Modified from Rasmussen AT: The principal nervous pathways: neurological charts and schemas with explanatory notes, ed 4, New York, 1952, Macmillan Co.)*

one, not only for touch but subsequently for pain and temperature as well. When the procedure is demonstrated to the patient, many simple responses are suitable, but probably the most useful is a simple "yes" when touched. Certain unsophisticated, neurotic, or malingering patients may respond "no" in a very revealing fashion.

One disadvantage to the testing of light touch with long-fibered cotton is encountered in areas of unusual hairiness. In this situation, modern modifications of Frey's hairs can be very useful; some neurologists prefer such a graded set of "hairs" in testing for appreciation of light touch throughout the body.

There is great variation in normal sensitivity to light touch, not only in various parts of the body in any one patient but also from one individual to another. The significance of such variation is not always apparent, but symmetrical comparisons and the responses with other modalities usually are of help. When a patient's attention fades and fluctuates during the examination so that variable responses are obtained with repetitions over the same region, one should consider the possibility of *"cortical sensory inattention"* from a parietal lesion on the opposite side. This "sensory inattention" pertains not only to light touch but to other modalities as well.

When the initial random testing has revealed an area of insensitivity to light touch, the borders of such an area can be outlined by testing from inside the area of loss toward the region of normal feeling. Perhaps it should be stressed again that the initial "random" survey of sensation only appears so to the patient. The examiner is actually making purposeful comparisons of any regions suggested by the history.

Superficial pain

In the peripheral nerves, fibers that subserve superficial pain are among the medium-sized and small medullated ones. These conduct less rapidly than the larger touch fibers but faster than the small unmyelinated fibers, which seem to carry poorly localized crude pain stimuli to the central nervous system. Compression of a peripheral nerve or its root is likely to damage the larger motor or touch fibers first, whereas chemical agents tend to affect the finer, less medullated fibers before the larger, medullated ones.

In the spinal cord, stimuli that are interpreted as superficial and deep pain as well as temperature are conducted cephalad by fibers that run in the lateral spinothalamic tracts (see Fig. 10-2). The fibers subserving deep pain are thought to lie closer to the midline than those for superficial pain and temperature. Within a few segments of their entrance into the spinal cord, fibers conveying pain and temperature make their primary synapse and cross the midline through the ventral commissure to the opposite lateral funiculus, where they join the medial aspect of the lateral spinothalamic tract (see Fig. 10-2). These anatomic details are important for two reasons: first, the crossing of the "pain and temperature" fibers in the anterior commissure (so close to the central canal) explains the dissociated sensory loss (of pain and temperature with preservation of touch) so characteristic of syringomyelia; second, the manner in which the most caudal contributions to the spinothalamic tract are pushed laterally by the incoming contributions from higher up results in a lamination of the tract, with the fibers from the lowest segments of the spinal cord most dorsolaterally placed on each side. This accounts for the "sacral" signs and symptoms that result from more or less superficial involvement of the lateral funiculus at even the highest level of the cord.

It might be well to point out, however, that these tracts are not necessarily arranged in compact bundles as represented in most anatomic diagrams and that considerable local diffusion may occur. It is also thought that an older and more diffuse system exists for the conduction of painful impulses (and possibly others) within the cord. These two factors, and the belief that some pain fibers may ascend without crossing, are undoubtedly responsible for some of the apparent inconsistencies in clinicopathologic correlation studies.

As with light touch, the test of superficial pain sensation should begin with a demonstration to the patient, who should be encouraged to answer "sharp" or "dull" with the least possible delay. Particularly in cases in which peripheral neuropathy or tabes dorsalis might be suspected from the history, the patient should understand that a change of answer from dull to sharp (or vice versa) is entirely in order if there is any reason for doing so. Unless prepared in this way, some reticent patients with *delayed pain appreciation* (occurring most often in the legs) will not acquaint the examiners with this important observation. Some examiners use the usual single or double pinprick of brief duration to test for delayed pain; others use a continuous boring pinprick. With either method, abnormal delays of 1 to 4 seconds in the appreciation of pain may be found.

After these preliminaries, the patient should close the eyes and the examiner should proceed initially in the same "random" fashion described for light touch. Any areas of sensory loss should then be outlined by testing from the abnormal area to the normal. It is of interest, when one is establishing a sensory level to pain in lesions of the spinal cord, to proceed not only from the abnormal to the normal region but also in a reverse direction, marking the level where pain appreciation disappears. The area between these lines will be narrow in the more completely destructive lesions but may be quite broad in less severe cases.

Temperature

It is suggested that in testing temperature appreciation, the metal disks be filled with the coldest and the hottest water available in free-flowing taps. This usually means water at about 10°C and 43°C. The outsides of the metal disks should be thoroughly dried and kept that way during the test. The stimulus used should, as usual, be the least one that produces a reliable response. By changing the duration of contact between metal disk and skin, considerable variation in strength of stimulus can be obtained. For some reason, temperature testing often gives a more consistent border of sensory loss than does pain testing.

In the initial survey, if areas of deficit are found, the borders may be more accurately determined by rolling the metal disk along the skin from the insensitive region to the normal one than by applying the metal disk at intervals.

Patients who overreact to many of the stimuli used in sensory testing are not unusual, and this is seen particularly in those with a significant emotional problem. It is also well to remember that in many older people and in others with poor peripheral circulation (especially in cold weather), the skin temperature of the hands and feet may be decreased enough to modify temperature responses considerably in an otherwise normal patient.

Tests for Deep Sensation
Joint sense (sense of position and passive movement)
Position and passive movements of the joints are appreciated through fibers located in the posterior fasciculi, and, along with vibration sense, joint sense is a good indicator of disturbances in this afferent tract (Fig. 10-3). It has been suggested that the afferent fibers for vibration and those for passive movement travel in slightly different parts of the cord, the fibers for vibration being located in the lateral funiculus and not being intermingled with the fibers conveying passive movement in the posterior funiculus. Such a concept allows explanation of a puzzling situation observed not infrequently in patients with the subacute combined degeneration of pernicious anemia and at times in patients with multiple sclerosis. In these instances, a lesion of the spinal cord brings about a striking loss in the appreciation of vibration but causes little or no disturbance in the identification of passive movement. Certain parietal lesions, on the other hand, may profoundly affect the appreciation of passive movement while leaving vibration sense almost intact, but this has a different explanation and will be discussed again.

Passive movement is tested in the lower extremities by vertical movements of the toes and in the upper extremities by similar movements of the thumbs and fingers. The digit is usually grasped by its lateral surfaces, but the dorsoventral surfaces may be used if they are held so firmly that the additional pressures needed to move the digit will not be apparent to the patient. Movement is confined to an upward or downward direction. Each move, however slight, should be identified by the patient with the single word "up" or "down" in relation to the previous stationary position (and not in relation to the neutral or midposition, as many patients tend to do). It is well for the first test movements to be large and easily identified, but once the idea is clear to the patient, the smallest detectable movements should be used. Quick jerks are more

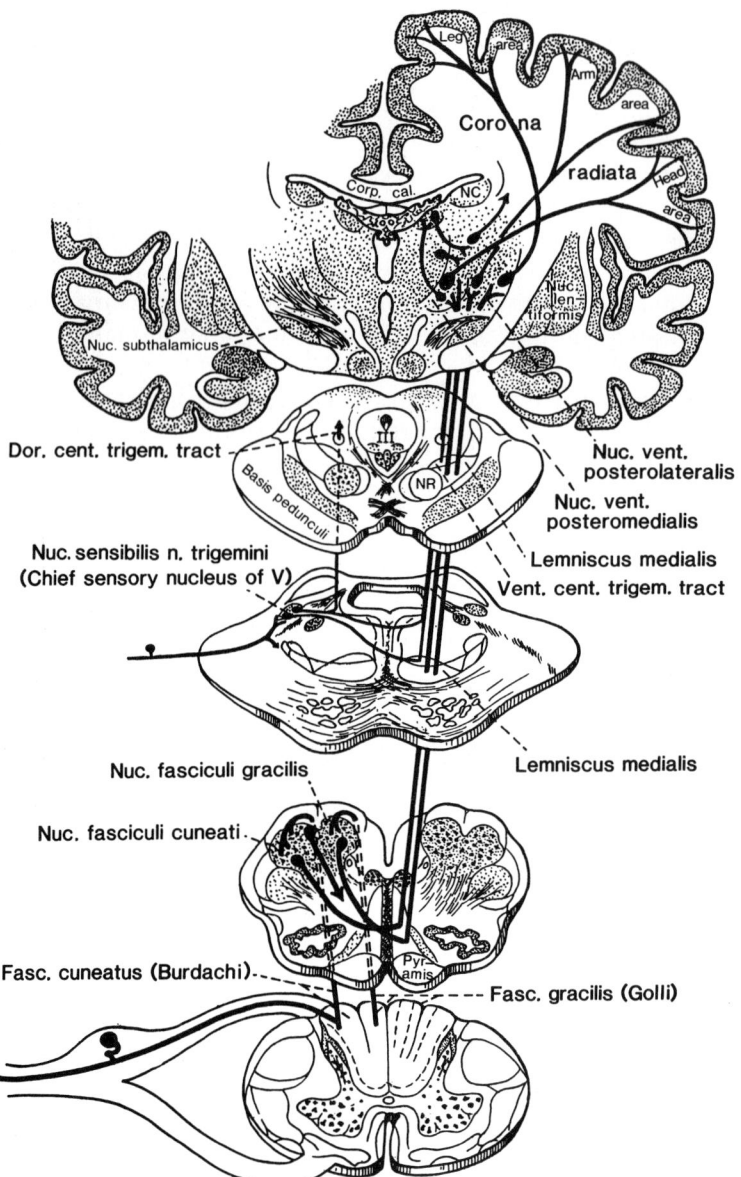

Figure 10-3
Tactile discrimination and deep sensibility (circuit to conscious center). *(Modified from Rasmussen AT: The principal nervous pathways: neurological charts and schemas with explanatory notes, ed 4, New York, 1952, Macmillan Co.)*

stimulating than slow movements, and an average middle speed should be used, as a rule. Very slow movement may be used in some instances as a refinement of the routine test.

The examiner should remember that when the whole digit is moved up or down, muscle and tendon stretch receptor organs attached in series to the joint are stimulated. In the case of finger movement, stimulation involves muscles in the forearm. Signs of distal proprioceptive peripheral nerve involvement might be missed. In the fingers, this problem can be overcome by maximally flexing the proximal interphalangeal joint and then testing proprioception by making movements across the distal interphalangeal joint.

Deep pain
Deep-pain sense is of particular interest in the peripheral neuropathies, tabes dorsalis, and some of the muscle diseases. Digital compression of slowly increasing severity is applied to various deep-lying structures. The evaluation of slight variations from the normal is not easy, but fortunately it is the extremes of hypersensitivity and hyposensitivity that are of most importance diagnostically. For the lower half of the body, the tendon of Achilles, calf muscles, and testicles are the regions usually tested, but the sensitivity of any weak or painful muscle may be of interest. In the upper extremity, the stretching of small finger joints into hyperflexion is a comparable test but is less often used. Patients with tabes dorsalis may tolerate maximal two-handed compression of the tendon of Achilles or calf muscles with complete equanimity.

When one is testing an unusually sensitive muscle, it is well to do so in a number of different areas and planes, with the possibility in mind that the tenderness may be linear and associated with a sensitive artery or vein rather than in the muscle itself. Increased warmth and a prominent venous pattern in a limb should suggest the possibility of local phlebitis.

Vibration
It is best to demonstrate the sensation of vibration to the patient by pressing the tuning fork to the sternum both during vibration and again when the fork is stopped (silent control application). The patient should respond to the testing by saying "buzzing" when vibration is felt and by saying "no" when only pressure is felt. When the procedure is understood, the patient should close the eyes and the test should begin. A running tap or other extraneous noise in the room helps to eliminate the auditory factor, and it is well to strike the fork before every application and stop it again with the hand for the control tests.

The bony points most conveniently tested in the lower half of the body are the dorsal aspects of the terminal phalanges of the great toes, the malleoli, the tibial tuberosities, and the anterior superior iliac spines. In the upper extremities, the terminal phalanges of the thumbs, the radial and ulnar tuberosities, the humeral epicondyles, the olecranon, and the acromial processes are readily available. The patient who identifies vibrations on one side of the skull, sternum, or symphysis pubis and not on the other is probably demonstrating a conversion reaction or malingering. It is customary to begin testing the peripheral areas first and to move centrally.

It seems advisable for the initial tests to be silent control applications. Some patients, particularly those with peripheral neuropathy or combined-system disease, may have a constant tingling sensation in the limbs peripherally that leads them to identify vibration when none is present. This may cause the unwary examiner to miss a severe loss in vibration appreciation unless the tests are controlled very carefully.

The vibration stimulus may be modified both by varying the force used to set the fork in motion initially and by noting the length of time that a vibrating fork is discernible to the patient while the fork "runs down." When a vibrating fork is no longer felt on one bony point but is still "buzzing" when tested at a comparable area on the other side of the body, a significant deficit is usually present if this difference is a consistent one.

A sharp gradient of vibration loss with a marked deficit peripherally and very little proximally suggests a lesion in the peripheral nerves. When the loss extends with little change from the peripheral joints to the girdle bones, a lesion in the spinal cord is more probable.

Since vibratory appreciation is seldom disturbed by lesions above the level of the thalamus and since passive movement requires some cortical participation for its recognition, a significant disturbance in the identification of passive movement with adequate appreciation of vibration favors a lesion above the thalamic level.

Tests for Combined Sensation (Two-Point Distinction, Traced-Figure Identification, and Stereognosis)

The ability to make these distinctions under normal conditions is a function of the cerebral cortex and is particularly related to activity in the parietal lobes. However, before a disturbance in these capacities can have any localizing significance, the basic sensory information from the region tested must be adequate. When the loss of deep and superficial sensation seems very slight in a limb but the ability to identify two points, traced figures, or familiar shapes is much impaired, the presumption of a cerebral lesion is strong but not absolute. In certain rare instances, lesions of both spinal cord and peripheral nerves have been the basis for just such findings. As a rule, other observations clarify the picture, however, and for the most part, the situation described should suggest the possibility of a lesion above the thalamus.

Two-point discrimination

Two-point discrimination is most readily carried out with a small pair of calipers or a compass. The variety shown in Figure 10-1 closely resembles the instrument devised by Dr. Gordon Holmes. Different regions of the body vary markedly in their capacity to distinguish two separate points of contact applied simultaneously at various degrees of separation. On the lips, for example, points within 2 or 3 mm of each other may be correctly identified as two points, whereas on the back, contacts 4 or 5 cm apart may be felt as one. Convenient areas for testing two-point distinction include the palms (where the average patient can distinguish points 8 to 15 mm apart), dorsa of the hands (20 to 30 mm) and feet (30 to 40 mm), fingertips (3 to 5 mm), dorsa of the fingers (4 to 6 mm), and shins (30 to 40 mm).

After the proper test responses have been demonstrated, the patient is asked to close the eyes and express the reaction to the stimulus by the word "one" or "two." Single and double points should be varied unpredictably during the test. When answers are consistently correct on a normal area of the body with minimal separation of the points, the comparable region is tested on the abnormal side. The same relation to the long axis of the limb or trunk is maintained on the two sides. This test may also be used to demonstrate a sensory level on the trunk.

Traced-figure identification

The inability to identify traced figures on the skin of one limb when superficial sensation is normal and the sensorium is intact usually indicates a lesion involving the contralateral parietal lobe.

The test is carried out with a pencil, swab stick, or other suitable marker. The digits 1 to 9 are convenient to use, but other obvious shapes or symbols may be tried. It is well to stand beside the patient and face the area to be tested, so that the traced numerals will have a familiar relationship to the patient. After the patient has watched one or two demonstrations, the rest of the test is conducted with the patient's eyes closed. The palm, fingers, and face are the areas most commonly tested.

Stereognosis

Stereognosis is the ability to identify an object by handling it. This is the one part of the sensory examination in which there is no preliminary visual demonstration. Any common object, such as a pocketknife, key, or pencil, may be used in the test, and coins of various denominations are particularly suitable. The abnormal side should always be tested first and then the normal side compared.

It has been said that the term "astereognosis" should not be applied when the hand under consideration shows any defect whatever in the appreciation of superficial or deep sensation. This is an attractive distinction for the purist, but such an unqualified astereognosis is practically never observed in our clinical experience. From the practical viewpoint, the term "astereognosis" is limited to situations in which an impaired ability to identify objects by palpation is associated with a sensory loss in the hands so slight that it is insufficient to account for the difficulty.

Double simultaneous stimulation

It has been observed that some patients who report normal, or almost normal, sensations in various parts of the body when these parts are separately tested are unable to do nearly so well when the same stimuli are applied to comparable areas simultaneously. Such patients are usually those with cerebral damage. A variety of terms have been used to describe a disturbance in the normal response to double simultaneous stimulation (DSS). These have included "extinction," "suppression," "repression," "perceptual rivalry," "tactile inattention," and "sensory eclipse." Of these, "extinction" seems to have won best acceptance. Current views favor a process of "delayed informational processing following cerebral damage" as an explanation for the phenomenon of extinction.

Any sensory stimulus, including visual and auditory stimuli, can be used for DSS. Although delicate refinements with carefully timed and modulated electric stimuli are available for laboratory research, the procedure in testing DSS at the bedside is a relatively simple one. Pinprick is usually the most sensitive indicator, but when patients are mentally slow or obtunded, simple finger contact may give helpful information. After closing the eyes, the patient is told to expect a sensation on either one side or both sides of the body. After the stimulation, the patient is asked to indicate the site of the stimulus or stimuli (they are always placed symmetrically) and their nature. Whenever only one stimulus is identified after two have been presented, the patient is again reminded that stimulation may be felt on only one side of the body or on both sides and the test is repeated. When pinprick is used, the two pins must be equally sharp.

If extinction is present, the stimuli on the involved side may be ignored entirely or the sharp stimulus may be consistently interpreted as dull. To allow for inequality of sharpness in the pins, the examiner should interchange them whenever such an "abnormality" is detected.

Unilateral abnormalities with DSS are found in patients with contralateral cerebral lesions and may be the only demonstrable sensory loss, although stereognosis, traced figures, joint position sense, and two-point discrimination also are likely to be impaired. Lesions of the parietal lobe are particularly likely to alter responses to DSS, but it has been claimed that in rare instances, injury to the internal capsule, the thalamus, or any part of its cortical projection may bring about such changes.

SENSORY SUPPLY (SEGMENTAL AND NEURAL)

Before a really adequate sensory examination can be carried out or interpreted, the examiner should have some knowledge of the distributions of the sensory dermatomes and peripheral nerves. This knowledge allows the margins of sensory loss to be tested with greater discernment as the examination is conducted. Although the distinction among lesions of the peripheral nerves, plexuses, nerve roots, and spinal cord is not always an easy one, differences in the distribution of sensory changes from such lesions may be quite distinctive. When these sensory abnormalities are considered along with the patient's complaints, reflex changes, and motor weakness, a pattern may be apparent on the basis of which confident localization can be made.

Figures 10-4 through 10-10 are included to illustrate these distributions of dermatomes and peripheral nerves, but it must be remembered that such patterns vary a great deal from patient to patient. These illustrations simply present the average arrangement from a large number of people tested over many years. Any individual patient may present certain minor differences, but the overall picture should conform.

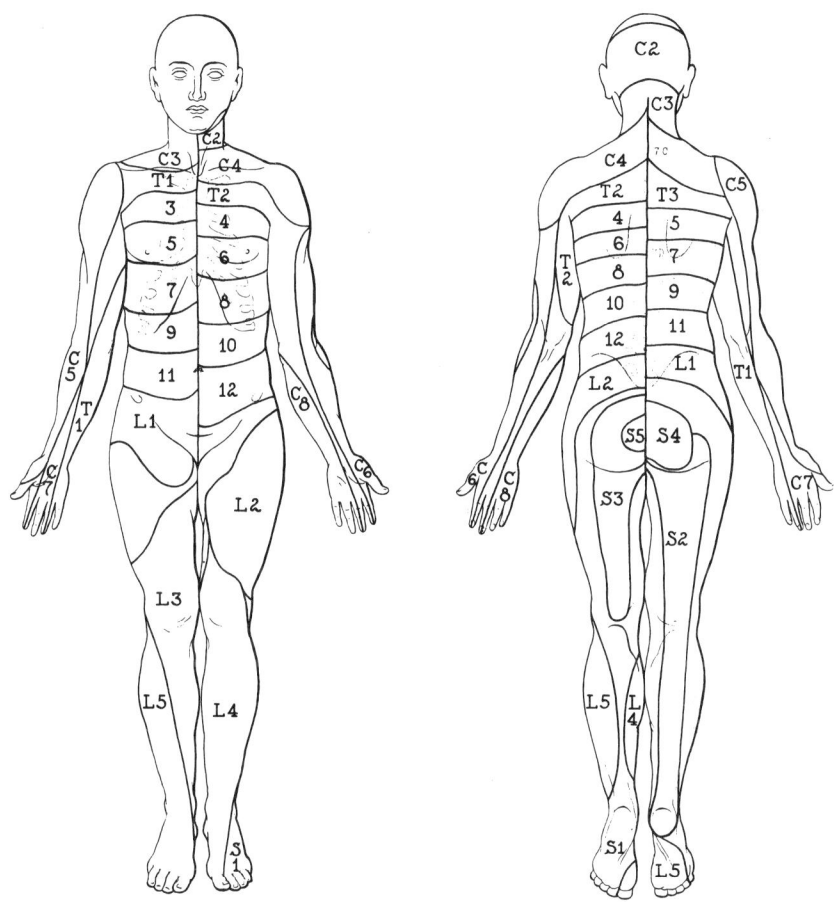

Figure 10-4
Distribution of the spinal dermatomes. The maximal extent of each dermatome is given. *(Modified from Ford FR: Diseases of the nervous system in infancy, childhood and adolescence, ed 3, Springfield, 1952, Charles C Thomas, Publisher. By permission of the publisher.)*

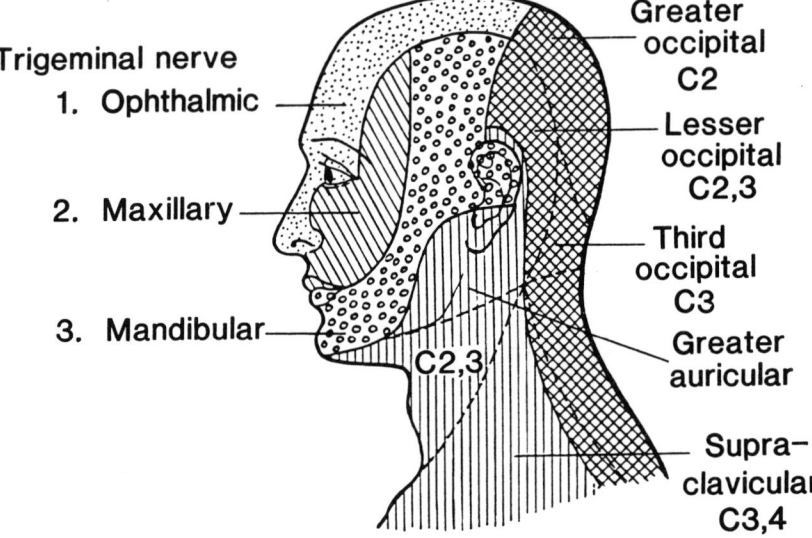

Figure 10-5
Distribution of cutaneous nerves to head and neck. *(Modified from Brash JC: Cunningham's text-book of anatomy, ed 9, New York, 1951, Oxford University Press. By permission of the publisher.)*

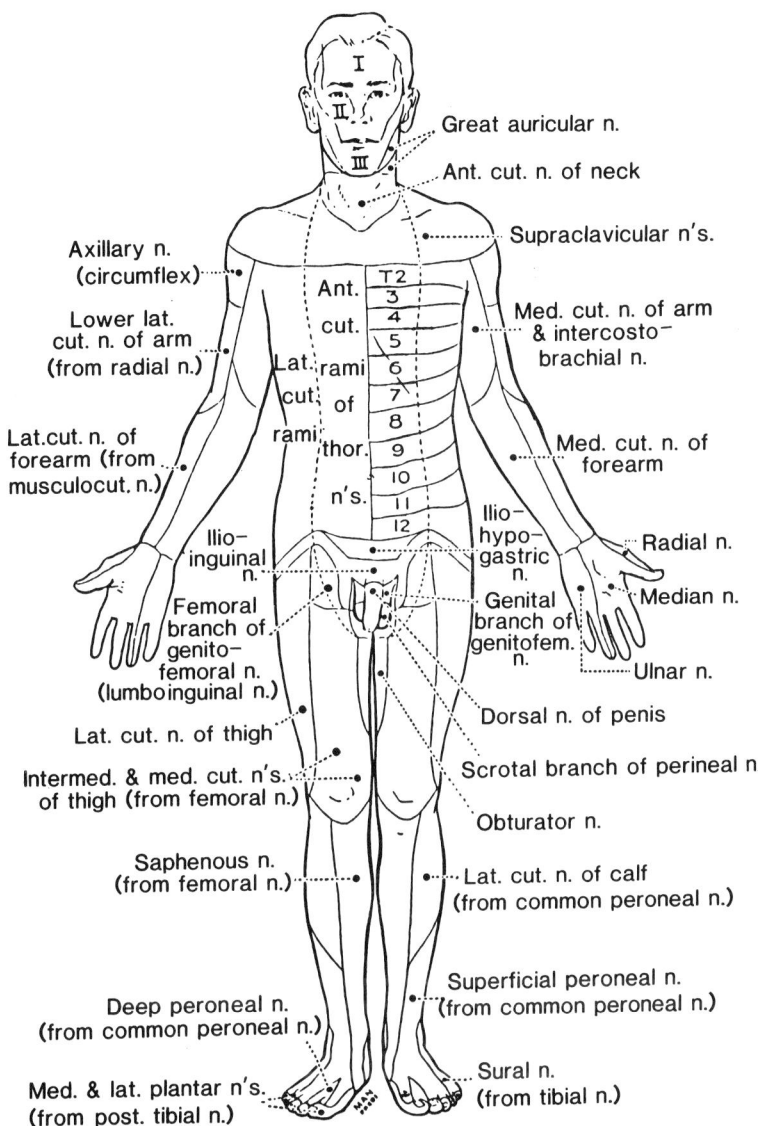

Figure 10-6
Cutaneous fields of peripheral nerves, anterior view. *(From Haymaker W, Woodhall B: Peripheral nerve injuries: principles of diagnosis, ed 2, Philadelphia, 1953, WB Saunders Co. By permission of the publisher.)*

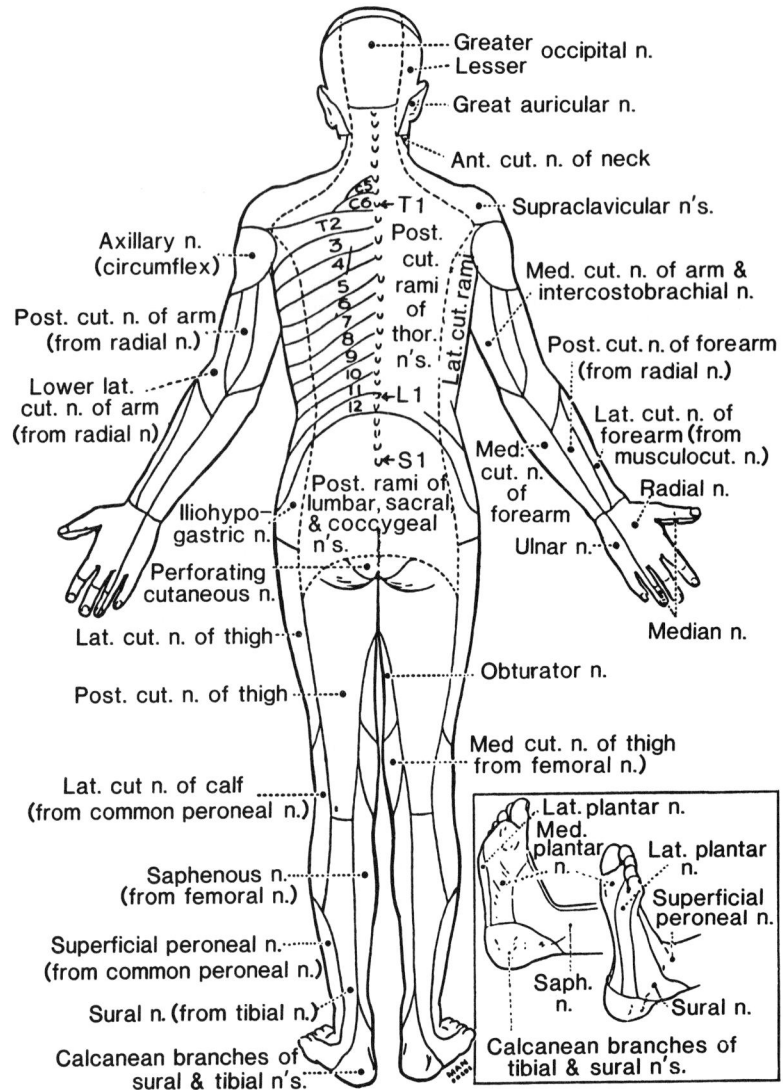

Figure 10-7
Cutaneous fields of peripheral nerves, posterior view. *(From Haymaker W, Woodhall B: Peripheral nerve injuries: principles of diagnosis, ed 2, Philadelphia, 1953, WB Saunders Co. By permission of the publisher.)*

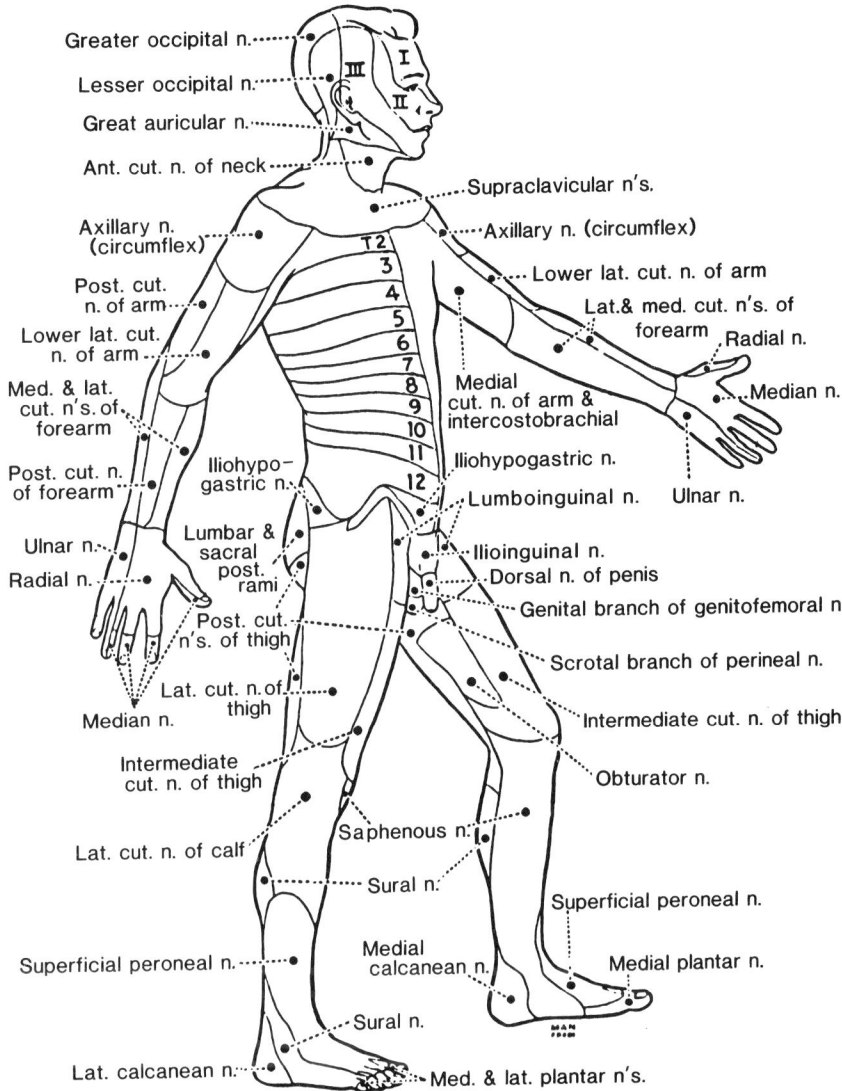

Figure 10-8
Cutaneous fields of peripheral nerves, side view. *(From Haymaker W, Woodhall B: Peripheral nerve injuries: principles of diagnosis, ed 2, Philadelphia, 1953, WB Saunders Co. By permission of the publisher.)*

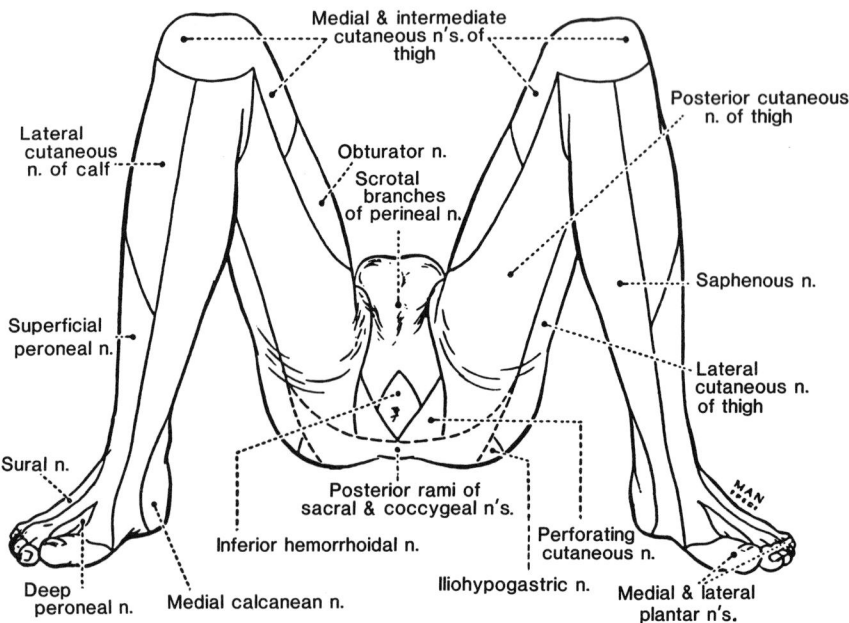

Figure 10-9
Cutaneous fields of peripheral nerves, perineal view. *(From Haymaker W, Woodhall B: Peripheral nerve injuries: principles of diagnosis, ed 2, Philadelphia, 1953, WB Saunders Co. By permission of the publisher.)*

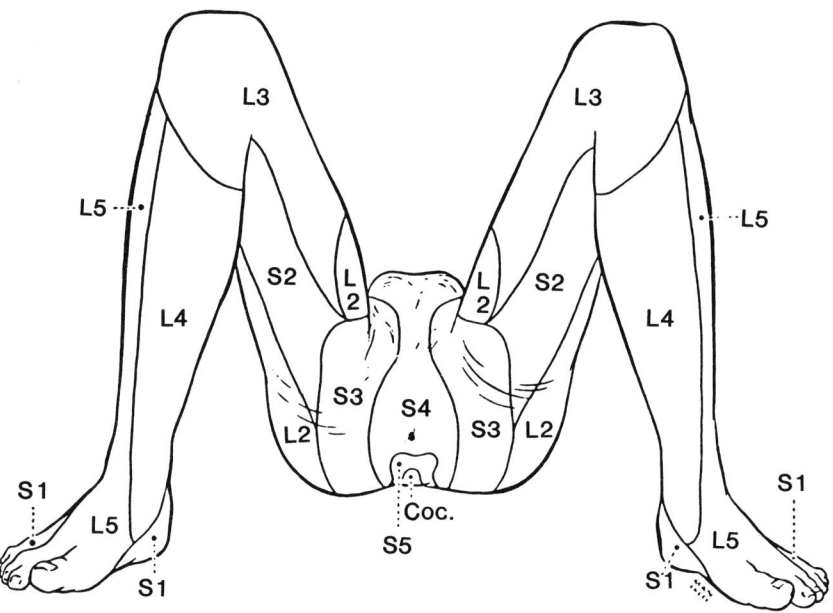

Figure 10-10
Location of dermatomes, perineal view. *(From Haymaker W, Woodhall B: Peripheral nerve injuries: principles of diagnosis, ed 2, Philadelphia, 1953, WB Saunders Co. By permission of the publisher.)*

Chapter 11

Autonomic Function

The autonomic nervous system is a primarily efferent system of nerve fibers with ganglia and plexuses outside the central nervous system innervating the blood vessels, heart, viscera, glands, and smooth muscles throughout the body. Afferent nerve fibers conveying impulses from these structures to the central nervous system are present in autonomic nerves such as the vagus and the splanchnic nerves as well as in peripheral somatic nerves. These visceral afferent nerve fibers are thinly myelinated or nonmyelinated, and the impulses they carry are related to visceral sensations, such as pain and distention, and to visceral reflexes underlying functions such as respiration, maintenance of blood pressure, and micturition. Their cells of origin are in spinal dorsal root ganglia and in certain cranial nerve ganglia. The visceral afferent fibers terminate in the spinal cord and brain stem on neurons subserving local visceral reflexes and on neurons forming secondary visceral tracts. In the spinal cord, these visceral tracts probably exist as multiple chains of neurons, crossed and uncrossed and not well defined into specific tracts, in the lateral columns of white matter near the ventral horns.

Anatomically, the autonomic nervous system consists of three divisions: a craniosacral (parasympathetic) outflow, a thoracolumbar (sympathetic) outflow (Fig. 11-1), and the enteric nervous system, located in the wall of the gastrointestinal tract (described later in this chapter). Arising from nerve cells in the midbrain, medulla oblongata, and the second, third, and fourth segments of the sacral spinal cord, the preganglionic parasympathetic fibers synapse in ganglia that are outside the central nervous system and located close to, or in, the structures they supply. The preganglionic sympathetic fibers arise from nerve cells in the intermediolateral column of gray matter in spinal cord segments T-1 through L-2, and they synapse in the two paravertebral sympathetic ganglionic chains and in the several prevertebral ganglia (celiac, superior and inferior mesenteric, and aortic). Preganglionic nerve fibers are myelinated; postganglionic nerve fibers are not.

The cranial portion of the parasympathetic outflow consists of nerve fibers carried in the third, seventh, ninth, and tenth cranial nerves. The

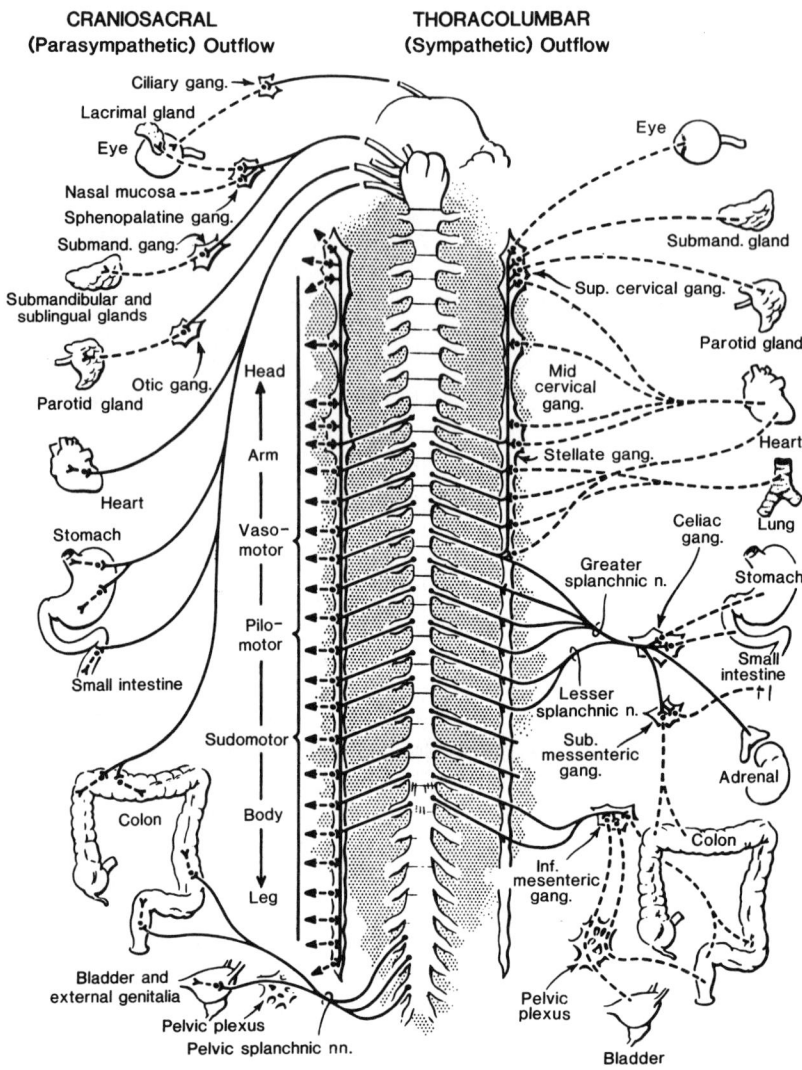

Figure 11-1
Diagrammatic representation of the autonomic nervous system. The thoracolumbar (sympathetic) outflow is shown to the right of the spinal cord. To the left of the cord are the gray rami arising from the paravertebral sympathetic trunk and, further to the left, the craniosacral (parasympathetic) outflow.

Edinger-Westphal nuclei, situated just in front of each oculomotor nucleus in the rostral portion of the midbrain, are the origin of preganglionic fibers that travel with the third cranial nerves. These fibers synapse in the ipsilateral ciliary ganglion in the orbit with the postganglionic fibers innervating the ciliary muscles and the sphincter pupillae muscle of the iris. The parasympathetic fibers are essential to the pupillary light and accommodation reflexes.

The superior salivatory nucleus, which lies near the nucleus of the facial nerve in the lower pons, gives rise to preganglionic fibers leaving the brain stem in the nervus intermedius portion of the seventh cranial nerve. They enter the facial canal but leave the facial nerve in the region of the geniculate ganglion. Some of these fibers enter the greater superficial petrosal nerve and proceed to the sphenopalatine ganglion, where they synapse with postganglionic fibers supplying the lacrimal gland and the nasal mucosa. Other preganglionic fibers travel with the chorda tympani to the submaxillary ganglion, where they synapse with postganglionic fibers supplying the submandibular and sublingual salivary glands.

The inferior salivatory nucleus, which is located in the rostral portion of the medulla, gives rise to preganglionic fibers that are contained in the glossopharyngeal nerve. These fibers synapse in the otic ganglion with postganglionic neurons supplying the parotid gland. The dorsal efferent nucleus of the vagus situated in the medulla gives rise to preganglionic fibers, which are distributed via the vagus nerves to ganglia in the cardiac and pulmonary plexuses, the esophagus, the stomach, and the intestines as far as the splenic flexure of the colon. These preganglionic fibers synapse with short postganglionic neurons that supply these viscera.

The sacral portion of the parasympathetic outflow arises from nerve cells located in the intermediolateral zone of gray matter of the second, third, and fourth sacral segments of the spinal cord. Preganglionic fibers from these cells leave the spinal cord with the corresponding sacral ventral roots and form the pelvic splanchnic nerves. These preganglionic fibers synapse with ganglia of the pelvic plexuses and mural ganglia of the bladder and large bowel distal to the splenic flexure. The sacral portion of the parasympathetic outflow is essential to bladder, bowel, and sexual function.

The thoracolumbar (sympathetic) outflow of the autonomic nervous system arises from nerve cells situated in the intermediolateral column of gray matter in the spinal cord, which extends over segments T-1 through L-2. Evidence that preganglionic fibers may also emerge from the remaining lumbar and sacral roots has not been substantiated in humans. Axons arising from these cells leave the spinal cord with the corresponding thoracic and upper two lumbar ventral roots to enter white communicating rami that connect with the two paravertebral chains of sympathetic ganglia. These ganglionic chains lie on either side of the vertebral column and consist of 3 cervical, 11 thoracic, and 4 to 6 lumbar ganglia. Gray communicating rami connect the paravertebral ganglia with each of the spinal nerves, carrying postganglionic sympathetic fibers for distribution to the entire body. In addition, some preganglionic sympathetic nerve fibers do not synapse in the paravertebral ganglionic chains; instead they pass through them to form the greater and lesser splanchnic nerves. These fibers synapse in the prevertebral ganglia (celiac, superior and inferior mesenteric, and aortic), from which relatively short postganglionic fibers pass to the viscera they innervate. The postganglionic sympathetic fibers supplying the head arise from the superior cervical ganglion on each side and travel upward on the surface of the internal and external carotid arteries to reach the glands, smooth muscles, and blood vessels of intracranial and extracranial structures. The musculus dilator pupillae of the eye and the smooth muscle fibers of the upper eyelid are supplied by postganglionic sympathetic fibers, and interruption of this sympathetic innervation results in Horner's syndrome (unilateral miosis, ptosis, and anhidrosis of the ipsilateral side of the face; ipsilateral anhidrosis occurs chiefly when the lesion is proximal to the bifurcation of the common carotid artery; lesions along the internal carotid artery cause anhidrosis restricted to the medial forehead and nasal bridge).

On a pharmacologic basis, the autonomic nervous system is still divided into a cholinergic portion and an adrenergic portion, depending on the distribution of the chemical transmitter substances, acetylcholine and norepinephrine. Acetylcholine is the transmitter substance at the synapses of all preganglionic autonomic nerve fibers, parasympathetic and sympathetic, as well as at the terminals of all postganglionic parasympathetic fibers. It is also the transmitter substance at the terminals of the postganglionic sympathetic fibers innervating sweat glands and the fibers causing vasodilatation of blood vessels in skeletal muscle. The transmitter substance at all other postganglionic sympathetic synapses is norepinephrine. Autonomic functions can be facilitated or inhibited by certain pharmacologic agents that act on transmission in autonomic ganglia or at effector sites innervated by postganglionic autonomic nerve fibers. Such agents affect the synthesis or release of the transmitter substance at the nerve terminal or interfere with the metabolism and removal of the transmitter substance at the synapse. They also may block receptor sites for the transmitter substance on the postsynaptic membrane of the postganglionic neuron or of the effector organ.

Recent evidence suggests a much more complicated pharmacology, with co-release of neuropeptide and classic neurotransmitters as well as release of adenosine phosphate as an inhibitory transmitter by enteric vagal efferent fibers (purinergic nerves).

RESPIRATION

A respiratory center, vital to the control of respiration, is located in the reticular formation of the pons and upper medulla, though it is not the sharply demarcated structure that the term implies. It is composed of a functionally integrated group of nerve cells and fibers that coordinate respiratory movements with the demands of body metabolism and circulation. The medullary respiratory center is said to be under the influence of the pontine center, situated near the midline at mid and upper pons levels. The neurons of both centers are stimulated by increasing carbon dioxide tension and hydrogen ion concentration in the blood as well as by a decrease in oxygen tension. The carotid body chemoreceptors are particularly sensitive to hypoxia and hydrogen ion excess, and impulses from these receptors travel via visceral afferent fibers of the glossopharyngeal nerves to terminate in the reticular formation of the pons and medulla. Stretch receptors in the lung underlie the Hering-Breuer reflexes, which are important to respiratory control, and their afferent pathways are in the vagus nerves. After interruption of both vagus nerves below the origins of the recurrent laryngeal nerves, with loss of the afferent impulses from the pulmonary stretch receptors, breathing becomes slower and deeper, the chest tends to assume a position of partial inspiration, and pauses often occur at the end of inspiration and expiration. If both vagus nerves are interrupted above the origins of the recurrent laryngeal nerves (which supply the muscles controlling the vocal cords), the larynx will no longer open with inspiration. Tracheostomy may be required because of the danger of asphyxia.

The muscles of respiration are innervated by somatic efferent nerve fibers arising from nerve cells in the ventral horns of cervical and thoracic spinal cord segments bilaterally. The diaphragm is innervated by the phrenic nerves (C-3, C-4, and C-5), whereas the intercostal and abdominal muscles are innervated by the intercostal nerves. Accessory muscles of respiration in the neck receive their innervation from cervical spinal cord segments. Descending nerve fibers in the anterolateral portions of the spinal cord modify the activity of the motor nerve cells in the spinal cord that innervate the muscles of respiration. These descending nerve fibers carry impulses from the respiratory centers of the brain stem for automatic breathing and from the cerebrum for the voluntary control and modification of breathing. Bilateral cordotomy can interrupt these fibers in the cervical region and interfere with respiration. Transection of the spinal cord above C-3 isolates the respiratory muscles from the brain stem and cerebrum and causes respiratory paralysis. Diseases such as myasthenia gravis, amyotrophic lateral sclerosis, poliomyelitis, and Guillain-Barré syndrome interfere with respiration by causing weakness of the respiratory muscles or by affecting their innervation.

Alterations in the rate and rhythm of respiration occur with disorders in the central nervous system, particularly those affecting the pons and medulla. Irregular or ataxic breathing, or weak inspiratory gasps, are especially associated with serious dysfunction of the lower part of the brain stem. Periodic respiration (such as the common Cheyne-Stokes variety) occurs with lesions at various levels in the brain. Cheyne-Stokes breathing is characterized by respiratory efforts that are weak at first and then become successively stronger before gradually diminishing again to the point of apnea to complete the cycle. At times, periodic breathing will consist of several full respiratory efforts interspersed with prolonged pauses rather than a gradual waxing and waning. Increasing intracranial pressure, when it becomes severe, can cause alterations in respiratory rhythm and rate, including periodic respiration, as well as bradycardia and a rising blood pressure.

TEMPERATURE CONTROL

Even during health, different parts of the body have different temperatures. A temperature gradient exists between the body core (the contents of the cranial, thoracic, and abdominal cavities) and the peripheral portions of the body, and, whereas the peripheral temperature fluctuates over a considerable range, the core temperature remains almost constant. Regulation of body temperature is dependent on the hypothalamus, which exerts its influence through the autonomic and somatic centers of the brain stem and the spinal cord. Muscle tone is a continuous source of heat, and the central nervous system can increase production of heat by the skeletal musculature through shivering. Activity in the sympathetic portion of the autonomic nervous system in response to cooling causes vasoconstriction of peripheral blood vessels, erection of hair (or "goose flesh"), and the secretion of epinephrine. In response to heating, sweating and cutaneous vasodilatation occur. Whereas vasoconstriction is due to increased impulses in postganglionic sympathetic fibers, vasodilatation is largely passive, the result of inhibition of impulses in sympathetic vasoconstrictor fibers.

Spinal cord lesions may be associated with important alterations in autonomic activity vital to the regulation of body temperature. Transection of the upper portion of the cervical spinal cord leads to falling body temperature unless it is artificially maintained. With transections in lower portions of the spinal cord, temperature regulation becomes increasingly more effective as larger portions of the sympathetic outflow remain under the influence of the brain. Below the level of a cervical or upper thoracic spinal cord lesion, neither sweating nor shivering occurs in response to changes in environmental temperature. If the spinal cord transection is below the first or second thoracic segments, thermoregulatory sweating or shivering can occur in upper portions of the body, with the lower border of this area clearly indicating the level of the spinal cord lesion. A sweat level can be identified from the transition from smooth dry skin to resistant moist skin by running the hand lightly upward over the body from below the level of the lesion. With complete spinal cord lesions, spinal reflex sweating can occur below the level of the lesion in response to bladder distention or noxious stimuli applied to the limbs or body below the lesion (such as scratching the foot or abdomen). Such reflex sweating is a component of the mass autonomic reflex discharge encountered with severe or complete transverse spinal cord lesions that leave an intact but isolated segment of the cord below, containing cell bodies for preganglionic sympathetic fibers. Afferent impulses coming into this isolated distal segment will produce these responses, the most serious and clinically significant being severe supine hypertension, which causes headaches and, rarely, intracranial hemorrhage.

REGULATION OF SKIN BLOOD FLOW AND VASOMOTOR FUNCTION

The angioarchitecture of the skin is unique. The highest temperature is about 1 mm below the skin, in the arteriolar complex. Superficial to it are the capillary loops and arteriovenous channels, and deep to it are the arteries and venae comites.

There are two types of skin blood flow (SBF): nutritive (SBFn) and arteriovenous (SBFav). SBFn is carried in capillaries 5 to 10 μm in diameter. These thin-walled microvessels supply oxygen and other nutrients to tissue. SBFav vessels, in contrast, are large in diameter (25 to 150 μm), are low in resistance, shunt blood from arterioles to venules at high flow rates, and are non-nutritive (that is, do not deliver oxygen to tissue). In human skin, SBFav can shunt blood to superficial skin to enhance heat loss, serving its key role in thermoregulation. Both systems contribute to thermoregulation, but SBFav is far more important. This is not surprising, because maximal capillary flow is 19 mL/100 g per minute, whereas minimal SBFav flow is 92 mL/100 g per minute. Some parts of the skin are very rich in SBFav. For instance, as much as 80% of finger blood flow is SBFav.

Rhythmic fluctuations in vasoconstrictor tone occur in the finger pulp, with an interval of 30 seconds to 2 minutes. The fluctuations are thought to be regulated by some central oscillator mechanism, but local mechanisms may also be present.

Autoregulation, the tendency to a stable blood flow despite varying blood pressures, is attained by regulation of arteriolar tone. Autoregulation is present for subcutaneous blood flow in humans and is lost in autonomic denervation in diabetes.

SBFn is richly innervated by both α- and β-adrenergic receptors, whereas SBFav is regulated by α-adrenergic receptors alone.

Vasoconstriction of SBFn is mainly mediated by vasoconstrictor reflexes, with norepinephrine and epinephrine as major neurotransmitters. Levels of regulation involve neural reflexes at the hypothalamic, spinal, and local levels. At the local level, important regulatory contributions are made by nonadrenergic mediators such as histamine, prostaglandins, vasoactive intestinal polypeptide, and other neuropeptides and by encephalinergic mediators.

Vasodilation is mediated by more complicated and less well understood mechanisms in humans. Several mechanisms are important in different situations. First, vasodilation may result passively by the release of vasoconstriction. Second, vasodilation may be active, occurring by the activation of cholinergic vasodilator fibers or as a result of sweat gland activity by the release of bradykinin, which causes vasodilation. Finally, vasodilation may also occur by noncholinergic mechanisms.

There are major regional differences in the behavior of SBF. Vasodilation of acral regions (the hands, feet, ears) is largely achieved by release of vasoconstriction and was previously considered to be purely vasoconstrictor. SBF to the forearm (and the cheeks, forehead, chin, neck, and trunk) is regulated by both vasoconstrictor and vasodilator fibers.

SBF is also regulated by arterial and venous baroreceptors, which are important in the maintenance of postural normotension. Standing or lower body negative pressure consistently results in vasoconstriction of the hand and forearm skin. When arterial pressure, especially pulse pressure, is reduced, the baroreflex arc is activated, and sympathetic efferent activation results in vasoconstriction of SBF, mainly SBFn, increasing total peripheral resistance. This response, in concert with the other limb of the baroreflex response (causing cardioacceleration), maintains postural normotension.

In addition to the above responses, there are other reflex and local regulatory mechanisms. A somatosympathetic reflex may be mediated by Aδ and sympathetic fibers. Three local axon reflexes are of interest. The first is the axon flare response. The second is the sudomotor axon reflex, mediated by sympathetic sudomotor C fibers and evoking bradykinin-induced vasodilation. The third is the venoarteriolar reflex, which is mediated by sympathetic C vasoconstrictor fibers. The receptor is situated in venules and the effector in the arteriole.

Several methods of measuring SBF are available. These include plethysmography, laser Doppler flowmetry, xenon clearance, and telethermography. Plethysmography measures the rate of volume increment of a digit or limb after release of a cuff that had occluded arterial inflow to a previously exsanguinated (by gravity) limb. The shape of the volume:time trace is an index of blood flow. Venous occlusion and mercury-in-rubber strain gauge types are in common use. Laser Doppler flowmetry is noninvasive and is capable of dynamically recording alterations in composite blood flow. The clearance of radioactive xenon from subcutaneous tissue can be used to assess SBF. Telethermography gives a topographic distribution of skin temperatures, usually in a color-mapped format.

Skin vasomotor reflexes, venoarteriolar reflex, and axonal flare responses have been used to study autonomic failure. The advantage of the postganglionic reflexes is the ability to localize autonomic failure to short segments of nerve. The disadvantages are that the vasomotor reflexes habituate and attenuate with aging and that they are not as sensitive an indicator of autonomic neuropathy as originally thought.

THE BLADDER

The micturition reflex is dependent on the integrity of the second, third, and fourth sacral segments of the spinal cord. Pressure receptors in the bladder wall are activated by rhythmic contractions of the smooth muscle fibers of the detrusor muscle, which become increasingly frequent as the bladder fills. Impulses from these receptors are transmitted via visceral afferent fibers to the sacral spinal cord, and, as their frequency increases, a conscious desire to urinate occurs. Efferent fibers of the micturition reflex arc arise from nerve cells situated in the intermediolateral zone of gray matter of the sacral spinal cord segments S-2 through S-4 and constitute the sacral portion of the parasympathetic outflow. These preganglionic fibers synapse in ganglia of the pelvic plexuses and in the wall of the bladder with postganglionic fibers that initiate the tetanic contraction of the detrusor muscle and bladder emptying. These fibers also innervate the internal sphincter of the bladder, which contains smooth muscle fibers arranged so that their contraction opens the sphincter. The external sphincter of the bladder, composed of striated muscle fibers, is innervated by somatic efferent nerve fibers in the pudendal nerves arising from ventral horn cells in the sacral spinal cord segments S-2 through S-4. Recent evidence suggests that control of the micturition reflex rests chiefly with cells in the pontine reticular formation that integrate and coordinate somatic and autonomic neural activity.

The sympathetic portion of the autonomic nervous system, primarily T-12 through L-2, also innervates the bladder and assists in maintaining continence and possibly detrusor relaxation during the storage phase of bladder function. Visceral afferent fibers arising from the peritoneal surface of the bladder and entering the lower thoracic portion of the spinal cord may transmit a sense of fullness.

When neurogenic bladder dysfunction is suspected, a careful neurologic examination to evaluate the integrity of the cauda equina, the spinal cord (especially its sacral segments), and, in some instances, the brain, is extremely important. The presence and distribution of sensory changes and signs of impairment of upper or lower motor neurons, particularly in the lower limbs, as well as alterations in reflexes provide clues to the location of a neurologic lesion. Impaired sensation in the sacral segments around the perianal area and over the posterior portion of the thighs must not be missed. The external anal sphincter is innervated by the sacral segments S-2 through S-4, and examination of anal sphincter tone, the anal reflex, and the ability to contract the sphincter voluntarily allows evaluation of those spinal cord segments that underlie the micturition reflex. Bladder distention can be identified by palpation and percussion of the lower part of the abdomen. The back, particularly the lumbar region, should be examined carefully for any evidence suggesting an abnormality of the spinal column, such as an alteration in its normal curvatures, paravertebral muscle spasm, bony tenderness to percussion, and overlying cutaneous anomalies, such as a hemangioma, a patch of hair, a sacral dimple, or a sinus.

GASTROINTESTINAL TRACT

The way the nervous system regulates motility in the gastrointestinal tract is unique. Autonomic regulation can be regarded as having an extrinsic neural component consisting of parasympathetic and sympathetic nervous systems and an intrinsic (enteric) nervous system component. The latter is made up of a huge number (10^8) of neurons arranged in plexuses interconnected by extensive nerve fiber bundles. This system has sensory mechanoreceptors and chemoreceptors, interneurons that integrate sensory input and control effector motor units. These units contain visceral motor neurons, the primary cells involved in the development of gut motility. The intrinsic system can function independently of the extrinsic and contains built-in or preprogrammed circuits that perform certain characteristic gut motility patterns (such as the peristaltic reflex and the cyclical, aborally propagating migrating motor complex of fasting). These circuits help determine the maximal contractile rate at different levels of the gut and the aboral movement of chyme. Extrinsic nerves can modulate lengthy sections of these preprogrammed circuits, especially in the stomach and distal portion of the colon. In general, the preganglionic vagal and sacral parasympathetic extrinsic nerves stimulate peristalsis, mediate sensation, and through purinergic inhibitory nerves cause relaxation of gastric and sphincter smooth muscle tone. The sympathetic nervous system acts as an "inhibitory brake" on motility, so that in its absence phasic and excessive uncoordinated segmental contractility occurs, sometimes associated with decreased colonic fluid reabsorption and watery diarrhea.

Common symptoms of neurogenic gastrointestinal dysfunction include dysphagia, gastroparesis, intermittent intestinal pseudo-obstruction syndrome, constipation, diarrhea, incontinence, and weight loss.

A variety of central and peripheral neurologic disorders may produce neurogenic gastrointestinal dysfunction. Common causes are neuropathies (due to amyloidosis, diabetes, inflammatory or immune-mediated paraneoplastic disorders, porphyria, or vincristine use); multiple sclerosis; traumatic, compressive, inflammatory, or infectious myelopathy; neurodegenerative disorders, including Parkinson's disease, multiple system atrophy, and pure autonomic failure; and structural lesions due to stroke or tumor of the brain stem and hypothalamus.

Testing of gastrointestinal autonomic function is described in section IX of Chapter 15.

CLINICAL EVALUATION OF AUTONOMIC NERVOUS SYSTEM FUNCTION

The Autonomic History

In addition to the neurologic and pertinent general medical histories, one needs an evaluation of orthostatic symptoms and vasomotor, sudomotor, pupillomotor, bladder, bowel, and sexual function.

Symptoms of orthostatic hypotension may be manifested as syncopal or near-syncopal episodes. More subtle symptoms should also be sought. The patient may feel faint only under conditions of orthostatic stress. Examples are orthostatic hypotension early in the morning, after meals, and with prolonged standing or exercise. The symptoms may not be a feeling of faintness but may be a feeling of tiredness or an aching tightness in the posterior head and neck muscles or even impaired cognition.

Vasomotor symptoms may initially be manifested as a feeling of coldness ("Doctor, I just can't keep my feet warm"). Later, there are color and trophic changes of the skin.

Generalized sudomotor failure is sought by asking if the patient sweats on a hot day or humid summer night or if clothes get moist. The presence of heat intolerance is sought (the patient feels hot, flushed, dizzy, dyspneic, and weak but does not sweat). Acral changes are best sought by direct questioning (ask the patient, "Are your socks [or hose] as moist as they used to be?" and then check for dampness). The patient's socks or hose should feel moist when taken off in your office. Secretomotor function should also be determined (ask about dry eyes and dry mouth).

Symptoms of pupillomotor disturbance should be sought. The patient may complain of blurring of vision or a glare in bright sunlight. These symptoms are usually related to difficulties with accommodation. Symptoms of erectile or ejaculatory failure should be sought. Symptoms of urinary incontinence, urgency, incomplete bladder emptying, weight loss, and unexplained vomiting, constipation, or diarrhea should be sought.

The Autonomic Examination

Full neurologic examination with particular attention to acral vasomotor and trophic changes and pupillary shape, size, and responses to light and accommodation should be done. The texture and dryness of the skin should be determined.

Blood pressure and heart rate should be checked in the supine and standing positions for 2 minutes in each position. A further recording at 5 minutes standing will infrequently demonstrate orthostatic hypotension. If the subject has an orthostatic reduction of systolic blood pressure of 30 mm Hg or of mean arterial blood pressure of 20 mm Hg, significant orthostatic hypotension is present. If there is a compensatory increase in heart rate, especially if marked, dehydration or other mechanisms of hypovolemia need to be ruled out. If orthostatic hypotension is not demonstrated in a patient who has symptoms of it, orthostatic stress tests can be done. One bedside method is to have the patient do 5 to 10 squats (depending on age) and then repeat the blood pressure measurements. Another stress is to retest the patient after use of one sublingual trinitroglycerin tablet. Bedside maneuvers such as eyeball pressure, carotid sinus massage, and Valsalva's maneuver with digital heart rate recordings are not recommended. Auscultation of the chest during slow deep breathing, however, frequently reveals little change in heart rate when autonomic failure is present.

Sometimes additional autonomic testing is warranted. The aims of autonomic testing are (1) to detect autonomic failure, (2) to determine the site of the lesion (preganglionic or postganglionic), and (3) to determine severity of the dysautonomia. Autonomic function tests are discussed in section IX of Chapter 15.

Chapter 12

Clinical Examinations for Selected Neurologic Problems

EXAMINATION OF THE COMATOSE PATIENT

The important components of consciousness are alertness, perception, short- and long-term memory function, and the ability to focus on tasks requiring alertness and attention. If any of these spheres is disrupted, consciousness becomes impaired. Normal consciousness requires stimuli from the pontine tegmentum, posterior hypothalamus, and thalamus projected to the cerebral cortex for processing. This nonspecific projecting system is called the "ascending reticular activating system."

In coma, the patient is not self-aware, does not speak, has no sleep-wake cycles, makes no purposeful movements, has closed eyes, and cannot be aroused. Important in the examination of the patient with impaired consciousness or coma is assessment of the size of the pupils and their response to light, position of the eyes at rest, oculocephalic reflexes and motor response, verbal response, and eye opening to any stimulus.

Often, additional laboratory tests are necessary to unravel the cause of coma. Mandatory tests are computed tomography (CT) scan; full chemical profile, which should include plasma glucose, electrolytes, arterial blood gas, and, if indicated, serum drug levels and toxicologic screening in plasma or urine. Electroencephalography and cerebrospinal fluid examination may be indicated as well. (In patients with "unexplained coma," magnetic resonance imaging may also be revealing.)

The Glasgow Coma Scale is used to grade the severity of coma in many institutions (Table 12-1). Although there is a tendency to add the scores, this should be discouraged, and only separate components of the Glasgow coma score should be communicated. The Glasgow coma score facilitates communication between nurses working in the unit, junior inexperienced physicians, and, particularly, non-neurologic staff. The scale is more useful than previously used "descriptive terms" of decreased level of consciousness, such as "somnolence," "confusion," and "semiresponsiveness."

Table 12-1   Glasgow Coma Scale

Eye opening	Spontaneous	4
	To speech	3
	To pain	2
	None	1
Best verbal response	Oriented	5
	Confused	4
	Inappropriate	3
	Incomprehensible	2
	None	1
Best motor response	Obeying	5
	Localizing	4
	Flexing	3
	Extending	2
	None	1

Before a detailed examination of a stuporous or comatose patient is done, steps should be taken to avoid permanent brain damage from potentially reversible disorders:

1. Possible hypoxia or hypercarbia or inability to protect the airway should be immediately managed by endotracheal intubation and, if indicated, mechanical ventilation. Hypotension should be avoided; if it occurs, the cause should be immediately identified. Hypotension very often indicates hypovolemia (for example, bleeding after trauma) and should not be attributed to a primary neurologic event.
2. When the cause of coma is unknown, it is useful to eliminate possible hypoglycemia with an intravenous injection of 50 mL of glucose after blood has been drawn for blood glucose determination. If narcotic intoxication is suspected, naloxone should be administered; if benzodiazepine intoxication is considered, flumazenil should be administered. Both drugs immediately counteract the effects of these agents that decrease the level of consciousness.
3. Thiamine should be administered intravenously if chronic alcoholism is suspected. Wernicke's encephalopathy seldom produces coma, but maintenance fluids of glucose administered in the emergency room may induce Wernicke's encephalopathy.
4. Otologic investigation is indicated if acute bacterial meningitis is suspected, and the spinal fluid must be examined immediately to rule out acute meningitis or encephalitis, both of which can be reversed after appropriate therapy. Antibiotic or antiviral therapy should be administered without delay if the possibility of infection is high.

After these immediate needs are met, assessment can proceed in a systematic manner. It is important to update history from relatives or witnesses, who may give valuable information about the circumstances of coma. A search of the patient's pockets may reveal drugs, and a wallet card or medical alert bracelet may indicate diabetes, epilepsy, or other medical conditions that could lead to coma. The skin should be searched carefully for abnormalities, such as the cherry red discoloration associated with carbon monoxide poisoning, generalized petechiae accompanying meningococcal meningitis, and petechiae associated with fat embolism located in the axilla and upper torso. Typical acne of the face may indicate long-term phenytoin administration. Evidence of injections should not be overlooked in coma of unknown cause. It is important to look for signs of battering or any other head injury, which may be identified by previous lacerations and scarring. Neurologic assessment then should concentrate on major clinical functions; level of consciousness is assessed by use of the Glasgow Coma Scale, and brain stem function is examined.

1. Level of Consciousness

The level of consciousness can be determined by applying painful stimuli, such as rubbing on the sternum and pressing on the supraorbital notch and temporomandibular joint. A standard pain stimulus is pressure with a blunt object, such as a pen or handle of a reflex hammer to compress the nail bed. Coma should be differentiated from a so-called locked-in syndrome. This condition results from abnormality in descending corticospinal and corticobulbar pathways at the level of the pons. Communication is possible only through vertical eye movement signals and blinking. Motor response and many brain stem reflexes are absent as well. In other words, the patient seems in a coma but is not.

Occasionally, patients fulfill the clinical criteria for brain death. Figure 12-1 is a guideline for the clinical diagnosis of brain death. The diagnosis can be made only after exclusion of confounding factors that mimic or partly mimic brain death, such as hypothermia, drug intoxication, the use of sedative drugs or neuromuscular blocking agents, and any other severe electrolyte abnormality or acid-base abnormality. Brain stem reflexes need to be tested carefully. In brain death, the pupils are fixed to light and in midposition, corneal reflexes are absent, oculocephalic responses are absent with ice water injection in both ears, pain does not produce facial grimacing, and no coughing is noted with tracheal suctioning. If brain stem reflexes and motor response are absent and apnea testing reveals no breathing efforts with a target P_{CO_2} of 60 mm Hg, the diagnosis of brain death can be made, and the patient is eligible for organ harvesting. The clinical diagnosis of brain death should be in doubt in patients with normal findings on CT scans or cerebrospinal fluid examination. Occasionally, however, patients with normal CT scan

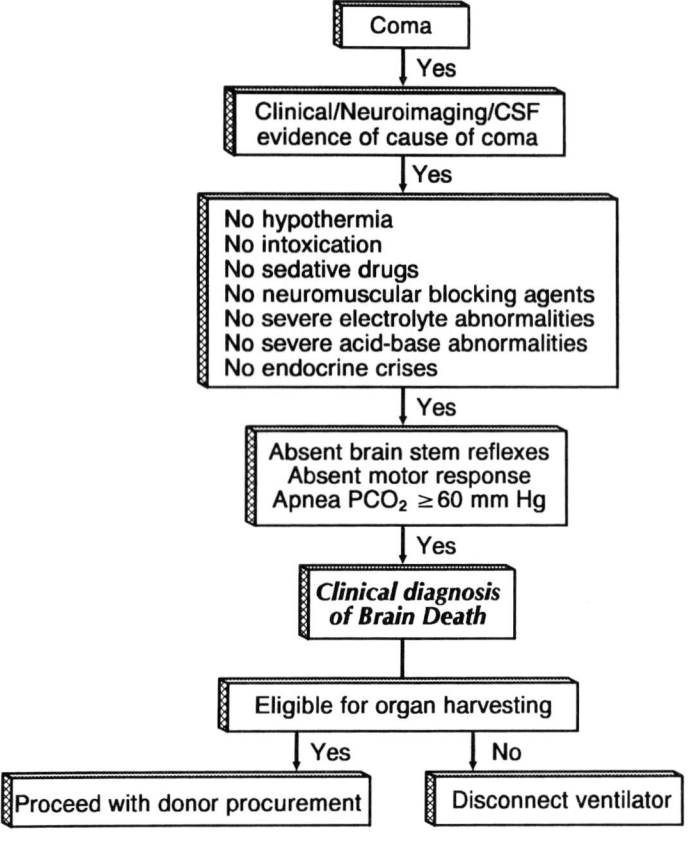

Figure 12-1
Flow chart for the clinical diagnosis of brain death. *(From Wijdicks EFM: Determining brain death in adults, Neurology, 45:1003–1011, 1995. By permission of the American Academy of Neurology.)*

findings have an ischemic-anoxic insult to the brain that results in brain death. In these patients, the clinical diagnosis of brain death should be made only if there is a high degree of certainty about the mechanism that led to brain death.

2. Pupils

Pupillary abnormalities are common in patients in coma and may localize. Midbrain damage leads to midpositioned pupils that are fixed to light. Pontine lesions, however, produce small (pinpoint) pupils. Unilateral pupillary dilatation may indicate compression of the third nerve as a result of uncal herniation through the tentorial notch or of stretching of the third nerve from displacement and torsion of the brain stem. It is important to recognize that the pupillary responses to light reflex remain normal in metabolic coma, often differentiating it from structural disease. The size of the pupils is often affected as well. Miosis often is seen in patients with metabolic encephalopathy; the light response should be present but may be very difficult to appreciate, even with a magnifying glass. Miosis may also occur with narcotic overdose (common reason). Pupils fixed in midposition are typical in brain death. Bilateral mydriasis may indicate anxiety, delirium, pain, seizures, or botulism; excessive magnesium; or overdose of atropine, norepinephrine, dopamine, or tetracycline.

3. Ocular Movements
Position of the eyes at rest often provides a diagnostic clue. Conjugate ocular deviation away from a paralyzed arm or leg is seen in a lesion of the cerebral hemisphere on the side to which the eyes are deviated. Conjugate ocular deviation toward the paralyzed arm and leg suggests brain stem disease. Roving eye movements often imply intact brain stem function. Skew deviation may occur in lesions of the brain stem and is often unmasked only after caloric stimulation with ice water. The oculocephalic reflexes are useful in determining abnormalities of ocular movements. The oculocephalic, or doll's eye, reflex is elicited by rapidly rotating the head from side to side (Fig. 12-2). In comatose patients with an intact brain stem, the eyes move conjugately in the direction opposite that of head rotation. In patients with brain stem involvement, the eyes do not move at all or ocular movement is not conjugate. Oculovestibular or caloric reflexes are studied by introducing 50 mL of ice water into the external auditory canal. The comatose patient with intact brain stem function responds with tonic, slow deviation of the eyes to the side of irrigation. In brain stem lesions, the caloric reflex is absent or ocular deviation is disconjugate.

4. Motor Responses
The motor responses are the most important component of the Glasgow coma score and need to be described carefully. These are localization to pain, pathologic withdrawal to pain, and extensor responses (Fig. 12-3). The use of terms such as "decorticate responses" or "decerebrate responses" is discouraged.

5. Respiratory Patterns
Figure 12-4 illustrates the respiratory patterns in comatose patients. They may have localizing significance, but in many patients a normal breathing pattern, hyperventilation, or agonal breathing is present. Cheyne-Stokes respiration (Fig. 12-4, *A*) implies diffuse involvement of the cerebral hemispheres from various causes but may also occur in patients with congestive heart failure and in normal patients. In occasional

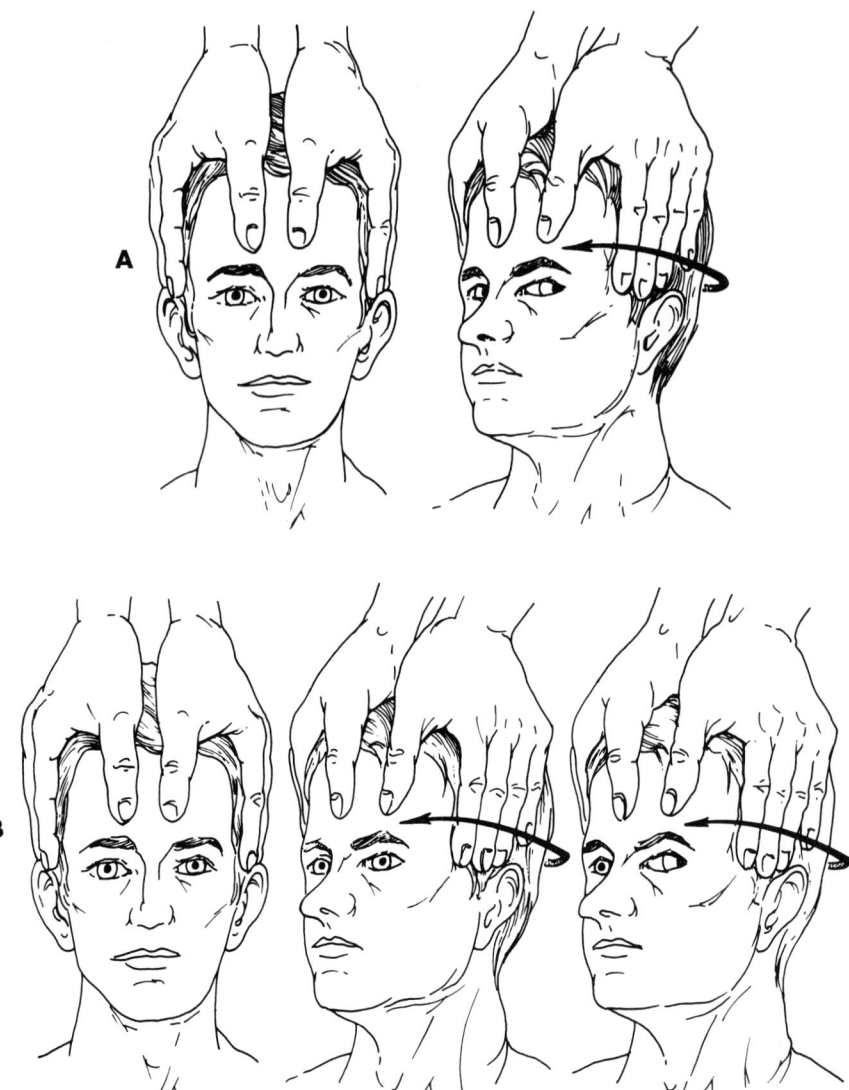

Figure 12-2
Oculocephalic reflexes with lateral rotation of the head to the right. **A**, Response of a comatose patient with intact brain stem function. The eyes move conjugately to the left. **B**, Response of a comatose patient with brain stem involvement. The eyes do not move or ocular movement may not be conjugate. (Additional cold or warm caloric testing may help in defining ocular abnormalities.)

Clinical Examinations for Selected Neurologic Problems

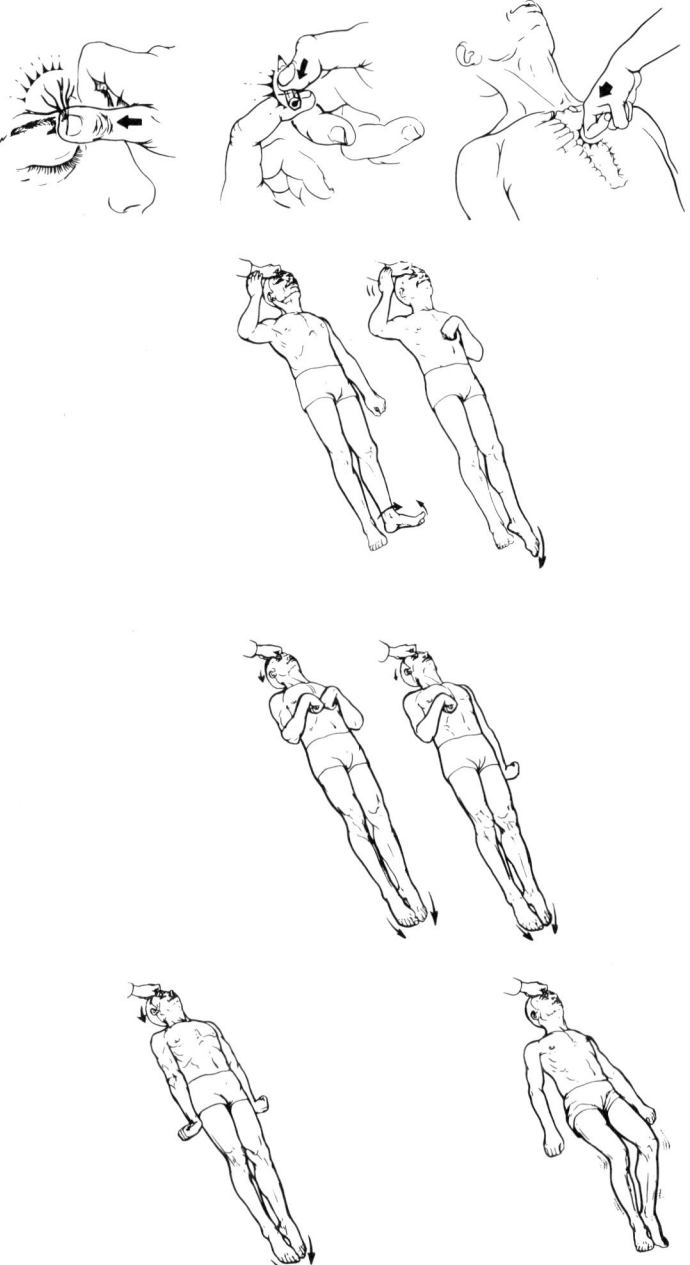

Figure 12-3
Typical motor responses after pain stimuli. *(From Plum F, Posner JB: The diagnosis of stupor and coma, ed 3, Philadelphia, 1980, FA Davis. By permission of the publisher.)*

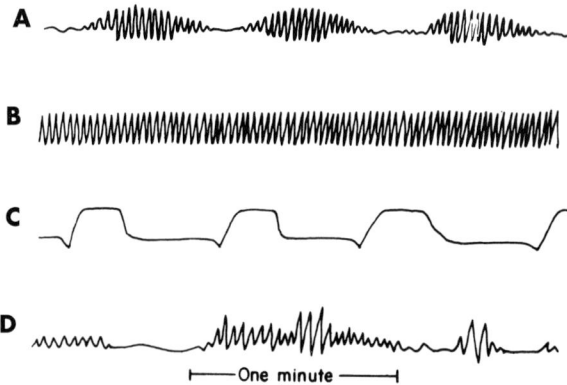

Figure 12-4
Respiratory patterns in patients with stupor and coma: **A,** Cheyne-Stokes respiration; **B,** Central neurogenic hyperventilation; **C,** Apneustic breathing; and **D,** Ataxic breathing. *(Modified from Plum F, Posner JB: The diagnosis of stupor and coma, ed 3, Philadelphia, 1980, FA Davis. By permission of the publisher.)*

circumstances, it can be interpreted as the first sign of herniation caused by pressure on the diencephalon. Central neurogenic hyperventilation (Fig. 12-4, *B*) is seen in patients with acute midbrain damage but more often is a compensatory response to metabolic acidosis. Apneustic breathing (Fig. 12-4, *C*) indicates a primary pontine hemorrhage or infarction. Ataxic breathing (Fig. 12-4, *D*) suggests involvement of the respiratory center in the medulla and is often a prelude to apnea and death. As noted previously, many of these respiratory abnormalities result in inadequate gas exchange, and the patient requires intubation and mechanical ventilation. Reducing the risk of an added hypoxemic insult to the brain is of great importance.

THE NEUROVASCULAR EXAMINATION

Careful and systematic examination of the vascular system, including the heart, should be an integral part of the neurologic examination, especially in patients with suspected cerebrovascular disease. All observations, however, must be cautiously interpreted in the context of the particular patient's problem, because arterial lesions are frequent and may correlate poorly with symptoms.

Inspection of the patient can be helpful. Prominent superficial temporal arteries, especially on one side, may be the result of collateral flow through these vessels to intracranial circulation compromised by proximal internal carotid artery occlusive disease. Horner's syndrome is at times seen with ipsilateral internal carotid disease (dissection, occlusion, or severe stenosis) in the neck.

Blood Pressure

Brachial blood pressure should be measured in both arms, at rest, with the patient in both recumbent and upright positions. A significant difference in blood pressure between the two arms indicates occlusive disease in the subclavian artery (or also, on the right, the innominate artery) on the side of the lower pressure. A significant decrease in the brachial pressure when the upright position is assumed, usually in excess of 40 mm Hg systolic and 15 mm Hg diastolic, indicates a decrease in autonomic vascular tone, often due to illness or medication. Many older patients who complain of dizziness or syncope have symptoms as the result of an orthostatic decrease in blood pressure. While recording the blood pressure on the change to the upright position, the examiner should note the response of the pulse; an absence of compensatory tachycardia indicates impairment of cardioaccelerator function. The brachial blood pressure also provides a basis for interpretation of the various measurements of the pressure in the ophthalmic arterial system.

In hypertensive disease, changes occur in the retinal vessels of both eyes. Severe occlusive disease of an internal carotid artery may reduce the pressure within the retinal vessels on that side, and the changes of hypertension in the ipsilateral fundus may be less severe than expected on the basis of the brachial blood pressure. Thus, asymmetry in hypertensive retinopathy is suggestive of internal carotid artery occlusive disease proximal to the eye.

Palpation

In addition to the examination of the abdominal aorta and major vessels to the lower extremities, arteries of particular importance include, on both sides, the superficial temporal, facial, and radial arteries. The presence of, absence of, or decrease or increase in the pulse (particularly for the superficial temporal arteries) and a comparison from side to side should be recorded. Although prominence of the pulse in the facial, supraorbital, and occipital arteries may give some support to the diagnosis of occlusive change in the internal carotid artery with compensatory collateral flow in the external carotid system, the reliability of observations is low. In cranial arteritis, tenderness, beading, or reduction in the pulse (one or more) of the temporal artery, although an inconstant finding, may be detected.

Palpation of the common and internal carotid arteries in the neck is discouraged. The risk of dislodging clot despite gentle palpation is not outweighed by the accuracy in detecting disease. The position of the common carotid artery behind the sternocleidomastoid muscle and its occasionally tortuous course make interpretation of its pulse particularly difficult. In addition, because of the close proximity of the internal and external carotid arteries, their pulses cannot be identified separately. If a pulse is felt above the bifurcation of the carotid artery, both arteries may be normal or one or the other may be stenotic or occluded.

The time of arrival of the radial pulse at the wrist should be noted. A tardy pulse on one side is indicative of occlusive changes in a proximal vessel, usually the subclavian artery. When subclavian obstruction is severe and proximal to the origin of the vertebral artery, the direction of blood flow may be reversed in the vertebral vessel, which thereby serves as a source of the blood supply to the ipsilateral upper limb.

Auscultation

The cranial vault and orbits, the neck over the carotid artery, and the supraclavicular and precordial regions should be auscultated. Particular attention should be paid to the carotid bifurcation and to the subclavian artery in the supraclavicular fossa. Auscultation is most easily performed by a rubber bell-type stethoscope, except that over the precordium, a stethoscope fitted with a diaphragm may be preferable. The patient may be in the supine or sitting position, with the head in the neutral position.

In many children, soft cranial or cervical bruits occur and are of uncertain importance. Bruits over the vault can be heard in children with increased intracranial pressure or with angiomatous malformations. Cranial bruits in adults are indicative of an arterial abnormality, including arteriovenous malformation or fistula, stenosis of an artery within the bony skull base, and abnormal collateral connections between the external and internal carotid systems. Rarely, bruits are heard only by the patient (so-called pulsatile tinnitus) or, in addition, by the examiner using a double–limbed stethoscope placed in the patient's ears; angiographic examination in these instances does not always disclose abnormalities, and the cause of these abnormal sounds is unknown and presumed to be due to an unusual vascular connection. Such bruits can be heard in patients with abnormal dural arteriovenous connections.

Auscultation over the orbit is performed by placing the stethoscope over the closed eye and instructing the patient to open the eyes: this maneuver tends to relax the orbicularis oculi and eliminate unwanted muscular sounds. Bruits heard over the one orbit may be the result of stenosis of the intracranial portion of the internal carotid artery or of excessive blood flow on the side of the bruit as compensation for severe occlusive disease of the proximal ipsilateral or opposite internal carotid artery. A continuous bruit may occur with a carotid-cavernous fistula.

Cervical auscultation provides a useful indicator of extracranial arterial abnormality. With the patient's head in a neutral position, the examiner places the stethoscope gently over each of the major vessels in the neck. Auscultation over the carotid bifurcation is of major importance. In most instances, bruits heard in this area are an indication of an underlying stenotic lesion with compromise of 40% to 50% or greater cross-sectional area. Lesser degrees of stenosis are seldom associated with turbulent flow sufficient to produce an audible bruit. A bruit can be heard over a normal carotid bifurcation when turbulent flow occurs from increased cardiac output or, rarely, in association with contralateral carotid occlusion. The bruit can arise from the origin of either the internal carotid artery or the external carotid artery, but since atherosclerotic changes are more common at the origin of the internal carotid artery, this is the usual site. When the internal carotid artery is occluded, atherosclerotic occlusive change in the ipsilateral external carotid artery may cause a similar bruit. Bruits resulting from moderate narrowing and roughening of the bifurcation are usually harsh and systolic, whereas high-pitched whistling-type bruits may be heard with more severe stenosis. In patients with internal carotid artery stenosis, the bruit may be heard along the internal carotid artery up to the angle of the jaw and may vary from short to long and from soft to harsh. Although bruits are systolic in timing, occasionally a diastolic component is also present and is usually predictive of severe stenosis. Although the location, intensity, pitch, radiation, duration, and timing of a vascular noise should be noted, the anatomic correlation and the clinical or pathological significance of all these variations are limited. A bruit that changes pitch or duration or that disappears or reappears from one examination to the next may be a reflection of either variation in systemic blood pressure or pathologic change at that site, including the occurrence of active thrombosis.

Transmitted murmurs from the heart may be a cause of cervical bruits. These should be audible diffusely along the length of the carotid artery in the neck and become softer more distally in the neck. Such bruits may also mask a localized carotid bruit.

Ocular Fundus

During the examination of the eye, one can see changes indicating possible vascular disease. The arteriolar changes of hypertension, the retinal changes in diabetes, and the large preretinal hemorrhages characteristic of subarachnoid hemorrhage are examples. Ischemic retinal changes include small cotton-wool patches (cytoid bodies) and retinal infarcts from an occluded retinal arteriole.

A careful search should be made for emboli. In occlusive disease of the internal carotid artery, particularly with ulcerated atherosclerotic plaques, bright yellow-orange refractile cholesterol emboli (Hollenhorst plaques) or, more rarely, white fibrin-platelet aggregates may be seen in retinal arterioles. The former do not obstruct blood flow; they lie at a bifurcation of a retinal arteriole and often move rapidly from one bifurcation to the next. The fibrin-platelet emboli often occlude the arteriole and produce temporary or permanent ischemia. They rarely move while being observed; in fact, the blood flow distal to them slows or stops and the red cells agglutinate, giving rise to a "boxcar" effect. Calcific emboli, usually from calcific aortic valves, may occlude an arteriole and produce retinal ischemia and a scotoma. Small retinal hemorrhages with a central white spot, the classic but nonspecific Roth's spots, are encountered in subacute endocarditis, leukemia, and other conditions.

Venous stasis retinopathy, consisting of microaneurysms, small round hemorrhages, and new vessel formation, is seen rarely in patients with chronic severe occlusive disease in the ipsilateral internal carotid artery. This change is similar to, but not the same as, diabetic retinopathy and is unilateral.

When the central retinal artery is occluded, the disk and retina become pale, the retinal arterioles become attenuated, and vision is permanently and severely impaired or lost completely.

A similar picture may be observed in the retina, including red blood cell agglutination, in those rare instances when the fundus is examined during a brief period of ischemia (amaurosis fugax); the abnormalities clear rapidly as the circulation is restored. Not all eyes show abnormalities during an episode of amaurosis fugax.

CLINICAL EXAMINATIONS IN SELECTED PAIN PROBLEMS

Pain is a subjective, unpleasant sensation produced by a wide variety of underlying conditions. The neurologist is increasingly regarded as an expert in the evaluation of a patient with pain and may be responsible for the short- and long-term management of some of these patients. The primary goal of a neurologic consultation is to diagnose or exclude a neurologic basis for the complaint. In addition, a competent neurologist should be able to recognize some non-neurologic conditions that occasionally present in an atypical fashion, such as angina pectoris, peptic ulcer disease, and pancreatic cancer.

Back pain is one of the most common problems seen by practicing physicians. Neurologists, therefore, must be intimately familiar with all disorders of the spinal column that may involve neural structures. Although most patients with back pain have muscular, ligamentous, or bony causes of pain, the neurologist should exclude serious disorders such as neoplasm, compression fracture, infectious processes, and ankylosing spondylitis.

Tests for Diagnosis of Pain Problems in the Lower Back and Lower Extremities

The examination actually begins while the history is being obtained with observation of the patient's overall appearance and demeanor. This should also include watching the patient arise and proceed to undress; ideally, the patient should also be observed walking without awareness of being watched, a technique that may be useful in suspected cases of conversion disorder or malingering.

The patient should then be viewed standing, facing away from the examiner, so that any spinal curvature, asymmetry of paraspinal muscles, scars, or skin lesions may be noted. Loss of normal lumbar lordosis may indicate paravertebral muscle spasm.

Flexion, extension, and lateral flexion should be observed, noting limitations, muscle spasm, and so-called corkscrewing or twisting motions, also seen with spasm and root irritation.

Having the patient point to the area or areas of pain may provide information additional to that gained from the patient's description.

Palpation for areas of tenderness in muscle and along the course of nerves should also be performed. It is useful to compare responses to palpation in the sciatic notch over the course of the sciatic nerve with those to palpation of the ischial tuberosities and areas of gluteal muscle mass. Rectal and vaginal examinations should be done to detect lesions along the course of the lumbosacral plexus or sciatic nerves within the pelvis. One should also palpate along the course of the sciatic nerve in the lower buttocks and posterior aspect of the upper thigh.

Palpation and percussion over the spinous processes may also elicit pain associated with bone lesions. Auscultation for bruits may be helpful in patients harboring abdominal aortic aneurysm or arteriovenous malformations of the spinal cord.

Straight leg raising test

With the patient supine, the examiner slowly lifts the relaxed, extended lower limb and the patient is asked whether, where, and when pain occurs. A positive test result reproduces the patient's sciatic pain. The test can be repeated while the patient is distracted or when the patient is sitting if one suspects nonorganic pain.

A "crossed" straight leg raising test is performed by elevating the unaffected lower limb. If the result also is positive, the likelihood of root compression from a protruded or extruded disk is increased.

These tests assess the lower lumbar roots L5 and S1, where most herniated disks occur. A "reverse" straight leg raising test should be performed with the patient prone and the leg flexed at the knee to assess the upper lumbar roots L2, L3, and L4.

Fabere (Patrick's) sign

Patrick's test (fabere sign) should always be performed to evaluate the possibility of hip joint disease. With the patient in the supine position, the heel of the lower extremity being tested is placed on the opposite knee. The knee on the side being tested is pressed laterally and downward as far as tolerated. The test result is positive if the range of motion is involuntarily restricted and accompanied by pain. Further evaluation includes medial and internal rotation, which may also be restricted by hip joint disease.

Kernig's sign
Although usually considered a classic sign of meningitis or meningeal irritation, Kernig's sign is also a corroborative finding of nerve root compression. With the patient supine, the examiner flexes the hip and then extends the knee to at least 135 degrees. The test result is positive if extension is limited and accompanied by radicular pain.

Tests for lumbar and lumbosacral joints
These tests may help differentiate musculoskeletal pain from root pain. With the patient supine, the examiner slowly flexes the hip and knee and presses below the knee toward the table and the head of the patient, attempting to passively flex the lumbar portion of the spine. A positive test result is indicated by limitation of flexion and pain, suggesting disease of lumbar or lumbosacral joints.

Psoas test
This is another maneuver designed to differentiate degenerative disk disease from degenerative joint disease. While the patient is prone, the examiner flexes the leg to 90 degrees and elevates the extremity, passively hyperextending the hip. Limitation and pain suggest disease in the psoas muscle itself, such as an abscess, or disease of the paraspinal soft tissues or lumbar vertebrae.

Tests for Diagnosis of Pain Problems in the Cervical Region and Upper Extremities
The preceding discussion of pain in the low back and lower extremities has covered many of the diagnostic difficulties related to pain in the cervical region and upper extremities. The same care is given to inspection and palpation of nerves and arteries, to palpation for abnormal masses, and to examination of joints as in the lower extremity. Gentle palpation of the cervical roots on either side of the sternocleidomastoid muscle may reveal undue tenderness, induration, or other abnormalities. In addition, auscultation for bruit in the supraclavicular and axillary spaces and palpation for cervical rib may aid in solving the problem of pain under consideration, and special tests (to be described) may be indicated by the nature of the problem.

Examination of cervical segment of the spinal column
The muscles of the cervical region are inspected and palpated for spasm, tenderness, and abnormal consistency. The motions of forward flexion, extension, and lateral flexion are performed as in the low back; in addition, tests of rotation to the extreme right and left are made.

Foraminal compression test of Spurling
Sometimes this test is of value in the diagnosis of a laterally herniated intervertebral disk in the cervical region. It is performed by applying downward pressure on the top of the head after the neck has been hyperextended and laterally flexed toward the extremity into which the pain extends. Aggravation of the pain under consideration is interpreted as a positive result.

Neck traction test
This test has about the same significance for diagnosis of cervical disk as the one described in the preceding paragraph. However, a positive result is signified by relief of root pain rather than by its aggravation. The test may be performed manually by the examiner, who, grasping both sides of the patient's head, exerts traction upward without inducing motion in the spinal column other than longitudinal stretching. This test can be performed by use of a halter under the chin and occiput. Traction can then be exerted by pulling on a rope attached to the halter and run through a pulley suspended above the patient.

Clinical tests for diagnosis of various thoracic outlet syndromes
Although we believe that the tests to be described frequently fail to distinguish between the normal and the pathologic and do not, as a rule, furnish evidence that is reliable in separating one type of thoracic outlet syndrome from another, they are described here, since occasionally they are of some help. An observation of an abnormal test result is rarely of value unless the maneuver also reproduces the patient's symptoms.

Adson's maneuver, or test
Adson's test is generally the most useful of this group of tests, since positive results are seldom obtained in normal subjects. It is of greatest value in deciding whether a cervical rib seen in roentgenograms or felt on examination accounts for the patient's symptoms. The test thus is an aid in selecting patients for surgical treatment. Opinions vary on its reliability in diagnosis of the so-called scalenus anticus syndrome.

The test is performed with the patient in the sitting position and hands resting in a natural and comfortable position on the thighs. The examiner palpates both radial pulses simultaneously as the patient rapidly and completely fills the lungs by deep inspiration. While holding the breath, the patient hyperextends the neck and then turns the head as far as possible toward one side and then the other. If the radial pulse on the affected side is decidedly or completely obliterated during the test while that on the unaffected side remains full or only slightly decreased, the result of the test is considered positive. During the same maneuver, a bruit often develops, which can be heard best in the supraclavicular space and may be accompanied by a palpable thrill in the subclavian artery.

Shoulder hyperabduction test
While the examiner is feeling the radial pulse, the relaxed upper extremity of the patient is slowly lifted laterally until the arm is in a position of full hyperabduction. Various degrees of posterior extension of the arm may be added to this maneuver of hyperabduction. The pulse decreases decidedly or disappears with maximal hyperabduction in most normal subjects and with only moderate degrees of abduction in some. If the pulse on the affected side is obliterated with greater ease than is usually the case in normal subjects, the test may have value in diagnosis of the "hyperabduction syndrome."

Shoulder bracing test
When the shoulders are braced backward in an exaggerated military position, the arterial pulses in the upper extremities can often be decreased markedly or obliterated in normal subjects and a bruit can be heard by auscultation in the region of the clavicle. Results of this test are, of course, positive in the "costoclavicular syndrome." Certainly, if the test should fail to obliterate the radial pulse, one would have evidence against the diagnosis of costoclavicular syndrome. We believe, however, that a positive diagnosis should be based on reproduction of the patient's symptoms in association with a positive reaction to the test.

Chapter 13

Examination of Infants and Children

Although the neurologic examination of infants and children is based on the same principles as those used in the neurologic examination of adults, the approach to the patient and the interpretation of findings can be entirely different. The pediatric patient is not merely a small adult but rather is a dynamic, developing individual, and the examination must be based and interpreted on a thorough knowledge of normal growth and development.

HISTORY

In addition to the usual elements of medical history, the physician should review carefully the prenatal, perinatal, and neonatal periods as well as document the development of the patient to the time of examination. By necessity, much of the history is obtained from parents or others close to the child. Care must be taken to distinguish between interpretive judgments by the historian and objective observations. The importance of interviewing the patient cannot be overemphasized, for even the very young child can often contribute valuable information.

Prenatal Period
The history should include the duration of pregnancy, maternal infection, exposure to radiation, drugs used by the mother during the pregnancy, signs of toxemia, maternal bleeding, and evidence of metabolic diseases. The mother's reaction to the pregnancy should also be assessed, for in situations of unwanted pregnancies, unsuccessful attempts at induced abortion may result in fetal damage. If the mother is infected by certain viruses (such as those causing rubella, herpes, and cytomegalic inclusion disease) or if she has toxoplasmosis *(Toxoplasma gondii)* or syphilis, embryopathies or fetal infection may result. It should be emphasized that these embryopathies or fetal infections often occur in the absence of overt clinical symptoms in the mother. Exposure to ionizing radiation early in pregnancy may result in fetal abnormalities. Certain

drugs may have teratogenic effects, and other drugs taken late in pregnancy may have a direct pharmacologic effect on the fetus and, subsequently, on the newborn.

Threatened abortion or maternal bleeding during pregnancy raises the question of placental or fetal abnormalities. Toxemia of pregnancy is associated with multiple pathologic states, including prematurity, placental insufficiency syndrome with intrauterine dwarfism, and neonatal hypoglycemia. Infants of diabetic or "prediabetic" mothers may have a high incidence of neonatal hypoglycemia and hypocalcemia, respiratory distress syndrome, and neonatal icterus. Infants born of mothers with hyperparathyroidism have a greater incidence of neonatal tetany. Those born of mothers with thyroid disease may exhibit cretinism, and infants born of mothers with hyperphenylalaninemia may be mentally defective. Mothers with myasthenia gravis may produce infants with neonatal myasthenia.

Birth and Neonatal Period
A history of maternal bleeding at term may suggest abruptio placentae or placenta previa, either of which may be the source of fetal hypoxia. Induction of labor may suggest a pathologic state of pregnancy. Cesarean section suggests either maternal or fetal pathology, and reasons for its selection should be investigated. Rupture of the membranes 24 hours or more before delivery predisposes the infant to infection. A prolonged, difficult labor may suggest fetal hypoxia or trauma; rapid, precipitous labor and delivery may be the first clue to subdural hematoma. Breech presentation may result in an increased incidence of fetal hypoxia or injury to the spinal cord. The size of the infant gives the clinician an idea of its maturity. Conventionally, the infant weighing less than 2,500 g at birth is considered premature. Strictly speaking, prematurity is confined to infants whose gestational age is less than 37 weeks, who weigh less than 2,500 g, and who are 47 cm or less in length. Thus, the infant who weighs less than 2,500 g but is delivered at term by gestational age is more properly designated "small for date" or an "intrauterine dwarf." The infant who, at birth, is hypoactive, hypotonic, apneic, or cyanotic and who requires intense resuscitative efforts is prone to neurologic sequelae. The same holds true for the infant in whom severe respiratory distress syndrome or significant neonatal jaundice develops, who has seizures, or who exhibits persistent somnolence or irritability.

Development
The activity of the pediatric patient varies with age. What is normal for an infant of 2 months may be pathologic for a 6-month-old infant. A thorough knowledge of the developmental norms and their variations is of importance in examining the patient and in interpreting the findings. The age at which various skills are acquired should be noted carefully.

Particular attention should be paid to the time that development slowed, ceased, or regressed. Such information gives the clinician insight into the onset of neurologic difficulties and the nature of the process at work. The following outline provides a general guide of developmental milestones. These milestones are variable; none in itself may be adhered to rigidly; rather, each should be interpreted in view of the whole picture.

1 Month:
  Spontaneous motor activity generalized
  Lifts head when prone; poor supine head control
  Beginning to regard surroundings
  Follows objects to midline
2 Months:
  Motor activity generalized
  Smiles and coos socially
  Follows objects past midline
3 Months:
  Follows well with eyes
  May wave at toy; beginning to regard hands
  Control of head good when prone and looking around
  Head control improved when in sitting position
  Moro's reflex disappearing
  Smiles; coos in more sustained fashion
4 Months:
  Beginning to reach for toys symmetrically
  Regards toys and may pull them to mouth
  Removes cloth from face
  Control of head good when sitting
  Plays with hands
  Laughs
6 Months:
  Reaches with either hand and begins to transfer objects
  Rolls over
  May sit briefly when placed in sitting position
  Laughs and plays with examiner
8 Months:
  Prehensile function palmar
  Sits alone
  Beginning to creep reciprocally
  Vocalizes with infantile rhythms and polysyllabic vowel sounds
  Regards self in mirror
10 Months:
  Crawls reciprocally
  Pulls up on rail
  May begin to cruise
  Uses thumb and index finger in opposition

May say "mama" or "dada"
Feeds self cracker and holds own bottle

12 Months:
  Walks with support
  Stands alone
  Places cube in cup; tries to build tower of 2 cubes
  May have 2 words besides "mama" or "dada"
  Begins to feed self with fingers

15 Months:
  Walks alone (toddles)
  Creeps upstairs
  4- to 5-word vocabulary
  Pats pictures
  Drinks from cup
  Beginning to feed self with spoon
  Makes wants known by pointing or vocalizing

18 Months:
  Walks well
  Sits in chair
  Throws a ball
  Climbs on furniture
  Stacks 3 to 4 cubes
  10-word vocabulary
  Begins to identify pictures
  Pulls toy on string
  May be toilet trained during day

2 Years:
  Runs well
  Negotiates steps one at a time
  Uses pronouns and 3-word sentences
  Feeds self with spoon
  Refers to self by name
  Toilet trained during day

2½ Years:
  Undresses self partially
  Attempts to put on socks
  Draws horizontal or vertical lines but does not cross them
  Refers to self as "I"
  Knows full name
  Helps to put things away

3 Years:
  Alternates feet going upstairs
  Pedals tricycle
  Builds tower of cubes
  Names drawings

Uses plurals and obeys propositional commands
   Feeds self well
   Buttons and unbuttons clothes and puts on shoes
4 Years:
   Runs and climbs well
   Walks downstairs alternating feet
   Hops on one foot
   Throws a ball overhead
   Attempts to catch ball or to kick it in the air
   Pedals tricycle rapidly
   Draws person with head, trunk, and arms or legs
   Counts 3 objects
   Names one or more colors
5 Years:
   Skips, alternating feet
   Draws a person
   Copies a square, cross, and circle
   Dresses and undresses without assistance
   Knows the names of 4 or more colors
   Counts to 10 or higher
6 Years:
   Draws person with hands and clothes
   Repeats 4 digits
   Knows morning and afternoon
   Knows right from left side

EXAMINATION OF INFANT

Much valuable information about the neurologic status of the infant is obtained by careful observation both when undisturbed and during playful stimulation. Many observations can be made as one obtains the history. The diagnosis of Down's syndrome, mucopolysaccharidoses, or Cornelia de Lange's syndrome is suggested by the phenotypic appearance of the patient. The symmetry or asymmetry of spontaneous movements should be noted. Persistent extension of the forearm in an infant with Erb-Duchenne paralysis is striking when compared with the normal opposite extremity. Similarly, in an older hemiparetic infant, the flexion posture and associated paucity of movement of the extremity also may be striking. Seizure activity, especially of the minor type, may be observed. Salaam seizures may be passed off as startle responses by parents, and other observers may dismiss "absence" spells in older children as "daydreaming." Finally, the responsiveness of the patient to parents, environment, and examiner should be noted and assessed in relation to age.

Neurologic examination of the infant includes a careful general physical examination. No rigid rules have been established for the order in which the examination is to be conducted except that the least disturbing part should be performed first and the more unpleasant ones saved until last. Thus, the physician should have a flexible and adaptable approach to the infant. Recognition of an abdominal mass in an infant with proptosis immediately suggests metastatic neuroblastoma. The appearance of acute hemiplegia in an infant with cyanotic congenital heart disease suggests an intracranial vascular occlusion, whereas in an older child the possibility of brain abscess may be more likely. Congestive heart failure in an infant with macrocrania should bring to mind the possibility of a large intracranial arteriovenous malformation. Often, the first clue to the diagnosis of tuberous sclerosis in the infant is the presence of achromic patches. Recognition of these may be facilitated by the use of a Wood's lamp. Café au lait spots may suggest neurofibromatosis and may afford an early indication of associated lesions. Neither of these cutaneous lesions may be evident in the neonatal period but may appear later. The nevus flammeus, usually in the trigeminal distribution, is present at birth in patients with Sturge-Weber syndrome. The neonate with Bloch-Sulzberger syndrome (incontinentia pigmenti) exhibits vesicular lesions that subsequently resolve, leaving the linear and whorl-like hyperpigmentation seen in affected older infants and children. Examination of the midline of the head and spinal column may reveal a dermal sinus with an underlying dermoid or a tuft of hair suggesting a diastematomyelia.

The newborn infant expresses little concern for the environment except as it is related to hunger, pain, and basic biologic needs. Much of the day is spent sleeping. When awake, the neonate may stare but does not follow with the eyes. The infant does blink at a bright light and respond to abrupt sounds. Vocalization is that of crying, and particular attention should be given to the quality of the cry, including its pitch, loudness, and duration. A high-pitched cry may be associated with intracranial disease. An unusually hoarse cry may denote a laryngeal abnormality. Drowsiness or irritability may be early evidence of intracranial disease. The older infant exhibits more awareness of the environs and may be tested by observing responses to simple objects such as a key ring, rattle, block, ball, mirror, and the like. Complete examination of social, adaptive, and language functions at one sitting is often impossible. Allowances must be made for circumstances such as fatigue, hunger, and intercurrent illness, which may modify the patient's responses.

Posture, Tone, and Muscle Strength

The normal term infant exhibits a general predominance of flexor tone in the extremities. Somewhat hypertonic, the infant, when disturbed, has generalized and symmetrical responses. The fists are clenched and the thumb is adducted into the palm. This attitude of the hands may be normal in the neonatal period, but subsequently it becomes less prominent, so that after 4 months such posture is abnormal and implies upper motor neuron deficit. The premature infant is generally hypotonic, and the degree of hypotonia is inversely proportional to gestational age. Careful assessment of the tone and posture of the infant is helpful in determining gestational age.* Hypotonia may be seen in the term infant depressed by drugs, sepsis, hypoxia, or hypoglycemia and in infants with Down's syndrome, cretinism, connective tissue disorders, anterior horn cell disease, or myopathies. Infants with an acute injury to the central nervous system, such as intracranial hemorrhage or spinal cord injury, have hypotonia, which may persist for weeks or months. After the neonatal period, hypotonia suggests connective tissue disorders, anterior horn cell disease, myopathies, neuropathy, or atonic diplegia. A persistent frogleg posture and reduced spontaneous activity in newborn or young infants may be caused by diplegia, paraplegia, or disease of lower motor neurons or muscles.

MOTOR RESPONSES

Extremities

Motor responses during the first 3 months are symmetrical and generalized but progressively become more purposeful. By 3 months of age, the infant follows objects with the eyes, relates well to the examiner, and is beginning to wave both hands at a dangling object. He or she kicks both feet simultaneously when excited. Consistent asymmetry of movement suggests unilateral neurologic deficit, such as hemiplegia or monoplegia. By 4 to 5 months of age, the infant should use either hand to remove a diaper placed over the face. An infant suffering from diffuse neurologic disease may ignore the diaper. The infant with hemiparesis or monoparesis persistently uses the same extremity to move the diaper, and if that extremity is restrained, the task is performed poorly or not at all with the opposite extremity. Reaching movements often have an athetoid quality, so that choreoathetosis is impossible to diagnose with certainty before the child is 6 months of age and extremely difficult to recognize before 12 to 18 months. Ataxia of the upper extremities is manifested by decompensation of movement on reaching for an object. Between the ages of 6 and 10 months, prehensile function becomes progressively more mature. By 7 months, the infant has generally mastered transferring objects from hand to hand. At 10 months, good opposition

---

*Koenigsberger MR: Judgment of fetal age: I. Neurologic evaluation. Pediatr Clin North Am 13:823–833, 1966.

of the thumb and forefinger is exhibited, and they are used to pick up small objects. Asymmetry of prehensile function, especially when associated with decreased use of the extremities, suggests hemiparesis.

Neck
Control of the head in the neonatal period is poor when the infant is in either the prone or the supine position. By 1 month of age, the infant is beginning to raise the head to look around when in the prone position, but in the supine position, control of the head remains poor. When the infant is pulled by the hands to the sitting posture from the supine position, there is a definite lag of the head. These functions improve, so that by 3 months of age, the infant exhibits excellent control of the head in the prone position and even raises the chest from the table surface. By 4 months of age, control of the head in the supine position is good, and when the infant is pulled to the sitting position, the head rises in the axis with the spine and the examiner senses a tightening of the shoulder girdle and arm muscles. Definite lag of the head after 4 months of age is abnormal and is a valuable clue to neurologic difficulty in the infant.

Ambulation
The 4-month-old infant pushes symmetrically with the feet when supported. Sitting begins by 6 months, and good sitting posture usually is achieved by 7 to 8 months. During the seventh month, the infant begins to propel the body in the prone position by squirming and then by dragging the lower limbs behind, and by the eighth or ninth month, reciprocal crawling begins. The infant begins to pull himself or herself up by furniture during the ninth month and travels along furniture by the tenth month. By 11 to 12 months, the child is walking with support. Most youngsters begin to walk without support between 12 and 14 months. Failure to walk by 16 months suggests neurologic or orthopedic disease. The spastic infant, when lifted under the arms, holds the lower extremities in rigid extension and crossed at the ankles. A patient with atonic diplegia, however, may exhibit flexion at the hips and knees when so supported. This has been referred to as "Foerster's sign." The infant with lower motor neuron deficit or myopathy may simply hang limply or exhibit less obvious weakness. The patient with atonic diplegia or flaccid paraplegia often propels the body in a sitting position, using the upper extremities and sometimes assisting with the lower, thereby scooting on the buttocks, whereas the spastic infant may persist in the commando crawl, propelling the body with the upper extremities and dragging the lower extremities behind.

The early gait of the toddler is wide-based and unsteady. Falling is frequent, and crawling is often resorted to when the toddler is in a hurry. By 15 to 16 months of age, the child toddles with assurance, and by 18 months, gait is steady. The child runs, using the upper extremities for balance and protection. Often, it is at the age of walking that families seek medical advice because of the infant's failure to walk, the asymmetry of gait, or the symmetrical peculiarity of gait.

Reflexes

Muscle-stretch reflexes are of limited help in the examination of the newborn. The quadriceps reflex is consistently present at this time. The biceps and brachioradialis reflexes are often elicited as brief responses, but this is not invariably so. The ankle reflex is generally not elicited in the newborn period but appears shortly thereafter. The triceps reflex is the last to appear but is consistently elicited by the sixth month. Muscle-stretch reflexes in the infant are normally brisk and somewhat hyperactive. Crossed adduction in response to tapping of the quadriceps tendon may be normal up to 7 months. Brief ankle clonus may be normal in the first weeks of life. Sustained ankle clonus, however, is abnormal at any age. Likewise, consistent asymmetry of muscle-stretch reflexes is abnormal at any age.

Abdominal and cremasteric reflexes are usually absent or not elicitable in the newborn, but they are usually elicitable by 2 to 4 weeks. The abdominal reflexes are difficult to obtain in the infant, since crying or abdominal distention may obliterate the response.

The *extensor toe reflex* is normally present in both premature and term newborn infants and persists until the end of the first year of life. Some believe that it may normally extend into the second year. In eliciting the plantar response, the examiner must take care to keep the stimulus on the lateral edge of the foot toward the fifth toe. A stimulus more medially placed brings into play the grasp reflex and invalidates the test.

Numerous reflexes have been described in the newborn and small infant, and no attempt will be made to review all of these. Rather, the reflexes most frequently used and those that have proved most useful to the authors will be discussed.

The *Moro reflex*, the best known of infantile reflexes, is elicited by supporting the infant in the supine position with neck slightly flexed and then dropping the head briefly and rapidly through an angle of about 30 degrees. The response consists of symmetrical abduction, extension and circumduction of the upper extremities, and extension followed by flexion of the lower extremities. It is present at birth in the full-term infant and generally disappears by 16 to 20 weeks of age. In the premature infant, it is easily elicitable and complete in the infant of 32 weeks gestational age. In the infant of 24 weeks gestational age, it is difficult to elicit, becoming more definite by 28 weeks. In the neonate depressed by drugs, hypoxia, or infection, the Moro reflex is depressed or sluggish and may be a prognostic sign in such cases. An asymmetrical Moro response suggests a brachial plexus injury, fractured clavicle, or, rarely, a hemiparesis. A hyperactive Moro reflex in the neonatal period may be associated with early kernicterus or hypocalcemia. A Moro reflex persisting beyond the fifth month suggests diffuse central nervous system dysfunction.

The *incurvation,* or *Galant's, reflex,* like the Moro reflex, is present normally from the day of birth, gradually wanes, and disappears by the third month. It is present in the premature infant of 24 weeks gestational age and thereafter. Persistence of the reflex beyond the third month suggests diffuse neurologic deficit. The reflex is elicited by stimulating the child's flank between the rib cage and the pelvic brim. Normal response is an incurvation of the trunk, ipsilateral to the stimulus.

The *tonic neck reflex* is less consistent and may vary from time to time in the same infant. It is elicited by placing the infant in the supine position and rotating the head to either side. The extremities ipsilateral to the direction of rotation extend, and the contralateral extremities flex. A persistent or obligate tonic neck response is abnormal at any age. Reproducible tonic neck responses in an infant more than 6 months of age are likewise abnormal and suggest a deficit in the pyramidal tracts and their connections at cortical and subcortical levels.

Sucking and rooting reflexes are primitive reflexes that are present from birth in all term and large premature infants. They may not be present if the infant has just been fed. The sucking reflex is elicited by stroking the lips, to which the infant responds by making sucking movements with the lips and tongue. A weak sucking reflex appears at about 28 weeks gestational age, becomes stronger by 32 weeks, and by 34 weeks is associated with synchronous swallowing movements. The rooting reflex is elicited by stimulating the cheek lateral to the mouth. The infant normally responds by moving the lips toward the stimulus. A minimal rooting reflex may be seen in the premature infant of 24 weeks gestational age, becoming progressively more apparent, so that by 32 weeks it is consistently elicitable. Infants depressed from any cause may exhibit diminution of these responses. The sucking reflex disappears about the fourth month and the rooting reflex about the third or fourth month. In the older child or adult, a persistent sucking response is indicative of diffuse brain disease.

Palmar and plantar grasp responses are elicitable from the day of birth. These differ from the forced grasp response seen in diseases of the pyramidal tract and the frontal lobes in older patients, because the normal palmar or plantar grasp of the newborn is a flexion response to sustained pressure against the proximal phalanges, whereas pathologic grasp is a response to a moving stimulus on the palmar or plantar surface. These responses are most striking in the neonatal period when the infant can support his or her weight with the palmar grasp and may be supported on a string by both hands and feet in the manner of a sloth. A feeble tonic flexor reaction usually is elicitable in the premature infant of 24 weeks gestational age, becoming progressively stronger, so that by

32 weeks gestational age, a consistently strong response is evident. The tonic flexor reaction of the fingers gradually disappears and is no longer consistently present after the fourth to sixth month, being gradually obscured by voluntary activity. The tonic flexor reaction of the toes gradually disappears between the sixth and the twelfth months. Absent plantar grasp may be the strongest clue to a deficit in L-5, S-1, or S-2 in the newborn infant with myelodysplasia.

Righting reflexes are present in the newborn during the first 4 months of life, after which time they fuse into voluntary movements. The neck-righting reflex is elicited with the infant in the supine position. Turning the head in either direction is followed by turning of the shoulders and then of the trunk to the same side as the head. Persistent, exaggerated, or obligate neck-righting reflex in older infants suggests diffuse cortical dysfunction. A vertical righting response may be elicited in the term newborn by holding the infant flexed over the examiner's arm with the buttocks against the examiner's body. Stimulation of the infant's feet with the hand should result in extension of the lower extremities against the hand and in subsequent extension of the infant's trunk and then the head. This particular response disappears within the first 2 months after birth. It begins to appear in the premature infant at 34 weeks gestational age but is not complete until 40 weeks or term. Asymmetry of the response that is clearly reproducible may suggest mild paresis or hemiparesis. Absence of the response suggests paraplegia or diplegia.

The term neonate normally exhibits a *primary walking,* or *steppage, reflex.* This is elicited by placing the infant's feet firmly on the examining table so that the primary standing position or vertical righting is exhibited. Then, by rhythmically advancing one shoulder and the other, the examiner can cause the infant to take definite steps characterized by dorsiflexion of the feet, so that the infant lights on the heel. Primary walking begins to appear in the premature infant at 34 weeks. At 36 weeks gestational age, the infant tends to exhibit a toe gait and at 40 weeks, a heel gait. This is an extension of primary standing and disappears during the first 2 months of life. *Placing reflex* may be elicited after about the tenth day of life by bringing the infant, held in the vertical position, to the edge of the table so that the dorsum of the foot touches the undersurface of the tabletop. Normally, the infant raises the foot, placing it on the tabletop in a stepping manner. Again, a persistently asymmetrical response suggests unilateral deficit, and a persistently absent bilateral response may suggest diplegia or paraplegia. These signs are present before abnormalities of deep tendon reflexes are detectable.

The *parachute response* is most helpful in detecting neurologic deficit in the upper extremities of the older infant. It is elicited by supporting the infant in the prone position and rapidly moving the head toward the examining table. The normal response is for the infant to extend the upper extremities and fan the palms toward the table's surface to break the descent. This response appears generally between 6 and 9 months of age and should be present universally by 1 year. It is inconsistently present after 2 years. A persistently asymmetrical response suggests hemiparesis or monoparesis. An absent or incomplete response before 1 year of age may not be significant, but between the ages of 12 and 24 months, it strongly suggests tetraplegia.

The *Landau reflex* normally is consistently present by the tenth month and is demonstrated by supporting the infant on the examiner's hand in the prone position. Normally, the infant tends to extend the neck, trunk, and lower extremities. Passive extension of the head exaggerates the extensor response, and flexion of the head results in flexion of the trunk and hips. The infant with diplegia, tetraplegia, or paraplegia does not exhibit the characteristic extension posture but, rather, tends to collapse over the examiner's hand. The infant with severe rigidity may exhibit an exaggerated extensor response. The reflex is gradually integrated into voluntary patterns of movement during the second and third years of life.

The Cranial Nerves

Examination of the cranial nerves is discussed in detail in Chapters 5 and 6. However, a summary of a few points specifically applicable to infants follows. The infant responds to certain olfactory and gustatory stimuli on the first day of life. The reaction to olfactory stimulation is grimacing. The symmetry of the grimace or cry or smile is also a test of seventh nerve function. The newborn infant reacts pleasurably to sugar and, generally, unfavorably to salt. The corneal reflex is present from birth but cannot be accurately quantified until the patient can communicate. The rooting reflex is dependent on cranial nerves V and VII, and the sucking response is dependent on cranial nerves V, VII, and XII. The tongue-retrusion reflex is present during the first few weeks of life and results when a firm object is placed in the infant's mouth. Normally, the tongue is used to attempt to expel the object. The gag reflex is present from birth. The facility with which the patient swallows, the quality of the cry, and the motility of the palate are clues to ninth and tenth nerve function. Function of the eleventh nerve is difficult to assess in the infant, although quality and symmetry of head control may afford some clues. Hearing is present from birth. It can be evaluated in the newborn only when the baby is quiet and content. A sudden auditory stimulus results in a start or even a Moro type of response and often is followed by a cry. A lesser stimulus may result only in blinking.

The newborn infant responds to bright light by blinking or grimacing. Ocular movements may be tested by the doll's eye reflex during the first 2 weeks of life. To carry out this test, the examiner gently rotates or tilts the infant's head. As this is done, the eyes appear to move in the direction opposite to the motion of the head. By 3 months, the infant will follow objects reasonably well with the eyes. In the older infant, visual fields may be tested by introducing objects from behind into the field of vision and noting the response to these. In examining the fundus of the newborn or small infant, the examiner should bear in mind that the optic nerve heads are physiologically pale as compared with those of the adult.

Examination of the Head

Observation, palpation, measurement, auscultation, percussion, and transillumination should be included. In the newborn, some degree of head molding is generally evident, and the sutures may be overriding or diastatic. Infants born by elective cesarean section or breech presentation show no evidence of molding. Molding resolves in the first few weeks of life. Caput succedaneum may be evident during the first few days of life and is simply edema of the scalp in the region of the presentation. Cephalohematoma, however, is the result of hemorrhage under the periosteum. The anterior fontanelle should be easily palpable in the newborn. The posterior fontanelle is generally palpable, but with severe molding and overriding at the sutures, it may be difficult to identify. The posterior fontanelle is the first to close and is normally not palpable after 6 weeks. The time of closure of the anterior fontanelle is variable and generally occurs between the ages of 10 and 20 months. Palpation of the fontanelle should be carried out with the infant quiet and in the upright position. In the older infant or child, the shape of the head may reveal clues to the nature of the underlying process. An elongated, narrow head may suggest prematurity or sagittal synostosis. A short, wide head with a flat brow is evidence of coronal synostosis. Trigonoencephaly is associated with synostosis of the metopic suture or hypoplasia of the frontal lobes. Bulging of a portion of the cranium may suggest underlying localized chronic pressure. A large head with a prominent brow, wide bitemporal diameter, and moderately enlarged occiput may indicate hydrocephalus with various etiologic aspects. A large head with an unusually prominent occipital shelf and a large posterior fossa may suggest Dandy-Walker syndrome.

Size of the head is of particular importance in infants, since this is a reflection of intracranial contents. The measurement of head size used in clinical medicine is the occipital frontal circumference. The figure generally accepted is the largest reproducible measurement. Serial measurements are of greater value than a single one, since they afford information on the rate of head growth as well as the head circumference at a particular time. Serial measurements may be plotted on a head-size graph, and single measurements may be compared against norms for the age. The mean head circumference has a normal variation of two standard deviations above and below the mean (Fig. 13-1). In children up to 2 years of age, it may be of value to compare circumferences of the head

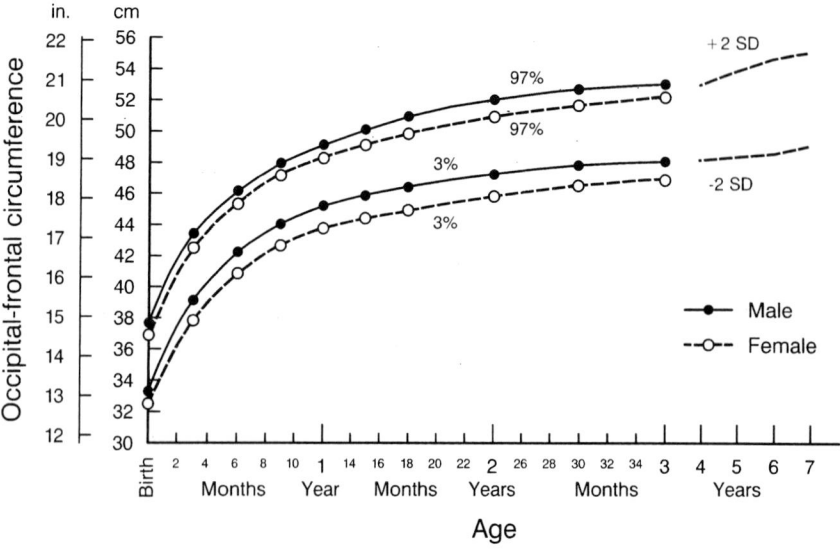

Figure 13-1
Normal head circumference for boys and girls through 3 years of age.

and chest. Circumference of the chest is measured at the nipple line. These two circumferences are normally similar up to 2 years of age, after which the circumference of the chest exceeds that of the head. The child with a head circumference of more than two standard deviations below the mean may be designated as having microcrania. This is generally synonymous with microcephaly. Exceptions would be individuals with turricephaly or heads elongated in the vertical dimension. On the other hand, the child with a large head (greater than two standard deviations above the mean) can only be designated as having "macrocrania." The underlying problem may be hydrocephalus from any cause, tumor, subdural hematoma, or a large brain. Further evaluation is necessary to define the nature of the macrocrania.

Transillumination of the head is accomplished by the use of a flashlight or high-intensity light fitted with a rubber adaptor so that light does not escape under the edges. The examination is carried out in a darkened room. The adaptor is applied to the head, and the light is turned on and moved over the head. In the infant, the area of the fontanelle may transmit more light than the surrounding areas. A more prominent halo is revealed around the light in a fair-complexioned infant than in a dark-complexioned infant. With a flashlight, a halo of more than 1 cm is considered abnormal, but with a high-intensity light, a halo of 2 to 3 cm may be normal, especially in the very young infant. Transillumination is useful in demonstrating subdural effusion, hygroma, chronic subdural hematoma, cerebral atrophy, porencephaly, arachnoid cysts, and hydranencephaly. The hydrocephalic head allows light to pass through if the cortical mantle is sufficiently thin. Edema of the scalp or effusion of clear fluid into the scalp may transmit light. Fresh subdural hematomas and cephalohematomas do not allow the passage of light.

Auscultation over the head of the normal infant or child sometimes reveals benign bruits. These are most commonly heard over the temporal regions and less often over the eyes. Loud, primarily systolic bruits may be heard in the presence of increased intracranial pressure from any cause. The bruits of arteriovenous malformations are generally prominent and have a machinery-like quality.

Sensory examination of the infant is difficult and can be carried out only in the quiet child. Several examinations may be required. Only pain and touch sensations can be appraised in the newborn and small infant. The examiner notes the infant's facial and motor responses to the stimuli. Gradation of response is most unreliable, and the examiner can hope only to establish whether the infant feels the stimulus. The infant with a lesion of the spinal cord and a sensory level deficit will consistently ignore the stimulus to the level of the deficit. Careful palpation of the skin of the patient with a cord lesion may reveal decreased sweating below the level of the lesion. In a child 12 to 18 months of age, one may be able to estimate vibratory sensation by noting the infant's response to the tuning fork when it is and when it is not vibrating.

EXAMINATION OF CHILDREN MORE THAN 2 YEARS OF AGE

The principles of conducting a neurologic examination of adults and children are the same, but the technique must vary for children, depending on their intelligence, social maturity, and emotional reactions. It is usually preferable to have the child's parents in the room during the examination. In general, the child should be allowed to move about freely before questioning begins or cooperation is requested. An attractive toy placed on the examiner's desk may gain attention and induce the child to come near the examiner. A small bell could serve this purpose, and it could also be used for gross hearing testing in infants and to obtain eye fixation when the ocular fundus is examined. Gait can be tested by having the patient go to one of the parents or to a person of the child's liking. Coordination can be tested by giving the patient objects to play with, such as a small toy or the examiner's reflex hammer or tuning fork. Strength can be tested by having the child pull or push, climb on a chair or the examining table, or get up off the floor. When examining the reflexes, it is important not to tap directly on the child's tendons but to place the left index finger (if the examiner is right-handed) on the tendon to be percussed. This simple maneuver may spare a breakdown in tears by a fearful child. Sensitivity to pain should not be tested until the end of the examination. If the patient is cooperative, the ophthalmoscopic test should be done early in the examination when the child is not tired; if the child is uncooperative and needs to be held, it should be done at the end. Stereognosis can be tested by having the patient feel and identify several objects in a paper bag without looking at them.

The following comments pertain to tests that are of particular importance in pediatric neurology. For the sake of brevity, certain tests mentioned are not described in detail because they are usually administered by clinical psychologists. It should be understood that these psychologic tests are an important adjunct to examination of the functions of the central nervous system. The following tests will be described: (1) spontaneous motor activity, (2) praxis (verbal commands and imitation), (3) lateral dominance or preference, (4) drawing, (5) articulation of sounds, (6) language, (7) auditory discrimination and memory, (8) reading and spelling, (9) calculation, (10) corporeal orientation, and (11) extracorporeal space orientation.

Spontaneous Motor Activity

Assessment of the quantity and quality of the spontaneous motor activity of a child may be helpful in understanding behavior. During the second and third years of life, normal children are constantly driven to explore their immediate environment. Compared with an older child or adult, toddlers are more active, but this is normal at their age. On the other hand, the hyperactive child of school age is often excessively aggressive, unable to sit still, and demanding of attention, disrupting the social order at home or in the classroom. This variety of hyperactivity is frequently associated with other neurologic symptoms, such as impulsiveness, clumsiness, short attention span, disorders of perception or of reading and writing, and subnormal intelligence. Observation in the examining room often confirms the parents' or the teacher's report of hyperactivity. Sometimes, because of the child's fear, the hyperactivity is not readily apparent to the examiner. When the patient becomes tired or bored, his spontaneous activity increases and may be characterized simply by frequent changes of posture or by more complex motor activity, such as walking or running about the room and climbing on furniture. No adequate method is known whereby the hyperactivity of children can be quantified. An adequate history from parents or teachers and the observations by the examiner are sufficient to establish the diagnosis. Checklist questionnaires designed to be answered by parents or teachers may facilitate obtaining the pertinent information.

Praxis

"Dyspraxia" means difficulty (awkwardness or clumsiness) in performing voluntary movements in the absence of weakness, spasticity, ataxia, and involuntary movements. It may affect all voluntary movements or only portions of the extremities. In a neonate, it may be developmental or secondary to an injury or a condition affecting the central nervous system, such as hyperbilirubinemia. Dyspraxia may be recognized by the parents of the preschool child but usually is not recognized until the child enters school. The teacher may observe that the child has trouble putting on an overcoat, tying shoelaces, or holding a pencil. The neurologic examination outlined for adults does not include appropriate tests for recognizing dyspraxia, and a systematic method of examining children is needed. Such an examination should include observation of the clumsy actions of the patient, some of which may be recognized if the child is asked (1) to follow certain commands or (2) to imitate certain movements.

1. Verbal commands

The examiner may use all or a portion of the following commands but should avoid demonstrating the action requested. The examiner may indicate right or left if the patient does not know. The following commands are classified according to the anatomic parts in action.

Eyes:
  Close your eyes
  Open your eyes
  Look to your right
  Look to your left
  Look up
  Look down
  Raise your eyebrows
  Frown
Mouth:
  Open your mouth
  Close your mouth
  Show your teeth
  Blow
  Pretend to kiss
Tongue:
  Put your tongue out
  Put your tongue up
  Put your tongue down
  Move your tongue to the right
  Move your tongue to the left
  Wiggle your tongue
  Pretend to lick an ice cream cone

Hands, arms:
  Make a fist with
  Make a cup with   } your right/your left hand
  Pretend to throw with
  Pretend to catch with
  Pretend to comb your hair
  Cup both hands together
Fingers:
  Snap your middle finger and thumb
  Spin a top
  Make an O with your index finger and thumb
  Make a V with your fingers
  Touch each finger with your thumb
  Unbutton/button your shirt
  Wind a watch
  Tie shoelaces
  Fold paper
  Place paper in an envelope
  String beads
Lower limbs:
  Walk straight
  Tandem walk
  Run
  Skip
  Stand on right foot
  Stand on left foot
  Hop on two feet
  Hop on your right/your left foot

2. Imitation

Praxis also can be tested with imitation tests in which spoken language plays only a small role. The tests require that the child imitate the examiner by placing fingers, hands, and arms to reproduce postures demonstrated by the examiner. The tests begin with simple gestures, such as holding out both hands with palms toward the child, and progress to much more complex gestures. For the sake of brevity the reader is referred to the detailed description of these tests in the monograph by Bergès and Lézine.†

Lateral Dominance or Preference

Lateral dominance means that one side of the body is used in preference to the opposite side. The preference may be limited to one hand, hand and foot, eye, eye and ear, or all these parts on the same side.

---

†Bergès J, Lézine I: *The imitation of gestures: a technique for studying the body schema and praxis of children three to six years of age.* Clin Dev Med 18:1–116, 1965.

Sometimes a subject is right-handed for a particular act but left-handed for another. For example, a child who is left-handed is taught to hold a spoon and to write with the right hand. Later, the child will be left-handed for throwing and batting but right-handed for eating and writing. Mixed preference is frequently found in children with acquired or developmental motor disorders but alone has no diagnostic significance.

To determine eye preference, it is sufficient to have the child sight through a paper tube or peek through a hole in a piece of paper held by the child with both hands. To determine hand preference, one may ask the patient to throw a ball or to deal cards. A simple method for toddlers is to hand five or six tongue blades to the patient, one by one, and ask to have them returned one by one. The child accepts and gives them with the preferred hand and stores them in the nonpreferred hand. To determine foot preference, getting the child to respond to the request to climb a step or to kick is sufficient.

Drawing

Children who are able to use pencil and paper should be asked to draw spontaneously. Drawing depends on the manual praxis of the child, but it is also an indication of intelligence and the experience acquired by the child in his cultural environment. One should look at the drawings for content, quantity of tracings or productivity, organization, and quality of figures. Although much has been said about analysis of personality, the use of drawings for this purpose is of doubtful value.

The child's intellectual maturity can be estimated with the Goodenough-Harris Draw-a-Person test, provided that there is no motor impairment of the drawing hand. With the aid of tables, the raw score is converted to a standard score with a mean of 100 for any age between 3 and 15 years. According to Harris, the test score parallels intellectual maturity determined by the Stanford-Binet test or Wechsler Intelligence Scale for Children and in part reflects the child's ability to form concepts.

The Bender Visual-Motor Gestalt test for children is widely used for patients 7 years of age or older. It consists of nine geometric figures to be copied with pencil on a single sheet of unruled paper. The cards are shown in a given sequence. In disorders of the central nervous system, the drawings may show simplification or fragmentation of figures, collision of one figure with another, rotation, incorrect number of units, perseveration, tremulous or poor line quality, and commas or dashes in the figures, all indicative of inadequate functional connection between motor and visual integration areas of the brain.

Articulation of Sounds

A child $2\frac{1}{2}$ to 3 years of age usually is able to produce a relatively complete repertoire of the speech sounds of the native language, but mastery of these sounds in words, particularly the consonant sounds, takes longer. The physician concerned about a child's communication skills will want to

Table 13-1 Ages in Years at Which 75% of Templin's Subjects Correctly Produced Given Consonants in the Initial and Final Positions

Consonant	Key Words	Age (yr) Initial Position	Age (yr) Final Position
h	*h*orse	3	—
w	*w*ater	3	—
m	*m*y, la*m*b	3	3
n	*n*o, ca*n*	3	3
ng	ri*ng*	—	3
f	*f*our, cal*f*	3	3
p	*p*ie, cu*p*	3	3
t	*t*oe, si*t*	3	3
k	*c*ome, ba*ck*	3	4
b	*b*oy, ru*b*	3	4
d	*d*og, re*d*	3	4
g	*g*irl, bu*g*	3	4
y	*y*ellow	3.5	—
r	*r*ed, ca*r*	4	3.5
sh	*sh*oe, bu*sh*	4	4
s	*s*ee, bu*s*	4	4.5
l	*l*ook, ba*ll*	4	6
j	*j*ump, bri*dge*	4	7
ch	*ch*air, wa*tch*	4.5	4.5
th (voiceless)	*th*umb, ba*th*	6	6
th (voiced)	*th*ere, smoo*th*	6	7
v	*v*ase, sto*v*e	6	6
z	*z*ipper, bu*zz*	7	7
zh	gara*ge*	—	7

Modified from Templin M: Certain language skills in children: their development and interrelationships. *Minneapolis, 1957, University of Minnesota Press. By permission of the publisher.*

elicit a sample of speech and to evaluate articulation skills, at least in general terms. The child may be asked to count to 20, tell about some action pictures, or tell about family and pets. The physician notes the degree of overall intelligibility and the adequacy of production of the consonants listed in Table 13-1. The examiner may go a step further and ask the child to repeat after him or her the key words listed in Table 13-1, noting the accuracy of their production; some sounds may be omitted, others distorted or slighted, and still others replaced by other consonants (for example, *w*abbit for *r*abbit, *f*umb for *th*umb). The physician may want to learn whether the child can imitate a model of specific sounds (in isolation rather than in words) on which the child makes errors in conversation. The object is to determine to what degree the child is stimulated when listening, watching carefully, and trying hard to imitate.

The tests of praxis for mouth and tongue may offer some indication of the reasons a child has trouble with specific sounds, revealing slow, incoordinate, or clumsy movement of the tongue and lips. In addition, one should note whether the upper anterior teeth are significantly misaligned, spaced unusually widely, absent, or located unusually with regard to typical tongue carriage, since the normal articulation of certain sounds (s, z, sh, f, v, th, and j) requires that the breath stream be directed sharply against a cutting edge. Audiometric testing may show that a child has trouble with those same sounds because of loss of hearing.

Language

The sample of conversational speech elicited by the physician yields useful information about the child's ability to handle language generally—vocabulary, grasp of the rules by which words are combined into phrases and sentences (syntax), and fluency. The physician can rate the following:

1. Number of different words used.—Does the child's vocabulary appear large, average, or meager?
2. Length of responses.—A preponderance of one-word "sentences" in a child 3 years of age or older suggests significant retardation in language skills.
3. Completeness and complexity of responses.—The older the child, the more complicated the syntax used. More modifiers, more phrases, and more subordinate clauses are used. The child, learning that pronouns change with case, abandons the sole use of "me" and uses "I," "me," "my," and "mine" differentially. Tense of verb and number of noun and pronoun are used accurately. The older child learns to transform certain sentences into other kinds of sentences (for example, declarative into interrogative and vice versa). And all of this is typically learned without formal teaching. The physician should note confusion in use of noun plurals, verb tenses, and case of pronouns; strange sequencing of words in sentences; and unusual difficulty in formulating negative and interrogative sentences. Children who have these problems, as well as those who have severe articulation problems or a tendency to alter the order of sounds within words they are asked to repeat, should be given a formal language evaluation. Test responses may suggest the presence of specific language disabilities that hinder them in comprehending oral language, in reading, or in speaking.
4. Fluency of speech.—Preschool children typically display substantial amounts of repetition and hesitation in their conversational

speech, especially when uncertain of what they want to say, when competing for attention, or when eager to report exciting events. Such nonfluency is typically easy, without self-consciousness, and should be considered normal. Of concern to the physician is an inordinate amount of repetition done tensely and with apparent struggle as the child appears to anticipate trouble and too carefully tries to avoid it. This development of an avoidant struggle reaction is termed "stuttering." Its appearance warrants investigation of the circumstances of its onset and the attitudes of the parents in trying to manage it.

For children who do not speak or who cooperate too poorly to permit the observations suggested in this and the preceding section, the physician (or the speech pathologist) may use a language counterpart of the Vineland Social Maturity Scale: The Verbal Language Development Scale. A language age can be estimated on the basis of information provided by a parent about a child's listening, speaking, reading, and writing activities.

Auditory Discrimination and Memory

Many children with problems in speech, reading, and spelling have particular difficulty in the discrimination of auditory signals, their retention in proper sequence, and their reproduction. This disability appears with sufficient frequency to warrant special observations by the examining physician.

1. Ask the child to reproduce two sounds: one high in pitch, one low; one loud, one soft; one long, one short. Then ask the child to reproduce more complicated patterns: high, low, high; loud, loud, soft; long, short, short; and so on.
2. Discrimination of speech sounds can be tested by asking the child whether two words are the same or different (stair-share, scare-stair, and others) or by displaying cards each picturing two words pronounced alike except for given sound elements and having the child point to the appropriate picture of the pair when the examiner says a word (car-star). Normative data on children 3 through 8 years of age on a 59-item test involving the latter task are available.
3. The digit span test from the Wechsler Intelligence Scale for Children or the Auditory-Vocal Sequencing Test of the Illinois Test of Psycholinguistic Abilities reveals difficulties in auditory retention and sequencing. Or the child can be asked to repeat sentences of increasing length, as in the sentence-repetition tasks of the Stanford-Binet Scale, Form L or M.
4. The ability of a child to fuse a sequence of separate sounds into a meaningful word may be related to articulatory skills and possibly

to other language capacities. It may be tested by presenting a series of two-phoneme (speech sound) words, one phoneme at a time, and then proceeding to three-phoneme and as many as five-phoneme words.

Words of Two to Five Phonemes

2	3	4-5
n-o	c-oa-t	p-ur-p-l-(e)
c-ow	b-oo-k	d-e-s-k
t-oe	r-igh-t	s-l-ee-p
s-ee	d-o-g	w-a-g-o-n
b-oy	s-i-t	t-a-b-le

Reading and Spelling

The physician who examines schoolchildren for whatever reason has a good opportunity of finding a dyslexic child. If the youngster is examined by a neurologist because of difficulty in learning, the neurologic examination should include testing the ability to read, write, and spell.

To test reading, any of the schoolbooks appropriate for the patient's grade level may be used if precaution is taken to use a book unfamiliar to the patient and without suggestive pictures.

Once the physician recognizes that the patient has reading disability, or dyslexia, the next step is to establish the patient's "reading age." There are many standardized reading tests designed for this purpose. Frequently they are administered by the clinical psychologist. Nevertheless, the neurologist should be familiar with Gray's Reading Paragraph or with the Wide Range Achievement Test and be able to "interpret" the test results.

Calculation

The examiner should test the preschool child's ability to count objects and the schoolchild's ability to add or subtract two digits mentally. The average 3-year-old child is able to count three objects and will show his or her age with the fingers when asked. The 4-year-old child is able to add 2 + 2 with fingers or objects. The Wide Range Achievement Test has been standardized for determining the proficiency of schoolchildren in doing computations.

Corporeal Orientation

During the first 2 years of life, the child gradually becomes aware of his or her own body and of its separation from the environment. The infant looks at and feels hands, mouth, feet, and other parts of the body and, while doing so, perceives with the hands the part touched while the touched part is stimulated by the exploring hand. Positions of the extremities as well as their movements and the effect of gravity are perceived. At 2 years of age, the child uses language and knows that parts of the body have names, so that he or she can associate with words not only what is seen but also what is felt as a part of the person.

1. Parts of body.—This simple test consists of asking the child to identify the part of the body to which the examiner points, such as an elbow or a wrist. The child also can be asked to name a particular part of his or her own body. The responses vary with mental age and with social and environmental conditions.
2. Finger agnosia.—Before the age of 2 years, children have "discovered" that they have fingers and toes but, of course, are not aware of their numbers. The concept of numbers 1 to 5 and 1 to 10 develops and grows in relation to the awareness of fingers. From ages 4 to 8 years, fingers are frequently used for counting, adding, and subtracting.

    The usual method of assessing finger localization in an adult consists in asking the patient to show a certain finger or to identify, by name or otherwise, a finger touched or pointed to by the examiner. Modification of this test consists of having the patient point to the finger in the drawing of a hand after the examiner has touched the patient's finger.
3. Right-left discrimination.—At 6 years of age, the average child knows the right and left sides of his or her own body. Between 9 and 11 years of age, the child has learned which is the right and which is the left side on the confronting person. Benton‡ designed tests of increasing difficulty to examine right-left orientation. The subject is asked to show consecutively left hand, right eye, left ear, and right hand, and then to touch the left ear with the left hand (double uncrossed command) and to touch the right eye with the left hand (double crossed command). The tests, first done with the eyes open, are repeated with the eyes closed. The child is then asked to point to a confronting person's right eye, left leg, left ear, and right hand and, finally, to use his or her right or left hand to point to the confronting person's right or left eye or ear. If handedness has been well established, a child will be able to tell which is the right hand simply by simulating the act of eating or throwing. Therefore, one should expect that the more right-handed or left-handed the child is, the better the child will be able to tell right from left. Right-left discrimination obviously correlates with mental age better than with chronologic age. Right-left discrimination may be impaired or delayed in children who are otherwise perfectly sound. More frequently, it is found in association with reading and writing disorders.

‡Benton AL: Right-left discrimination. Pediatr Clin North Am 15:747–758, 1968.

Extracorporeal Space Orientation

The child learns to move about and to manipulate objects before a symbolic representation of space is acquired. During the second year of life, as this new process begins, it is aided by the child's exploratory activity. It is as usual to find a 2-year-old child trying to put a solid object into an empty box as it is to see this child climbing on furniture.

Many tests are available to study a child's spatial orientation. The Seguin Form Board, designed as a test of intelligence, consists of 10 different flat geometric figures, each one to be fitted into a recess on a board. The time used and the correct placement are recorded. Children 2½ years of age or older can be tested.

Although these tests are considered to depend on motor coordination, they also reveal other functions, such as visual, tactile, and kinesthetic perception. More important yet, they show how the subject integrates all these forms of perception to create a symbolic representation of space. Matching shapes, geometric figures, or pictures of objects and recognizing orientations of geometric figures in spaces, such as in Frostig Developmental Tests of visual perception, the Kohs block design, and the Goldstein-Scherer Stick Test, are additional ways to explore the child's concept of bidimensional space. The child's ability in tridimensional space orientation can be explored with building blocks by asking the subject to copy a structure such as a three-cube or a six-cube pyramid.

SUMMARY

The unique aspects of the pediatric neurologic history and physical examination have been emphasized in this chapter. Detailed discussions of the cranial nerve, motor, sensory, autonomic, and muscle functions and evaluation of these as well as specific neurodiagnostic testing techniques are found in subsequent chapters. Selection of appropriate tests is predicated on collation and formulation of the findings from a carefully elicited history and physical examination into a working diagnosis. The rationale and nature of the indicated test or tests should be explained to the patient and parents insofar as possible so that they know what to expect. Appropriate sedation should be arranged for tests in which sufficient discomfort or anxiety might be involved. Care must be taken to avoid scheduling tests in such a way that one test would adversely affect the next; for example, a test requiring sedation or much discomfort and anxiety should not immediately precede neuropsychologic testing.

PART TWO

Diagnostic Procedures

Chapter 14

Neuroradiologic Procedures

Radiology has become an indispensable part of neurologic practice. Modern neuroradiologic techniques allow the clinician to instantly test hypotheses of localization and facilitate the arrival to accurate diagnosis. Many radiologic procedures in the past were labor-intensive, uncomfortable for the patient (for example, pneumoencephalography), and hampered by poor sensitivity and specificity. By comparison, most modern neuroradiologic techniques are much more convenient for patient and clinician and possess astonishing diagnostic accuracy.

Neuroradiologic studies applied to unique clinical situations are best undertaken after consultation with the neuroradiologist. Acquaintance with the clinical aspects of the case enables the radiologist to select the optimal technique for the examination and assists in the interpretation of the neuroradiologic findings. The importance of clear communication between clinician and radiologist about the goals of a particular study cannot be overemphasized.

When a study of one neuroanatomic region fails to reveal a suspected lesion, the clinician should consider the possibility that the lesion is located in a different region. For example, lesions of the spinal cord often lie higher than their clinical signs suggest, and more than a few parasagittal frontal lobe meningiomas have been discovered only after fruitless examination of the spinal canal. Also, when a radiologic study fails to show a suspected lesion, the clinician should question whether the proper imaging plane or technique was selected. For instance, if one suspects a medial temporal lobe lesion, coronal images of the temporal lobes with thin cuts should be obtained rather than transaxial images alone.

Accurate interpretation of neuroradiologic studies requires a sound knowledge of the anatomic features of the imaged region. For example, the inexperienced examiner may misinterpret the middle meningeal groove on skull roentgenograms as a fracture. The artifacts of a particular imaging modality also need to be considered. For instance, magnetic resonance imaging (MRI) is potentially fraught with artifacts that in some cases strongly resemble pathologic lesions. An example of such an artifact is a motion-induced linear abnormality located in the central spinal cord that could be mistaken for syringomyelia. The neurologist and radiologist must obviously be aware of such pitfalls before making diagnostic conclusions.

When imaging studies are examined, a definite routine should be followed so that no region is overlooked. For example, examination of a magnetic resonance image of the head should begin with the sinuses and proceed to the subcutaneous regions, calvarium, investing membranes, sella, brain parenchyma, and, finally, the ventricular system. The order in which this is done is not so important so long as all regions are evaluated in a systematic manner.

In this chapter, we introduce the radiologic techniques most widely used in current neurologic practice. The limitations and merits of each imaging modality are discussed, along with application of the technique in a variety of common neurologic disorders. The technique, advantages, and disadvantages of the radiologic procedures most commonly used and the clinical disorders in which they are useful are summarized in Table 14-1.

PLAIN ROENTGENOGRAPHY

Spine Roentgenography

Morbid conditions of the spinal column or within the spinal canal may require a variety of neuroradiologic studies for adequate evaluation. Plain roentgenograms are usually obtained first, because they can provide diagnostic information quickly and economically. Descriptions of some of the abnormalities found on spine roentgenography in various diseases of the spine follow.

Developmental anomalies

Spondylolysis and spondylolisthesis are easily recognized on lateral and oblique views of the spine. Spina bifida is usually of no diagnostic significance by itself but may be associated with other congenital anomalies that are of clinical importance. Syringomyelia is sometimes associated with widening of the spinal canal. Diffuse widening of the spinal canal, scoliosis, kyphosis, and multiple vertebral anomalies suggest diastematomyelia, a condition that is proved by the visualization of a bony septum in the midsagittal plane of the vertebral canal. Spinal dysraphism, seen most commonly in the lower thoracic and lumbar areas, is often associated with a meningocele or a myelomeningocele within the spinal canal. Conversely, the spinal canal may be found to be developmentally narrow, predisposing the patient to symptomatic spinal stenosis. Such narrowing may be seen in achondroplasia but may also occur in a general, regional, or localized manner in otherwise normal persons.

The Klippel-Feil deformity can be identified on cervical spine roentgenography as occipitalization of the atlas, failure of posterior fusion of the upper cervical segments, or fusion of two or more cervical vertebrae.

Table 14-1 Summary of the Common Neuroradiologic Modalities

Imaging Modality	Technique	Advantages	Disadvantages	Clinical Indications
Plain radiographs, spine and skull	Exploits differences in the penetration of x-rays through different tissue constituents	Widely available Inexpensive	Limited sensitivity and specificity Does not visualize neural or soft tissues	Trauma Certain developmental abnormalities Spinal stenosis Tumors Inflammatory conditions
Myelography	Spinal canal opacified to display lesions impinging on it and its contents	Readily demonstrates and localizes a variety of spinal lesions	Hospital-based, labor-intensive Complications possible Certain contraindications Sacral canal inadequately evaluated	Certain developmental anomalies Spinal stenosis Disk herniation Spinal tumors Leptomeningeal metastases Spinal cord AVM
Angiography	Opacification of the cerebral vasculature	Procedure of choice for most CNS vascular diseases	Hospital-based Certain contraindications and complications Requires specialized facilities	Occlusive cerebrovascular disease CNS AVMs (including spinal) Aneurysms Certain tumors Sinus thrombosis Cerebral vasculitis
Computed tomography	Image determined by the relative penetrability of tissue components to intersecting x-ray beams	Widely available, inexpensive Excellent visualization of skull base, brain, and ventricles Sensitive for acute intracranial blood Short image acquisition time Sensitive for detection of most large intracerebral lesions Can augment myelography	Contrast agents potentially toxic Poor discrimination of cord, roots, and posterior fossa Multiplanar imaging inferior to MRI Resolution inferior to MRI Susceptibility to bone artifacts	Trauma Hydrocephalus Tumors CNS infections Stroke Intracranial hemorrhage Disk disease Spinal stenosis

Continued

Table 14-1　Summary of the Common Neuroradiologic Modalities — cont'd

Imaging Modality	Technique	Advantages	Disadvantages	Clinical Indications
Magnetic resonance imaging	Scans reflect tissue-dependent relaxation properties after imposed magnetization	Superior anatomic resolution Can determine certain tissue components No ionizing radiation Convenient multiplanar imaging Directly visualizes neural tissues and disks	Slow image acquisition Expensive Limitations in certain patients Claustrophobia	Congenital malformations Diseases of the spinal cord White matter diseases Low-grade gliomas Epilepsy CNS infection
Radionuclide imaging (SPECT and PET)	Radiolabeled compound penetrates or is selectively taken up by particular regions in the brain	Allows assessment of neurochemical activity and function of various neuroanatomic structures	Poor anatomic resolution Technically demanding Not widely available Clinical utility not established for many disorders	Epilepsy surgery patients Certain degenerative disorders (PD, Alzheimer's)

AVM, arteriovenous malformation; CNS, central nervous system; MRI, magnetic resonance imaging; PD, Parkinson's disease; PET, positron emission tomography; SPECT, single-photon emission computed tomography.

Cervical spine roentgenograms can also demonstrate ribs in patients with symptoms of thoracic outlet syndrome.

Metabolic and endocrine disorders

Osteopenia is a common finding on spine roentgenography and may be due to a variety of underlying causes, such as osteoporosis, chronic use of corticosteroids, disuse, and malnutrition. Roentgenographic evidence of early changes in osteoporosis includes diffuse demineralization of the vertebral bodies with sharply demarcated borders. Compression fractures, a common complication in such patients, can be readily identified on plain roentgenography.

In acromegaly, the appearance of the spinal column may be normal, but the anteroposterior diameter of the vertebral bodies may be increased and massive spur formation may be evident. In diabetes mellitus, spine roentgenography often reveals diffuse hypertrophic spurring of the vertebral end plates, a condition commonly referred to as "diffuse idiopathic skeletal hyperostosis" (or "DISH").

Inflammatory conditions
Osteomyelitis of the spinal column may be detectable by demineralization or new bone formation or both. Infections of the vertebral interspaces also may be recognized roentgenographically by destruction of the bony margins of the adjacent vertebral end plates. Paravertebral abscesses may produce a fusiform shadow next to the vertebral bodies. MRI and gallium radionuclide studies are superior to roentgenography in sensitivity and specificity and should be considered if vertebral osteomyelitis is truly suspected.

Rheumatoid spondylitis is manifested by marginal destruction of the sacroiliac joints, formation of syndesmophytes, and destructive changes of the intervertebral articular surfaces. Of particular importance in the neurologic evaluation of patients with rheumatoid arthritis is the recognition of atlantoaxial dislocation and basilar invagination of the odontoid process on cervical spine radiographs. These anomalies result from disruption of the transverse odontoid ligament by rheumatoid arthritis and are best appreciated on lateral flexion and extension views of the cervical spine.

Degenerative conditions
The radiologic manifestations of degenerative diseases of the spine include narrowing of intervertebral spaces, hypertrophic changes of adjacent vertebral end plates, and, occasionally, Schmorl's nodes, which are radiolucent abnormalities within the vertebral body due to invagination of the neighboring nucleus pulposus. The mere presence of such changes does not prove their causal relationship to a patient's clinical symptoms and signs. However, when viewed in the light of the clinical evidence, these changes may provide a valuable clue to diagnosis and help rule out alternative pathologic conditions, such as metastatic or infectious disease of the spine. Herniated, uncalcified intervertebral disks cannot be demonstrated on plain roentgenography; MRI, computed tomography (CT), or myelography is usually necessary to demonstrate herniated intervertebral disks and their relationship to the neighboring neural structures. Spinal stenosis is a degenerative disorder of the spine resulting in compression of the spinal roots or cord due to ligamentous hypertrophy, osteophytic spur formation, and disk degeneration and prolapse. In the cervical area, spinal stenosis can be suspected when the sagittal diameter is less than 13 mm. In the lumbar area, such measurements are not so reliable. When spinal stenosis is seriously considered in the diagnosis, CT or MRI is usually necessary.

Traumatic conditions
Traumatic lesions of the spinal column, such as fractures and dislocations, are important indications for spine roentgenography. Complete radiographic studies are required to establish the site, type, and extent of the lesion if one exists. Flexion and extension views may need to be cautiously used in certain situations when ligamentous disruption is

suspected. CT is often necessary to identify fractures of the pedicles and laminae. A complete discussion of emergency room radiology of the spine is beyond the scope of this book.

Neoplasia of the vertebral column and spinal cord
CT, MRI, or myelography is required to establish the diagnosis in most neoplastic conditions of the spine. Nevertheless, primary and secondary tumors of the spine commonly produce abnormalities on spine roentgenography of which the clinician must be aware. Metastatic disease of the spine may be manifested by radiolucent osteolytic or radiopaque osteoblastic abnormalities. Metastatic epidural spinal cord compression typically occurs as the direct extension of neoplastic tissue from contiguous bony metastatic lesions. Such lesions frequently are located in the pedicles and best appreciated on anteroposterior views of the spine. In primary tumors of the spinal cord, one may see erosion of the pedicles or laminae and scalloping of the posterior surface of the vertebral bodies. Spinal canal enlargement, as evidenced by increased interpedicular distance, is often seen, especially with large congenital tumors of the cord. Occasionally, calcification is present in these tumors and may be identifiable on the roentgenogram. Neurofibromas often lead to enlargement of the intervertebral foramen; this finding is best appreciated on oblique views of the affected spinal region.

Miscellaneous conditions
Other conditions readily identifiable on routine spine roentgenography are Paget's disease, osteomalacia, osteitis condensans ilii, and various forms of bone dysplasia.

Roentgenography of the Skull
Newer neuroimaging procedures, such as CT and MRI, have largely replaced the skull roentgenogram in the radiologic evaluation of intracranial diseases. For the most part, skull roentgenograms are superfluous in the diagnosis of intracranial disease. They do remain useful in the evaluation of intrinsic skull lesions and, occasionally, in trauma cases. Despite the limited usefulness of skull roentgenograms, the clinician should be aware of diagnostic abnormalities that can sometimes be seen on them. Some of these abnormalities are discussed below.

Neoplastic disease
Increased intracranial pressure from an intracranial mass lesion may be suggested by demineralization of the posterior clinoid processes in an adult and separation of the cranial sutures in a young child. Shift of the normally present pineal calcification away from the midline should prompt an aggressive evaluation for an intracranial neoplasm. Craniopharyngiomas and oligodendrogliomas sometimes give rise to

calcification visible on the skull roentgenogram. In some superficial intracranial lesions, such as meningiomas, destructive and proliferative changes can occasionally be seen in the neighboring skull. Erosion of the internal auditory meatus may be a sign of an acoustic neuroma. Similarly, pituitary tumors may produce enlargement of the sella once sufficient size is reached. Erosion of the clinoid processes and dorsum of the sella may be apparent on the skull roentgenogram, as may erosion of the floor of the sella. Primary and metastatic tumors of the skull may result in osteolytic (as in multiple myeloma) or osteoblastic (as in metastatic prostate carcinoma) alterations. Benign hemangiomas of bone may simulate metastatic malignant lesions.

Traumatic lesions

Roentgenograms are sometimes helpful in head trauma but have been replaced by CT because of the ability of the latter to simultaneously evaluate the intracranial structures. Penetrating or puncture wounds of the face or skull (no matter how small) should always be examined roentgenographically to identify an unsuspected foreign body. Sometimes a "scout" skull roentgenogram facilitates identification of these objects, which if small enough might be missed on CT if thick transaxial cuts are used. Fractures may be seen on the skull roentgenogram, but basilar skull fractures are more consistently identified on CT. A fracture that passes through the groove produced by the middle meningeal artery should alert the physician to the possibility of an epidural hemorrhage; if a fracture is in the neighborhood of the mastoid or paranasal sinuses, the patient may be at risk for meningitis.

Congenital anomalies

Of the vast number of congenital anomalies of the skull, only a few examples of the more common ones will be considered here. In craniosynostosis, the sutures of the skull close before the brain has fully developed. This results in malformation of the skull, the exact configuration depending on the particular sutures that closed prematurely. The convolutional markings on the inner table of the skull caused by cortical gyri are often accentuated in such cases. In infants, the skull roentgenogram may be helpful in differentiating cephalohematoma from meningocele, since in the latter, a defect in the underlying bone should be identifiable. In hydrocephalus, one may see separation of the sutures and thinning of the cranial bones, particularly in the vicinity of the suture lines. The microcephalic skull is small, and the sutures are well visualized (as opposed to craniosynostosis, in which the sutures are not well visualized).

Lateral roentgenograms of the skull are helpful in suspected cases of basilar invagination. In such patients, the foramen magnum may be small and irregular in outline, with the odontoid process displaced upward into it. In addition, thinning of the bony floor of the posterior fossa and congenital anomalies of the cervical portion of the spinal column may be evident. To delineate this malformation clearly, MRI and CT are usually required. The "tram-track" calcifications of Sturge-Weber syndrome are usually demonstrable on the skull roentgenogram as well.

Inflammatory lesions
Osteomyelitis of the skull may be manifested by destructive and proliferative changes on the skull roentgenogram. Certain long-standing infectious diseases of the brain give rise to changes on skull roentgenography as well. Old abscesses, tuberculomas, gummatous lesions, and the lesions of toxoplasmosis and cysticercosis can on occasion give rise to areas of calcification on the skull roentgenogram. Clearly, however, these conditions are best evaluated with CT or MRI.

Metabolic and endocrine diseases
Roentgenograms of the skull may provide either the initial clue or confirmatory evidence of metabolic and endocrinologic diseases. Paget's disease produces thickening of the cranial bones and base of the skull; a patchy increase in the density and thickness of the bone is characteristic, and basilar invagination may develop. Fibrous dysplasia may result in both sclerotic and cystic lesions. Symmetrical calcification in the basal ganglia and the dentate nuclei may be associated with hypoparathyroidism. Acromegaly may result in enlargement of the sella turcica and frontal sinuses, thickening of the calvarium, and mandibular enlargement.

MYELOGRAPHY

General Aspects
Myelography is performed by first introducing a radiopaque substance into the subarachnoid space and then proceeding with fluoroscopy of the spine. The purpose of myelography is to demonstrate lesions in the spinal intradural or extradural compartments. MRI has replaced myelography in the evaluation of some diseases of the spine, but myelography remains the definitive procedure for many disorders. Myelography is more specific in the diagnosis of vascular diseases of the spinal cord and more sensitive (when used with CT) in the diagnosis of cervical and lumbar disk disease.

In myelography, the lumbar route is used almost exclusively; occasionally, the substance must be introduced in the cervical region when access to the lumbar area is not possible. Contraindications to myelography cannot be stated categorically. Many conditions, such as infections of the lumbar vertebrae, xanthochromic spinal fluid, adhesive arachnoiditis, anticoagulant therapy, and suspected complete spinal block, have been regarded as contraindications to myelography, but none of them is absolute. There is no convincing evidence to indicate that myelography aggravates degenerative or demyelinating diseases of the spinal cord.

Intraspinal disease is demonstrated on myelography by an alteration of the flow of contrast medium in the subarachnoid space. In myelography, the opacified subarachnoid space or spinal canal is commonly referred to as the "contrast column" and the radiolucent filling defect caused by the spinal cord is termed the "central zone." Pathologic conditions resulting in gross structural changes of the vertebral canal, intervertebral connective tissues, spinal cord and roots, and meninges and blood vessels are usually identified by myelography. CT has greatly enhanced the localizing ability, sensitivity, and specificity of myelography.

Myelography is indicated whenever a spinal lesion is suspected and surgical treatment is being seriously contemplated. In addition to locating space-occupying intraspinal lesions, myelography can be useful in the detection of vascular abnormalities, arachnoiditis, and congenital anomalies such as tethered cord and diastematomyelia. Some of these congenital disorders are perhaps best evaluated by noninvasive studies such as MRI. During myelography, the entire spine should be imaged fluoroscopically for several reasons. For example, in the evaluation of metastatic disease of the spine, multiple lesions are often present, and the clinical effects of one lesion may be masked by others. Also, when imaging the entire spine, one may occasionally identify a significant asymptomatic lesion. It is not unusual for an asymptomatic spinal meningioma to be identified during complete myelographic evaluation performed for a focal disk herniation.

It is usually best to defer lumbar puncture if myelography is planned. Spinal fluid can be obtained for analysis at the time of the myelogram in such cases. This avoids the unnecessary discomfort of multiple lumbar punctures. Also, on occasion, lumbar puncture collapses the thecal sac, causing subsequent myelographic attempts to be unsuccessful.

Complications

Significant complications of myelography are fortunately rare. Myelographic contrast media can produce a variety of adverse effects on the nervous system. Mild irritative effects, such as transient pains in the legs, low-grade fever, and increased cell count and protein concentration in the spinal fluid, may follow myelography. In rare instances, seizures occur. Arachnoiditis was a relatively common complication of the oil-based myelographic contrast agent iophendylate (Pantopaque) but is fortunately rare with modern contrast materials. After puncture of the thecal sac, herniation can occur if high-grade spinal compression is present. Rarely, tonsillar or tentorial herniation occurs during myelography if an unsuspected space-occupying intracranial lesion is present.

Fortunately, the intracranial imaging modalities currently available usually identify such conditions in advance.

Pathologic Findings

Narrowing or obstruction of the spinal canal by a space-occupying lesion is demonstrated by displacement of the contrast column. The contour of this defect depends on the relationship of the lesion to the meninges and spinal cord. It is helpful to anatomically categorize the lesions seen on myelography relative to the structures outlined by the contrast column; for example, it is usually possible to categorize such lesions as extradural, intramedullary, or intradural-extramedullary (Fig. 14-1). Although such localization is usually possible, it is sometimes inaccurate. Localization is greatly enhanced by using anteroposterior and lateral views and cross-sectional CT.

Classifying myelographic lesions anatomically can facilitate differential diagnosis, as summarized in Figure 14-1. The differential diagnostic considerations for each type of lesion are discussed below. These

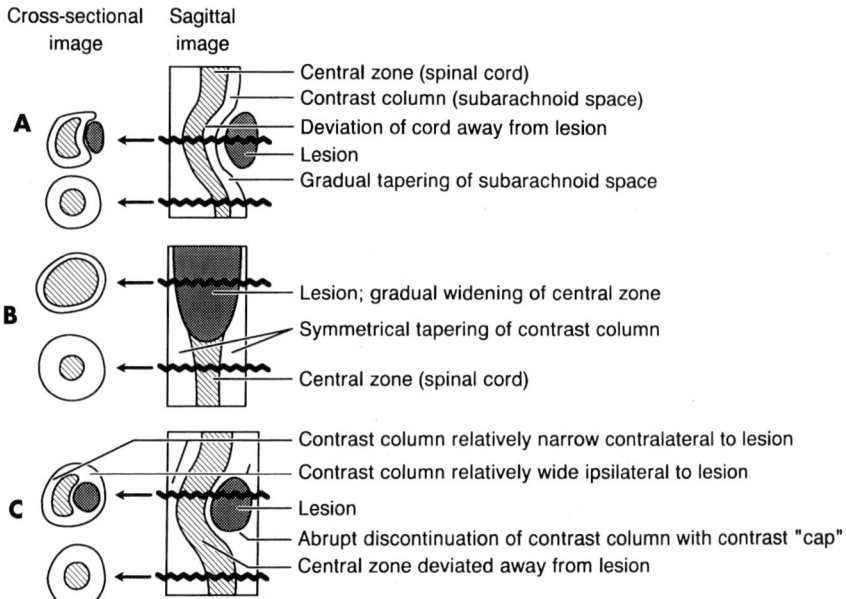

Figure 14-1
Myelographic localization. Lesions identified on myelography can often be categorized in accordance with their location within the three spinal compartments illustrated here: **A**, the extradural compartment; **B**, the intramedullary compartment; and **C**, the intradural-extramedullary compartment.

diagnoses are for illustration and are not meant to be exhaustive. In addition, some histopathologic lesions occur in more than one of the basic anatomic compartments. For example, lipomas, usually localized to the intramedullary region, sometimes appear as an extradural defect.

Extradural defects (see Fig. 14-1, *A*) characteristically exhibit gradual tapering of the contrast column. The defect is usually confined to one or two vertebral levels and is maximal at the center. Extradural lesions in the cauda equina often give rise to a serrated appearance at the interface between lesion and contrast column due to the rounded, tubular morphology of the nerve roots draped over the lesion. In addition, the interface between lesion and contrast column is often not sharp in extradural lesions. Examples of pathologic lesions that produce extradural defects on myelography are herniated disks, spinal stenosis, and epidural spinal cord compression due to destructive malignant and infectious vertebral lesions.

Intramedullary lesions (see Fig. 14-1, *B*) are characterized by gradual widening of the central zone (that is, spinal cord) within the contrast column. The opaque contrast column on either side of the central zone gradually tapers until it is obliterated by the intramedullary lesion. Examples of lesions that cause intramedullary defects are intrinsic spinal cord tumors, such as ependymomas, gliomas, and hemangioblastomas; acute transverse myelitis; syrinxes; and spinal cord arteriovenous malformations.

Intradural-extramedullary lesions (see Fig. 14-1, *C*) lie within the subarachnoid space. They are characterized by an abrupt discontinuation of the contrast column giving rise to formation of a concave "cap." Intradural-extramedullary lesions lead to deviation of the central zone away from the lesion. As a result, the contrast column on the ipsilateral side of the lesion is wide relative to the contrast column on the contralateral side. The most common pathologic lesions causing intradural-extramedullary filling defects are meningiomas and neurofibromas of the spine. Leptomeningeal metastatic lesions also reside in the intradural-extramedullary space. However, they usually appear as nodular thickening of the cauda equina and surface of the central zone rather than discrete solitary lesions.

CEREBRAL ANGIOGRAPHY

Cerebral angiography is a method of roentgenologic visualization of the cerebral vascular system by injection of radiopaque material into the cerebral arterial bloodstream. If angiography is to yield optimal results, the radiologist must be thoroughly familiar with the clinical problem and the exact nature of the suspected lesion.

Methods, Contrast Media, and Complications

Various techniques have been used in cerebral angiography. Femoral artery catheterization with selective arterial injection is the current standard. Selective arterial catheterization is the method of choice when visualization of a region supplied by a specific vessel is under consideration, such as in the evaluation of carotid occlusive disease. Aortic arch injection with simultaneous four-vessel angiography is usually inferior to selective arterial catheterization. Unless the dye load is significantly increased and x-ray time extended, the intracranial circulation is suboptimally visualized.

A complete angiogram includes the arterial, capillary, and venous phases and is obtained by making rapid, successive roentgenographic exposures after injection of the contrast medium. The arterial phase outlines the characteristics of the surface of the brain, whereas the venous phase demonstrates the deep cerebral structures.

Cerebral angiography is not a harmless procedure. Excessive radiation to patients and personnel must be avoided. Contrast media also may be irritative and toxic. An unpleasant warm sensation is common during angiography; the patient needs to be warned of this before injection. Contrast media are potentially nephrotoxic; therefore, the benefits of the procedure must be weighed thoughtfully before angiography is performed in a patient with preexisting renal insufficiency. Minor side effects of cerebral angiography are pain during the injection and tenderness at the puncture site after the procedure. Occasionally, vomiting occurs; therefore, the patient should have nothing by mouth on the day of the examination. Convulsions are rare; if they occur, they often are focal and affect patients otherwise predisposed to seizures. Transitory paralysis of the recurrent laryngeal nerve and Horner's syndrome have been reported. Arterial wall dissection, arterial rupture, and intra-arterial thrombosis are rare complications; however, their gravity prevents angiography from being a routine screening neuroradiologic procedure.

Because of the potential risks, it is imperative that angiography be reserved only for patients in whom it is likely to provide needed information not obtainable by other procedures. Cerebral angiography is the definitive procedure for visualization of the cerebral arterial and venous system. The angiographic findings in a variety of neurologic conditions are discussed below.

Cerebrovascular Disease

Saccular aneurysms, arteriovenous malformations, tumors of blood vessels, and occlusive vascular disease lend themselves well to angiographic demonstration. Angiography furnishes information about the approximate size, type, and location of such lesions and allows assessment of the adequacy of collateral circulation and the associated normal cerebrovascular anatomy; all are essential factors in clinical decision making.

Angiography is the radiologic study of choice for the diagnosis of cerebral aneurysms. Angiography should be performed in any sufficiently stable patient with nontraumatic subarachnoid hemorrhage in whom surgical intervention would be considered. The resolution of angiography is such that aneurysms even only a few millimeters in diameter can be reliably detected. Vasospasm, a common and significant complication of subarachnoid hemorrhage, can also be reliably demonstrated by angiography. Several points need to be emphasized when angiography is done in patients with subarachnoid hemorrhage. First, a thrombosed cerebral aneurysm may be missed on angiography. Second, a causative vascular lesion is not always identifiable in patients with spontaneous subarachnoid hemorrhage. Third, four-vessel angiography is essential in the evaluation of subarachnoid hemorrhage because multiple aneurysms are common in such patients. And fourth, opposing radiologic views are important in subarachnoid hemorrhage angiography to help differentiate aneurysms from aberrant vascular loops and to more ably identify aneurysms that might not be demonstrable on a particular view.

Angiography is very important in the evaluation of patients with certain cerebrovascular malformations. The major types of cerebral vascular malformations are arteriovenous malformations, cavernous malformations, capillary telangiectasias, and venous malformations. Arteriovenous malformations are readily demonstrated on angiography, as is the anatomy of their major arterial feeding vessels and draining veins. In some cases, an arteriovenous fistula may be identified. Venous malformations are characterized by radially oriented venous channels, referred to as the "caput medusae," feeding into a large draining vein. Capillary telangiectasias and cavernous malformations are not visible on angiography because of their small caliber and slow flow, respectively, and are referred to as being angiographically "occult." In Sturge-Weber-Krabbe disease, the abnormal vessels are often so minute that angiography does not demonstrate them.

In clinical neurology, angiography frequently is an aid to diagnosis of symptoms produced by occlusive disease in the intracranial and extracranial cerebral vessels. Vascular occlusion is evidenced by the nonfilling of the involved artery. Arterial plaques are revealed by defects in the opaque column of contrast medium in the vascular lumen. Nonfilling of an artery is not always indicative of an occluded vessel but may be the result of faulty angiographic technique. Angiography allows visualization of the intracranial portions and proximal origins of the vertebral and carotid arteries, areas not reliably accessible by noninvasive imaging techniques. Angiography is essential for definite diagnosis and for optimal selection of patients for carotid endarterectomy. It is also necessary in confirming complete occlusion in patients without flow on carotid Doppler ultrasonography, because false-positive results can occur with the latter technique.

Angiography is also important in the diagnosis of cerebral vasculitis. Angiography has significantly limited sensitivity and specificity in this disease, however, and biopsy is often necessary. Angiographic diagnosis of vasculitis is hampered because vasculitis often affects vessels with lumina below the resolution of angiography and the diagnostic abnormalities can be mimicked by other diseases (such as leptomeningeal metastatic lesions and arteriosclerosis).

Mass Lesions
Angiography is no longer a primary tool in the diagnosis of intracranial neoplasms. However, the clinician may encounter neoplastic changes when angiography is performed for other purposes and needs to be aware of them. An expanding intracranial lesion displaces the adjacent brain substance and its vessels. Blood vessels normally present may be uncurled or straightened by a tumor. A sound working knowledge of normal cerebral angiography is essential for the identification of such vascular irregularities. Some neoplasms exhibit neovascularity, which has a distinctive appearance on angiography. Newly formed blood channels in a neoplasm differ from normal vessels in their course, in their irregular caliber, and by the occasional presence of abnormal arteriovenous connections. In contrast to vascularized expanding lesions, lesions with a diminished vascular supply, such as cysts, certain gliomas, abscesses, and hematomas, can be signaled by abnormal vessel displacement and by a region devoid of, or abnormally poor in, blood supply.

Craniocerebral Trauma
Angiography can be used to detect extracerebral intracranial hematomas; however, it has been replaced by CT and MRI for this purpose. Nevertheless, the clinician should become familiar with the typical angiographic appearance of such lesions. In subdural hematoma, the blood vessels are displaced away from the calvarium on the anteroposterior projection, leaving an avascular region, and the insular vessels are compressed from above. The anterior cerebral artery is usually shifted across the midline. Epidural hematomas show similar abnormalities. Intracerebral hematomas are manifested by displacement of certain vessels, analogous to the effect of intracerebral neoplasms discussed above. Carotid artery dissection, an often overlooked neurologic complication of craniocervical trauma, has a characteristic appearance on angiography: a tapering intraluminal stenosis beginning 2 to 3 cm distal to the carotid bifurcation; on occasion, a demonstrable intimal flap; pseudoaneurysm formation; a double lumen; and a "string sign" (that is, an extended narrowing of the carotid artery, usually ending where the carotid enters the skull).

COMPUTED TOMOGRAPHY

CT allows convenient, safe, and detailed visualization of the intracranial contents. The same technique can also be applied to the orbits, the sinuses and nasopharynx, and the spinal canal—all structures of potential importance in neurologic patients. CT of the thorax, abdomen and pelvis, and even the limbs can be useful to search for such conditions as neuromas, tumors of the thymus gland, and tumors compromising neural structures, such as the large plexi and nerves, and can aid in the search for a primary neoplasm in patients in whom paraneoplastic disorders are suspected.

Theory

The basic mechanism of CT relies on the varying transmissibility of intersecting x-ray beams through the components of the anatomic structure being imaged. A computer calculates the resulting x-ray absorption coefficients (density) at each intersecting point. The acquired digital data are then displayed in analog form on a screen and can be photographed. These data can be stored on magnetic disks and tape for future regeneration and analysis. Substances that deflect x-ray radiation (such as calcium) give rise to an opaque or "high attenuation" (bright) image, whereas substances allowing free passage of x-ray radiation (such as fat and spinal fluid) yield a lucent or "low attenuation" (dark) image.

CT scans of the head are usually performed in the horizontal plane or with 20-degree angulation toward the feet (the orbitomeatal line) (Fig. 14-2). For most clinical purposes, slices of 10-mm thickness are adequate, but in special situations, slices as thin as 1 mm can be acquired to focus on minute anatomic detail.

Examination of the head by CT reveals, in addition to the calvarium, the ventricular system and cerebrospinal fluid cisterns, pineal gland, falx cerebri, and gray and white matter. Details of the cerebral and cerebellar sulci can also be seen. Resolution within the spinal canal is not good enough to dispense with myelography in the evaluation of many intraspinal conditions, but CT cuts at selected sites during myelography greatly enhance the information obtained from that study. Bony narrowing and ligamentous hypertrophy within the spinal canal can be reliably detected by CT, making it a useful diagnostic study for spinal stenosis.

Contrast Enhancement

Iodinated contrast dye improves the identification of certain normal and abnormal intracranial structures. Hypervascular structures, such as the choroid plexus, the falx, and major vessels, become more opaque with contrast administration. Contrast also improves the detection of many

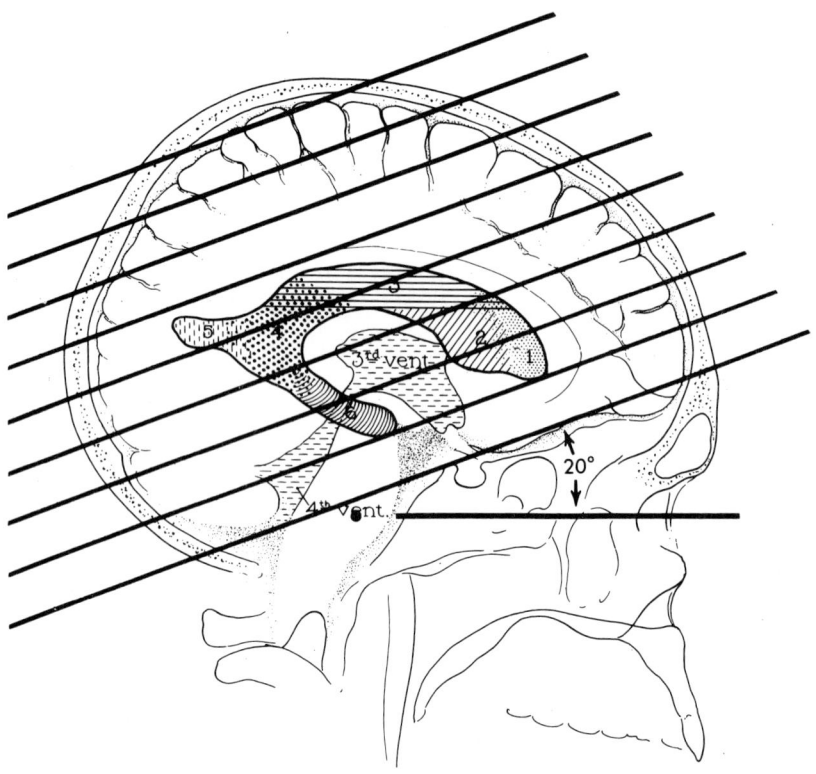

Figure 14-2
Orientation of the transaxial plane in computed tomography imaging. The transaxial images on computed tomography are oriented at a 20-degree angle from the horizontal, following the orbitomeatal line.

pathologic lesions, such as meningiomas, metastatic lesions, malignant brain tumors, and arteriovenous malformations. Intravenous contrast medium increases the risk of the procedure, however. Patients with impaired myocardial or renal function may be susceptible to the osmotic load imposed by contrast administration. Minor allergic reactions to the iodine-containing contrast material are common. Fortunately, severe anaphylactic reactions and delayed reactions resulting in shock are rare.

Clinical Applications

CT has had a major impact on the practice of neurology and neurosurgery. Many varieties of intracranial pathologic conditions can be safely and rapidly visualized by the technique, bypassing the need for dangerous invasive methods. A negative scan may be just as helpful as a positive study in the evaluation of patients with common neurologic conditions, such as chronic headache, brain injury, and organic brain syndromes. Although less sensitive than MRI, CT offers a convenient and relatively inexpensive alternative for patients in whom the suspicion of a significant intracranial lesion is low. The relative advantages and disadvantages of CT and MRI are summarized in Table 14-1. The following discussion focuses on the use of CT in the evaluation of a variety of neurologic conditions.

Cerebrovascular disease

CT is extremely useful in the diagnosis of intracerebral hemorrhage. It is superior to MRI in the detection of acute intracranial bleeding. CT has great reliability in the detection of freshly extravasated blood, which appears as a focal or diffuse intracranial area of increased attenuation (or opacity). The distinction between infarction and hemorrhage is readily made by CT at any time within the first week after the ictus. Such information is essential for therapeutic decision making. Subarachnoid blood is also readily detectable on CT, particularly within a few days of the hemorrhage. Blood in such cases is usually seen in the extracerebral cisterns, sulci, and, in some cases, the ventricles. Certain caveats need to be remembered about CT and subarachnoid hemorrhage. The sensitivity of CT for subarachnoid blood decreases considerably within a few days after hemorrhage. Also, small hemorrhages may be missed by CT. Therefore, if a few days have elapsed between ictus and CT scanning or if CT fails to confirm a highly suspicious case of subarachnoid hemorrhage, spinal fluid examination must be performed to definitively rule the diagnosis in or out.

Cerebral infarcts, especially large ones, can be seen within 24 hours on CT scans in some cases. Early findings in large cortical infarctions include increased attenuation of the cortical and subcortical gray matter, obliteration of normal sulcal markings ipsilateral to the infarct, midline shift of intracranial contents away from the infarct, and patchy areas of decreased attenuation within the ipsilateral cortical white matter. Some infarcts are initially isodense to the surrounding parenchyma and do not appear as areas of altered density for several days. Peak detection of brain infarction by CT occurs between 7 and 10 days after infarction.

Most infarcts are eventually detectable by CT, although sequential scanning may be necessary in some cases. Posterior fossa strokes are more difficult to visualize on CT than supratentorial infarcts because of obscuration by artifacts arising within the complex bony anatomy of the region. MRI is often necessary to demonstrate infarcts in the posterior fossa. Some brain infarcts demonstrate gyral enhancement after contrast administration because reactive hyperemia is induced by the vascular occlusion; this selective gyral enhancement may occur without a discrete area of decreased density and be the only CT evidence of the infarction. Initially bland infarcts in the brain may become hemorrhagic.

This complication is readily detectable on CT imaging, and a repeat CT scan should be considered if unexpected deterioration occurs in a patient suffering a stroke, particularly if anticoagulants or thrombolytic agents have been administered.

Larger infarcts often produce cerebral swelling, resulting in distortion or displacement of the ventricular system. This mass effect can be present as early as the day of the ictus but usually becomes maximal 4 to 5 days after stroke onset. It may persist for a few weeks after the stroke. The distinction between cerebral infarct and glioma may be difficult in this situation. Serial scans may help determine the kind of lesion in uncertain situations.

Arteriovenous malformations appear as ill-defined areas of calcification on unenhanced CT scans but are readily identifiable with contrast administration. Venous malformations are likewise identifiable on contrast-enhanced CT. Cerebral aneurysms are occasionally identified on CT scans, but this is exceptional. CT is not a good screening test for unruptured cerebral aneurysms.

Neoplasms

Both primary and secondary brain tumors are demonstrable by CT. MRI is more sensitive for smaller lesions. Most neoplasms appear as areas of decreased density or more commonly as areas of mixed or mottled density and are often surrounded by a zone of decreased density corresponding to edema. Some metastatic lesions may be hemorrhagic and appear as areas of increased density in relation to the surrounding brain parenchyma. The distinction between primary and metastatic brain tumors by CT rests mainly with the multiplicity of the latter. A single large metastatic mass may be indistinguishable from a primary brain tumor or cerebral abscess. Occasionally, when intracranial tumors or other masses are not directly visualized, their presence may be suspected by the finding of a shift of the normal intracranial landmarks, dilatation or deformity of the ventricular system, or obscuration of the ipsilateral sulci.

Extra-axial intracranial tumors, such as meningiomas, acoustic neuromas, pituitary tumors, and metastatic tumors in the meningeal spaces, are often detectable by CT; however, contrast enhancement is required for reliable detection. Thin slices and slices in the coronal plane are useful in the evaluation of pituitary and parasellar lesions. As with all radiographic techniques, the more clinical information given to the radiologist, the better the yield of the study. In the case of tumors of the vertex or base of the skull, the area of interest may not be visible on routine CT scanning unless a specific request is made. A negative CT scan does not exclude a low-grade infiltrating glioma. Sequential scans or MRI are often necessary for detection of these lesions.

Trauma

The high sensitivity for acute intracranial bleeding, wide availability, and rapid image acquisition times make CT ideal for the evaluation of patients with head trauma. It is sensitive and specific for the detection of subdural and epidural hematomas. CT is superior to skull roentgenography in the detection of basilar skull fractures as well. Some aspects of the CT evaluation of intracranial hematomas need to be pointed out, however. A subacute or chronic hematoma may become isodense to the underlying brain parenchyma, obscuring its presence. A ventricular shift may indicate such an isodense hematoma, but bilateral isodense clots may not lead to midline shift. Abnormally small ventricles and the lack of apparent sulci over the convexity (because of the overlying hematoma) are other indirect features that may suggest bilateral isodense subdural hematomas. In uncertain cases such as these, MRI can be extremely useful.

Degenerative disorders and hydrocephalus

CT is of value in the investigation of dementia, hydrocephalus, and many degenerative conditions that affect the nervous system. In the evaluation of dementia, CT serves as a tool to help rule out certain potentially treatable causes of dementia, such as subdural hematomas, hydrocephalus, and intracranial neoplasms (for example, meningiomas). There are no pathognomonic findings on CT—or with MRI, for that matter—in the diagnosis of the degenerative dementias. In such diseases, one may see large ventricles and widened cerebral cortical sulci or cerebellar fissures indicative of cerebral or cerebellar atrophy. These findings must not be overinterpreted, however.

CT is very valuable in the diagnosis of hydrocephalus. The ventricular system is exquisitely demonstrated on CT. CT makes it possible in most cases to differentiate obstructive from nonobstructive hydrocephalus. Follow-up in patients with shunts is facilitated by CT as well. Occasionally, the distinction between secondary ventricular enlargement due to cerebral atrophy and communicating or normal pressure hydrocephalus is difficult. Widened cortical sulci and sylvian fissures suggest the former, whereas moderate enlargement of the ventricles with little cortical atrophy usually indicates normal pressure hydrocephalus.

Inflammatory and infectious diseases

Cerebral abscesses give rise to a characteristic "ringed" appearance after contrast administration. Smaller abscesses visible on MRI may be missed on CT, but contrast-enhanced CT shows most clinically significant abscesses. Enhancement of the leptomeninges is sometimes visible in meningitis, and occasionally unenhanced CT scanning shows increased attenuation in the sulci if the subarachnoid space contains abundant inflammatory cells. Toxoplasmosis and cysticercosis give rise to cysts and calcified lesions readily visible on CT. CT is insensitive in the diagnosis of most inflammatory demyelinating diseases.

Toxic and metabolic disorders

CT usually serves to rule out alternative causes in patients presenting with toxic-metabolic central nervous system disorders. However, some toxic-metabolic disorders give rise to characteristic CT changes. For example, carbon monoxide poisoning often leads to selective necrosis of the globus pallidus; this is evident on CT as replacement of the globus pallidus by foci of decreased attenuation. Hypoparathyroidism occasionally is associated with calcification of the basal ganglia; however, one should not place too much emphasis on this finding in adults, because basal ganglia calcification is a fairly common finding in this population. Conversely, basal ganglion calcification is always significant in children and can occur in a number of disorders, such as mitochondrial cytopathies.

Diseases of the spine

As mentioned earlier, CT is mainly useful in the myelographic evaluation of spine diseases. When used without myelography, however, CT allows detailed evaluation of the basic anatomic substructures of the vertebrae. Unfortunately, the soft tissues, disks, and neural structures within the spine are inadequately visualized by CT in most cases. In general, MRI is more sensitive and gives more specific information about diseases of the spine, as does myelography. CT is helpful in certain traumatic spine conditions and is useful as a screening test for patients with spinal stenosis.

MAGNETIC RESONANCE IMAGING

MRI produces images of greater anatomic detail than CT does and also provides information on tissue characteristics. Magnetic resonance images are obtained by placing the patient within a uniform magnetic field. Radiofrequency pulses are then applied in a direction perpendicular to the magnetic field. Hydrogen nuclei (protons) absorb this energy and are deflected from their alignment induced by the magnetic field into a higher energy state. As the nuclei return from this stage of excitation to the rest state, a signal is emitted that is detected by a receiver. These signals are then assimilated in analog form into a diagnostic image.

Diagnostic MRI strategies take advantage of the different magnetic relaxation properties of various components within tissues. MRI findings are often described in terms of signal intensity detected at various time intervals after pulse delivery. Such signals, depending on the time at which they were detected after pulse delivery, are described as being either T1- or T2-weighted. A complete discussion of the engineering and physics aspects of MRI is beyond the scope of this book. In general, tissues that are rich in protons (such as water) produce high signal intensity on T2-weighted images and reduced signal intensity on T1-weighted images. Therefore, spinal fluid and edema appear bright on T2-weighted and dark on T1-weighted images. Fat has the opposite characteristics: it has increased signal (appears bright) on T1-weighted images and decreased signal (appears dark) on T2-weighted images. As a result, MRI is particularly suited for neurologic conditions that lead to alterations in the normal makeup of neurologic tissue. One should consult textbooks on MRI for a more detailed discussion of the signal characteristics of various tissue constituents and the effect of different MRI techniques on them.

MRI has various advantages over CT. These are summarized in Table 14-1. Because the proton densities of spinal fluid, bone, and neural tissue differ significantly from one another, each is easily distinguishable on MRI. Calcified structures such as the skull are basically canceled out by MRI; therefore, neural structures lying adjacent to bone (such as the posterior fossa and spinal cord) can be demonstrated in exquisite anatomic detail on MRI without the significant bony artifact sometimes encountered on CT. Like CT, MRI allows multiplanar imaging; in general, this is more readily available on MRI. Unlike CT, MRI does not use ionizing radiation and does not require iodinated agents; both of these factors reduce the relative risk of MRI. In addition, the resolution of MRI is superior to that of CT and allows the identification of smaller lesions, leading to higher sensitivity.

On the other hand, MRI has certain disadvantages. MRI is impractical for most emergency and trauma purposes, primarily because of the longer image acquisition time relative to that of CT. Also, MRI is not as sensitive in the detection of acute hemorrhage. Claustrophobia is a significant problem, also. Some patients actually require anesthesia for MRI to be performed. MRI is contraindicated in patients with pacemakers and other ferromagnetic materials in the body, such as shrapnel, iron filings in the eyes, and many aneurysm clips. Although MRI is nearly equivalent to myelography in many intraspinal diseases, the need for immobility and the slow scan time may make it impractical in patients with suspected spinal cord compression, since many of them have bony pain that prevents them from lying still for a long period. Also, bony anatomy is poorly demonstrated on MRI.

Clinical Applications

There are several clinical indications for MRI, which is becoming the diagnostic study of choice for many diseases. MRI techniques are rapidly expanding as well and should lead to even more favorable diagnostic abilities in the future. The use of MRI in various neurologic disorders is discussed below.

Cerebrovascular disease

MRI is very sensitive in the detection of ischemic lesions and is helpful in delineating the neuroanatomic extent of cerebral infarcts. It is superior to CT in the detection of infarcts in the posterior fossa because of the relative lack of artifacts in this region on MRI relative to CT. Small ischemic lesions (e.g., lacunar infarcts) are readily identifiable on MRI. MRI is also very sensitive in detecting hemosiderin, a substance indicative of previous cerebral hemorrhage. Hemosiderin detection helps identify cavernous arteriovenous malformations, capillary telangiectasias, and old hypertensive hemorrhages and aids in the diagnosis of amyloid angiopathy. MRI is not sensitive in detecting subarachnoid blood, however.

A variety of vascular abnormalities can be detected on MRI. Because moving fluids produce dark low-signal "flow voids" on MRI, the technique is highly sensitive in the detection of patent pial arteriovenous malformations. (It is important to point out here that dural-based arteriovenous malformations are frequently missed on MRI, however.) Likewise, loss of a normal flow void can signify occlusion of a carotid artery, venous sinus, or one of the major cerebral arteries and is an extremely helpful finding. Moderate-to-large cerebral aneurysms are sometimes visible on MRI. However, cerebral angiography is the study of choice in the search for symptomatic cerebral aneurysms. Nevertheless, MRI performed for another purpose on occasion detects an asymptomatic cerebral aneurysm.

Neoplasia

MRI is superior to CT in the detection of low-grade neoplasms, small neoplasms, and cerebral metastatic lesions, primarily because of differences in resolution. The anatomic extent of the tumor and its relationship to eloquent cortex is delineated more precisely by MRI than by CT. These factors are critical for surgical planning in patients with such lesions. Gadolinium contrast-enhanced MRI is also quite helpful in diagnosing leptomeningeal and dural metastatic tumors of the brain and spinal cord. Epidural spinal cord compression can be reliably detected by MRI as well. In addition, MRI is the initial procedure of choice, for the most part, in the diagnosis of primary tumors of the spinal cord. As in myelography, it is helpful to attempt to categorize such spinal lesions by location relative to the spinal cord and dura (see Fig. 14-1).

Epilepsy

MRI is more sensitive than CT in detecting relevant lesions in patients with epilepsy. Low-grade glial neoplasms below the resolution of CT can usually be detected by MRI. Several studies have demonstrated the superiority of MRI in detecting such tumors. MRI is very sensitive as well in the diagnosis of non-neoplastic epileptogenic lesions, such as cavernous arteriovenous malformations, cerebral malformations, contusions, strokes, and hamartomas. MRI has become as integral as electrophysiologic studies in the management of patients with refractory epilepsy.

MRI is particularly helpful in the evaluation of localization-related (partial) epilepsy. Lesional disease is more common in this type of epilepsy than in the primary generalized epilepsies. Proper technique must be observed, however, and the clinician must be certain that the area suspected of giving rise to the seizures is imaged properly. For example, to evaluate the temporal lobes, thin coronal sections are required. Significant lesions in the temporal lobe may be missed if transaxial images alone are used.

MRI is integral in the selection of patients for epilepsy surgery. In fact, the identification of a resectable epileptogenic lesion on MRI imaging is one of the most important factors in choosing patients for epilepsy surgery. The proximity of such epileptogenic lesions to regions of functional cortex can often be determined by MRI as well. A variety of MRI techniques are being developed to expand MRI's role in the preoperative evaluation of patients with epilepsy. Computerized hippocampal volumetry is an example of such a technique. Patients with focal hippocampal atrophy as measured by MRI hippocampal volumetry in general have an excellent outcome after epilepsy surgery.

Demyelinating diseases

MRI is very sensitive in the detection of white matter diseases, such as the leukodystrophies and multiple sclerosis. In multiple sclerosis, demyelinating plaques appear as focal areas of increased signal intensity in the white matter on T2-weighted images. Acute or subacute plaques sometimes become enhanced with gadolinium. Classic MRI abnormalities in multiple sclerosis include elliptoid periventricular white matter lesions oriented perpendicular to the ependyma, "notching" of the corpus callosum on sagittal brain images, and focal areas of increased T2 signal in the middle cerebellar peduncles. Spinal cord plaques are often detectable by MRI as well.

The practitioner is warned not to place too much emphasis on MRI when diagnosing multiple sclerosis, especially if other confirmatory findings are lacking. Small areas of increased T2 signal of uncertain significance are a common finding on MRI and do not always indicate a pathologic condition. Overinterpreting such lesions in a patient with atypical symptoms and no other corroborating findings may lead to an erroneous diagnosis of multiple sclerosis. Likewise, occasional patients with otherwise definite multiple sclerosis lack typical MRI abnormalities.

Inflammatory and infectious conditions
Brain MRI is extremely sensitive in the diagnosis of herpes encephalitis. Herpes encephalitis typically produces an area of increased T2 signal in the medial temporal lobe or lobes. Encephalitis due to other infectious agents does not give rise to this characteristic appearance. MRI is not very useful in the diagnosis or management of bacterial meningitis. MRI can sometimes show gadolinium enhancement of the meninges in chronic tuberculous or fungal meningitis. In cases of chronic meningitis of unknown cause, biopsying such an area of meningeal enhancement may yield a particular etiologic agent. Although cerebral abscesses are usually visible with CT, MRI is more sensitive because of its ability to detect smaller lesions. It is unclear whether MRI offers any significant advantages over CT in the diagnosis of toxoplasmosis or cysticercosis. MRI is also helpful in the diagnosis of transverse myelitis and neurosarcoidosis.

Degenerative diseases
Contrast-enhanced CT is usually adequate in ruling out alternative causes of dementia in patients with suspected Alzheimer's disease. Most degenerative disorders lack reliable specific MRI abnormalities. MRI offers certain advantages over CT in diagnosing dementia, however. For example, hippocampal atrophy, as detected by computerized MRI hippocampal volumetry, correlates with disease severity in patients with Alzheimer's disease. In addition, patients presenting with focal cortical degenerative disorders are best evaluated with MRI so that small yet potentially significant lesions in the area of cortical dysfunction can be excluded. A few degenerative central nervous system disorders, such as Hallervorden-Spatz disease and Huntington's disease, have relatively characteristic MRI abnormalities. MRI is also helpful in the diagnosis of certain dementing disorders of children, such as the leukodystrophies and mitochondrial disorders.

Congenital abnormalities
The anatomy of the neuronal migrational disorders can be exquisitely demonstrated by MRI. Spinal dysraphisms and their associated neurologic tissue anomalies can be precisely evaluated as well. The anatomy in cases of hydrocephalus can be readily demonstrated. In addition, with the use of certain computer software, spinal fluid flow can be measured noninvasively by MRI. This technique may help in the diagnosis of normal pressure hydrocephalus in the future. Arnold-Chiari malformations are readily demonstrated by MRI as well, and MRI is useful in identifying syringomyelia.

MRI ANGIOGRAPHY

MRI angiography (MRA) takes advantage of the normal signal void produced on MRI by moving blood. Computer software available on most modern MRI machines can re-create the additive flow voids detected during MRI scanning into a representative image of the cerebral vasculature. The advantage of a noninvasive means of visualizing the cerebral vasculature is obvious in light of the potential complications of selective cerebral angiography discussed previously. An enormous variety of MRA techniques have been developed, each with its own particular advantages and disadvantages. It is imperative that neuroradiologists involved in the study be aware of the limitations of the particular technique used on their MRI machine before interpreting the results. For example, the maximal intensity projection technique may lead to overestimation of stenosis.

MRA is helpful in the evaluation of occlusive cerebrovascular disease. It is usually reliable in detecting reduced flow within the major extracranial and intracranial cerebral arteries. Smaller intracerebral arterial branches are less reliably visualized by MRA. Some MRA artifacts, however, give the erroneous appearance of a significant stenosis. Therefore, clinical correlation is always advised when interpreting MRA. Intravascular thrombosis can usually be identified by MRA. MRA is extremely sensitive and specific in the diagnosis of venous sinus thrombosis.

MRA has promise in the detection of intracerebral aneurysms but has not yet replaced standard angiography. Aneurysm detectability depends on the location of the aneurysm, its size, and the flow within it. Giant aneurysms and fusiform aneurysms may be poorly visualized by MRA because of the slow flow occurring in them. Giant aneurysms, however, are usually readily detectable on standard MRI. More importantly, aneurysms less than 0.5 cm in diameter are not reliably visualized by current MRA techniques. In two studies, MRA was able to detect only about 50% of aneurysms less than 0.5 cm. Carotid aneurysms, especially those in the carotid siphon, are particularly difficult to detect because of turbulent flow in that region. It is hoped that improved techniques will allow MRA to become a more reliable screening tool for cerebral aneurysms.

Cerebral angiography remains the definitive diagnostic technique in the evaluation of cerebral arteriovenous malformations. Pial arteriovenous malformations can be visualized by MRA but not in as great anatomic detail as by standard cerebral angiography. Dural arteriovenous malformations (dural arteriovenous fistulae) are not reliably demonstrated by MRA but are reliably seen on standard angiography. Cavernous malformations, readily visible on standard MRI, are usually not detectable on MRA because of their extremely slow blood flow. In contrast, MRA can often demonstrate the typical angiographic anatomy of venous malformations, especially when gadolinium is used.

RADIONUCLIDE IMAGING

Radionuclide imaging is beginning to find use in clinical applications. PET (positron emission tomography) and SPECT (single-photon emission computed tomography) allow noninvasive in vivo assessment of a number of properties not assessable with structural imaging, including cerebral blood flow, the function of particular neuroanatomic structures, and the quantity of various neurochemicals and neurotransmitter receptors in particular disease states. The kind of information obtained depends on the radionuclide used. The interested reader is referred to appropriate texts for a detailed discussion of the various radionuclide agents currently available.

Radionuclide imaging has shown potential value in the diagnosis of Alzheimer's disease and Parkinson's disease. PET and SPECT both have localizing value in patients with intractable partial epilepsy. At present, the main limitations of radionuclide imaging are expense, limited availability, and poor anatomic resolution.

FUTURE PERSPECTIVES

The biggest advances in neuroradiology in the near future are likely to be improvement of MRA resolution and accuracy, refinement of a technique referred to as "magnetic resonance spectroscopy" (which allows in vivo assessment of cerebral metabolism), and improvements in radionuclide imaging. Novel MRI sequences are likely to further improve sensitivity and specificity, and new techniques may reduce artifacts that still limit the usefulness of MRI in some areas. It is hoped that techniques can be developed to lessen the image acquisition time for MRI as well. CT technology continues to advance and has led to reduction of troublesome bony artifacts. Neuroradiologic procedures will undoubtedly contribute even more to neurologic clinical practice in the future as these improvements occur.

Chapter 15

Clinical Neurophysiology

Diagnostic studies of the nervous system are broadly subdivided into biochemical, immunologic, imaging, and physiologic testing. Physiologic testing of the nervous system defines alterations in function that may not be visualized by imaging procedures. Although physiologic testing may take a variety of forms, electrophysiologic studies are the most widely applied for assessing function of the central and peripheral nervous systems, particularly of the cortex and the motor and sensory systems. These studies make up the area of clinical neurophysiology.

The major areas of study in clinical neurophysiology are electroencephalography (EEG; spontaneous activity of the brain recorded from the scalp), electromyography (EMG; spontaneous and voluntary activity recorded from muscle), nerve conduction studies (stimulus-induced responses recorded from peripheral nerve and muscle), and evoked potentials (stimulus-induced responses from the sensory systems). Each of these will be described separately in the following sections.

SECTION I: ELECTROENCEPHALOGRAPHY

The electroencephalogram (EEG) may be viewed as an extension of the neurologic examination in the evaluation of aspects of cerebral function not always accessible to conventional clinical testing. The EEG, in use at the Mayo Clinic since 1936, basically involves recording of the spontaneous electric activity of the brain from the scalp and activity elicited by activation procedures. The test has the advantage of being safe and relatively painless, and it can be undertaken on patients of any age. It is most helpful when the clinician understands the proper indications for using it and is aware of its limitations.

Recording Procedure and Preparation of Patient

For the standard recording, small metal disks containing conductive gel are attached to the scalp and earlobes by means of collodion and according to a system of measurements (Fig. 15-1). Each disk forms the terminal end of a

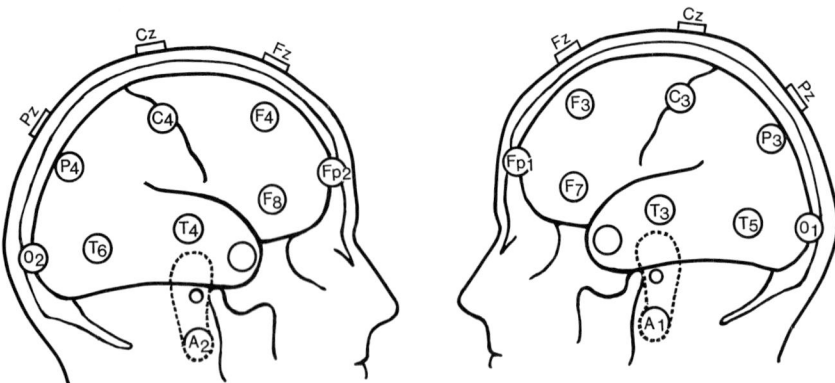

Figure 15-1
Placement of routine electrodes according to the International 10-20 System.

flexible wire (lead), and each lead is connected separately to the recording instrument (electroencephalograph). The test lasts 30 to 60 minutes during wakefulness, longer if recording during sleep is also necessary.

The amplitude of EEG activity recorded by the scalp electrodes is generally about 10 to 60 μV and needs to be amplified about 1 million times before a tracing can be made on a moving sheet of paper. Usually, the EEG is sampled simultaneously from 16 or 21 pairs of electrodes (derivations) in selected combinations (montages).

The activity from each derivation requires a separate channel of amplification and is recorded on paper or digitally. Because of the great amplification necessary to view the EEG activity, the instruments used for recording are extremely sensitive and require expertly trained technical personnel to operate them. Moreover, many kinds of extraneous electric signals can contaminate the tracing and render it illegible unless they can be identified and eliminated. Interference from other electric apparatuses often causes difficulties when an attempt is made to record the EEG at the patient's bedside, particularly in intensive care units. Thus, assurance of reliable results is generally greater if the recording can be made in the EEG laboratory. Even in the laboratory, however, artifacts in the recording are commonly generated by the patient from movement of the head, body, eyes, or tongue and from muscular contraction. Satisfactory recordings may be difficult to obtain, therefore, from patients who are uncooperative or anxious or who have severe movement disorders. In these instances, sedation may be necessary. However, reassuring the patient in advance about the innocuous nature of the EEG test helps to allay anxiety and facilitates the recording.

Ordinarily, little advance preparation of the patient is needed. The use of greasy hair cream or metallic hair spray should be avoided before the test; mealtimes need not be altered. A few patients, however, may need to forgo sleep and meals for 24 hours for purposes of EEG activation.

Special Electrodes

Scalp leads, in addition to those in the standard positions of the International 10-20 System, are placed in regions selected for the individual patient to help localize an abnormality or to add more nearly complete coverage of the scalp surface when an abnormal discharge has not been discovered.

Nasopharyngeal leads are sometimes added to help assess activity originating from the basal surface of the frontotemporal regions. The main disadvantages of the nasopharyngeal leads, however, are the considerable number of artifacts often associated with their use and the discomfort they cause in some patients.

In certain patients for whom surgical treatment of seizures is contemplated, specially designed electrodes are implanted within the substance of the brain in advance for recording from selected regions (depth EEG), or a grid of electrodes is implanted subdurally. Also, in patients undergoing surgery for seizures, special leads are used for recording from the pial surface of the exposed brain to help delineate the epileptogenic region (electrocorticography).

Normal EEG Activity

The EEG is a composite of several different types of activity, each of which is characterized by the factors of frequency, amplitude, quantity, morphology, reactivity, variability, topography, and phase relationships. The frequency bands of EEG activity are known as the delta (less than 4 Hz), theta (4 to 7 Hz), alpha (8 to 13 Hz), and beta (13 Hz or more) bands. The most characteristic feature of the normal EEG of an adult during relaxed wakefulness is the alpha rhythm, which occurs over the posterior regions of the head while the eyes are closed (Fig. 15-2).

Judgments of normality for the various types of activity depend greatly on the age and state of alertness of the subject at the time of the recording. Complex changes in EEG patterns occur throughout life, although in most persons the longest period with the least variability usually occurs between the ages of 20 and 60 years. Appreciable changes from the patterns during wakefulness occur at all ages with drowsiness and the different stages of sleep (Fig. 15-3).

During these same ages, and particularly in childhood, rhythms that the EEG comprises differ greatly among normal subjects. Therefore, for each person, an important assessment is the degree of similarity (symmetry) of rhythms recorded from the two sides of the head (Fig. 15-4). This principle is no different from the one used in the practice of clinical neurology, placing great emphasis on the comparison between the two sides of the body in the same patient for evaluating alternate motion

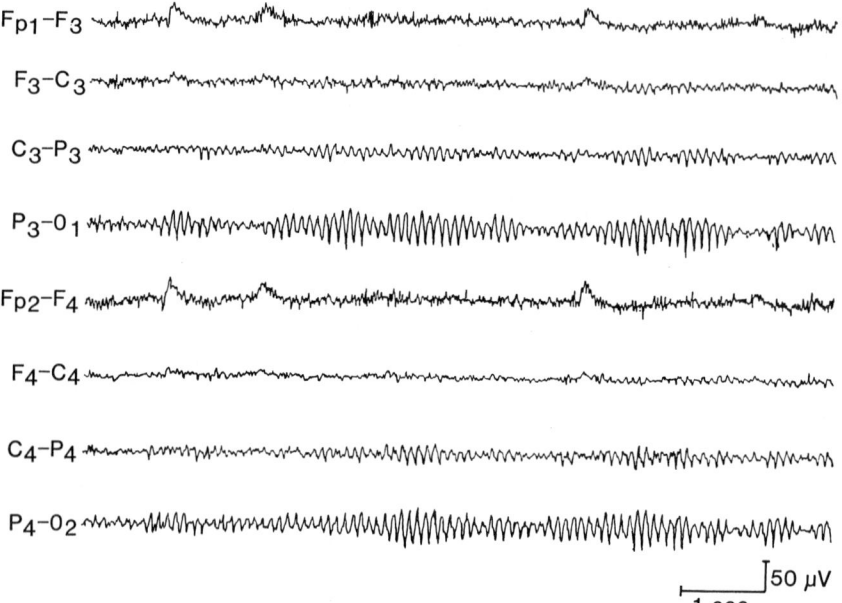

Figure 15-2
Normal EEG from adult patient during wakefulness with eyes closed. Alpha rhythm is maximal over the occipital regions (channels 4 and 8).

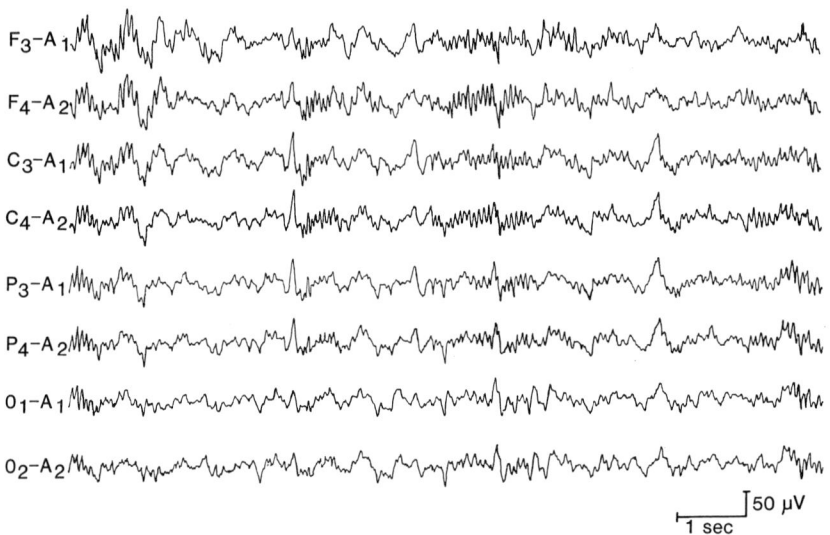

Figure 15-3
Normal EEG of 15-year-old patient during sleep (stage 2) showing sleep spindles and V waves (maximal in upper four channels) and diffuse slow waves.

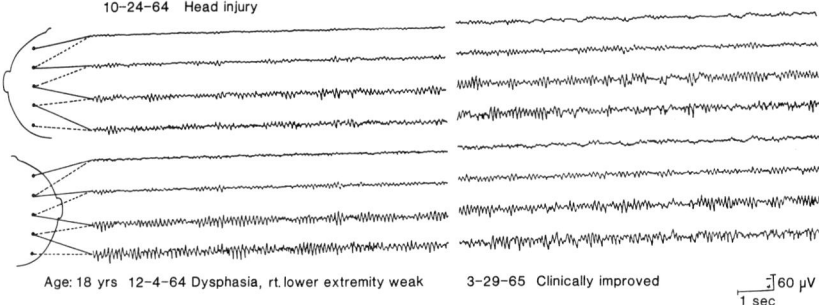

Figure 15-4
Left tracing (Dec. 4, 1964) shows asymmetrical alpha rhythms, attenuated on left side after head injury. *Right tracing* (Mar. 29, 1965) shows symmetrical alpha rhythms later during recovery.

rate, size of limbs, sensation, and reflexes, to mention only a few examples.

Abnormal EEG Activity
Classification

Thorough knowledge of the range of normal EEG activity is essential for recognition and visual analysis of abnormal patterns of activity constituting a departure from an expected pattern at a given age and level of alertness. Some EEGs may be judged abnormal because they contain aberrant frequencies. Other types of activity are abnormal because of distinctive and deviant wave configurations (Fig. 15-5). Furthermore, EEG abnormalities may vary in magnitude or degree of severity (grade), in distribution (location) over the surface of the head, and in their dynamic physiologic properties (type) (Fig. 15-6).

A classification system of EEG activity, based on these principles, has been used at the Mayo Clinic for many years and is outlined in Table 15-1. It has proved useful for the following reasons: (1) it provides an abbreviated summary of the EEG, which is convenient for conveying the results to clinicians; (2) it provides a means of dividing EEGs into major groups according to important electrophysiologic criteria for subsequent retrieval and review; (3) it provides a means of helping to achieve uniformity in the assessment of records by several different interpreters; and (4) it provides a means for quickly checking the evaluations of an EEG by students, technicians, or residents.

The Mayo EEG Classification System is based on the descriptive variables already mentioned. The categories of abnormality (Asymmetry, Dysrhythmia, Delta, and so forth) are classified in three parts: grade of severity, location over the head, and type. It will be seen from Table 15-1 that a general distinction exists between the two major classes of abnormal

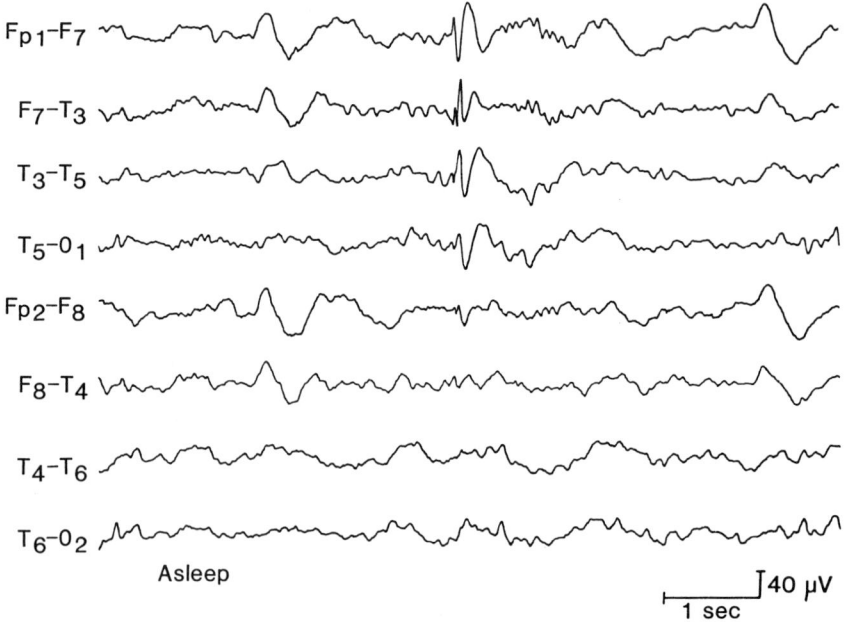

Figure 15-5
Focal spike discharge in left temporal lobe *(upper four tracings).*

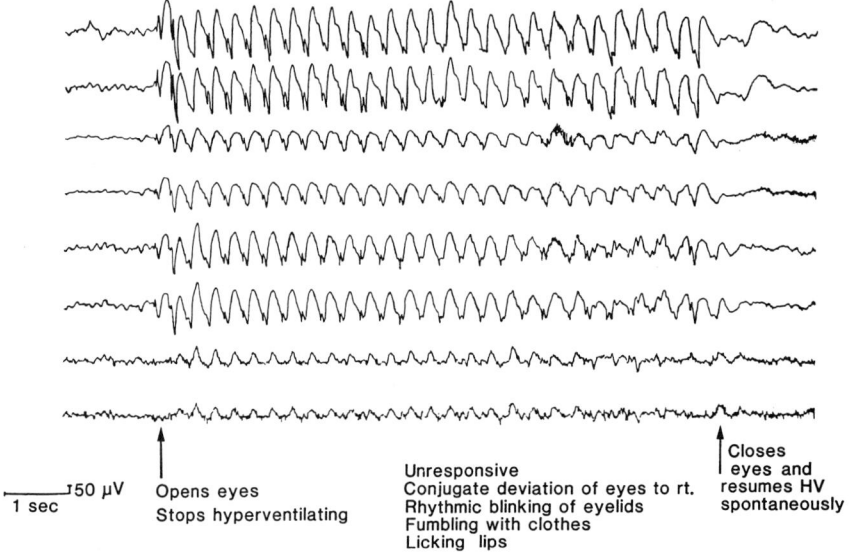

Figure 15-6
EEG of 17-year-old patient during hyperventilation *(HV)*, showing activation of diffuse 3-Hz spike-wave paroxysm and "absence" seizure. Derivations from above downward: (1) F_{p1}-A_1, (2) F_{p2}-A_2, (3) T_3-A_1, (4) T_4-A_2, (5) C_3-A_1, (6) C_4-A_2, (7) O_1-A_1, (8) O_2-A_2.

Table 15-1 Mayo Classification System of EEG Abnormalities

	Classification of Abnormality		
Category	Grade	Location	Type
Asymmetry (consistent)	I (25%–50%) II (50%–75%) III (>75%)	Regional or hemispheric	Amplitude, frequency, or reactivity (awake or asleep)
Dysrhythmia*	I (<30 µV) II (30–60 µV)	Focal, bilateral, or diffuse Same	Nonspecific Mainly nonspecific; also minor projected or minor photic activation
	III (>60 µV)	Same	Mainly distinctive waveforms (type specified); also major projected, photicactivation, recorded seizures, and nonspecific
Delta*	I (<30 µV) II (30–60 µV) III (>60 µV)	Focal, bilateral, or diffuse	Polymorphic or quasi-rhythmic
Suppression	I partial II	Localized or diffuse	Abnormal attenuation
	III complete	Diffuse	Electrocerebral inactivity

See text for definitions.

activity, "Dysrhythmia" and "Delta." These terms were chosen arbitrarily to designate briefly the difference between abnormal patterns that are pliable, that is, those capable of changing from time to time either spontaneously or by external stimuli (Dysrhythmia) and those that are fixed and persistent throughout the recording (Delta). The specific definitions for Dysrhythmia and Delta in this classification system merit emphasis, since the term "dysrhythmia" has been used in many different ways in EEG, and the term "delta" is used most widely for a particular frequency band (see earlier discussion). Nevertheless, these two terms have been retained because of the familiarity generated by long usage at this institution.

Activation procedures

Activation procedures are used to elicit abnormal EEG activity, which may not be manifested spontaneously. Most of these procedures, however, also elicit patterns of activity in EEGs of normal subjects that differ from the patterns present spontaneously during relaxed wakefulness and that need to be differentiated carefully from patterns having definite pathologic significance.

Hyperventilation for 3 minutes is used routinely for most patients able to cooperate well enough to carry out the procedure. It is most effective for activating diffuse spike-wave paroxysms in the EEG and generalized nonconvulsive absence seizures (petit mal) (see Fig. 15-6). Hyperventilation also may activate focal abnormalities and partial seizures less frequently. The procedure is not carried out if the patient has had a recent subarachnoid hemorrhage, cardiac infarction, or severe pulmonary disease or if the referring physician indicates some other medical contraindication by checking the "omit hyperventilation" item on the referral form.

Another activation procedure that is used routinely is photic stimulation. Repetitive brief flashes of light are generated by an electronic apparatus and are delivered at frequencies ranging from 1 to 30 Hz. This procedure evokes responses over the occipitoparietal regions in most subjects (photic driving or photoentrainment). The most frequent abnormal response to photic stimulation is the diffuse paroxysmal discharge composed of spike-wave complexes—the "photoparoxysmal" response (previously called "photoconvulsive")—which may be accompanied by minor seizures manifested by "absence" or myoclonus. Another response that may be associated with myoclonus of the facial muscles is called the "photomyogenic" response (previously called "photomyoclonic"). This response is not accompanied by abnormal paroxysmal EEG activity, and it occurs more frequently in asymptomatic subjects and nonepileptic patients than does the photoparoxysmal response.

As part of the standard EEG, the patient is also asked to scan a standard picture to elicit normal "lambda waves" that arise from the occipitoparietal regions and to scan a standard geometric pattern to elicit paroxysmal discharges that may occur in some epileptic patients who have pattern-sensitivity.

An activation technique used frequently, but not routinely, is recording the EEG during sleep. This procedure is most useful for recording paroxysmal abnormalities in patients who have epileptic seizures. Sleep may activate generalized and focal epileptogenic EEG abnormalities. The patient should be deprived of sleep the night before the test because sleep in the laboratory is thereby facilitated and because sleep deprivation itself sometimes causes activation. Some patients, however, have difficulty falling asleep during the daytime in the strange environment of the laboratory without the aid of a hypnotic medicament. For this purpose, a substance such as chloral hydrate may be administered orally if the referring physician has indicated approval.

The EEG Report

The standard EEG report consists of three parts: (1) the abbreviated diagnostic classification, (2) a detailed narrative description of the contents of the tracing, and (3) an interpretation of the EEG findings in light of the individual clinical problem. The more specific the question asked by the referring clinician when requesting an EEG, the more specific and pertinent the interpretation of the individual findings by the electroencephalographer can be and, therefore, the greater the contribution to the solution of the individual diagnostic problem.

It has been customary to indicate in red on the diagram of the head on the EEG report sheet the approximate location of focal abnormalities of the Delta category. This marking has emphasized the expected reliability of the findings and has given the clinician a rapid indication of the location and extent of the lesion, which, it should be noted, may not coincide exactly with the red area in the diagram. The abnormal EEG activity arises from injured but viable cortical neurons and not from the pathologic lesion itself. Furthermore, no distinction of the pathologic type of lesion is intended, since a red diagram may represent a neoplasm, infarct, abscess, hemorrhage, or other localized process.

EEG and Clinical Correlates
General principles

Before proceeding with a discussion of the applications of the EEG for clinical diagnosis, let us return to the concept of abnormalities mentioned previously. Assessing the clinical significance of these EEG abnormalities requires considerable judgment. For example, the general population shows a 10% to 15% incidence of diffuse Dysrhythmia, grade I, and 2% to 3% incidence of diffuse Dysrhythmia, grade II. Although these types of nonspecific EEG abnormalities may occur as so-called constitutional variations in asymptomatic persons, indistinguishable changes also may be produced by many different diseases. Furthermore, merely because the EEG abnormality is termed "nonspecific," it should not be construed as being insignificant, since, in some circumstances, it may be of great clinical importance. Any disease process afflicting cerebral neuronal function is capable of producing nonspecific EEG abnormalities.

Basic distinctions, however, need to be drawn between diseases affecting primarily localized areas of the brain and those that affect the brain more diffusely. All types of localized EEG abnormalities are highly significant, in general, since they occur only rarely in asymptomatic persons. Nevertheless, a focal abnormality in one EEG cannot distinguish the pathologic type of lesion, and, therefore, a single EEG should not be used in attempting to differentiate a neoplasm from an infarct or an abscess.

The EEG is a dynamic physiologic process involving dimensions of time and space conjointly (spatial-temporal biodynamics). Viewing the EEG in this way helps one to understand the clinical and pathologic correlations more clearly and to apply the EEG more appropriately for diagnosis.

With regard to the spatial dimension, the *extent* of the lesion is of fundamental importance. A lesion may not produce an EEG abnormality until it attains sufficient size to be detected by standard scalp recording. The *density* of the lesion, or the concentration of its effects on adjacent cortex, also plays a role in the production of EEG changes. Local pressure from a concentrated mass generally produces focal EEG abnormality more readily than a neoplasm, even a highly malignant one, which infiltrates among neurons more diffusely. Another important factor is the *location* of the lesion. In conventional scalp recording, potential fluctuations constituting the EEG are derived from neuronal activity of only the most superficial cortical layers over the convexity of the cerebral hemispheres, and disturbance of deeply situated structures affects the EEG only indirectly. Thus, a brain tumor located superficially creates a focal electric disturbance readily, whereas a tumor of similar size situated deeply seldom does. Tumors situated near the base of the skull or in the posterior fossa generally produce little or no EEG abnormality unless they encroach on the midline ventricular axis (third ventricle, aqueduct, fourth ventricle), obstruct the flow of cerebrospinal fluid, and cause increased intraventricular pressure. In this way, pressure on diencephalic nuclei that have widespread connections to the cortex can produce bilaterally synchronous EEG abnormalities (projected rhythms) distant to the site of the lesion.

In the temporal dimension, one needs to consider the cross section in time at which the EEG is obtained during the *evolution* of the lesion. An EEG recorded at a very early stage in the development of a neoplasm may be normal, but a focal abnormality may be present in a tracing obtained at a later time. Sequential recordings from the same patient, therefore, are often helpful diagnostically. Multiple EEGs also increase the likelihood of recording intermittent abnormalities that occur infrequently. The type and magnitude of EEG abnormality also depend on the age of the patient at the time a disease occurs. Some types of EEG abnormality are expressed only during a particular stage of *maturation.* Finally, the *rate of development* of the lesion and the *balance* between destructive and reparative forces influence the EEG activity. For example, a rapidly expanding neoplasm typically produces very slow polymorphic and highly persistent delta activity (Fig. 15-7), in contrast to a slowly growing tumor, which may produce, as the only EEG manifestation, a focal spike indistinguishable from the effects sometimes caused by scar formation (Fig. 15-8).

Examples of diagnostic applications

Some examples of the usefulness of the EEG for clinical diagnosis will be considered according to major disease categories.

Neoplastic diseases

The EEG can provide important information for diagnosis of brain tumor by demonstrating a focal abnormality when clinical suspicion has been low. This situation may occur when the symptoms are vague or nonspecific and when the results of neurologic examinations are normal or minimally abnormal. Most often, these circumstances are encountered with neoplasms arising in the frontal or temporal lobes (see Fig. 15-8).

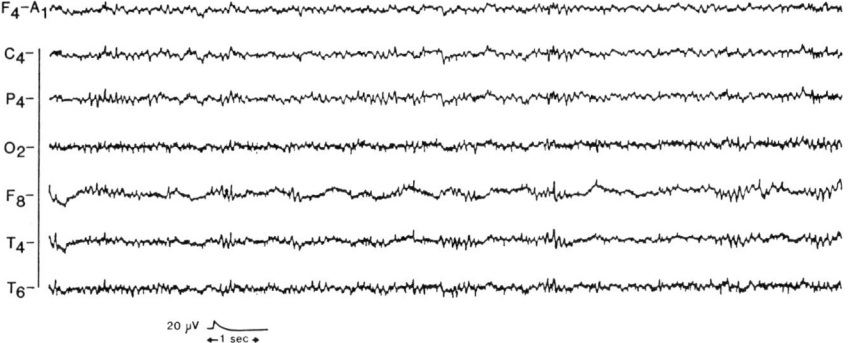

Figure 15-7
Focal polymorphic delta activity, maximal in electrode F_8, recorded from 48-year-old patient with brain tumor in right middle fossa.

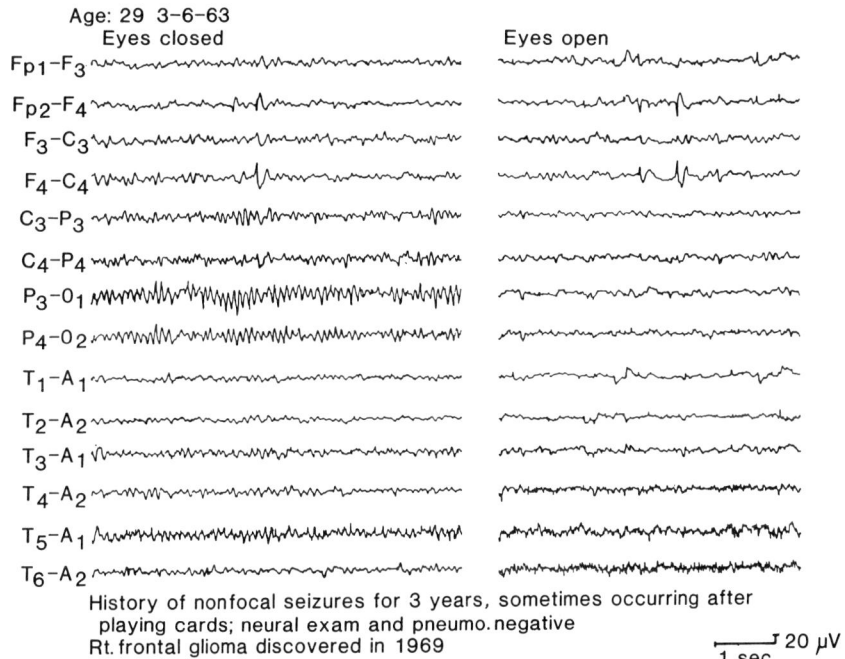

Figure 15-8
Focal sharp waves (spikes) recorded from right frontal region (electrode F_4) as the first EEG manifestation of infiltrating neoplasm in right frontal lobe.

Sequential recordings may help to establish the progressive nature of a lesion. When early tracings are normal or when they are abnormal but nonfocal, the subsequent appearance of focal abnormality or an increasingly severe focal disturbance strongly suggests neoplasm.

Sometimes a single recording may suggest the likelihood of an expanding lesion if there is a definite discrepancy between the nature of the EEG findings and the time course of the disease. For example, the conjunction of focal and bilateral projected abnormalities recorded on the EEG of a patient with a chronic illness simulating a degenerative type of disease should lead one to be highly suspicious of intracranial tumor (Fig. 15-9).

The EEG may help in distinguishing between a supratentorial and an infratentorial location of a tumor when clinical manifestations may make the distinction difficult. Symptoms of a lesion involving the cerebellum, for instance, can resemble closely those of a lesion situated in a frontal lobe, whereas the EEG manifestations from lesions in these two locations are almost always different (normal or nonfocal Dysrhythmia in the former and focal frontal Delta in the latter).

After a surgical procedure for supratentorial brain tumor, reliance is usually placed on imaging techniques for assessing the postoperative course of the patient and the possible recurrence of the tumor. Nevertheless, the EEG can be a valuable adjunct, since it may detect pathophysiologic changes before anatomic alterations appear and may alert the clinician to the appearance of epileptogenic discharges. For this purpose, it is important to obtain a tracing shortly after operation to serve as a baseline for comparison with subsequent EEGs, since EEG alterations usually occur from the surgical procedure and resultant skull defect (in-

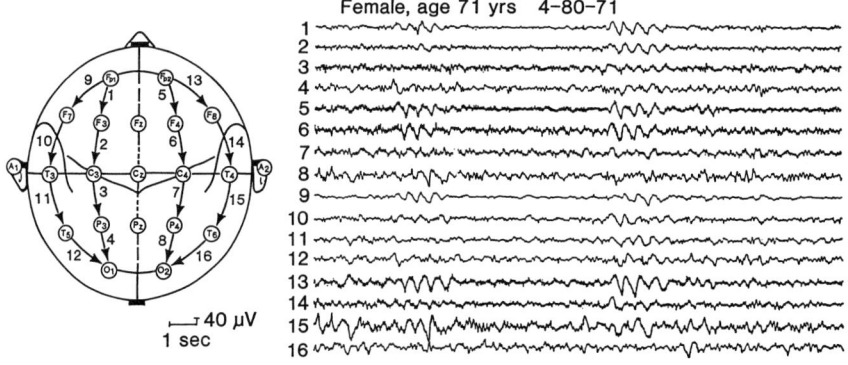

Figure 15-9
Persistent focal polymorphic delta activity maximal in right posterotemporal region (channels 15- and 16), and intermittent bursts of rhythmic delta activity (projected rhythms) distributed diffusely.

creased amplitude of activity from leads overlying the craniotomy site) and render the postoperative EEG different from the preoperative record. EEGs also are helpful in the assessment of the effects of radiation or chemotherapy that may be used for treatment of an intracranial malignancy (Fig. 15-10).

By the time of operation, the EEG is abnormal in approximately 96% of patients with supratentorial primary or metastatic brain tumors, and the abnormality is helpful for localization in approximately 87% of primary brain tumors and in 81% of metastatic neoplasms. On the other hand, EEGs are normal in approximately 45% of tumors situated in the cerebellopontine angle and in 18% of those situated in the midline of the posterior fossa, in a cerebellar hemisphere, or in the third ventricle.

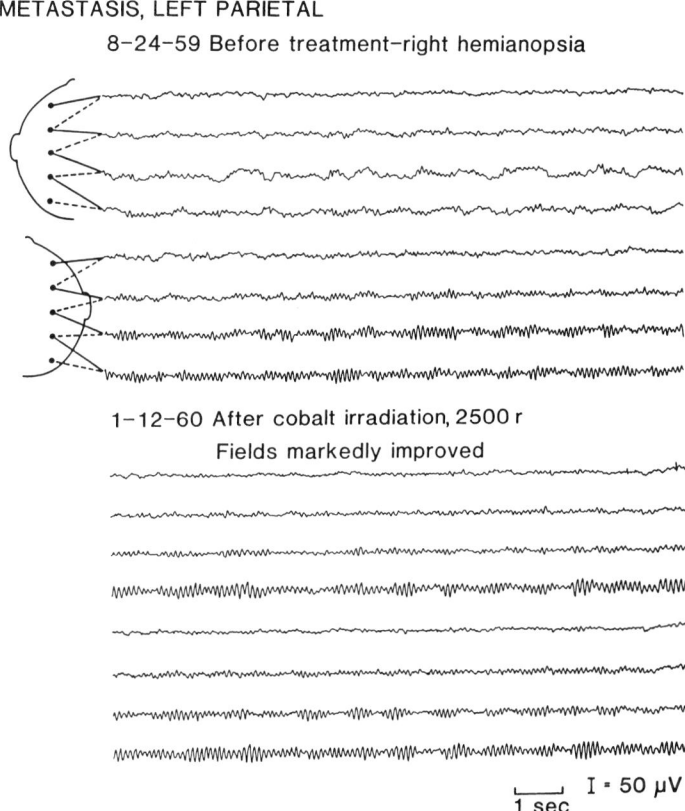

Figure 15-10
EEG from a 21-year-old patient with metastatic brain tumor (Ewing's tumor) showing focal polymorphic delta activity and attenuation of alpha activity in left parieto-occipital region (channels 3 and 4, *upper segment*). After cobalt irradiation *(lower segment)*, abnormal delta activity is no longer present and is replaced by normal alpha rhythm.

Vascular diseases

The general principles for the use of the EEG for diagnosis and localization also apply to cerebrovascular lesions. Intracerebral hemorrhage produces EEG abnormalities similar to those caused by brain tumor. A large and acute cerebral infarction often produces similar manifestations (focal Delta and bilateral projected Dysrhythmia), frequently before anatomic changes can be demonstrated by imaging techniques; however, in contrast to the abnormalities caused by a neoplasm, abnormalities shown by sequential EEGs during the resolution of an infarction usually diminish progressively (Fig. 15-11). Within a few hours or days after an acute cortical infarction, the EEG sometimes contains periodic lateralized epileptiform discharges (see Fig. 15-11), and these are frequently associated with clinical seizures. However, these discharges also result from many other types of lesions and should not be considered pathognomonic for cerebral infarction.

One should recognize that a small infarct involving the internal capsule usually produces little EEG abnormality, even when it is acute and when it is accompanied by severe motor paralysis. This circumstance should not be surprising, however, if one considers that severe neurologic deficits can be caused by a minute lacunar lesion in this region and that the EEG shows abnormality infrequently with a small lesion situated deep to the cerebral surface.

The EEG may be helpful diagnostically in comatose patients who have cerebrovascular lesions involving the brain stem. Infarction or hemorrhage involving the central core of the brain stem in the region of the pontomesencephalic junction can be associated with an EEG containing predominant alpha activity and resembling the EEG of normal wakefulness (alpha pattern coma) but lacking normal reactivity.

The EEG almost always is normal after a transient ischemic attack of primary cerebrovascular origin. Therefore, a focal Delta abnormality recorded between attacks indicates a more permanent structural lesion as the cause of the symptoms, and a focal spike discharge suggests epileptic seizures rather than transient ischemic attacks.

The EEG is usually normal between attacks of vasovagal syncope, and the changes during the attacks are almost always distinguishable from the EEG abnormalities recorded during epileptic seizures.

Traumatic and anoxic conditions

The EEG is usually abnormal when recorded soon after a head injury that is severe enough to cause more than momentary unconsciousness and that is associated with significant retrograde amnesia or neurologic deficit. Acute EEG abnormalities may be focal or diffuse and may vary considerably in magnitude. Abnormalities may be recorded more frequently from children than from adults after rather minor head injury. Mild nonfocal EEG abnormalities recorded after a head injury are not

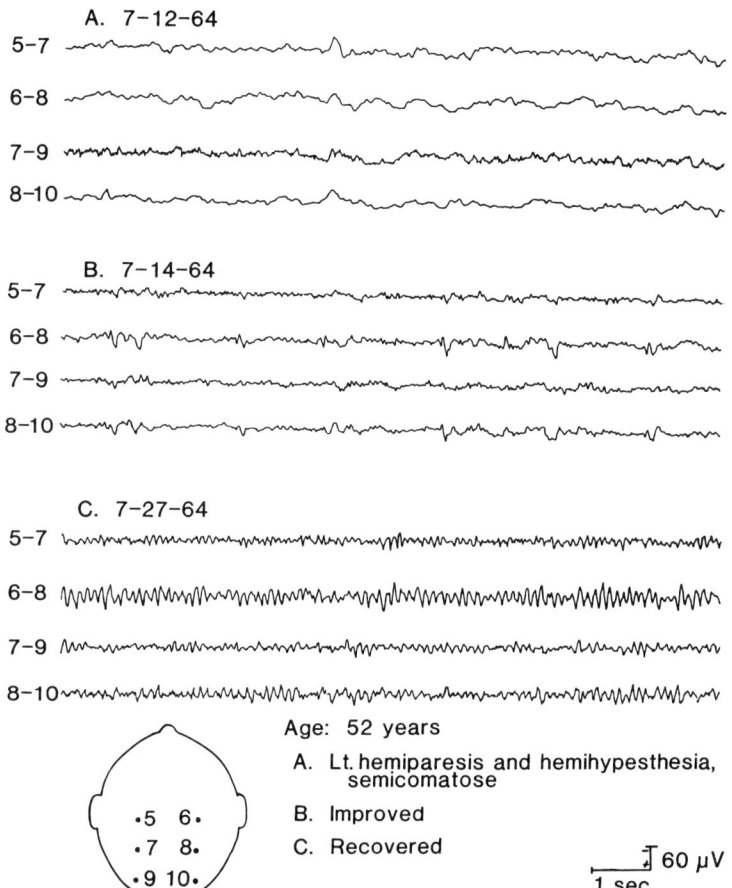

Figure 15-11
EEG samples from patient during recovery from stroke involving right hemisphere. **A,** First EEG shows focal delta activity in right parieto-occipital region (channels 2 and 4). **B,** Second EEG made 2 days later shows periodic lateralized epileptiform discharges in same area. **C,** Third EEG made 2 weeks later when the patient had recovered no longer shows abnormal activity, and alpha rhythms have appeared but are enhanced on the right side. Electrode designations: 5, left anterior parietal; 6, right anterior parietal; 7, left posterior parietal; 8, right posterior parietal; 9, left occipital; 10, right occipital.

necessarily related to the trauma, and well-formed diffuse spike-wave complexes usually are unrelated. Interpretation of many types of EEG abnormalities is difficult because of the usual lack of a pretraumatic tracing for comparison.

In contrast to the usefulness of the computed tomography scan, the EEG is most helpful when sequential recordings can be obtained. A relationship between EEG abnormalities and head trauma can be established more confidently if the abnormalities gradually decrease parallel to clinical recovery. Frequently, however, the EEG and clinical improvement do not occur concomitantly, and new EEG abnormalities, such as focal spikes, may appear long after head trauma as manifestations of chronic scar formation (Fig. 15-12). An increasingly severe focal abnormality after head injury indicates an expanding lesion, such as an intracranial hematoma.

The EEG does not provide reliable data for distinguishing between subdural hematoma and cortical contusion on the basis of abnormalities manifested within about 2 weeks after head trauma.

Although the EEG is seldom reliable for clinical prognosis after head injury, it is frequently helpful in one circumstance. In a patient rendered comatose by head trauma or by disease, the EEG may exhibit patterns that are usually recorded during normal sleep (spindle-coma) and cyclic sleep changes in prolonged recordings made overnight. Frequently, the sleep patterns can be reversed to waking patterns by administration of methylphenidate hydrochloride (Ritalin), and the level of alertness is also greatly improved. These sleep patterns and cyclic changes usually indicate a favorable prognosis for clinical recovery.

Cerebral hypoxia produces diffuse nonspecific slow-wave abnormalities that may be reversible. More severe hypoxia may cause residual EEG abnormalities that may be paroxysmal and may be associated with

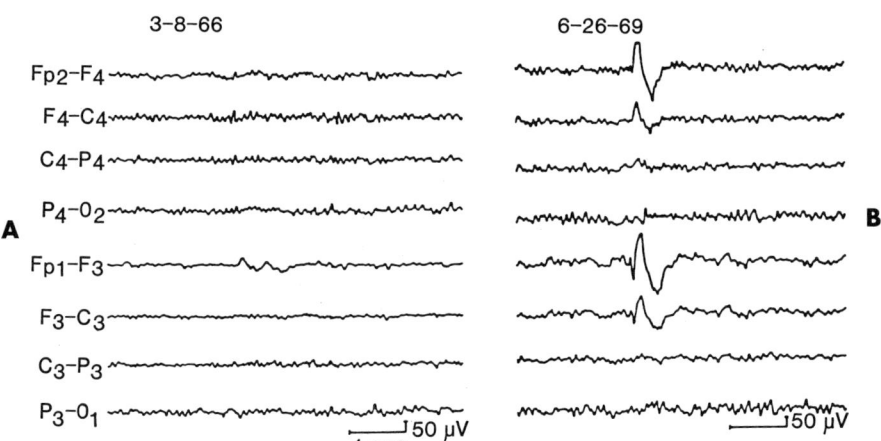

Figure 15-12
EEGs from 17-year-old patient who sustained a head injury in November 1965; seizures developed subsequently. **A**, First EEG shows minimal focal slow-wave abnormality in left frontal area (F_{p1}) and attenuation of background rhythms over left hemisphere. **B**, Second EEG made 3 years later shows recovery of background activity on left side and development of epileptiform abnormality (sharp wave) in left frontal region (F_{p1} and F_3) that is transmitted to the right side (F_{p2}, F_4) secondarily.

myoclonus. Profound and prolonged anoxia, whether due primarily to cardiovascular disease or secondarily to severe neurologic disease, causes electrocerebral inactivity (suppression, complete and generalized) associated with irreversible coma or death.

Inflammatory diseases
Most inflammatory diseases of the central nervous system that affect the EEG produce predominantly diffuse and nonspecific slow-wave activity, regardless of the type of causative agent. Establishing significant cerebral electric disturbance may be important, however, since mental symptoms frequently constitute prominent features of these conditions, and sometimes, early in the course of the disease or in the chronic phase, there may be doubt as to whether the symptoms are primarily emotional or whether they have an organic basis. When the dominant EEG abnormality is focal, an abscess should be suspected. Herpes simplex encephalitis, however, may cause focal slow-wave EEG abnormalities and periodic lateralized epileptiform discharges. Occasionally, the EEG can suggest a specific diagnosis, for example, from the characteristic stereotyped periodic complexes that occur with subacute sclerosing panencephalitis.

Jakob-Creutzfeldt disease is another condition in which periodic diffuse EEG complexes can be highly important for diagnosis, especially if they are associated with myoclonus. In contrast to the periodic complexes that occur with subacute sclerosing panencephalitis, however, typically the duration of each complex is shorter and the interval between complexes is shorter.

Toxic, metabolic, degenerative diseases
EEG abnormalities resulting from most toxic, metabolic, or degenerative diseases consist of diffuse slow waves with different degrees of severity, and generally these changes do not have distinctive features. Since many of these disorders produce cerebral dysfunction, the EEG can be useful for documenting organic disease when the origin of the symptoms is doubtful clinically.

In some circumstances, the EEG can provide helpful diagnostic information for the type of disorder. Some hypnotic or ataractic medicaments produce an increase in beta activity and, after withdrawal, a photoparoxysmal response to photic stimulation. These drugs, taken in large enough doses to cause semicoma or coma, produce a characteristic pattern in the EEG that can indicate a toxic origin of the coma with a high degree of reliability (Fig. 15-13).

Another distinctive diagnostic syndrome occurs during an intermediate stage of hepatic encephalopathy. The typical syndrome comprises clinical obtundation and the following features in the EEG: (1) reduction or loss of normal background rhythms and (2) broad triphasic waves that are bilaterally symmetrical and synchronous and have frontal predominance, positive polarity of the intermediate phase, and a time lag

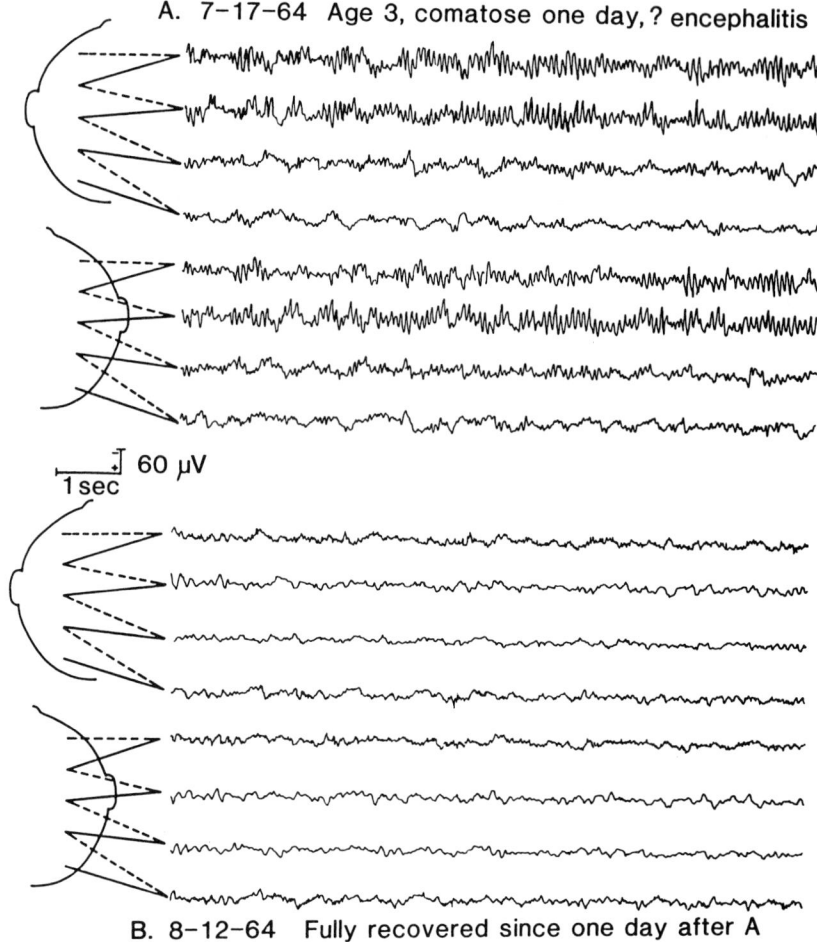

Figure 15-13
A, EEG from 3-year-old comatose patient with barbiturate intoxication. Note continuous 12-Hz rhythm in leads over the frontal regions (channels 1, 2, 5, and 6) and diffuse delta activity. B, EEG from same patient after recovery, showing normal activity for the patient's age.

between anterior and posterior regions of the head (Fig. 15-14). If all these criteria are fulfilled, the EEG is highly suspicious for hepatic encephalopathy. It should be emphasized, however, that not all triphasic waves in the EEG are caused by hepatic disease and that some patients with hepatic encephalopathy do not necessarily exhibit the typical electroclinical syndrome.

Patients with uremia, uremic patients undergoing hemodialysis, and

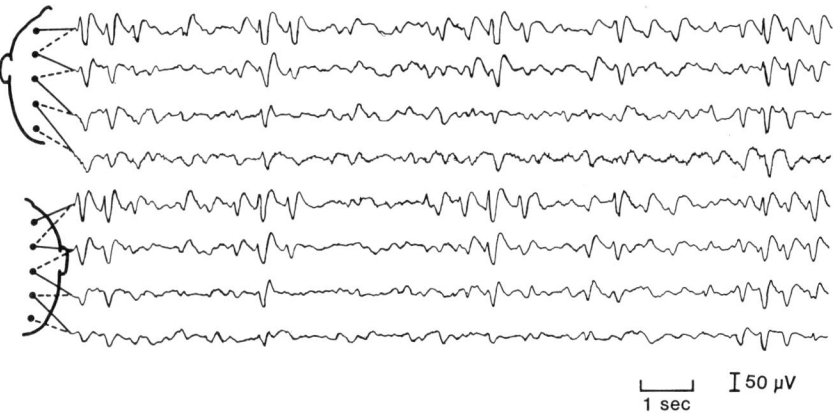

Figure 15-14
EEG from 69-year-old patient with hepatic encephalopathy. Note absence of alpha activity and the presence of diffuse slow waves and triphasic waves maximal in frontal regions (channels 1 and 5).

patients with hyponatremia may exhibit paroxysmal spike-wave discharges and photoparoxysmal responses in addition to the more common slow-wave abnormalities. Patients with hypoglycemia frequently have an exaggerated slow-wave response to hyperventilation.

No attempt will be made to cover all the diverse EEG changes that can occur with the many different types of congenital cerebral malformations or the degenerative disorders that occur at later stages of life.

Convulsive disorders
Seizures are only symptoms and can be caused by many different disorders, although frequently their cause cannot be determined. Nevertheless, one of the most important uses of the EEG is for diagnosis of epileptic attacks.

Some types of interictal EEG patterns are termed "epileptiform," since they have a distinctive morphology and appear in a high proportion of EEGs from patients with seizures but rarely in records from asymptomatic persons. Examples of such patterns include certain types of sporadic spikes, sharp waves, and spike-and-slow-wave complexes (see Fig. 15-5, 15-6, 15-8, 15-11, and 15-12). These EEG patterns allow prediction of clinical convulsive disorder with a high degree of probability. Not all types of spikes or spike-wave patterns, however, have similar implications. The 14- and 6-Hz positive spike bursts, the so-called small sharp spikes or benign sporadic sleep spikes, "wicket spikes" (wicket waves), the "psychomotor variant" pattern (rhythmic temporal theta of drowsiness), and the 6-Hz spike-wave complexes have no definite significance for diagnosis of epilepsy. Furthermore, the significance of some EEG discharges depends on the age of the patient at the time of recording. Some types of spike activity may appear transiently during childhood, especially in the occipital and central areas, without overt clinical manifestations, whereas similar activity in a record from an adult would have a higher correlation with clinical seizures.

The relationship between particular symptoms and interictal EEG abnormalities, therefore, is not absolute but rather is an association of varied probability, dependent on the nature of the symptoms and the character of the different EEG patterns. The most convincing proof of the epileptic nature of particular clinical symptoms or behavior is obtained if they occur during the EEG recording at the same time as a definite ictal EEG abnormality. This may be the only way to establish the nature of the disorder if the patient cannot or will not relate symptoms adequately, if an attack has not been observed, or if the attack seems atypical.

The absence of epileptiform discharge in a single EEG does not exclude a convulsive disorder. It should not be surprising that a normal EEG can be recorded from a patient who has had definite clinical seizures, since seizures are by their very nature transient events and may leave no clue to their presence in any examination performed between attacks. Similarly, occasional paroxysms in the EEG may be missed unless the recording is prolonged or frequently repeated.

The EEG helps to establish whether seizures originate from a limited area of the brain (focal, partial) (see Fig. 15-8 and 15-12) or involve the brain as a whole from onset (generalized, holoencephalic) (see Fig. 15-6) — an important distinction because of the different possible causes of these two basic types of epilepsy and because the clinical manifestations of both types may be similar or identical.

Focal delta activity in the interictal period usually indicates an underlying structural lesion of the brain as the cause of the seizures. However, focal delta activity in the EEG may be a transient aftermath of a partial seizure (analogous to clinical Todd's paralysis) and may not necessarily denote a gross structural lesion. This kind of postictal abnormality, however, usually subsides within 2 or 3 days.

The EEG can make an important contribution to the diagnosis in a patient who is obtunded or semicomatose when prolonged epileptiform discharges with only brief interruptions are recorded, signifying nonconvulsive status epilepticus. Only rarely is the EEG unaltered during a true epileptic seizure.

Ancillary Techniques in EEG

The techniques and principles of EEG need not be reserved for amplifying and recording cerebral potentials. They can be used to measure many other kinds of biologic activity. In patients with poorly defined spells of impaired cerebral function, simultaneous recording of the electrocardiogram with the EEG can help differentiate cardiogenic from epileptic origins. Monitoring of EMG potentials or of movement by means of an accelerometer may be helpful in correlating peripheral motor manifestations with abnormal cerebral activity during some seizures. The gross appearance of the muscle activity recorded from scalp leads in the standard EEG also may be sufficient to identify the distinctive rhythmic and periodic bursts of facial myokymia. This characteristic activity is an important diagnostic clue to intracranial disease, since the EEG itself is usually normal and facial myokymia is likely to be associated with intrinsic lesions of the lower part of the brain stem. Finally, the same general methods of recording and analysis can be applied to ocular potentials for electroretinography, electro-oculography, and electronystagmography.

This section has emphasized the use of EEG as a practical diagnostic procedure. Proper application of knowledge already available can provide information helpful to the clinician about many patients suffering from many different diseases. The electroencephalographer needs to strive continually to maintain the highest possible standards of quality, to ensure reliability of the test data, and to implement improvements whenever they are needed. No routine procedure, however accurate, suffices for every patient. Traditionally, electroencephalographers at the Mayo Clinic have held the conviction that optimal clinical application of EEG entails adapting and modifying the standard test appropriately to derive the maximal amount of beneficial information about each patient's specific medical problem. When new problems are encountered, new means of solving them need to be devised. One patient came to the Mayo Clinic because her parents thought she was acting obstinately by dropping her schoolbooks as she went out the front door on her way to school. During the EEG examination, she exhibited myoclonus of her upper extremities from photic stimulation and marked photoparoxysmal responses in the trace. These findings indicated a convulsive mechanism, triggered by change in illumination, that explained her otherwise obscure symptoms. Such light-induced seizures may be greatly diminished by the wearing of dark glasses. Another patient came to this clinic because of his peculiar behavior, particularly when he was in the presence of his father. Much of the time he seemed withdrawn and restless. Testing in the EEG laboratory revealed that absence attacks and myoclonus, associated with paroxysmal spike-wave complexes in the recording, could be induced by viewing geometric patterns. Some of these patterns resembled closely the striped ties and checkered jackets that his father was fond of wearing. This patient suffered from an uncommon type of convulsive disorder in which seizures are induced by visual pattern, not from a psychologic conflict in relation to his father as had been suspected initially. The clinician should inquire about any afferent precipitation of seizures and inform the EEG laboratory about any suspected precipitants so that appropriate testing can be performed. In this way, the alert physician may make important observations that may help one to understand the neurophysiologic mechanisms of a patient's symptoms and may lead to discovery of new adjunctive measures of treatment.

The EEG in Infants and Children—Normal Patterns
Ten or more channels of EEG recording are needed in infants to record EEG activity and other physiologic variables important for determining the state of the infant. These include respiration, electrocardiogram, eye movement, and chin myogram. The recording should be long enough to record the stages of wakefulness and sleep.

Premature infant
In infants less than 32 weeks of conceptional age (CA; age since the first day of the mother's last menses), the EEG shows an intermittent or discontinuous pattern, bursts of mixed frequency activity alternating with long quiescent periods (Fig. 15-15). There is little or no reactivity or spontaneous variability. The wake and sleep states are not well differentiated. After CA 32 weeks, there is a difference between the wake and sleep states, with two types of sleep states: *active* sleep and *quiet* sleep. The active sleep stage is analogous to rapid eye movement sleep in the adult and is characterized by slow rolling or rapid eye movements, body twitches, facial grimaces, a decrease in

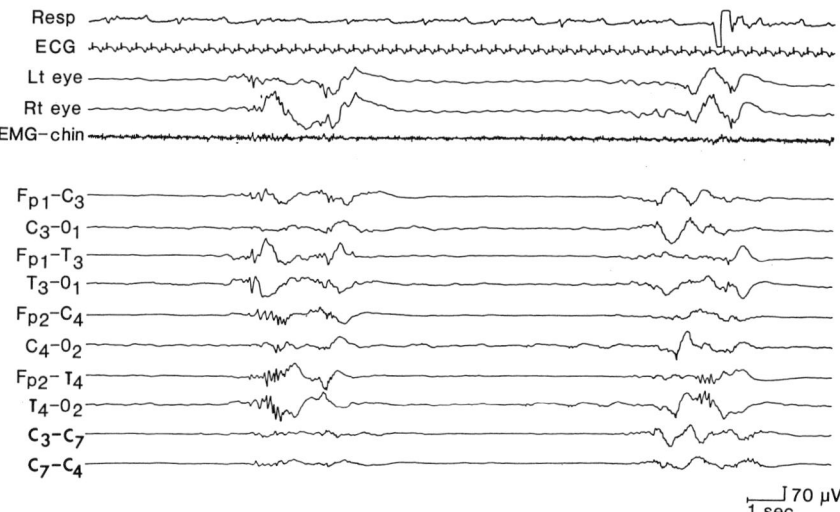

Figure 15-15
Recording from a normal premature infant. The first five channels are used to monitor respirations, electrocardiogram, eye movement, and chin myogram. The next 10 channels represent the EEG activity during quiet sleep, with an intermittent pattern consisting of slow waves, focal sharp transients, and the delta brush pattern.

muscle tone, and irregular respiratory rates. Quiet sleep is similar to non–rapid eye movement sleep and is characterized by decreased eye and body movements, tonic muscle activity on the chin myogram, and more regular respirations.

After CA 32 weeks, the EEG shows two patterns: a discontinuous pattern and a more continuous one. The wake state and active sleep state show the continuous patterns, whereas a discontinuous pattern consisting of intermittent bursts of mixed sharp and slow waveforms alternating with a quiescent or flattened background is present during quiet sleep. As the infant matures, the periods of activity lengthen and the periods of quiescence decrease in duration. Between CA 32 and 38 weeks, the EEG shows activity that is characteristic of premature recordings: the "delta brush" pattern, occipital dominant slow waves, anterior slow waves, and multifocal sharp transients.

The delta brush pattern consists of slow delta waves with superimposed low-amplitude fast activity ranging from 8 to 20 Hz. This pattern becomes less prominent as the infant matures, and it disappears by CA 40 or 41 weeks. Multifocal sharp transients consist of random sharp-contoured waveforms occurring in various locations over the two hemispheres, often maximal over the anterior head regions. In the premature infant, they are present during wakefulness and sleep but are more frequent and prominent during sleep. The sharp transients become less prominent as the infant matures and disappear first in the wake tracing in the term infant and then in the sleep recording by 4 to 6 weeks after birth.

Full-term infant

The characteristic EEG patterns of full-term infants are seen by about CA 38 weeks. Four types of EEG patterns are evident: a low-voltage irregular pattern, a mixed pattern, a high-voltage slow-wave pattern, and a "tracé alternant" pattern. The first three patterns consist of continuous, but irregular, amorphous activity in the theta and delta range that varies in amplitude from a low-voltage to a high-amplitude slow-wave pattern. The continuous low-voltage pattern is present during wakefulness and active sleep. The mixed pattern is present during drowsiness and active sleep. The high-voltage slow-wave pattern is present during quiet sleep. The tracé alternant pattern consists of bursts of mixed-frequency slow and sharply contoured waveforms ranging up to several seconds in duration and alternating with a low-voltage irregular pattern of less than 10 seconds in duration, similar to the discontinuous pattern in the premature infant. This disappears by about CA 45 or 46 weeks to be replaced by a continuous slow-wave pattern that becomes the dominant pattern of quiet sleep.

In infants, photic stimuli induce evoked responses of longer latency (150 to 200 msec) than the 30 to 50 msec in adults. They are best seen with single flash stimuli or very low flash rates, and they rapidly fatigue with repeated stimuli.

Childhood

The waking EEG follows a sequential change in frequency in childhood (Table 15-2). During the first 3 or 4 months of age, rhythmic 4- to 6-Hz activity that does not attenuate is seen predominantly over the central regions. At 3 months of age, 3- to 4-Hz activity that reacts to eye opening becomes evident over the occipital regions. By 5 or 6 months, a fairly well-developed 5- to 8-Hz rhythm is present over the central regions, and 5- to 6-Hz activity with reactivity to eye opening appears over the occipital head regions. After 6 months of age, better developed rhythmic activity is present over the posterior head regions, and after 1 year of age, this begins to resemble the alpha rhythm.

At 2 to 5 years, there is a further development of the central and occipital rhythms, with the central activity having a frequency of 7 to 10

Table 15-2   Changes in Normal EEG Activity With Maturation

Age	EEG Aspect	State of Patient During Recording		
		Awake	Drowsy	Asleep
<1 mo	Amplitude	Low	No change	Slight increase, tracé alternant
	Frequency and type	Delta and theta	No change	No change
1 mo–1 yr	Amplitude	Increased to high	Same	Same
	Frequency and type	Delta and theta	Sustained, rhythmic	Spindles asynchronous; long duration
1–5 yr	Amplitude	High	Same	Same
	Frequency and type	Theta, alpha increased, delta decreased	Rhythmic, bursts or sustained	Spindles synchronous; asymmetrical
6–10 yr	Amplitude	Decreased to moderate	Attenuation or bursts	Decreased V and spindles
	Frequency and type	Alpha increased, theta decreased, delta decreased or absent	Increased rate of rhythmic slow waves	Synchronous and symmetrical
11–20 yr	Amplitude	Moderate or increased	Attenuation or anterior rhythmic theta	Decreased V and spindles
	Frequency and type	Alpha, theta minimal, posterior delta		

Hz and the occipital alpha activity having a frequency of 6 to 8 Hz. There is also a progressive decrease in the amount of activity in the slower frequency ranges.

From 6 to 16 years, there is a progressive increase in the frequency of the alpha activity, with adult frequencies of 9 to 10 Hz attained by 8 or 9 years. In older children and adolescents, there are posterior 2- to 3-Hz slow waves of youth interspersed with alpha activity that reacts to eye opening. In younger children, *hyperventilation* often precipitates rhythmic, high-voltage, 2- to 3-Hz slow waves that are maximal over the posterior head regions. In older children and adults, the amplitude is usually maximal over the anterior head regions. In those less than 10 years of age, the photic driving response is seen best at flash frequencies of less than 10 Hz. After 10 years of age, the driving response occurs up to frequencies of 15 to 20 Hz.

EEG Abnormalities in Infants

The EEG in infants must be interpreted with caution because of the variability of maturation. Because of the absence of organized rhythmic activity, a greater degree of structural abnormality is required to be manifested as an EEG abnormality. Definite abnormalities that are seen in infants' recordings include

1. A flat or inactive tracing.
2. A persistent low-voltage tracing beyond the first week of life.
3. A true burst suppression pattern. This needs to be differentiated from the discontinuous pattern of premature infants and the tracé alternant pattern of quiet sleep.
4. A focal suppression of activity or a persistent asymmetry of activity.
5. An invariant pattern that shows no change with sleep and wake states and no reactivity.
6. A persistent or continuous diffuse or focal delta or theta slowing that shows no lability or variability.
7. Paroxysmal epileptiform abnormalities occurring throughout the recording during both wake and sleep states. This occurrence needs to be differentiated from the benign multifocal sharp transients that can be seen during sleep in the newborn infant. Ictal seizure discharges in infants consist of the sudden occurrence of a repetitive sequence of abnormal waveforms having a different morphologic appearance from the background activity. The seizure discharges can be variable and may consist of spikes, sharp waves, slow waves, or rhythmic alpha, beta, theta, or delta waveforms (Fig. 15-16). The seizure discharges are usually focal or lateralized to one hemisphere but can migrate from one location in the brain to the other. There may be a discordance between the location of the ictal discharges and the clinical manifestations of the seizure. Electrographic seizure discharges can occur without an apparent clinical accompaniment and vice versa.

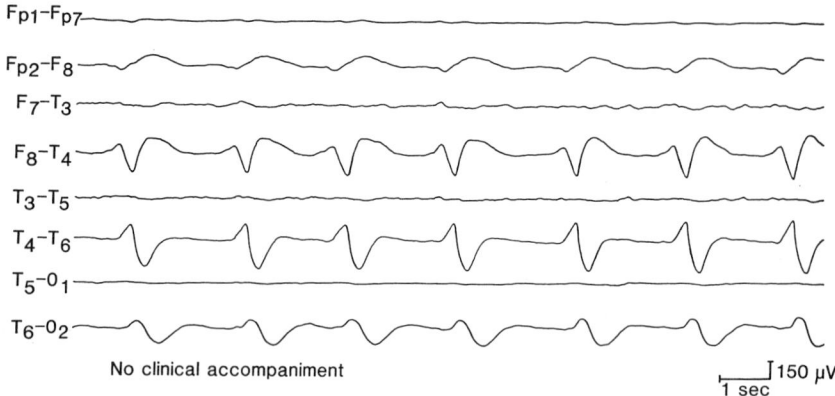

Figure 15-16
Electrographic seizure discharge consisting of repetitive sharp waves over the right temporal (T_4) region in an 8-day-old infant.

EEG Abnormalities in Children

Children's EEGs show abnormalities similar to those in adults. The two main types of abnormalities are slow waves and epileptiform discharges.

Children's EEGs often show more prominent slow-wave abnormalities than are seen in adults; they may take longer to resolve, and the slow-wave abnormalities often have a maximal expression over the posterior head region. The degree of the abnormality is related to the age of the child at the onset of the disease, the more severe EEG changes occurring in the younger child.

Almost all types of epileptiform patterns can be seen in children. Hypsarrhythmia, the 3-Hz spike and wave, the slow spike and wave, and centrotemporal spikes are the common or unique types. *Hypsarrhythmia* refers to a high-voltage, arrhythmic EEG pattern with a chaotic admixture of continuous, multifocal spike- and sharp-wave discharges and widespread, high-voltage, arrhythmic slow waves (Fig. 15-17). This EEG pattern often occurs in association with infantile spasms and mental retardation and usually indicates a severe disturbance of cerebral function. The findings are not associated with a specific disease entity but reflect a severe cerebral insult, usually occurring before 1 year of age. In about half the patients, the cause is unknown; in the others, hypsarrhythmia may result from perinatal or postnatal insults, encephalitis, congenital defects, or the metabolic derangements that occur in the young child. Patients with hypsarrhythmia often have myoclonic jerks or infantile spasms. The myoclonic jerks are often associated with generalized, high-amplitude spike and wave or sharp-wave complexes in the EEG. Of longer duration, infantile spasms consist of tonic flexion or extension of the neck, body, and extremities, with the arms flung outward, that may last from 3 to 10 seconds. The EEG

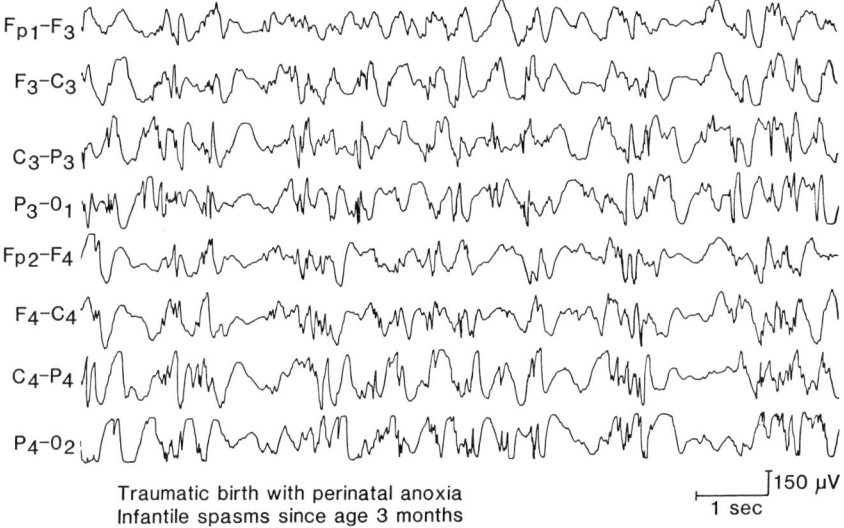

Figure 15-17
Hypsarrhythmic pattern in a 7-month-old child, showing the mixture of high-amplitude spikes, sharp waves, and slow waves.

accompaniment of an initial high-amplitude spike- or slow-wave complex (or both) followed by abrupt decrease in the amplitude of activity has been referred to as an "electrodecremental pattern."

The *3-Hz spike-and-wave pattern*, consisting of stereotyped bilaterally synchronous and symmetrical, repetitive 3-Hz spike-and-wave discharges, is often associated with absence, or "petit mal," seizures. It is most often seen in children between the ages of 3 and 15 years and is enhanced by hyperventilation and hypoglycemia. The bursts are often associated with a clinical accompaniment consisting of staring, brief clonic movements, motor arrest, or unresponsiveness.

The sharp- and slow-wave complexes of the *slow spike-and-wave pattern* occur at a frequency of 1 to 2.5 Hz in serial trains and are usually generalized and symmetrical (Fig. 15-18). The slow spike-and-wave pattern occurs in children between 1 and 6 years of age who have some type of underlying organic disease. Most of these patients are mentally retarded and have poorly controlled seizures. The combination of mental retardation, severe convulsive disorder, and the slow spike-and-wave pattern has been referred to as the Lennox-Gastaut syndrome.

The *central midtemporal spike* of childhood is a broad, high-amplitude, diphasic, blunt spike followed by a slow wave over the central and midtemporal areas (Fig. 15-19). From 60% to 70% of the children with this spike discharge have focal seizures consisting of clonic movements of the side of the face or hand or tingling of the side of the mouth,

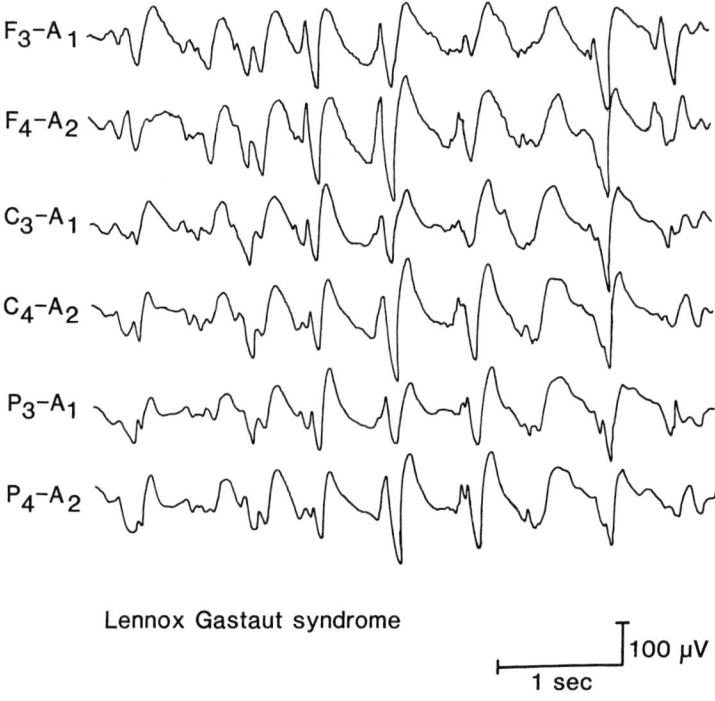

Lennox Gastaut syndrome

Figure 15-18
Generalized slow spike-and-wave discharges in a 4-year-old girl with seizures and mental retardation (Lennox-Gastaut syndrome).

tongue, cheek, or hand; motor speech arrest; and excessive salivation. These seizures have been called "benign rolandic epilepsy of childhood," "sylvian seizures of childhood," and "rolandic epilepsy of childhood." The seizures are often nocturnal and may progress to a generalized seizure. The seizures are easily controlled by anticonvulsants and disappear by 12 to 14 years of age.

In some conditions unique to children, the EEG shows a characteristic pattern. In *subacute sclerosing panencephalitis,* the EEG pattern shows generalized, periodic, and stereotyped complexes, reoccurring every 4 to 15 seconds, often associated with a jerk or spasm. Subacute sclerosing panencephalitis affects children between 5 and 15 years of age with a progressive deterioration in intellect and behavior.

In the *HHE* (hemiconvulsions, hemiplegia, and epilepsy) *syndrome,* described by Gastaut, the infant or child has a series of seizures or hemiconvulsive status during an acute febrile illness, with a residual hemiparesis. Later, chronic epilepsy develops. The EEG in the acute stage shows frequent or continuous spike or spike-and-wave discharges over the involved side. In association with the hemiparesis, there is a persistent attenuation of activity over the affected side. Later, focal, multifocal,

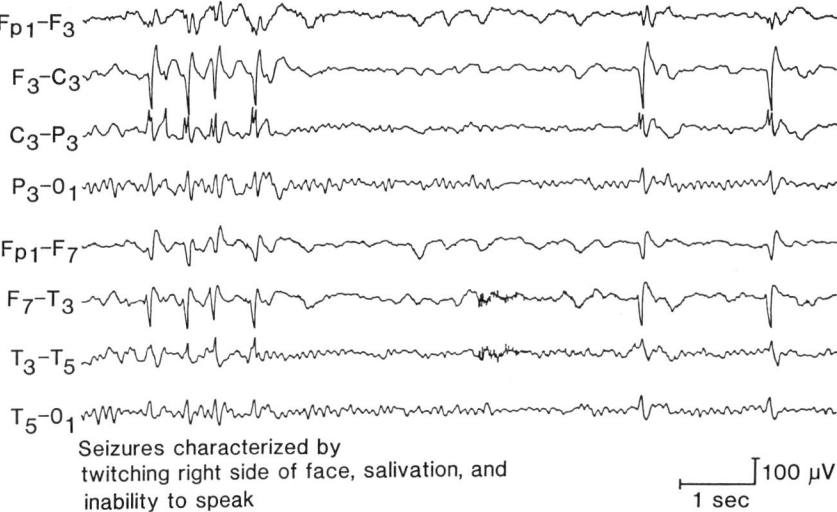

Figure 15-19
Left-sided centrotemporal spikes in a 9-year-old boy with benign sylvian seizures of childhood.

or bilateral epileptiform discharges emerge over either hemisphere, often with a reduced amplitude over the involved side.

Prolonged Monitoring

Patients with intractable focal seizures are sometimes candidates for surgical removal of the area of abnormality. Precise identification of the area of brain from which the seizures are arising is needed to proceed to surgery. This is best accomplished by recording a number of the clinical seizures. This often requires prolonged monitoring over a number of days, sometimes with a need to reduce or stop anticonvulsant medications if the seizures are not occurring often enough. Prolonged monitoring is usually performed with video monitoring recorded on tape with the simultaneous EEG to allow precise correlation of the EEG abnormalities with the clinical features. Overnight monitoring can be accomplished with automated, computer-controlled systems for detecting abnormal discharges. These procedures are performed in the hospital or in a setting with immediate nurse or physician availability.

Ambulatory EEG Monitoring

Ambulatory electroencephalographic monitoring (A/EEG) is the recording of an EEG in a freely mobile patient outside the EEG laboratory. This procedure is analogous to Holter monitoring for the ambulatory recording of an electrocardiogram.

Technical aspects

Eight channels of EEG are recorded continuously on a four-track, 1/8-inch magnetic tape cassette similar in size to that used in home stereo systems or for dictation. The recording instrumentation is encased in a small, lightweight box attached to a belt or a shoulder strap. About 12 disk electrodes are affixed with collodion to the scalp for A/EEG. The electrocardiogram may be recorded from chest electrodes by use of one of the eight EEG channels. The analog electrical signals are digitized and multiplexed (with tape management and time information included) to be stored on four tracks of tape.

At the completion of the study, the cassette is played through a computer that translates the four tracks of tape into eight channels of EEG data that can be reviewed at 20 or 60 times the recording speed. Reviewal is done on a video screen, and simultaneous audio and video monitoring of electrical activity helps identify epileptiform activity or seizures. The section of the recording containing evidence of a spell, a seizure, epileptiform activity, or other abnormalities is written out on oscillograph chart paper for further review by an electroencephalographer. Patients receive a diary to record the time of symptoms. Pressing a button on the recorder marks the position of each spell on the tape.

Clinical aspects

The main indication for performing A/EEG is to determine whether an unusual or vague "spell" is a seizure. Syncope, migraine, transient ischemic attacks, behavioral problems, and symptoms related to cardiac arrhythmia may be confused with epilepsy. The spells should occur at least once a day to be recorded during 24 hours of continuous monitoring. A/EEG is helpful for recording spells that occur predominantly at unusual times, with specific events or activities, with stress, or with a combination of factors. For example, amnestic, nonconvulsive seizures may be associated with either generalized 3-per-second spike-and-wave patterns or focal epileptiform activity from the temporal or frontal lobes. Another use of A/EEG is to supplement prolonged recordings in the EEG laboratory by extending the recording time from the 8-hour working day to an additional 16 hours. Some patients have their A/EEG done on an inpatient basis if anticonvulsant medication dosages are reduced and status epilepticus is a possible complication. Some seizures, especially those associated with generalized spike-and-wave patterns, may have minimal clinical accompaniment. A/EEG for 24 hours while the patient is in a natural environment may provide additional information about the abundance of epileptiform activity. This information is desirable before anticonvulsant treatment is modified.

For more than half the patients, some useful information is obtained. The more frequent the spells, the greater the chance of them being recorded during A/EEG. The yield depends on the type of patient selected by the clinician. The absence of electrographic seizure activity during a spell does not exclude a seizure disorder, since surface electrodes may not record some of the mesial temporal, basal frontal, or deep midsagittal seizure discharges. Also, the eight-channel recording does not sample all the electrode sites recorded in the routine EEG.

Quantitative Analysis of Spontaneous EEG

Digital computers may be used to extract information from the spontaneous EEG that is not readily obtainable with conventional visual analysis. Also, computer analysis, by allowing key EEG features to be quantitated, facilitates comparison of serial EEGs on the same subject or comparison of subject groups in scientific investigations using EEG. Because of the increasing availability of inexpensive but powerful digital computers, sophisticated analytic methods are becoming more widely used in the practice of clinical EEG. However, the most common use of digital processing techniques in routine EEG may be simply to make the process of obtaining, storing, retrieving, and viewing an EEG record easier.

All modern computer methods involve first digitizing the EEG, that is, sampling the continuous voltage changes at a fixed rate and converting the measured voltage at each sampling time to a digital number, "analog-to-digital conversion." For routine spontaneous EEG, a sampling rate of 100 to 200 samples per second and a sampling accuracy of 1 part in 1,024 to 1 part in 2,048 are generally adequate. Note that the signal sampled is the amplified and filtered signal produced by the analog electronics of the EEG machine, not the extremely weak signal picked up by the scalp electrodes directly. The digitized voltages may be stored by the computer in various forms, may be manipulated by computer programs, and, after reconversion to analog form, may be displayed on a screen in the form of a continuous curve.

Simple forms of processing include montage reformatting and digital filtering. *Montage reformatting* involves subtracting data samples from two channels (derivations) sharing a common reference to give a third derived channel. Thus, if channel 1 represents the potential difference between electrode A and electrode R (the reference) and channel 2 represents the potential difference between electrode B and electrode R, channel 1 minus channel 2 represents the potential difference between electrode A and electrode B. This type of reformatting allows the electroencephalographer to bring out important EEG features and to analyze the spatial distribution of patterns of brain electrical activity. *Digital filtering* involves a type of time-averaging of the EEG signal that removes activity of unwanted frequencies while preserving desired activity unchanged. This may be used, for example, to remove certain artifacts from the record.

The mathematical technique of *spectral analysis* allows the EEG signal to be decomposed into a set of sine waves of specific frequency, amplitude, and phase. The amplitude of each component sine wave may then be plotted as a function of its frequency. Often, the *power* (amplitude squared) is plotted against frequency; this type of plot is a *power spectrum* and is a useful way to demonstrate slight differences in the preponderance of waves of different frequencies and slight shifts of frequency. The clinical significance of these changes must be determined in terms of what frequencies are normal or abnormal in a given age group.

Other types of analysis occasionally used are *cross-correlation*, which evaluates the degree of similarity between two different sources recorded simultaneously, and *autocorrelation,* which compares activity from one area of the head at different times. *Coherence analysis* determines the dependence of the correlation coefficient on the EEG frequency. Cross-correlation and coherence analysis may help in studies of the spatial properties of EEG activity, such as in determining the source of abnormal epileptic activity. Autocorrelation analysis is especially suited to reveal periodic components in the EEG and is analogous to spectral analysis.

Finally, computer methods for displaying the spatial features of EEG activity over the surface of the head are becoming more widely used. One method plots the distribution of equipotential lines superimposed on a diagram of the head at one instant of time. Another method includes both power spectral and spatial analysis and plots the power (amplitude squared) in each of several frequency bands (for example, delta or alpha) as a color or gray-scale map on a head diagram. The resulting map has the appearance of a low-resolution CT scan and may be helpful in visualizing the location of an abnormal focus of slow waves. The method is unfortunately sensitive also to artifacts and must be used with caution when the EEG contains artifacts.

EEG Monitoring During Surgery

An EEG can be used to assist the surgeon in three major areas: carotid endarterectomy, cardiac surgery, and epilepsy surgery. All three of these present difficulties not encountered with standard, diagnostic EEG recording because of both the striking effects of anesthesia on the EEG and the many sources of artifacts in the operating room. Clamping is needed to perform a carotid endarterectomy, but it may result in significant cerebral ischemia and stroke. Scalp-recorded EEG slowing can identify cerebral ischemia before stroke occurs. EEG slowing begins to occur with blood flow less than 15 mL/100 g per minute and occurs in some degree in up to 25% of cases. More severe EEG changes develop when cerebral blood flow decreases to 5 mL/100 g per minute or lower, a rate that occurs in 2% to 4% of all patients. The EEG slowing occurring as a consequence of carotid clamping can thus be used to identify patients in whom shunting will eliminate the risk of hemodynamic stroke during surgery.

Cerebral ischemia can also be detected during cardiac surgery if the EEG activity has not been altered by the profound hypothermia and changes in P_{CO_2} levels that are so often present. Newer methods of studying digitally processed EEG signals may enable EEG monitoring to be used more effectively during cardiac surgery.

Corticography and depth recording in association with epilepsy surgery can more precisely identify the source of the interictal abnormality seen with routine recordings and can identify foci that were not seen with surface recordings. These acute intraoperative recordings are helpful in planning the extent of the surgical procedure, but this decision ultimately is based on the integration of intraoperative findings with the preoperative EEG (interictal and ictal) and neuroimaging studies.

SECTION II: ELECTROMYOGRAPHY

Electromyography is a component of electrodiagnostic medicine consisting of recording the variations of electric potential or voltage detected by a needle electrode inserted into skeletal muscle. This electric activity is displayed on an oscilloscope or monitor and played over a loudspeaker for simultaneous visual and auditory analysis. In normal resting muscle, no electric activity is detected, but during voluntary contraction, the action potentials of motor units appear. In disorders of the motor unit, electric activity of various types may appear in the resting muscle and the action potentials of motor units may have abnormal forms and patterns of activity. Abnormalities of the EMG serve as objective criteria of dysfunction of the motor unit. These abnormalities may characterize the nature of the disease process and its location in the neuron, neuromuscular junctions, or muscle fibers.

EMG is an extension of the neurologic examination. It does not provide a clinical diagnosis of the patient's illness. There are no waveforms that are pathognomonic of specific disease entities. The EMG results must be integrated with the results of other tests, the clinical examination, and the clinical history in arriving at a diagnosis.

The value of EMG to clinical neurology is based on the quality of help it affords in selected problems. A survey of some of the common clinical applications of EMG will indicate the scope of its usefulness.

Survey of Clinical Uses of EMG
Detection of disease in the motor unit

At times, the clinician has difficulty deciding whether muscular wasting, paralysis, or some other type of motor dysfunction is the result of

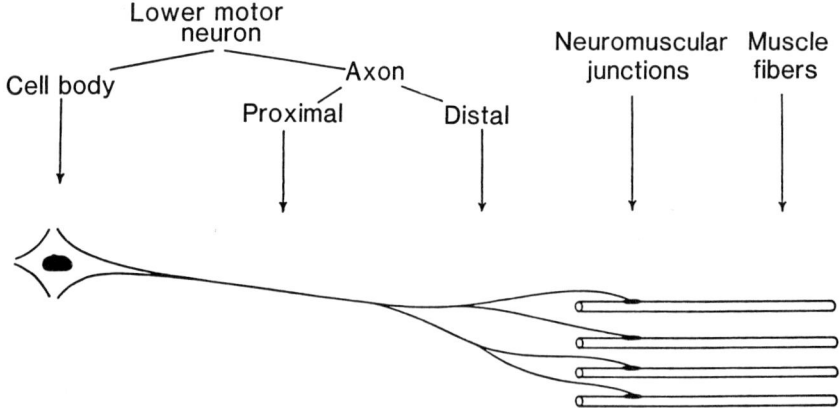

Figure 15-20
The motor unit. The number of muscle fibers innervated by a single neuron varies from a few fibers in muscles of precision, such as the extraocular muscles, to several hundred in powerful muscles, such as the quadriceps.

disease of the motor unit (Fig. 15-20) or is attributable to pain, a conversion reaction, disuse, or a central nervous system disorder. Under such circumstances, clinical tests may be difficult to evaluate, and EMG evidence of normality or unequivocal abnormality of the motor unit is of utmost importance.

Similarly, in the early stages of disease or when disease is mild, EMG may present the only objective evidence of dysfunction of the motor unit.

Diagnosis of primary muscle disease

Occasionally the clinician encounters difficulty in determining whether weakness of muscle results from primary muscle disease or is secondary to a nerve disorder. Fortunately, the EMG picture of primary muscle disease often is strikingly dissimilar to that of denervation secondary to axonopathy or neuronopathy. That distinction frequently can be made unequivocally by EMG, even though the clinical picture is not clear. EMG may be an important aid in determining the type of primary muscle disease. For example, spontaneous activity or myotonic discharges may occur in some disorders but not in others. On this basis, the occurrence of spontaneous activity in polymyositis may serve to differentiate this condition from thyrotoxic myopathy but not from muscular dystrophy. Myotonic discharges in hyperkalemic periodic paralysis may differentiate this condition from other forms of periodic paralysis. In general, however, the ability to identify specific myopathies on the basis of EMG alone is, as yet, limited.

Detection of defects in transmission at the neuromuscular junction

The EMG may provide evidence of a defect in transmission at the neuromuscular junction and, consequently, be of value in the diagnosis of myasthenia gravis and Lambert-Eaton myasthenic syndrome. Similar defects in transmission may be detected in other diseases, particularly those of the anterior horn cells, such as amyotrophic lateral sclerosis. However, in the latter, the transmission defect, in contrast to the situation in myasthenia gravis, is associated with other EMG evidence of disease of the motor cells.

Diagnosis of disease of the lower motor neuron

EMG is of particular value in the diagnosis of disease of the lower motor neuron. EMG evidence of denervation is often present unequivocally at a time when clinical evidence of denervation is lacking. Furthermore, this evidence can be obtained in the presence of upper motor neuron disease, pain, and other factors, such as hysteria, that may make it difficult to reach reliable conclusions from the clinical examination. Further, the needle electrode can examine individual muscles whose weakness on clinical testing may be obscured by the action of synergists. Thus, EMG may not only aid in detection of disease of the lower motor neuron but also define the distribution and relative number of the affected neurons. With this information, the methods of deduction habitually used by the clinician are applied in furthering diagnosis and understanding of the problem. Is the pattern of denervation that which results from a lesion of a nerve root, plexus, peripheral nerve, or segment of the spinal cord? If so, is more than one segment, nerve root, or peripheral nerve involved? Is the process localized, diffuse, or widely disseminated?

In addition to supplying information to answer these questions, EMG techniques may aid in differentiating diseases of the anterior horn cells from those that affect primarily the peripheral nerve and in differentiating physiologic block of conduction from axonal destruction of the nerve.

In comparison with other tests used in the diagnosis of peripheral nerve lesions, EMG excels not only in detection of minimal denervation but also in detection of minimal residual innervation and the earliest evidence of reinnervation, both of which are important to the management of nerve lesions. EMG evidence of reinnervation frequently precedes clinical evidence of return of function by several weeks.

The Electromyograph

The essential components of the electromyograph are an electrode system, an amplifier, a monitor, and a loudspeaker. Two types of needle electrode are commonly used: the concentric (coaxial) needle of Adrian and Bronk and the monopolar (unipolar) needle. The diameter and length of the needle electrode are selected to meet the needs of the specific muscle tested. The most commonly used needles range in diameter from 24 to 26 gauge and in length from 35 to 65 mm. The monopolar needle consists of a solid steel needle that is coated except at its tip (about 0.2 mm) with an insulating plastic. An electrode on the skin surface serves as a reference electrode. The concentric electrode consists of an insulated wire, usually platinum, cemented in a hypodermic needle. The wire is bare at its tip, which is flush with the bevel of the needle. Variations in electric potential or voltage between the uninsulated tip of the central wire (exploring electrode) and the bare needle shaft (reference electrode) are amplified, displayed on the monitor, and played on the loudspeaker.

Since the fluctuations of voltage in skeletal muscle occur at frequencies in the audible range, they may be translated to sound waves by connecting the output of the amplifier to a loudspeaker as well as to the monitor. The characteristic sounds produced by different waveforms are often of more value than the visual picture for identification of action potentials of different types.

Permanent records may be made by photographing the trace from the oscilloscope, by storing the electric signal on magnetic tape, using a suitable tape recorder, or by storing the signal in a digital computer. Tape-recorded signals have the advantage that they may be played back just as they occurred at the original examination. With the development of digital electromyograph instruments, the signals can be digitized and stored for later detailed analysis and quantitative measurements.

Origin of Electric Activity of Muscle

The electric activity detected in EMG is produced by muscle fibers and may be referred to as "muscle action potentials." Occasionally, unique potentials occur when the needle electrode is in contact with motor end plates and injures the small intramuscular nerve terminals, but potentials from other structures, such as sensory receptors, have not been identified with certainty in clinical EMG.

The action potential of a normal muscle fiber originates at the motor end plate, its appearance being triggered by the arrival of a nerve impulse at the neuromuscular junction. The action potential sweeps down the muscle fiber in both directions from the motor end plate at a velocity of about 4 m/sec, initiating excitation-contraction coupling in the muscle fiber. Contraction of the fiber begins after an interval of about 1.0 msec. The contraction itself produces no electric activity.

In a normal muscle, the muscle fibers are organized into functional units, called "motor units," each of which consists of a single lower motor neuron and all the muscle fibers that are innervated by its branches. During voluntary contraction, all the muscle fibers innervated by a single lower motor neuron act together, their individual action potentials summating to produce the larger action potential of the motor unit.

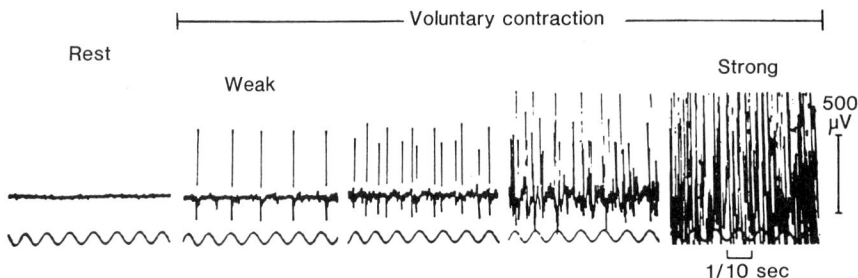

Figure 15-21
EMG of normal biceps brachii muscle. The records are photographs of the tracing on the cathode-ray oscilloscope. In this and other figures, an upward deflection is caused by a change of voltage in the negative direction at the needle electrode.

In normal muscle at rest, the motor units are inactive and no electric activity is detected ("electric silence," Fig. 15-21). During a weak voluntary contraction, only a single motor unit may be active in the vicinity of the needle electrode. Its action potential recurs as the muscle fibers of the motor unit contract in a semirhythmic fashion at a rate of 5 to 10 times per second. As voluntary effort increases, the rate at which the motor unit fires increases and other motor units are recruited, each acting rhythmically and independently, to increase the strength of contraction. During a strong contraction, many motor units are active. Their rhythmically recurring action potentials are so numerous that one cannot be distinguished from another. The resulting record is called an "interference pattern."

There is some variation of size and form of the motor unit action potentials in a single muscle and of the average size and form of action potentials in different muscles. Motor unit action potentials recorded in muscle of the extremities are most commonly diphasic or triphasic waves (Fig. 15-22, *I* and *J*) with a duration of 3 to 15 msec and an amplitude of up to 4 mV (most often between 0.2 and 2.0 mV). They produce a thumping or knocking sound over the loudspeaker.

Procedure of the Examination

There is no completely "routine" procedure for EMG that would allow the examination to be performed by a technician and later to be satisfactorily interpreted by the clinician, as is the case in electrocardiography and EEG. There are at least two reasons for this. First, it would not be feasible to examine in a set order all the muscles that might be involved in the various neuromuscular disorders. Muscles must be selected for examination according to the problem presented by the individual patient. The electromyographer must understand the diverse clinical

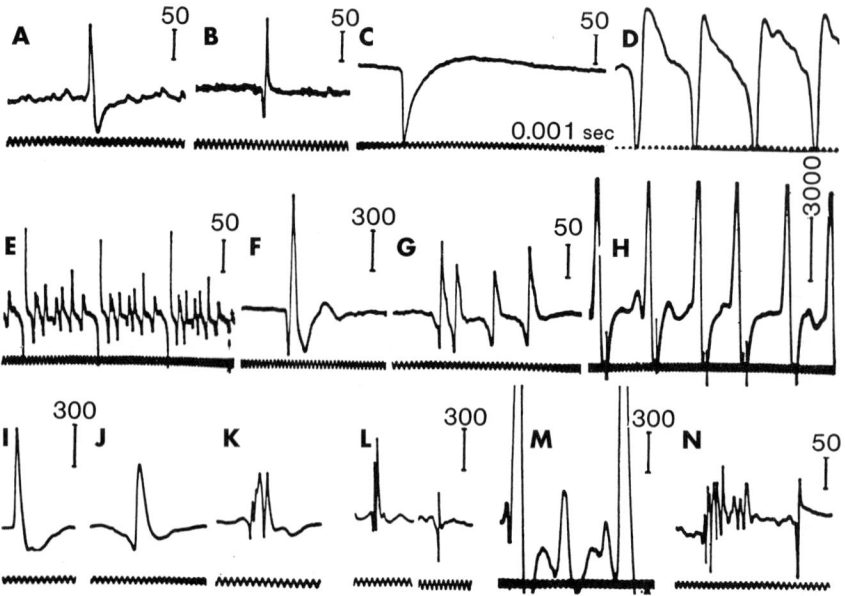

Figure 15-22
Muscle action potentials in EMG: **(A)** end plate noise (small negative deflections) and an associated muscle fiber spike from normal muscle; **(B)** fibrillation potential and **(C)** positive wave from denervated muscle; **(D)** high-frequency discharge in myotonia; **(E)** complex repetitive discharge; **(F)** fasciculation potential, single discharge; **(G)** fasciculation potential, repetitive or grouped discharge; **(H)** synchronized repetitive discharge in muscle cramp; **(I)** diphasic, **(J)** triphasic, and **(K)** polyphasic motor unit action potentials from normal muscle; **(L)** short-duration motor unit action potentials in progressive muscular dystrophy; **(M)** large motor unit action potentials in progressive muscular atrophy; **(N)** highly polyphasic motor unit action potential and short-duration motor unit action potential during reinnervation. Calibration scales are in microvolts. All time scales are 1,000 cycles per second.

problems that may be encountered, so that he or she can plan the examination and, during the examination, frequently modify this plan to obtain necessary information with the least discomfort to the patient. Second, the electric activity of muscle is greatly affected by what the patient does, by what the electromyographer does, and by the position of the electrodes at the moment when records are made. Interpretation in the light of these variables is most satisfactorily done at the time of the examination. It is essential that the electromyographer be thoroughly familiar with the anatomic arrangement and innervation of the skeletal muscles as well as with the nature of neuromuscular disorders and the significance of various forms of abnormal electric activity.

A preliminary history and neurologic examination are indispensable

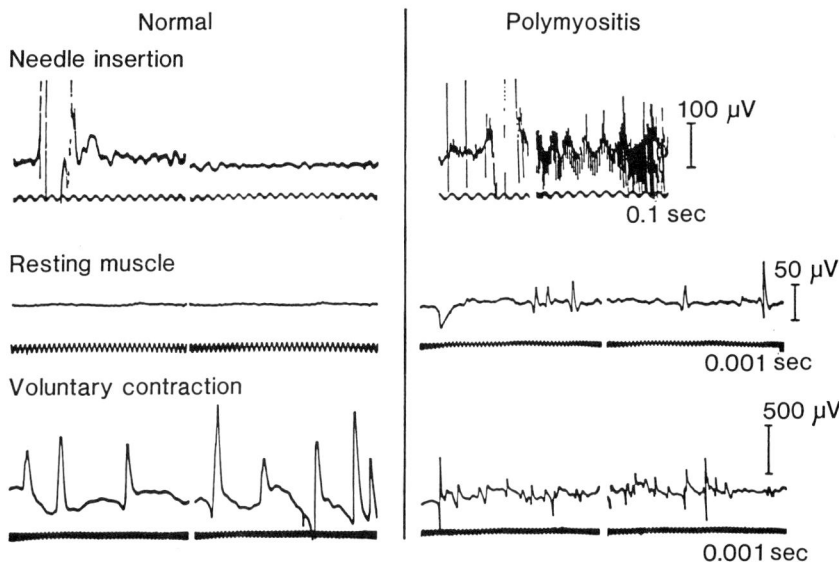

Figure 15-23
EMG activity in normal muscle *(left)* and in myositic muscle *(right)*. (From O'Leary PA, Lambert EH, Sayre GP: Muscle studies in cutaneous disease, J Invest Dermatol 24:301–310, 1955. By permission of Williams & Wilkins.)

for planning, as well as interpretation, of the EMG examination. With this information, the electromyographer is able to examine first those muscles obviously or most probably affected by the disease to determine the nature of the process. Other muscles are then examined as may be necessary to establish the distribution of the disease.

The examination itself is conducted with the patient lying in a comfortable position. The needle electrode is inserted into the muscle and is advanced by steps to several depths of the muscle. In each area observations are made of (1) the electric activity evoked in the muscle by insertion and movement of the needle, (2) the electric activity of the resting muscle with the needle undisturbed, and (3) the electric activity of motor units during voluntary contraction (Fig. 15-23). Several insertions of the needle into different parts of a muscle are necessary for adequate analysis of its electric activity. The time required for the examination varies considerably from a few minutes for examination of a single muscle to an hour or more for more extensive examination of many muscles.

The EMG examination, although not without some discomfort, is usually well tolerated by the patient. In fact, satisfactory examinations can be carried out on infants and usually on young children. Most often, insertion of the needle causes much less pain than was anticipated. Routine use of sedatives or local anesthetics is not necessary.

The after effects of the examination are minimal. Slight tenderness of the muscle in the area examined may be present for several hours. Direct damage to muscle fibers by the needle during an extensive needle examination can result in an increase in creatine kinase. If needed, the level of this enzyme should be determined before EMG.

Needle electrodes should not be inserted into muscles in which a muscle biopsy may be done. Abnormalities produced by the needle electrode may cause errors in interpretation of the biopsy. Similarly, intramuscular injections, biopsies, surgical procedures, or extensive probing with a needle electrode may account for abnormalities in a subsequent EMG as a result of damage to nerve and muscle fibers.

Criteria of Abnormality in the EMG

Abnormality of the EMG is indicated by one or more of the following criteria: (1) an unusually prolonged discharge or an absence of any discharge of electric activity in the resting muscle in response to insertion of the needle electrode, (2) the occurrence of spontaneous electric activity in the relaxed muscle, and (3) the presence of abnormalities of shape, size, number, rhythm, or recruitment of the motor unit action potentials observed during voluntary contraction. An increased mechanical resistance to insertion or movement of the needle electrode suggests an increase in relative amount of collagen in the muscle.

Abnormal response of the muscle to mechanical stimulation by insertion or movement of the needle electrode

Action potentials evoked by injury to muscle and nerve fibers during insertion or movement of the needle electrode have been called "insertion" potentials (Fig. 15-24). In normal muscle, insertion of the needle electrode generally evokes only a brief discharge of electric activity that lasts little longer than the actual movement of the needle. Occasionally, a more prolonged discharge occurs when the needle electrode is in the end plate zone ("end plate noise"; see Fig. 15-22, *A* and 15-24), but this can be differentiated from the abnormal activity seen in neuromuscular disease.

Several types of abnormal muscle fibers respond to insertion of the needle with prolonged repetitive activity. They continue to discharge impulses rhythmically for long periods after the needle has come to rest. This is particularly true of (1) denervated muscle fibers, (2) muscle fibers in myotonia, (3) muscle fibers in early stages of degeneration (possibly also during regeneration), and (4) muscle fibers in certain myopathies, for example, glycogen storage diseases. The insertion potentials observed in these conditions are of two types, which almost always coexist. One is a diphasic or triphasic wave (spike) of short duration; the other is a larger potential called a "positive wave," or "positive sharp wave."

In denervated muscle, the spikes and positive waves evoked by

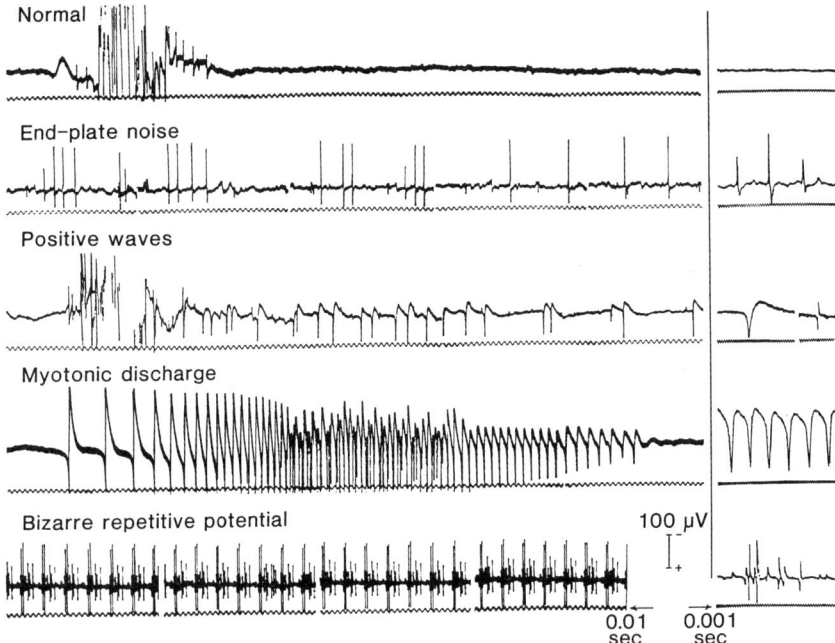

Figure 15-24
Insertion potentials, electric activity evoked by insertion of a needle electrode into muscle. *Normal*, a brief discharge of electric activity lasting little longer than the movement of the needle. *End-plate noise* and associated muscle fiber action potentials, electric activity evoked when the needle is in contact with motor end plates and irritates small intramuscular nerves. *Positive waves*, a form of fibrillation potential, evoked in denervated muscle. A myotonic discharge in myotonia congenita. Complex, or *bizarre, repetitive potential* in myositis. The time signal is 100 cycles per second. Details of the form of the various action potentials are shown in Figure 15-22 in photographs taken with a more rapid time base.

needle insertion (see Fig. 15-22, *B* and *C*) usually occur with a regular rhythm at frequencies of 1 to 10 per second, continuing for several seconds to several minutes after the needle has come to rest. This activity resembles the action potentials of fibrillation, which occur spontaneously in denervated muscle, and frequently the distinction between activity evoked by insertion of the needle and that which may be spontaneous is difficult to make and at best is arbitrary. However, abnormal insertion activity may be evoked in denervated muscle when spontaneous fibrillation is not observed, particularly between 8 and 14 days after nerve injury, just before the appearance of spontaneous fibrillation, and in chronically denervated muscle.

Insertion activity is particularly striking in myotonia congenita and myotonic dystrophy, in which prolonged trains of spikes and positive waves in great profusion, sometimes synchronized in unusual forms, are evoked by the slightest movement of the needle. The discharges occur at a high frequency (see Fig. 15-22 *D*), up to 120 per second, and usually have a characteristic quality, waxing and then waning in both frequency and amplitude. The sound produced over the loudspeaker has been compared with that of a dive bomber. It is the marked tendency for muscle fibers in myotonia to continue firing repetitively after stimulation, which is the basis of the myotonic phenomena observed in the clinical examination. Myotonic discharges are also observed in myopathy with acid maltase deficiency in adults and in infants (Pompe's disease) and often are found in the hyperkalemic form of periodic paralysis.

Abnormal insertion activity is evoked from muscles in which degeneration of muscle fibers is occurring. In some instances, spikes and positive waves occur at relatively low frequencies, resembling the activity commonly seen in denervated muscle; in other instances, these potentials occur at high frequencies, resembling more the activity seen in myotonia. The amount of abnormal insertion activity is usually minimal in slowly progressive muscular dystrophies but may be considerable in more rapidly progressive conditions such as polymyositis. The increased insertional activity that occurs rarely as a normal variant in individuals with hypertrophied muscles and in some families can be differentiated from diseases with increased insertional activity by its widespread distribution and the lack of abnormalities of the motor unit potentials.

Another type of abnormal activity observed occasionally is a complex repetitive discharge that does not wax and wane as myotonic discharges do (see Fig. 15-22, *E* and 15-24). This occurs strikingly in the Schwartz-Jampel syndrome, occasionally may occur in progressive muscular dystrophy and polymyositis, but also may be seen in other chronic disorders of muscle and nerve.

A marked reduction or absence of insertion activity occurs when muscle fibers are severely atrophied or replaced by fibrous tissue or fat or when they become inexcitable, for example, during severe paralysis in familial periodic paralysis.

Spontaneous electric activity

Although no electric activity is detected in normal muscle when the muscle and the needle electrode are at rest, several types of electric activity may be found in voluntarily relaxed muscles of patients with neuromuscular disorders (Fig. 15-25). In diseases that affect the motor unit, fibrillation potentials associated with spontaneous contraction of individual muscle fibers, fasciculation potentials associated with spontaneous contraction of motor units or bundles of muscle fibers, and repetitive potentials associated with muscle cramps may occur. In certain diseases of the central nervous system, action potentials of motor units

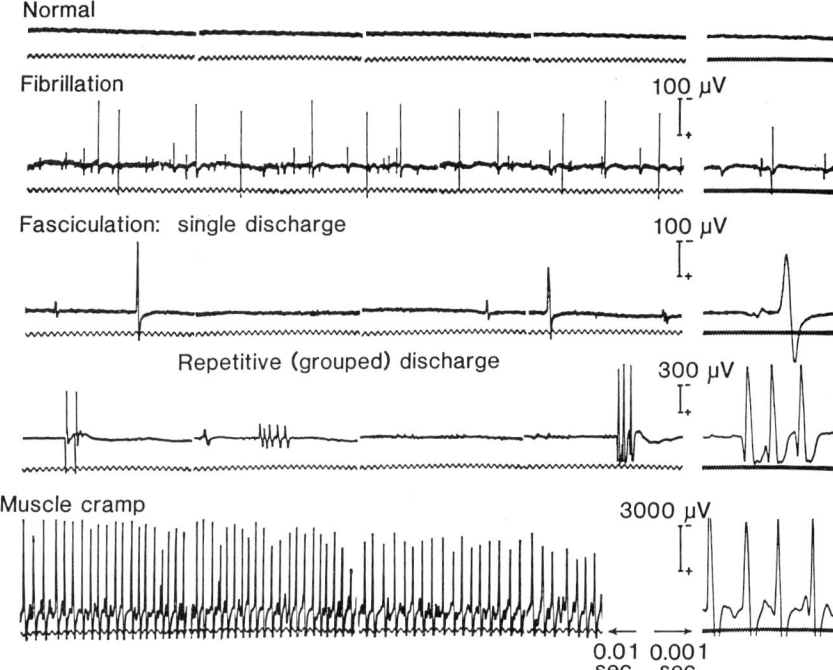

Figure 15-25
Spontaneous electric activity in voluntarily relaxed muscle. *Normal*, no electric activity. The slight irregularity of the baseline is "noise" inherent in high amplification. *Fibrillation*, action potentials of fibrillation in denervated muscle. *Fasciculation, single discharge* type, from a person with "benign" fasciculation. *Fasciculation, repetitive* or *grouped discharge* type, from a person with myokymia. *Muscle cramp*, a high-frequency synchronous discharge of a large number of muscle fibers.

occur in association with involuntary movements and with contractions, such as tremor and rigidity.

Fibrillation

A distinction must be made between use of the term "fibrillation" in EMG to describe the activity of denervated muscle fibers and an older use of the term in clinical neurology to describe twitches of muscles visible through the intact skin. For the latter, which represent the spontaneous contraction of motor units or bundles of muscle fibers with intact innervation, the term "fasciculation," as proposed by Denny-Brown and Pennybacker, is more appropriate.

A muscle fiber that is not innervated, either because it is recently regenerated or because it has lost its innervation, undergoes spontaneous, rhythmic contractions. Although these contractions can be observed as a delicate, fine flickering of light reflected from the surface of an exposed muscle, they are not visible through the intact skin. Each of the contractions of a denervated muscle fiber is associated with a muscle fiber action potential. These regularly firing action potentials are called "fibrillation potentials." The appearance of recorded fibrillation potentials varies with the location of the needle electrode. The presence or absence of fibrillation can be determined only by inserting a needle electrode into the denervated muscle to detect the fibrillation potentials.

Fibrillation potentials are the smallest muscle action potentials observed in EMG. This is consistent with the view that they are the action potentials of single muscle fibers. Fibrillations may be recorded as either a triphasic spike potential or a positive waveform potential. They are usually brief diphasic or triphasic waves with an initial positive spike followed by a negative spike (see Fig. 15-22, B). The latter, most commonly, has an amplitude of 25 to 200 μV and a duration of 0.5 to 1.5 msec. The potential characteristically recurs with a regular rhythm (2 to 10 per second), although occasionally the rhythm may be irregular or interrupted or the rate may be rapid (up to 30 per second). Over the loudspeaker, the potential produces a sharp "clicking" sound. When present in large numbers, fibrillation potentials produce a sound like that caused by wrinkling crisp tissue paper. The positive waveform of a fibrillation begins with a sharp positive deflection of 25 to 200 μV followed by a slow return to baseline with or without a broad, low negative phase of up to 30 msec duration. Positive waveform fibrillation potentials can be readily differentiated from other types of positive waveforms, since they have the same slow, regular firing pattern as the spike form of fibrillation potentials.

Fibrillation potentials may be found in any disease that causes degeneration of lower motor neurons. The lesion may affect primarily the anterior horn cells, nerve roots, plexuses, or peripheral nerves. The occurrence of fibrillation potentials in nerve lesions is considered evidence of healthy denervated muscle fibers. Further details about the occurrence of fibrillation are found in the section "Sequence of Abnormalities of the EMG After Nerve Injury."

Fibrillation potentials are not found when atrophy is the result of simple disuse or when weakness is the result of disease of the central nervous system that does not affect lower motor neurons.

Although fibrillation potentials have been considered by some to be pathognomonic of lower motor neuron disease, potentials for the most part indistinguishable from those of denervated muscle are found commonly in polymyositis and dermatomyositis and occasionally in progressive muscular dystrophy. Because fibrillation potentials are found in some myopathies, their occurrence, by itself, cannot be used to differentiate neuropathic from myopathic diseases. The associated abnormalities of the EMG, particularly the character of the motor unit activity, and correlation of the EMG findings with the clinical examination are more important in making this differentiation.

Fasciculation

Fasciculations are twitches of portions of muscle and are visible through the skin or mucous membrane. They represent the spontaneous contraction of a motor unit or a bundle of muscle fibers and are accompanied by action potentials that are comparable in size to those of the motor unit. EMG may aid in the detection of fasciculation, since the action potentials of fasciculation may be observed when no twitches are visible, particularly when the patient is obese or when the fasciculation occurs deep in the muscle. EMG is also useful for the classification of fasciculations. Accordingly, they may be divided into two general groups: (1) those with a single action potential (see Fig. 15-22, *F*) and (2) those with a repetitive action potential (grouped motor unit discharge) (see Fig. 15-22, *G*).

The fasciculation with a single action potential is the commoner of the two types. Twitches of this type are brief and usually occur sporadically at rates of 1 to 30 per minute. They are found in normal persons. They occur also in irritative or compression lesions of the lower motor neuron, where they may be limited to muscles innervated by the affected nerves and thereby aid in localization of the lesion. Similar fasciculations are found occasionally in peripheral neuropathy, but they occur very commonly in anterior horn cell diseases such as amyotrophic lateral sclerosis and progressive muscular atrophy. In degenerative diseases of the lower motor neuron, an increased proportion of the fasciculation potentials may be polyphasic potentials and spikes of relatively long duration.

The fasciculation with a repetitive action potential is observed much less frequently than that with a single potential. It is a brief tetanic contraction of a motor unit that is more prolonged than the twitch associated with a single potential. Such discharges may occasionally be found with irritative or compression lesions (ischemia) of the lower motor neuron (such as nerve root compression, carpal tunnel syndrome, and hemifacial spasm) and in certain metabolic disorders (tetany, uremia, thyrotoxicosis) but infrequently in anterior horn cell disease. Similar twitches may be observed in otherwise normal persons. When they are numerous and relatively prolonged, they produce an undulation of the surface of the muscle, a condition called "myokymia" (see Fig. 15-25). Not infrequently in the conditions mentioned in this paragraph, motor unit discharges during voluntary contraction may have the same form (grouped discharges) as the action potentials associated with the twitches.

Thus far, attempts to distinguish, on the basis of their action potentials, between fasciculations that are "benign" and those that are associated with degenerative diseases of the lower motor neuron have not been rewarding. Fasciculations by themselves are not evidence of degeneration of the lower motor neuron. This diagnosis depends on the finding of fibrillation potentials in at least some of the fasciculating muscles. The significance of fasciculations must be determined from associated EMG and clinical findings.

Muscle cramps

In common muscle cramps, a more or less continuous high frequency discharge of motor units (up to 150 per second) involves a large part of the muscle (see Fig. 15-22, *H*). The discharge continues despite voluntary effort to relax the muscle. Eventually it becomes intermittent and stops. The discharge can be initiated by strong voluntary contraction of the muscle when it is in a shortened position and can be stopped by passive stretching of the muscle. Muscle cramps of this type may occur in such conditions as salt depletion and amyotrophic lateral sclerosis and in otherwise normal persons. The peripheral origin of such cramps is demonstrated by the fact that nerve block or spinal anesthesia prevents voluntary induction of a cramp, but a cramp can still be induced by repetitive stimulation of the nerve distal to the block.

The involuntary muscle contraction in rigidity and spasticity and in muscle spasm, as well as in postural contractions of muscle, is associated with asynchronous activity of motor units like that observed in a voluntary contraction. On the other hand, the delay in relaxation of a willed movement in myotonia is associated with spontaneous repetitive activity of individual muscle fibers, the action potentials resembling those of fibrillation rather than those of motor unit activity. In neuromyotonia, prolonged bursts of high frequency motor unit firing occur as a result of spontaneous activity in motor axons. The rate of firing (up to 200 per second) is often so rapid that only a fraction of the muscle fibers of the motor unit can respond and action potential of the unit decreases in size. In still another form of contraction disorder, delay in relaxation of a willed movement has no associated electric activity but is due to abnormality of calcium uptake by the sarcoplasmic reticulum. Electromyography is useful in differentiating the various forms of contraction abnormality.

Abnormalities of the motor unit action potential

Details of the duration, amplitude, and shape of motor unit action potentials are studied during a minimal voluntary contraction in which only a few motor units are active (Fig. 15-26). With increasing strength of contraction, the number of motor units recruited relative to the strength of contraction is determined, and finally during effort to produce a maximal contraction, the total amount of motor unit activity is estimated (Fig. 15-27).

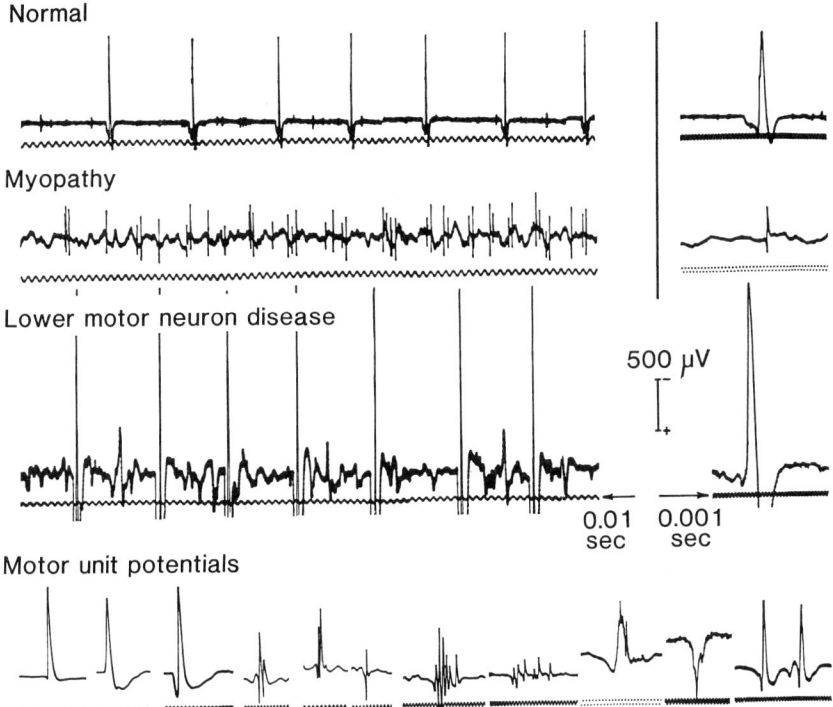

Figure 15-26
Motor unit action potentials during weak voluntary contraction (m. biceps brachii) in a *normal* person, in progressive muscular dystrophy *(myopathy)*, and in amyotrophic lateral sclerosis *(lower motor neuron disease)*. Action potentials on the *left* are recorded with a slow time base (time signal is 100 cycles per second). Action potentials on the *right* are recorded with a more rapid time base (time signal is 1,000 cycles per second).

Because of the wide variety in duration, amplitude, and shape of the action potentials of motor units in normal muscle, it is necessary to examine in a random fashion a large number of potentials in several areas of a muscle and in several muscles in different stages of the disease to determine whether a change in the mean value of these variables has occurred. Quantitation of motor unit potentials may be necessary for reliable evaluation. Careful study is rewarding, since differentiation of neurogenic and myogenic lesions usually depends on recognition of changes in the size and number of motor unit action potentials.

Form of the motor unit action potential
Although motor unit action potentials in normal muscle are most commonly diphasic or triphasic waves with a single negative spike, about 5% of the potentials, depending on the muscle studied, may be

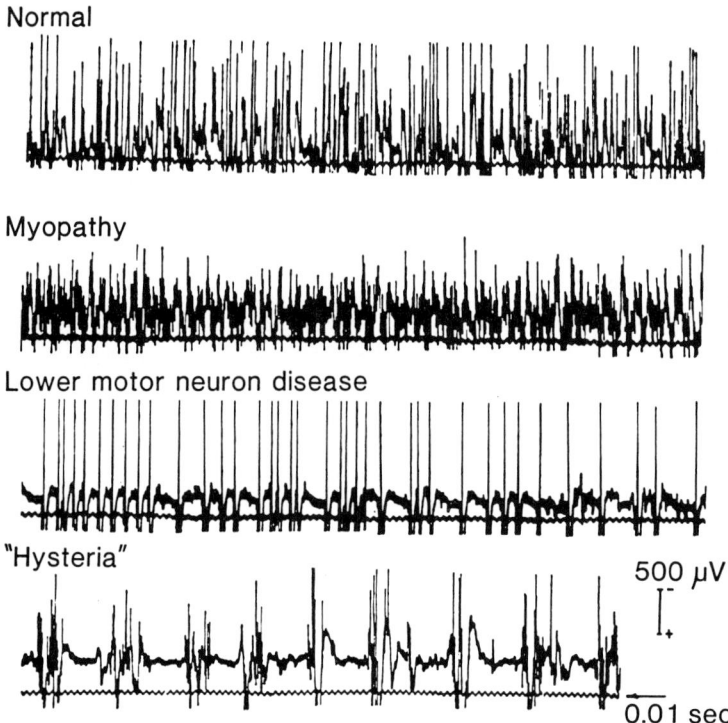

Figure 15-27
Motor unit action potentials during maximal voluntary contraction (m. biceps brachii). Compare with Figure 15-26. The record labeled *"Hysteria"* illustrates the irregular grouping of motor unit potentials associated with a tremorous contraction in a hysterical type of muscle weakness.

polyphasic, having four or more phases and two or more negative spikes (see Fig. 15-22, *K*). Spike components that are not fully separated are called "turns" but have a similar significance. Polyphasic potentials are the result of temporal dispersion of the action of separate groups of fibers of the motor unit, probably due mainly to differences in conduction time through the various branches of the lower motor neuron.

In many neuromuscular diseases, an increase in proportion and complexity of polyphasic potentials may occur as a sign of abnormality of motor units. The conditions in which this may occur form three groups: (1) primary muscle diseases, such as progressive muscular dystrophy, polymyositis, and myasthenia gravis; (2) degenerative diseases of the lower motor neuron, particularly in disease of the motor cells, such as amyotrophic lateral sclerosis; and (3) reinnervation of muscle after nerve injury or neuropathy. Complex motor unit action potentials with an increase in turns may occur as the earliest sign of reinnervation of muscle, in which case they have been called "reinnervation potentials," or action potentials of "nascent" motor units. These potentials have a low amplitude (less than 500 μV) and vary in complexity from potentials having two or three sharp spikes to highly polyphasic potentials (see Fig. 15-22, N) having as many as 15 spikes and a duration of more than 20 msec. They produce a characteristic "chugging" sound over the loudspeaker.

Size of the motor unit action potential
A reduction in the mean duration and amplitude of motor unit action potentials occurs characteristically in primary diseases of muscle and in other conditions in which the number of active muscle fibers in the motor unit is reduced. Other factors also may be involved. The action potentials that consist mainly of sharp spikes and polyphasic potentials (see Fig. 15-22, L) have been described as "disintegrated" or as being of a "myopathic type." Over the loudspeaker the short duration of the spikes of these action potentials causes a higher pitched sound than that produced by normal action potentials.

An increase in the duration and amplitude of motor unit action potentials occurs most frequently and is most marked in diseases that affect the anterior horn cells, such as poliomyelitis, amyotrophic lateral sclerosis, progressive muscular atrophy (see Fig. 15-22, M), Charcot-Marie-Tooth disease, syringomyelia, and tumors that affect the anterior horns. The amplitude of the action potentials observed during a weak contraction in these diseases is frequently 10 times the amplitude of action potentials of normal muscle. The large size of these action potentials is related to the large number of muscle fibers that contract more or less synchronously as functional units, as is evidenced by the occurrence of gross "contraction fasciculation" when these units are active. The large unit may represent a large normal motor unit whose action has been uncovered by selective destruction of the small motor units that usually initiate the contraction in normal muscle. On the other hand, histologic evidence suggests that as some motor neurons degenerate, the denervated muscle fibers are reinnervated by sprouts from the remaining axons, resulting in enlarged motor units. Early during reinnervation following nerve injury, the action potentials of immature motor units have a low amplitude and are sharp spikes and polyphasic potentials that may resemble the potentials seen in myopathies.

Number of motor unit potentials
In diseases of muscle in which the number of muscle fibers that function in each motor unit is reduced, the number of motor units that must be active to produce a contraction of a certain strength is greater than would be the case in normal muscle. In these diseases, the total number

of potentials associated with maximal effort may not be appreciably less than normal until many motor units have lost all their muscle fibers and the loss of strength is marked.

In diseases affecting the lower motor neuron, whole motor units are lost or become inactive, so that the principal feature is a decrease in total number of motor units active during maximal effort.

Rate of firing of motor units
The rate at which a motor unit fires increases with strength of contraction during voluntary effort. However, a single motor unit seldom is observed to fire at a rapid rate (more than 10 to 15 per second) in normal muscle, because, as the strength of contraction increases, additional motor units are recruited and their action potentials interfere with observation of the potential of a single unit. When the number of motor units remaining in a muscle is reduced, this interference is decreased, so that the activity of single motor units may be observed during strong volition. Under these circumstances, a rapid rate of firing of motor units is assurance that the patient is making a strong effort to contract the muscle, even though the contraction is weak. In the case of upper motor neuron lesions, hysterical paralysis, or limitation of contraction due to pain, the amount of motor unit activity associated with the weak contraction is usually like that of a weak contraction of normal muscle, with the motor units firing at a slow rate.

Rhythm of motor unit activity
The rhythm of activity of motor units in most conditions is regular. In fatigue and frequently in the hysterical type of motor dysfunction, the rhythm may be irregular, the motor units tending to fire in poorly synchronized groups, producing an irregular or tremorous contraction (see Fig. 15-27). In tremors, the motor unit potentials occur in more or less regularly spaced groups.

In latent tetany, motor units discharge rhythmically during voluntary contraction, but frequently each discharge is double or triple (Fig. 15-28). This phenomenon occasionally may be observed in certain other conditions but only to a minor degree in normal muscles.

Fatigue of motor units
Most often, fatigue during voluntary contraction of a muscle is associated with a progressive decrease in the number of active motor units without an appreciable change in the size of their action potentials. In some diseases, however, a progressive decline in amplitude of the potential occurs during continued contraction, as fewer and fewer muscle fibers of the motor unit respond to the nerve impulse (see Fig. 15-28). This may be seen in myasthenia gravis, particularly when weakness is marked, and, in some instances, in progressive muscular atrophy, amyotrophic lateral sclerosis,

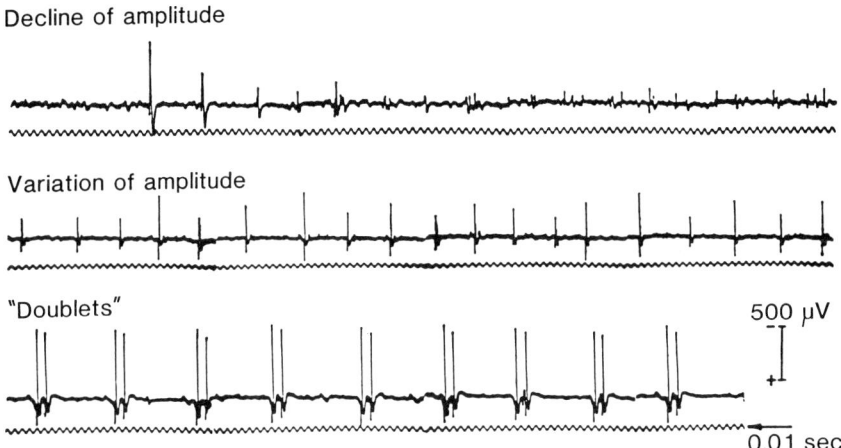

Figure 15-28
Motor unit action potentials during weak voluntary contraction. *Decline in amplitude* and *variation in amplitude* of motor unit action potential during continued contraction in presence of defect of neuromuscular conduction, as in myasthenia gravis. *"Doublets,"* rhythmic double discharge of a motor unit in tetany.

poliomyelitis, and syringomyelia. Occasionally in these diseases and during the early stages of reinnervation of muscle, motor unit action potentials are found to vary in amplitude and form from moment to moment. Variation in amplitude of the motor unit action potential is prominent in the Lambert-Eaton myasthenic syndrome.

With careful observation after a period of rest, a characteristic decline in amplitude of motor unit action potentials can be seen in myotonia congenita. The action potential reaches a minimal amplitude in 5 to 30 seconds and then recovers despite continued contraction.

Sequence of Abnormalities of the EMG After Nerve Injury
Successful use of EMG in the diagnosis of nerve lesions requires an understanding of the sequence of changes in the EMG after nerve injury. This sequence may be divided into three parts: the period immediately after nerve injury when degeneration of the nerve is occurring, the period of denervation after degeneration of the nerve is complete, and the period of reinnervation.

Immediately after injury to a nerve, the only abnormality of the EMG is an absence (complete paralysis) or a reduction (partial paralysis) of motor unit activity during voluntary effort to contract the muscle innervated by the damaged nerve. The insertion activity is normal, and no fibrillation potentials are present. The latter, which would be evidence of denervated muscle fibers, do not appear until the nerve has degenerated. Unfortunately, immediately after nerve injury neither EMG nor any other electrodiagnostic test can determine whether the injured nerve fibers are only reversibly blocked or are irreversibly damaged. The value of EMG at this time is in detecting minimal residual innervation, which may not be evident on clinical examination. The presence of a few motor unit potentials in a severe nerve injury indicates that at least a few nerve fibers are still intact. If anomalous or accessory innervation of the muscle can be excluded, evidence of some intact innervation may justify conservative treatment.

The earliest evidence of degeneration of the nerve is failure of the nerve to respond to electric stimulation below the site of injury. This usually occurs 3 to 4 days after injury. The earliest significant abnormality of the EMG usually appears 8 to 14 days after injury and consists of a transient appearance of fibrillation potentials after insertion or movement of the needle electrode (abnormal insertion activity).

Spontaneous fibrillation does not occur until 2 to 4 weeks (average, 18 days) after the nerve has been damaged. The shorter the length of nerve between the site of injury and the muscle, the earlier the spontaneous fibrillation begins. After a root lesion, fibrillation occurs earlier in paraspinal muscles than in limb muscles. Once spontaneous fibrillation has occurred, fibrillation usually can be found until reinnervation occurs or until the muscle fibers become markedly atrophic or degenerate. In partially denervated muscles, fibrillation potentials have been detected more than 20 years after the original injury or illness. However, in completely or nearly completely denervated muscle, fibrillation gradually decreases in amount and, in some instances, may be difficult to detect after 1 year. Abnormal insertion activity usually persists.

There are several reasons, therefore, why fibrillation may not be present in a muscle that is thought to be partially or completely denervated:

1. Sufficient time (2 to 4 weeks) for degeneration of the nerve may not have elapsed.
2. Damage to the nerve may not be so severe as to have caused degeneration (neurapraxia).
3. The temperature of the muscle may be low or its circulation poor. In this case, heat, massage, galvanic currents, and administration of neostigmine or edrophonium chloride (Tensilon) may be used in an attempt to stimulate fibrillation.
4. Severe atrophy or degeneration of the muscle fibers may have made them inactive.
5. Reinnervation may be in progress.

When reinnervation begins, there may be a reduction in the amount of fibrillation potentials. However, the earliest positive evidence of reinnervation is the appearance during voluntary effort of low-amplitude motor unit action potentials, many of which are highly polyphasic, others of which are diphasic or triphasic spikes of short duration (see Fig. 15-22, *N*). These may be present several weeks before there is clinical or other evidence of recovery of function. Appearance of a few polyphasic motor unit potentials, particularly when reinnervation apparently has been delayed, is a source of encouragement to the patient and is a justification for continued conservative treatment. However, serial examinations are necessary to determine whether reinnervation is progressing. As reinnervation progresses, motor unit activity increases in amount and the form of the action potentials becomes more normal.

Location of Lesions Affecting the Lower Motor Neuron

Electromyography can aid in the diagnosis of lesions affecting the lower motor neuron by determining whether evidence of denervation, in particular the presence of fibrillation potentials, is distributed widely or is confined to muscles innervated by a particular segment of the spinal cord, a root, plexus, or peripheral nerve.

Damage to a single nerve root causes denervation only in muscles that receive innervation from that root (Fig. 15-29). Electromyographic localization of the lesion depends on the finding of fibrillation potentials only in those muscles of the extremity that receive innervation from the anterior primary division of the spinal nerve and in the paraspinal muscles that receive innervation from the posterior primary division of that nerve. Similarly, trauma, infections, or tumors of the spinal cord that damage anterior horn cells cause fibrillation potentials to appear in muscles innervated by the segments involved. However, in some instances, when anterior horn cells are involved, fibrillation may be minimal and the extent of involvement may be indicated by the occurrence of large motor unit potentials.

When a lesion affects a nerve plexus or a peripheral nerve, fibrillation potentials are found in muscles innervated by the portion of the plexus or by the peripheral nerve that is damaged but not in the paraspinal muscles, as is the case in root or spinal cord lesions, and not in other muscles of the extremity innervated by other nerves.

It may be established, on the other hand, that evidence of denervation is distributed widely, as in polyneuropathy or degenerative diseases of the anterior horn cells of the spinal cord. Early in the course of degenerative diseases of the spinal cord, such as amyotrophic lateral sclerosis, the clinical evidence of degeneration of lower motor neurons may be limited to one extremity or a portion of it and thus suggest the diagnosis of a surgical lesion, such as tumor of the spinal cord or protrusion of an intervertebral disk. In such cases, EMG can contribute to the diagnosis by demonstrating that abnormalities characteristic of denervation are not limited to muscles supplied by only a few segments or roots and, consequently, are not the result of surgical lesions mentioned above.

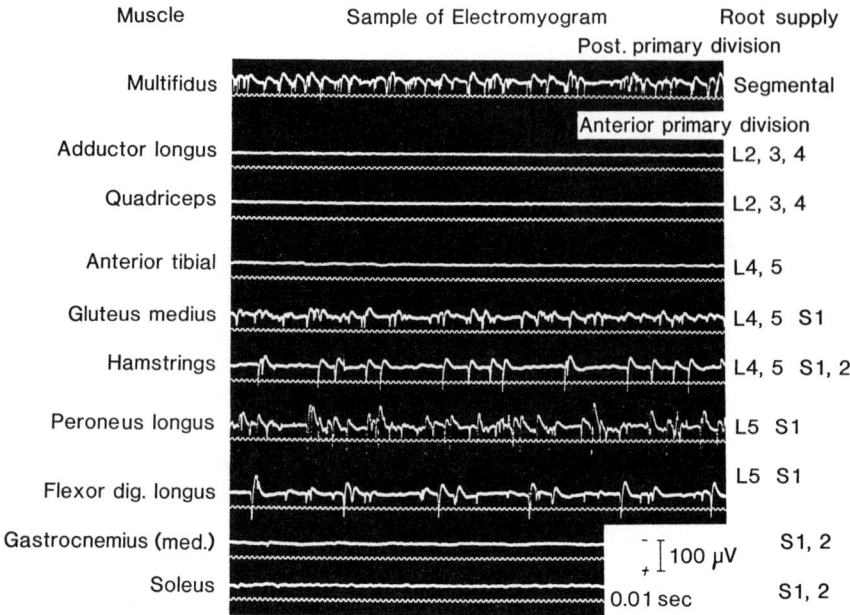

Figure 15-29
Electric activity after needle insertion in relaxed muscles of patient with a fifth lumbar root lesion. Fibrillation, predominantly positive waves, occurred in muscles innervated by this root. The anterior tibial muscle may in some persons be innervated exclusively by the fourth root. (From Lambert EH: Electromyography. In Youmans JR, editor: Neurological surgery: a comprehensive reference guide to the diagnosis and management of neurosurgical problems, vol 1, Philadelphia, 1973, WB Saunders Co., pp 358–367. By permission of the publisher.)

Differentiation of Primary Muscle Disease From That Secondary to Denervation

The character of the motor unit activity during voluntary contraction is usually the most useful aspect of the EMG for differentiating predominantly myopathic from predominantly neuropathic diseases. In myopathies, weakness is associated primarily with a decrease in size rather than a decrease in number of motor unit action potentials. The number of action potentials relative to the strength of contraction actually may be greater than normal. It should be recalled, however, that degeneration or blocking of conduction of some nerve terminals or neuromuscular junctions, as well as muscle fiber disorders, can decrease the size of motor units. In disease of the peripheral nerves and the motor cell of the lower motor neuron, the motor unit action potentials often are larger than normal as well as decreased in number.

This differentiation, though simple to make in most instances, can tax the ingenuity of the electromyographer. In any case, the pattern and degree of the abnormalities in all aspects of the electric activity of the muscle, including the insertion activity, the occurrence of fibrillation and fasciculation, and abnormalities of the motor unit action potentials, must be correlated with measurements of nerve conduction velocity and tests of neuromuscular transmission, as well as with the degree of weakness and atrophy of the muscles examined and with information about the duration and course of the disease, before conclusions are drawn.

Single Fiber Electromyography

Single fiber electromyography (SFEMG) records single muscle fiber action potentials of all types, including spontaneous activity such as fibrillation potentials and complex repetitive discharges. It has been applied primarily clinically in the recording of voluntary activity generated by motor units.

SFEMG enhances the recording from a small number of muscle fibers near the electrode while suppressing the activity of more distant fibers. There are two essential steps in this enhancement, both equally important. The first is the suppression of activity from more distant fibers by filtering low-frequency components of the electric signal. A 500-Hz filter effectively eliminates the contribution from fibers more than half a millimeter distant. The second step involves the use of a small recording surface (25 μm), which reduces the number of muscle fibers in direct contact with the electrode to one or two and decreases the effective distance over which the recordings from individual muscle fibers can be made to approximately 200 μm. The combination of these two techniques permits recording from individual muscle fibers that are within 200 μm of the electrode as biphasic potentials with rise times from positive to negative peak of less than 300 μsec, durations of 1.3 msec, and amplitudes up to 25 mV.

The recordings obtained with SFEMG can be accurately measured and quantitated. The ability to quantitate SFEMG measurements is one of the major advantages of this procedure. The small size of the active recording electrode results in some disadvantages, especially the need for extremely precise localization and holding of the electrode in a specific location while a series of measurements is made. Reliable SFEMG is therefore highly dependent on the electromyographer's skill at manipulation and control of the needle electrode. This skill is much like that required for the quantitation of motor unit potentials with standard concentric needle electrodes, and the electromyographer with the latter skill can usually perform SFEMG as well.

Since the recordings made in SFEMG are derived from the same potentials that make up the standard motor unit potentials, they can be directly related to motor unit potentials, but they include variables not commonly assessed on standard needle EMG. Four types of measurement are typically made during SFEMG: fiber density, jitter, blocking, and duration. Each of these is altered just as standard motor unit potentials are in a variety of neuromuscular disorders. Their abnormalities can provide important clues in the identification of specific diseases.

Fiber density

An SFEMG recording in most areas of normal muscle records an action potential from only one muscle fiber in a motor unit, since only one fiber is found within 200 μm of the electrode in most areas of a muscle. Single fiber potentials are under voluntary control and have the typical pattern of firing of motor unit potentials. At any one recording site, there may be 5 to 10 such potentials recorded from the different motor units whose muscle fibers are in the recording area as the effort of voluntary contraction is increased and as additional motor units are recruited. Approximately 60% of recording sites in normal muscle have such single potentials, but the percentage varies with the age of the patient and from muscle to muscle. At some locations, two single fiber potentials are recorded together, time-locked to each other. Such potential pairs may have intervals up to 10 msec between them (interpotential interval) but are usually within 3 msec of each other and commonly overlap to produce a notched potential. The interpotential interval between single fiber potentials from a motor unit has only a slight variation, the jitter (see below). Pairs of potentials are found in approximately 35% of sites, and three or more time-locked potentials are found in the remaining small percentage of recording sites.

Fiber density is the mean number of single fiber potentials recorded from motor units in 20 or more different recording sites. Normal fiber density ranges from 1.3 to 1.8 in normal individuals less than 70 years of age. Fiber density reflects the density of muscle fibers in one motor unit within the recording area and corresponds most directly to the number of notches seen on standard motor unit potentials (a feature of the motor unit potential sometimes called "complexity"), since each of these notches usually represents a separate fiber contributing to the motor unit potential. Fiber density has an indirect relationship to the percentage of polyphasic motor unit potentials, since in a polyphasic potential a phase may include more than one notch or turn. Satellite potentials seen in standard recordings also are recorded as separate single fiber potentials on SFEMG.

Since fiber density is directly related to the number of muscle fibers in an area that are innervated by a single motor unit, it increases with any disorder that results in histologic grouping of muscle fibers. Grouping is most common in neurogenic disorders with reinnervation, and increased fiber density is therefore seen in a large number of disorders of peripheral nerve or anterior horn cell. It is particularly striking early in the course of reinnervation, when the differences in conduction along regenerating nerve terminals result in marked asynchrony of firing of newly reinnervated muscle fibers and dispersion of the single fiber potentials. However, some grouping of muscle fibers may also be seen in myopathies as a result of fiber splitting or fiber regeneration after necrosis. Increases in fiber density are therefore also seen in a number of myopathies. Thus, while fiber density can quantify the severity of some diseases and their evolution, it cannot be used to differentiate the two broad categories of neurogenic and myopathic diseases.

Jitter

When two or more single fiber potentials are recorded from a single motor unit, the interpotential interval between them shows a small fluctuation called "jitter." This fluctuation is the result of end plate potential variation at the neuromuscular junction and is also seen at other synapses. The amount of neurotransmitter (acetylcholine at the neuromuscular junction) released varies from moment to moment and results in synaptic potentials (end plate potentials at the neuromuscular junction) of varying size. A lower amplitude end plate potential has a slower rise time to peak and reaches threshold later than a higher amplitude end plate potential, so that the interval of time from the action potential in the nerve terminal to the action potential in the muscle fiber varies by up to 50 μsec. Two single fiber potentials with no jitter are either time-locked by ephaptic (electric) activation of each other or recorded from a single fiber that has been split or otherwise distorted.

The normal muscle jitter of under 70 μsec varies with the age of the patient and with the muscle from which the recording is being made (Fig. 15-30). The normal mean jitter in the most commonly recorded muscle, the extensor digitorum communis, for individuals less than 60 years of age is between 18 and 34 μsec, with an upper limit of normal for jitter in potential pairs of 55 μsec. In normal muscle, the jitter is not identifiable on standard needle EMG.

Since jitter results from fluctuations in end plate potential amplitudes, any disorder that results in a reduction in the end plate potential will cause an increase in jitter. This is most often seen in disorders of neuromuscular transmission, such as myasthenia gravis, but may also be seen in disorders with ongoing reinnervation or regeneration, such as amyotrophic lateral sclerosis and polymyositis. Abnormalities of jitter, therefore, are not diagnostic of specific disease of the neuromuscular junction but must be considered in relation to findings obtained with standard electrophysiologic recordings.

Blocking

In a normal muscle, the end plate potential always reaches threshold and initiates a single fiber action potential; therefore, when multiple single fiber potentials are found, they occur with each discharge of the motor unit potential. However, if an end plate potential does not reach threshold or if conduction fails in a nerve terminal, one or more single fiber potentials would be missing with some discharges of the motor unit. These potentials are blocked. Blocking is measured as the percentage of discharges of a motor unit in which a single fiber potential is

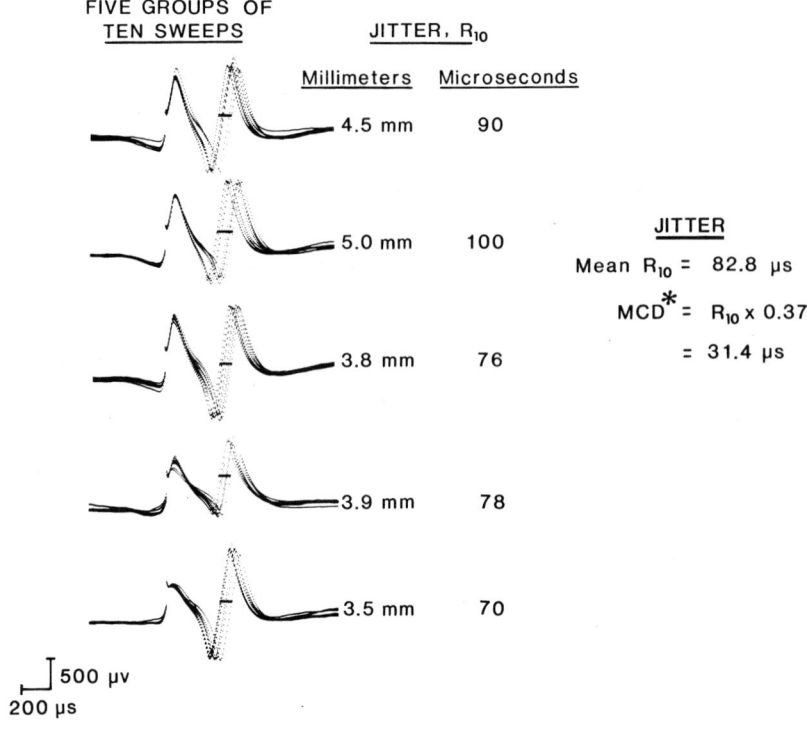

Figure 15-30
Manual measurement of jitter in single fiber electromyography (recording extensor digitorum). *MCD, mean consecutive difference. (Method of Stalberg E, et al: EEG 31:429, 1971.)

missing. A normal motor unit would have no blocking, whereas a motor unit in which a single fiber potential did not fire half the time would have 50% blocking (Fig. 15-31). Some elderly individuals may have normal occasional blocking in some muscles.

Blocking is usually due to inadequate neurotransmitter release. It is therefore most commonly seen in disorders of neuromuscular transmission, such as myasthenia gravis, and is evidence of a defect severe enough to be associated with weakness. As with jitter, however, it can occur in other disorders in which neuromuscular transmission may be impaired, such as amyotrophic lateral sclerosis, polymyositis, and ongoing reinnervation. It is not a reliable criterion of a specific disease. For blocking to be considered evidence of a disorder such as myasthenia gravis, it should be found in the absence of other electrophysiologic signs of neurogenic or myopathic disease. Blocking is also manifest on standard needle EMG, in which the blocking of individual muscle fibers

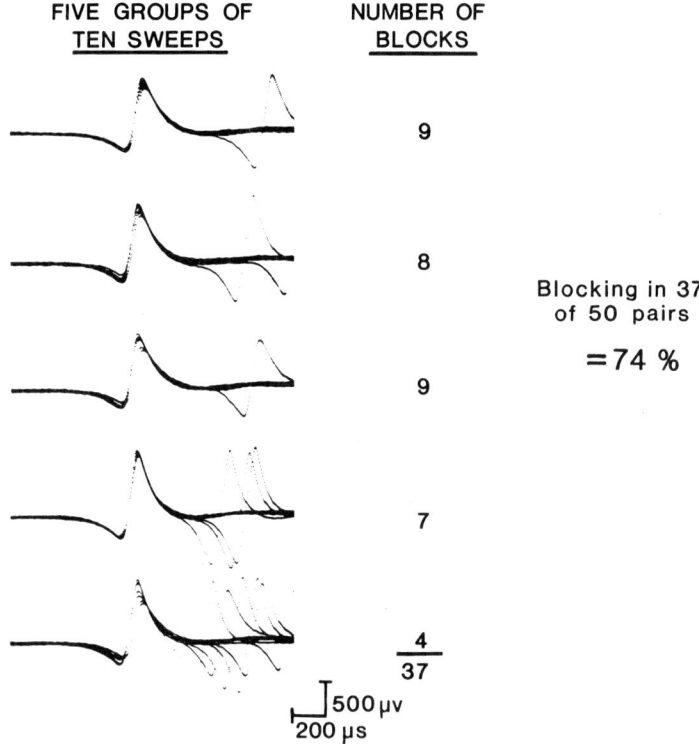

Figure 15-31
Manual measurement of blocking in single fiber electromyography (recording extensor digitorum).

in the motor unit potential is seen as a moment-to-moment variability in the motor unit potential. It should be expected, then, that whenever blocking is present on SFEMG, motor unit potential variability will be seen and the presence of motor unit potential variability on standard needle examination will be associated with blocking on SFEMG.

Duration

The interval between the first and last potentials of multiple single fiber potentials recorded from a motor unit has been measured as duration or mean interspike interval. The duration is the total time from the first to the last potential averaged for all multiple potentials recorded, whereas the mean interspike interval divides the duration by the number of single fiber potentials in each discharge. The mean interspike interval and duration might be expected to increase with any phenomenon that increases dispersion in the time of activation of individual single fiber potentials and reduces their synchrony of firing, such as differences in conduction in nerve terminals, spread of the sites of end plates along muscle fibers, or differences in conduction velocity among muscle fibers because of differences in diameter. Duration is therefore nonspecific but can provide useful evidence of abnormality of peripheral nerve or muscle.

Summary
SFEMG is a very sensitive method for identifying and quantitating a variety of disorders of peripheral nerve or muscle. The changes seen with SFEMG are nonspecific and must always be assessed in conjunction with standard electrophysiologic tests. The precise quantitative measurement of small numbers of muscle fibers within a motor unit is particularly useful for identifying a mild degree or early stage of disease, especially in disorders of neuromuscular transmission before they are manifest on standard electrophysiologic tests. In most of the disorders in which there are electrophysiologic abnormalities on standard testing, SFEMG will show changes that are not specific. SFEMG can also provide quantitative measures that can be followed during the course of a disease.

Recording Abnormal Movements
Voluntary and involuntary muscle activity can be recorded with electrodes placed on the skin. It is sometimes helpful to record this activity from several muscle groups synchronously to compare activity in antagonist muscle pairs and to compare the sequence of activation of muscles. This technique can be used to analyze tremors and other involuntary movements, many of which have characteristic patterns of muscle activation. In addition, it may be helpful to record muscle activity in myoclonus. The timing and duration of the bursts of muscle activity are useful in identifying the generator of myoclonic jerks.

SECTION III: NERVE CONDUCTION STUDIES

Conduction in Motor Nerve Fibers
Observation of the muscle contraction and measurement of the size of the muscle action potential produced by electric stimulation of peripheral nerves are useful as tests of function of the peripheral neuromuscular system. The presence, absence, or reduction of innervation often can be determined without need for cooperation by the patient. Conduction velocity can be measured as a test of function of the peripheral nerve. The location of a conduction block or segmental slowing of conduction can often localize a lesion along a nerve. Abnormal fatigability may be detected by repetitive stimulation of the nerve, and anomalous innervation may be detected by observing the responses of muscle to stimulation of a nerve.

Recording electrodes are placed on the skin over the motor point of a muscle (active electrode) and over the tendon of the muscle (reference electrode). Stimulating electrodes are placed on the skin over the nerve at the point to be stimulated. A brief pulse of electricity, strong enough to produce a maximal response of the muscle, is applied once to produce a twitch of the muscle or repetitively to produce a tetanic contraction. The response of a muscle innervated by the nerve can be observed visually or by palpation, or it can be measured by recording the compound muscle action potential (CMAP) with the recording electrodes (Fig. 15-32). The action potential is amplified and displayed. A stimulus artifact appears on the record at the moment of stimulation of the nerve, and after several milliseconds, the action potential of the muscle appears. The delay between stimulus artifact and action potential is the conduction time of the impulse along the nerve and across the neuromuscular junction. The CMAP represents the summation of the potential of all the muscle fibers that respond to stimulation of the nerve. Its magnitude is determined, in part, by the number of fibers that respond, but it varies with the position of the electrodes on the muscle, temperature, and the strength of the stimulus. Comparison of the responses to values obtained from normal subjects determines whether there is an abnormality. Comparison of the action potentials of corresponding muscles on the two sides of the body may aid in establishing the presence of a unilateral lesion. Serial records of the action potential may serve as an index to the progress of denervation in peripheral nerve disorders or of reinnervation after nerve injury or to progression or regression of degenerative diseases.

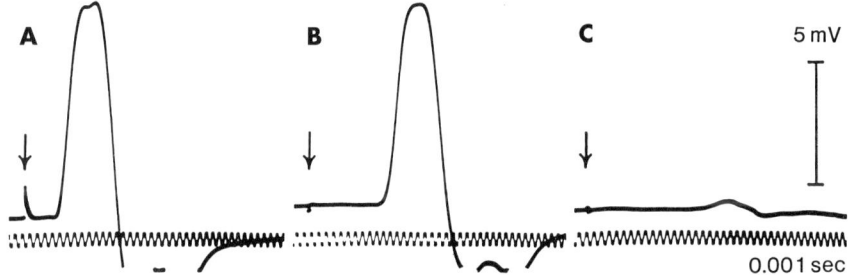

Figure 15-32
Location of the site of a block of nerve conduction. The action potential of the hypothenar muscles was recorded as an indication of the response to maximal stimulation of the ulnar nerve. A normal response occurred when the nerve was stimulated at the wrist **(A)** or at the elbow **(B)**. A greatly diminished response was obtained when the nerve was stimulated 11 cm or more above the elbow **(C)**. Surgical exploration revealed compression of the nerve at a point 10 cm above the elbow as the cause of paralysis of voluntary contraction. The stimulus artifact is indicated by the *arrow*. Time scale is 1,000 cycles per second.

Excitability of the Peripheral Neuromuscular System

In patients with paralysis that might be attributed to an upper motor neuron lesion or a conversion reaction, it is often desirable to establish simply whether or not the peripheral neuromuscular system is excitable. This can usually be done by stimulating the peripheral nerve in question. A normal response of muscles innervated by the nerve indicates that the cause of paralysis is proximal to the point stimulated, either in the proximal portion of the lower motor neuron or at a higher level in the central nervous system. If there is a lesion of the lower motor neuron proximal to the point of stimulation, a normal response indicates that wallerian degeneration has not occurred. The lesion in this case may be one that has caused only a functional block of conduction (neurapraxia). This may occur in acute inflammatory polyradiculoneuropathy (for example, Guillain-Barré syndrome) or as a result of mechanical pressure. On the other hand, the lesion may be more severe but so recent that wallerian degeneration has not yet progressed to the point that the nerve is inexcitable. The peripheral nerve may remain excitable for 2 to 3 days after an acute injury, becoming inexcitable before the appearance of fibrillation potentials in the muscle.

An absent or reduced response of the muscle may be caused by (1) inexcitability of the nerve at the point stimulated, (2) impaired nerve conduction below the point stimulated, (3) impaired neuromuscular conduction, or (4) inability of the muscle fibers to respond. Further tests are required to differentiate these conditions.

In some instances, it may be possible to locate the site of a conduction block by demonstrating that a response is obtained when the nerve is stimulated below, but not when it is stimulated above, the suspected lesion (see Fig. 15-32). This test is easy to perform at such common sites of pressure as the elbow (ulnar nerve) or head of the fibula (peroneal nerve) but may require needle electrode stimulation at sites less accessible to stimulation.

Magnetic stimulation of the central nervous system may similarly help localize damage to the motor system along its central pathways.

Conduction Velocity of Motor Nerves

The conduction velocity of motor nerve fibers is reduced in certain diseases that affect peripheral nerves. This is evident in the EMG record of the response to nerve stimulation as (1) an increase in conduction time from the point of stimulation to the muscle (distal latency), (2) an increase in conduction time between two stimulation sites on the nerve, (3) an increase in the latency of the F waves due to action potentials traveling antidromically up motor nerves to the anterior horn cells and then back to the muscle, or (4) an increase in duration of the action potential of the muscle due to an increased temporal dispersion of the action of individual muscle fibers when the conduction time is not

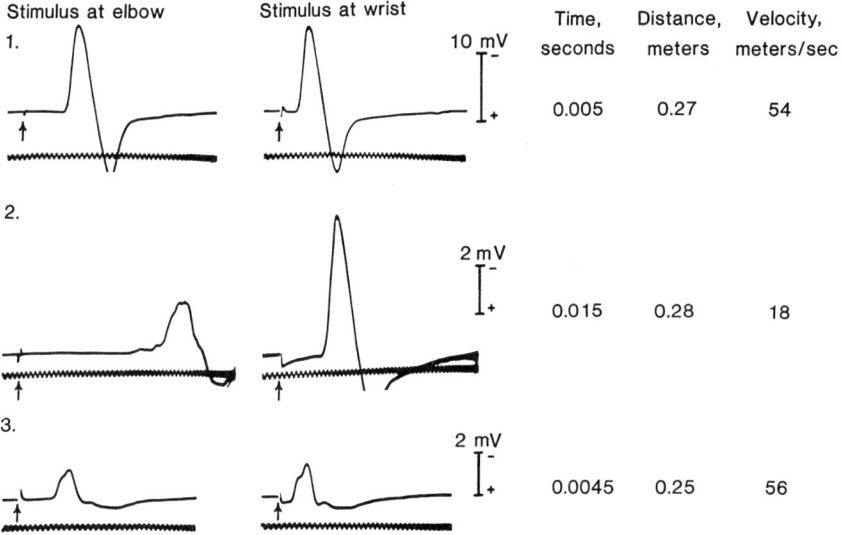

Figure 15-33
Measurement of conduction velocity of the ulnar nerve in a normal person (1), in chronic polyneuropathy (2), and in dermatomyositis (3). The action potential of the hypothenar muscles was recorded as an indication of the response to stimulation of the ulnar nerve at the elbow and at the wrist. The *arrows* indicate the stimulus artifact. The time scales are 1,000 cycles per second. The conduction time, conduction distance, and conduction velocity of the nerve impulse between elbow and wrist are indicated in columns on the right. The conduction time between elbow and wrist is the difference between conduction time from elbow to hand and wrist to hand.

uniformly decreased in all nerve fibers. Measurements of the conduction time, the duration of the action potential, the F-wave latency, and the conduction velocity between two points on a nerve are frequently of value in the diagnosis of neuropathies (Fig. 15-33).

No slowing of conduction velocity is observed in conditions such as polymyositis and progressive muscular dystrophy. In diseases that affect anterior horn cells, such as amyotrophic lateral sclerosis and progressive muscular atrophy, conduction velocities are within the normal range in more than 90% of patients, and rarely are they less than 75% of the average normal conduction velocity for the nerve tested. A marked slowing of conduction velocity, to between 5% and 60% of the average normal velocity, is found only in conditions that affect the peripheral nerve. Thus, a marked slowing may be found (1) during regeneration of nerve after nerve injury or neuritis, (2) in chronic neuropathies or polyneuropathies, particularly in primarily demyelinating disorders, including Guillain-Barré syndrome and certain rare hypertrophic neuropathies, (3) in Charcot-Marie-Tooth atrophy of the neuropathic type (hereditary motor-sensory neuropathy, type I), and (4) in areas of chronic nerve compression—for example, in the carpal tunnel in carpal tunnel syndrome.

The low conduction velocity observed during reinnervation of muscle after a nerve injury or neuropathy is related directly to the small diameter of the regenerating nerve fibers. Significant slowing of conduction in neuropathies is associated with segmental demyelination. The moderate slowing of conduction velocity observed in some patients with progressive muscular atrophy and other primarily axonal neuropathies may be due to selective destruction of the large-diameter, fast-conducting motor nerve fibers, so that only the slower-conducting motor fibers remain in the nerve; to secondary demyelination; and to decrease in diameter of axons.

Temperature of the nerve and age of the patient affect conduction velocity and must be considered in determining the significance of low values. Conduction velocity of nerves at birth is about half of adult values, by age 3 to 5 years increases to adult values, and after age 20 to 30 years slows progressively, becoming on the average from 5 to 10 m/sec slower by age 80. Because conduction velocity decreases with temperature ($Q_{10}=1.5$), it is necessary to warm cold extremities before study and to monitor temperature during the study to prevent cooling.

Late Responses

Stimulation of peripheral motor nerve fibers causes electrical impulses to travel proximally (antidromically) as well as distally (orthodromically). The orthodromically conducted impulse excites the muscle and produces the *M wave,* or direct response, which is used in standard calculations of amplitude and conduction velocity. The antidromic impulse travels proximally in the motor nerve fibers to the anterior horn cells in the spinal cord. When this impulse invades the axon hillocks, some anterior horn cells respond by depolarizing and producing an action potential. This action potential travels back down the motor nerve fibers and activates the muscle fibers innervated by the firing anterior horn cells. The resulting late response can be recorded from the muscle and provides a measure of conduction velocity in the most proximal parts of the peripheral nerve. The response is known as the *F wave.* Repeated stimulation of the motor nerve may cause different anterior horn cells to fire. As a result, the F wave varies slightly in its latency, morphology, and polarity (Fig. 15-34). F waves can be elicited in many motor nerves.

A second type of late response is the *H reflex.* This can be elicited in the soleus and forearm flexor muscles but not in other muscles in normal adults at rest. This response differs from the F wave in that the impulses traveling proximally are conducted in sensory axons rather than in motor nerve fibers (see Fig. 15-34). The impulses traveling in sensory

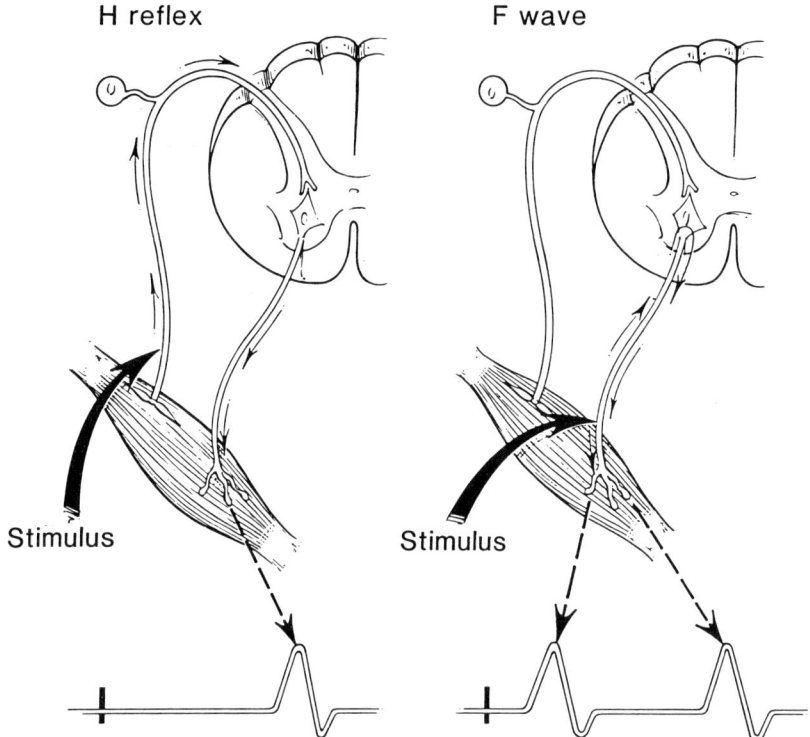

Figure 15-34
Schematic diagram of the origin of two types of late responses, an H reflex and an F wave.

axons stimulate anterior horn cells by way of synapses within the spinal cord. The H reflex can be differentiated from the F wave because the H reflex is greatest in amplitude at low levels of stimulation and decreases in size with increasing stimulus intensity. F waves are best seen with supramaximal nerve stimulation. The H reflex provides information about proximal conduction and may be used in the diagnosis of some radiculopathies.

When the nerve to an actively contracting muscle is stimulated, there is a brief pause in the electrical activity and the force of contraction of the muscle. This pause lasts for about 100 msec after the nerve is stimulated and is called the *silent period*. With small adjustments to the intensity of the stimulus and the effort of contraction, a brief burst of electrical activity occurs in the middle of this silent period. The origin of this burst is unclear, but it may be generated in a long loop pathway that includes the brain. This late response is seen about 50 msec after the stimulus. It has been called the "long loop reflex," the "C response," and the "M_2/M_3 response" by different authors. It is elicited most easily in contracting hand muscles. Some patients with disorders such as myoclonic epilepsy have this long loop response at rest. This is thought to be due to stimulus sensitivity of the hyperexcitable cortex or brain stem.

Motor Unit Number Estimates

Neurogenic disorders make up the largest proportion of peripheral neuromuscular diseases. The primary abnormality in many of these is a loss of axons or motor neurons. Needle electromyography, as described, can make judgments about the number of motor units still active in a muscle, but it cannot give numerical data like amplitude and conduction velocity measurements. A number of methods utilizing nerve stimulation and CMAP recording have been developed to provide such an estimate, referred to as motor unit number estimate (MUNE).

MUNE uses the same stimulation and recording methods that are used for the standard nerve conduction studies described earlier in this chapter. The methods are modified to allow an estimate of the size of the average single motor unit potential (SMUP) recorded on the surface. The size (amplitude or area) of the CMAP is known from standard conduction studies. Dividing the size of the CMAP by the size of the average SMUP gives an estimate of the total number of motor units in the muscles being tested.

The method is highly dependent on an adequate sample of the motor units in the muscle, particularly if there are units of different sizes (Fig. 15-35). The method becomes increasingly reliable as the number of motor units decreases. If fewer than 10 motor units remain, each can be individually counted to give an absolute value for the MUNE.

The average size of the motor units may be estimated by four different methods, each with its unique advantages. The methods are therefore complementary. The first method, and the simplest if the MUNE is markedly reduced, is a direct count by making small changes in the stimulus intensity just above threshold. This results in all-or-none increments for each new unit activated. The second method measures the average size of reproducible F waves. The third method averages a surface recording triggered by motor unit potentials recorded by an intramuscular needle. The fourth method estimates the MUNE from the variance of a sequence of CMAPs tested at axonal thresholds.

MUNEs are particularly valuable in defining the extent of loss of motor units in chronic neurogenic processes in which the loss of axons has been masked by reinnervation from collateral sprouting from intact motor units. MUNEs can also provide documentation of the rate of serial changes in a progressive disease.

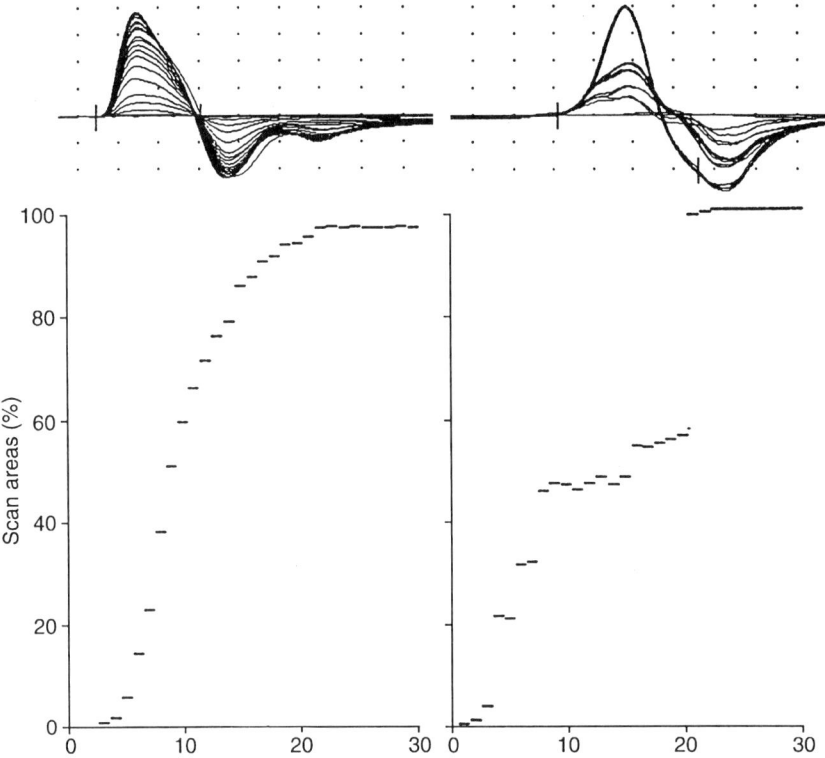

Figure 15-35
Normal *(left)* and abnormal *(right)* scans showing the compound muscle action potential recorded from thenar muscles in response to 30 stimuli with equal increments between threshold and maximum. In the normal subject, there is a sigmoid curve of small steps. In the neurogenic patient, there are marked irregularities, particularly a single large, all-or-none step at a high stimulus intensity along with the small, lower threshold steps. (From Daube JR: Estimating the number of motor units in a muscle, J Clin Neurophysiol 12:585–594, 1995. By permission of the American Electroencephalographic Society.)

Repetitive Stimulation

Abnormal fatigability of the peripheral neuromuscular system can be revealed by recording a CMAP during repetitive stimulation of a peripheral nerve. A decline in the amplitude or area of sequential CMAPs may be observed as progressively fewer muscle fibers respond to the stimuli that a normal muscle could endure for long periods. Repetitive stimulation of motor nerves has been used chiefly in the diagnosis of myasthenia gravis. In this disease, a characteristic progressive decline in amplitude of the first few responses is revealed at a stimulation rate of 2 per second (Fig. 15-36). The abnormality is characterized by the way it is altered after a brief contraction of the muscle. Three seconds after a

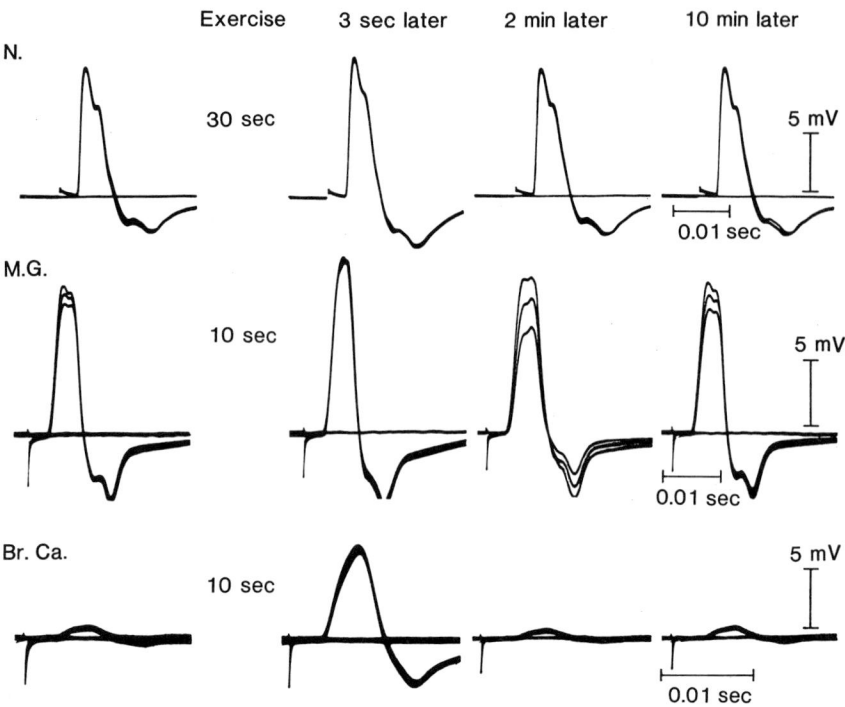

Figure 15-36
Effect of exercise on the action potential of the hypothenar muscles evoked by maximal stimulation of the ulnar nerve at the wrist. The response of the rested muscle *(record on left)* is compared with responses 3 seconds, 2 minutes, and 10 minutes after the end of a maximal voluntary contraction of the muscle. Each record consists of three superimposed action potentials evoked at a rate of 3 per second. N. designates responses of a normal subject, M.G. responses of a patient with generalized myasthenia gravis. In the rested muscle, a progressive decline of amplitude occurs during stimulation at a rate of 3 per second. Three seconds after exercise, this defect is repaired and there is some increase in the amplitude of response (post-tetanic facilitation). Two minutes after exercise, the defect is more marked than it was initially. At 10 minutes, the response is returning to its original level. Br. Ca. indicates a patient with the myasthenic syndrome associated with a small cell bronchogenic carcinoma. The slight progressive decline in amplitude of response during stimulation at a rate of 3 per second that occurred in the rested muscle is not evident in the reproduced record. There is marked post-tetanic facilitation 3 seconds after exercise, but a depression of the response is seen 2 minutes after exercise. (*From Lambert EH, et al: Myasthenic syndrome occasionally associated with bronchial neoplasm: neurophysiologic studies. In Viets HR, editor: Myasthenia gravis [The Second International Symposium Proceedings], Springfield, 1961, Charles C Thomas, Publisher, pp 364–410. By permission of the publisher.*)

10-second strong voluntary contraction, the amplitude of the initial response is increased and the progressive decline of amplitude during repetitive stimulation is diminished or absent (postactivation facilitation). Two to 4 minutes later, the defect reappears and is more severe than it had been in the rested muscle (postactivation exhaustion). The defect is repaired by drugs such as neostigmine and edrophonium chloride.

Although occasionally in myasthenia gravis the characteristic response to repetitive stimulation may be demonstrated in muscles that are not clinically weak, this is not always true. Care must be taken to test muscles most probably affected by the disease. Therapy should be withheld for several hours before the test unless weakness is definite. The test can be performed on cranial muscles and on muscles of the extremities that are supplied by nerves accessible to stimulation.

Although the pharmacologic tests described in Chapter 17 under "Myasthenia Gravis" are usually reliable and relatively simple to perform in the clinic, EMG tests for myasthenia gravis are a useful objective demonstration of the defect. They may be of particular value when the results of the other tests are equivocal or when an objective test is desired.

EMG tests are invaluable for diagnosis of the Lambert-Eaton myasthenic syndrome and for differentiating this condition from myasthenia gravis (Fig. 15-37). In the myasthenic syndrome, the initial action potential evoked in the rested muscle by a single maximal nerve stimulus is greatly reduced in amplitude. A transient further reduction may occur during stimulation at a low rate (0.2 to 10 per second). Striking postactivation facilitation, sometimes preceded by a transient decrement, occurs during stimulation at higher rates. Postactivation facilitation is 2 to 20 times greater than that in myasthenia gravis.

Unusual fatigability of the peripheral neuromuscular system can be demonstrated in other diseases. It may be found occasionally, but not regularly, in weakened muscles of patients with poliomyelitis, amyotrophic lateral sclerosis, and progressive muscular atrophy. This increased rate of fatigue and decrement with repetitive stimulation are observed during reinnervation of a muscle. A prominent decrement in amyotrophic lateral sclerosis is indicative of a poorer prognosis. The defect in these conditions is repaired to some extent by neostigmine or edrophonium chloride, but administration of these drugs seldom causes significant clinical improvement. In myotonia, a characteristic decrease in amplitude of the action potential, different from that of myasthenia gravis, is associated with the development of the myotonic contraction during repetitive stimulation of the nerve. Demonstration of these phenomena has not been of particular value in diagnosis.

Serial observation of the muscle twitch evoked by single nerve stimuli may be of value, especially in periodic paralysis. Phenomena occurring

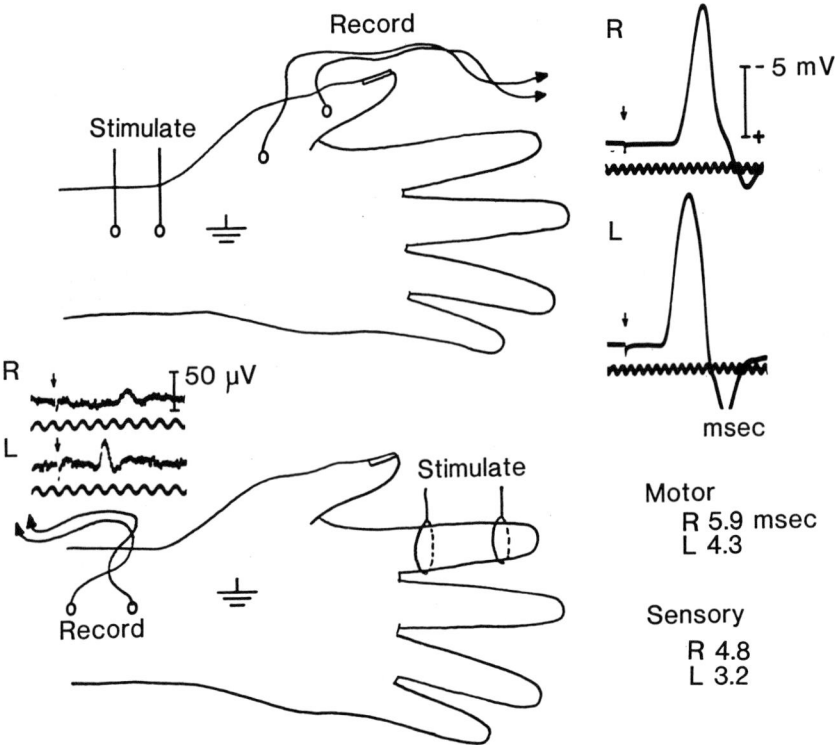

Figure 15-37
Latency of muscle and nerve action potentials in right carpal tunnel syndrome. Nerve action potentials evoked by stimulation of digital nerves in index finger are detected by surface electrodes over median nerve at wrist. The action potentials of thenar muscles evoked by stimulation of the median nerve at the wrist are recorded by surface electrodes over belly and tendon of abductor pollicis brevis. Latency of both responses (to start of muscle action potential and to peak of nerve action potential) is prolonged on the right side.

after exercise of the muscle and the paralysis produced by intra-arterial injection of epinephrine (in the hypokalemic form) may be useful in diagnosis.

Conduction in Sensory Nerve Fibers

Conduction in afferent nerve fibers is studied by recording the action potential evoked in a cutaneous nerve by a maximal electric stimulus. In cutaneous nerves such as the digital, radial, and sural nerves, the nerve action potential can be recorded consistently in healthy persons by electrodes at standard positions along the course of the nerve. The small triphasic action potential, usually less than 50 μV in amplitude, represents the action potential of large myelinated fibers. Components resulting from the small delta and the unmyelinated C fibers cannot be identified. The action potential, similarly recorded from mixed nerves such as the ulnar, median, and peroneal nerves, is composed predominantly of impulses in large afferent fibers that conduct at a velocity slightly higher than that of the motor fibers.

Reduction in amplitude, increase in duration, slow conduction (see Fig. 15-37), and absence of the nerve action potential are criteria of abnormality. Often, abnormality of the nerve action potential is a more sensitive indication of involvement of the large myelinated fibers than are tests of conduction in motor fibers. The cutaneous nerve action potential may be small, absent, or delayed in neuropathies even though the neurologic examination reveals little or no sensory deficit. The sensory nerve action potential is normal in myopathies. It is normal in diseases of the anterior horn cells, such as amyotrophic lateral sclerosis and infantile muscular atrophy, even though some slowing of conduction in motor fibers may occur in these conditions. The cutaneous nerve action potential is preserved in the presence of lesions proximal to the dorsal root ganglion; for example, it may be preserved despite loss of sensation after avulsion of the root.

Cranial Nerve Conduction Studies

The trigeminal, facial, and spinal accessory nerves are easily accessible for study in the EMG laboratory. The facial nerve can be directly stimulated at the angle of the mandible with percutaneous stimulating electrodes while recording is done with surface electrodes over the quadratus labii superioris group of muscles beside the nose. Measurements obtained 5 to 7 days after the onset of Bell's palsy or other acute injury to the facial nerve have been clinically useful in assessing prognosis.

Trigeminal nerve function can be studied by eliciting the jaw jerk in standard fashion with a reflex hammer designed to trigger a sweep on the oscilloscope. By recording over both masseter muscles simultaneously, the latencies of the masseter reflexes can be measured and compared. This may help localize lesions involving the motor root of the trigeminal nerve.

The trigeminal and facial nerves as well as their central connections can be studied by means of the blink reflex. This test is performed by stimulating the supraorbital nerve while recording from the orbicularis oculi muscles bilaterally (Fig. 15-38). Normally, an early ipsilateral (R1) response is obtained, followed by a later response that is bilateral (R2). Lesions involving the trigeminal nerve produce a prolongation or absence of the R1 response as well as the contralateral and ipsilateral R2 responses. Facial nerve lesions may produce prolonged or absent R1 and ipsilateral R2 responses, whereas the contralateral R2 response is normal.

The response can also be abnormal in lesions interrupting the central connections of the reflex arc. It has been reported by several

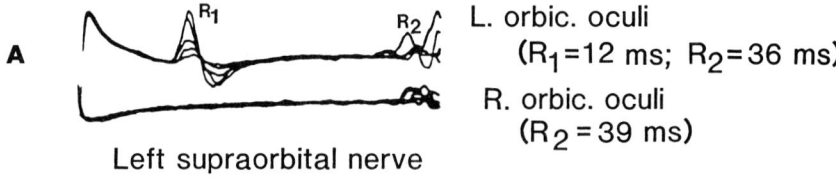

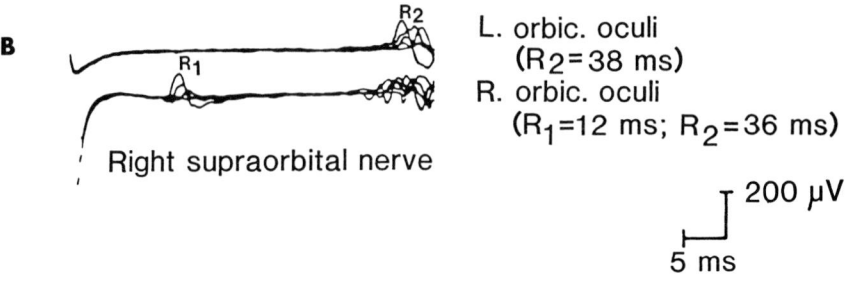

Figure 15-38
Responses obtained following supraorbital nerve stimulation in a normal subject recorded from both orbicularis oculi muscles simultaneously. Results were obtained **(A)** after left supraorbital nerve stimulation and **(B)** after right supraorbital nerve stimulation. The latencies represent the earliest deflection from the baseline. R_1, early response; R_2, late response.

investigators that the R1 response is prolonged in approximately 50% of patients with multiple sclerosis who do not have clinical signs of brain stem disease and is often prolonged with acoustic neuroma.

Spinal accessory nerve function can be assessed by recording a CMAP from the trapezius muscle while stimulating the nerve in the posterior triangle of the neck. This nerve can be stimulated for repetitive stimulation studies when a disorder of the neuromuscular junction is suspected.

SECTION IV: SURGICAL MONITORING

The brain, spinal cord, cranial nerves, spinal roots, and peripheral nerves can be injured during a variety of surgical procedures. Damage occurs by mechanical trauma or ischemia and frequently produces pain, functional disability, and cosmetic deformity. Electrophysiologic measures of ner-

Table 15-3 Modalities Used to Monitor Cranial and Peripheral Nerve Function During Surgery

Electromyography
Compound muscle action potentials
Compound nerve action potentials
Auditory evoked potentials
Visual evoked potentials
Somatosensory evoked potentials
Motor evoked potentials

vous system function help to avoid or minimize damage by providing information about the location and functional status of sensory and motor pathways within the central and peripheral nervous systems. Useful information is also obtained about the mechanism of injury when functional information is fed back to the surgeon immediately. Signals evoked by electrical, mechanical, or metabolic stimuli can be used to monitor the nervous system during surgery (Table 15-3).

Surgical Monitoring Techniques
Electromyography

Monitoring of EMG activity during surgery is best performed with fine wire electrodes placed in the muscles of interest preoperatively. With two wires in each muscle, continuous recording of EMG activity is accomplished with the same equipment and variables as those used in standard needle EMG. A variety of electrical discharges generated by muscle are observed and can be distinguished by differences in morphology, pattern of activation, and firing frequency of the action potentials. Table 15-4 lists the major types of muscle potentials encountered during intraoperative EMG monitoring. The most important activity is the neurotonic discharge. Neurotonic discharges represent high frequency bursts of motor unit potentials, which are generated in response to mechanical or metabolic irritation of the nerve that innervates the muscle. The occurrence of neurotonic discharges alerts the surgeon to the location of the peripheral nerve being stimulated and to the potential for nerve damage should the stimulation continue. Some potentials recorded during surgery are not generated from muscle action potentials and are artifacts. The most common artifacts are potentials generated by electrode movement or by an external electrical source. Equipment and fluorescent lights in the operating room also can produce electrical artifacts. Because of electrical interference, EMG activity cannot be monitored while the surgeon is using cautery.

Table 15-4 Types of Electromyographic Activity Recorded During Surgery

Activity	Frequency	Pattern	Morphology
Neurotonic discharge	50–200 Hz	Short burst or long trains	Single or groups of MUP
MUP activity	10–15 Hz	Semiregular and continuous	Normal MUP
Fibrillation potentials	1–5 Hz	Regular and continuous	Small single muscle fiber action potential
Movement artifact	Intermittent	Irregular	Triangular

MUP, motor unit potential.

Neuromuscular blocking agents may affect EMG recordings. In the ideal situation, a short-acting agent is given during induction of anesthesia and neuromuscular transmission returns to normal before critical stages of the surgical procedure take place. Although the absence of a blocking agent increases the possibility of unwanted movement during surgery, adequate levels of narcotic and inhalation anesthesia can sometimes eliminate this movement. At times, additional agents, such as fentanyl and midazolam, are needed to reduce background muscle contraction and the associated motor unit potentials. If additional protection against movement is desired, neurotonic discharges can still be recorded when a constant infusion of short-acting, nondepolarizing neuromuscular blocking agent is titrated to produce a 75% reduction of the baseline CMAP recorded over either a cranial or an extremity muscle.

Compound muscle and nerve action potentials

Compound action potentials recorded from muscle or nerve represent the temporal and spatial summation of individual muscle fiber or axonal action potentials recorded in response to direct stimulation of a nerve. The stimulus is usually electrical, but occasionally a more natural stimulus is used (for example, the nerve action potential [NAP] recorded directly from the auditory nerve in response to a click or tone-burst stimulus applied to the tympanic membrane). Either the stimulating or the recording electrode (at times, both) may be applied directly to the nerve within the operative field by the surgeon. These techniques help locate and identify nerves, locate lesions along the course of a nerve, and estimate the amount of nerve damage that occurs during the course of surgery.

Auditory evoked potentials

The auditory nerve can be monitored during surgery with brain stem auditory evoked potential (BAEP), electrocochleography (ECoG), and recordings of the NAP directly from the auditory nerve. Stimulation methods are similar for BAEP, ECoG, and auditory NAP recordings. Several types of ear inserts are available to deliver the stimulus. Some systems incorporate an external ear canal recording electrode into the earphone. Molded or foam inserts can be sealed in place with water-impermeable bone wax and tape. Square wave clicks of 100 to 200 μsec in duration are typically used as a stimulus. Placement of a short polyvinyl tube between the transducer and the ear insert reduces stimulus artifacts by producing a delay between the artifact and the arrival of the click at the tympanic membrane. Alternating click polarity (condensation and rarefaction) can also reduce stimulus artifacts; however, this cannot be used if one is interested in the cochlear membrane potential of the ECoG, because this potential changes polarity with a change in stimulus polarity. Stimulus intensities ranging from 60 to 80 dB SL (above the patient's own hearing threshold) are delivered to the monitored ear with white masking noise of 40 dB below that intensity delivered to the contralateral ear. The latter is essential to prevent stimulation of the contralateral ear through bone conduction. Reported rates of stimulation vary from 10 to 30 Hz. Stimulus rates that are fractions of 60 Hz may cause synchronization of the stimulus with 60-Hz artifacts and should therefore be avoided.

The BAEP is recorded from an electrode placed on the mastoid or external ear or within the external ear canal and referenced to an electrode at the vertex of the scalp. Adequate resolution of the five major waves of the BAEP typically requires averaging of 500 to 1,000 stimuli. This takes 1 to 2 minutes to accomplish. Wave I of the BAEP is generated in the most peripheral (lateral) portion of the cochlear nerve within the auditory canal. Wave II is generated either in the proximal (medial) portion of the auditory nerve near the brain stem or in the adjacent cochlear nucleus. Waves II through V are generated in the brain stem between the cochlear and inferior collicular nuclei and are recorded as far-field responses at the vertex electrode.

Recording of the ECoG requires placement of a monopolar needle electrode through the tympanic membrane into the soft tissue covering the bony promontory of the middle ear. With a reference needle electrode in the skin of the pinna or over the mastoid, near-field potentials can be recorded from the cochlear membrane and the lateral segment of the auditory nerve. Stimulus and recording values are similar to those described for BAEP, with the important exception that ECoG requires averaging of only 20 to 50 stimuli, thereby providing the surgeon with rapid feedback on the functional status of the cochlea and auditory nerve. The ECoG consists of two major waveforms: (1) the cochlear microphonics (CM) potential generated from the cochlear membrane and spiral ganglion and (2) the N1 potential, which is analogous to wave I of the BAEP.

The auditory NAP is recorded directly from the auditory nerve in response to an acoustic stimulus delivered to the external ear. It represents spatially and temporally summated NAPs within the auditory nerve. The recording electrode consists of a thin malleable silver wire with a small cotton pledget sutured onto a 2-mm segment of exposed tip. The electrode is placed onto the auditory nerve under direct vision after the cerebellopontine angle has been exposed. A small needle electrode in the subcutaneous tissue of the wound serves as the reference. When a click or tone-burst stimulus is delivered to the ipsilateral ear, a well-defined 10- to 30-μV potential can be recorded with only minimal or no averaging.

Comparison of auditory evoked potential techniques

Each of the three major techniques of auditory evoked potential (AEP) monitoring has distinct advantages and limitations. BAEPs are simple and noninvasive, can be used to monitor auditory function during the entire surgical procedure, and can monitor the entire segment of the auditory system at risk during posterior fossa surgery, from the cochlea to the inferior colliculus. BAEP monitoring appears to be a more sensitive indicator of damage to the auditory pathway than ECoG, because preservation of wave V of the BAEP at the end of surgery is associated with preservation of useful hearing in most cases. BAEP monitoring may be limited by low amplitude, poorly defined waveforms on preoperative baseline studies in patients with acoustic tumors, relatively long signal acquisition time that may prevent rapid notification of the surgeon about potentially reversible changes, and relatively low specificity compared with other AEPs.

The limitations of BAEP have led some investigators to use ECoG for intraoperative auditory nerve monitoring, particularly in patients with acoustic neuromas in whom waves II through V of the BAEP may be absent despite useful hearing. High-amplitude, reproducible CM and N1 potentials can be defined within several seconds in most patients, providing the surgeon with immediate feedback on the function of the auditory nerve. Preservation of the N1 potential has a high predictive value for preservation of gross hearing postoperatively. Most of the limitations of ECoG are technical. The proper placement of the electrode is invasive and time-consuming and requires experience. ECoG is also less sensitive than other AEPs. Patients have had hearing loss after surgery despite preservation of N1 during surgery. This occurs when the injury involves the proximal portion of the auditory nerve (near the brain stem) that does not contribute to the N1 potential.

The recording of an auditory NAP from an electrode placed directly on the eighth nerve in the posterior fossa is the most sensitive monitoring technique available. This technique provides a real-time monitor of auditory nerve physiology from the cochlea to the brain stem. Because of the limited space within the posterior fossa in patients with acoustic tumors, the use of direct auditory NAP monitoring is restricted to those with small tumors or to those undergoing microvascular decompression or sectioning of the fifth, seventh, or eighth cranial nerve. Some variation in the amplitude of the response occurs when the electrode is moved or momentarily covered with cerebrospinal fluid. This technique requires diligent cooperation and participation of the surgeon to be successful.

Pathophysiologic correlations
Mechanisms that produce a change in AEPs include stretch, compression, ischemia, and transection of the auditory nerve or the brain stem. Mild traction during cerebellar retraction produces a stable increase in the latency of wave V with no significant change in the ECoG. Moderate traction or contusion of the nerve may produce a reproducible change in the latency and amplitude of wave V, N1, and the auditory NAP. The magnitude of change considered to be significant is still a matter of debate. We consider an increased latency of 1.0 msec or more or a 50% reduction in amplitude significant enough to alert the surgeon. The surgeon must interpret the changes in the context of the surgical circumstances at that moment and options for the remainder of the procedure. Changes in the position of the cerebellar retractor or in the surgical dissection can result in reversal or stabilization of the AEP abnormalities. At other times, the BAEP is gradually lost despite efforts to modify the dissection. Severe contusion or transection of the auditory nerve causes a loss of wave V and the NAP. The N1 potential may be spared if the cochlear blood supply is preserved and the lateral portion of the auditory nerve is not injured. Avulsion of the nerve from the cochlea or interruption of the internal auditory artery results in rapid, irreversible loss of all AEPs and hearing. Even though changes in AEPs are not always reversible, correlation of AEP changes with surgical events helps to determine mechanisms of hearing loss. This information can be used to modify surgical techniques with the hope of preventing the recurrence of similar mistakes and improving the rate of hearing preservation over time.

Somatosensory evoked potentials
Somatosensory evoked potentials (SEPs) are recorded over the peripheral and central nervous system after electrical stimulation of a mixed or cutaneous peripheral nerve. The responses recorded represent activity in the proprioceptive system that is generated peripherally by myelinated, fast-conducting cutaneous and muscle afferent fibers of large diameter. Within the central nervous system, the SEP represents activity in the pathway between the dorsal column and the medial lemniscus, the ventroposterior lateral nucleus of the thalamus, and the frontoparietal cortex of the contralateral cerebral hemisphere. The spinocerebellar pathways in the lateral columns of the spinal cord and collaterals to the spinal cord gray matter also contribute to the SEP. With digital averaging equipment, electrodes placed over the peripheral nerve, spine, and scalp record

reliable potentials, ranging from 1 to 50 μV, that can be followed during surgery. The median or ulnar nerve in the upper extremities and the tibial nerve in the lower extremities are stimulated with surface electrodes. Recordings are made over the sciatic nerve at the buttock, the cervical spine, and the cerebral cortex. Surface electrodes are used to record cerebral potentials. Peripheral and spinal potentials are recorded with needle electrodes placed next to the peripheral nerve or bony lamina of the spine. Nasopharyngeal or esophageal electrodes are used to record spinal potentials during cervical spine surgery. Occasionally, sterile electrodes are placed on or next to the spinal cord in the surgical field.

Changes in the amplitude and latency of the SEPs recorded during surgery are produced by damage to the portions of the nervous system that generate them; by alterations in physiologic variables, such as anesthesia and blood pressure; and by excess noise at the site of recording. Changes related to noise and physiologic variables can be differentiated from those related to pathologic changes by paying close attention to technical aspects of the recording, by recording potentials at multiple sites that are both proximal and distal to the area at risk for injury, and by determining the effect of anesthesia and other variables on the SEP during parts of the operation that do not risk injury to the nervous system.

Motor evoked potentials

The motor system can be monitored by a number of modalities during surgery. EMG and CMAP monitor the peripheral motor axon. Motor evoked potentials (MEPs) measure the response of the motor axon or muscle to a stimulus applied to the central nervous system. The stimulus can be applied to either the motor cortex of the contralateral frontal lobe or the spinal cord. The cortex of the brain can be stimulated through the intact skull with high-voltage electrical or magnetic stimulation. Magnetic stimulation produces less discomfort than electrical stimulation in the awake patient because the high resistance and capacitance of the skull and scalp are bypassed. Magnetic stimulation may also be safer in the anesthetized patient because there is a lower risk of electrical hazard. Both electrical and magnetic stimulation of the cortex produce multiple descending volleys of action potentials in the corticospinal and other motor pathways that summate temporally and spacially on the anterior horn cells of the spinal cord. In the awake patient, a large proportion of the lower motor neurons within the cervical and lumbar segments of the cord are activated by the descending impulses, producing a well-defined CMAP in limb muscles. Unfortunately, all general anesthetics and induction agents significantly suppress the excitability of motor neurons at the cortical, brain stem, and spinal levels. As a result, it is difficult or impossible to record reliable transcortical electrical or magnetic MEPs during surgery unless special anesthetic regimens (for example, narcotic anesthesia) are used.

MEPs can also be recorded from limb muscles after stimulation of the spinal cord. The response is less susceptible to the depressant effects of anesthetics and very reliable. Stimulation is applied either directly to the spinal cord or indirectly through electrodes in the esophagus and over the laminae of the cervical spine. Unlike the case with SEPs, averaging is not necessary to record reliable MEPs over limb muscles. In addition, a constant infusion of neuromuscular blocking agent can be used to minimize patient movement without interfering with the ability to record reliable MEPs during surgery.

Visual evoked potentials

Visual evoked potential (VEP) monitoring has been reported to be of benefit in patients undergoing surgery for aneurysms or tumors in the vicinity of the optic nerve or chiasm. Despite the widespread use of VEPs in routine neurologic practice, the role of this technique in intraoperative monitoring has yet to be defined.

The difficulty in recording reliable VEPs intraoperatively is in part due to the use of an inadequate stimulus. Flash stimuli can be delivered through closed eyelids by a light-emitting diode array mounted on the interior surface of small goggles or by fiberoptic cables transmitting light through a contact lens. Care must be taken to avoid injury to the cornea with the latter technique. The VEP recorded after a flash stimulus is more variable and less quantitative than pattern reversal VEPs. Stimulation and recording requirements are similar to those used for standard VEPs performed in the nonoperative setting. The rate of stimulation used is usually 1 to 2 Hz. A single-channel recording with an O_z-C_z montage, a low filter of 5 Hz, a high filter of 100 Hz, a 500-msec sweep, and an average 200 to 300 stimuli is usually adequate.

The normal VEP consists of three major peaks (negative, positive, negative) with average latencies of 75, 100, and 135 msec, respectively. Because the VEP is a mid- to long-latency evoked potential, its amplitude and latency vary considerably with temperature, blood pressure, hypoxemia, inhalation anesthetics, barbiturates, and other central nervous system depressants.

Applications of Surgical Monitoring Techniques
Cranial nerve monitoring

Cranial nerves II through XII are monitored with one or more of the modalities outlined previously. The equipment used must be able to simultaneously record free-running EMG activity, CMAPs, and evoked potentials. This requires multiple channels (four to eight) that can be run at different sweep speeds, amplifications, and filter settings; be triggered by various stimuli or be free-running; and be averaged when necessary. The various modalities used to monitor different cranial nerves are outlined in Table 15-5. The types of surgery monitored are classified by location and the nerves at risk.

Table 15-5 Surgical Monitoring of the Cranial Nerves

Cranial Nerve	EMG	CMAP	NAP	Evoked Potential
II				?VEP
III, IV, VI	+	+		
V	+	+	?	?
VII	+	+		
VIII			+	AEP
IX, X, XI, XII	+	+		

AEP, auditory evoked potential; CMAP, compound muscle action potential; EMG, electromyography; NAP, nerve action potential; VEP, visual evoked potential; +, definite utility; ?, questionable utility.

Middle fossa surgery
Surgery in the region of the orbit, supraorbital ridge, cavernous sinus, or petrous portion of the temporal bone risks injury to the oculomotor nerves. Examples are tumors such as meningiomas, lymphomas, carcinomas, and pituitary adenomas and vascular lesions such as carotid and ophthalmic aneurysms. Especially in the case of neoplasms, the normal anatomy is distorted, making it difficult to locate and identify the oculomotor, trochlear, and abducens nerves. These nerves are monitored with EMG and CMAP. Intramuscular electrodes are placed after the patient has been anesthetized. Two nichrome wires are placed in the medial rectus muscle to monitor the oculomotor nerve, in the lateral rectus muscle to monitor the abducens nerve, and in the superior oblique muscle to monitor the trochlear nerve. If the neurophysiologist is unfamiliar with the technique of needle insertion into the extraocular muscles, an ophthalmologist can be of assistance.

Once the wires are inserted and connected to the amplifier, free-running EMG activity is monitored continuously for the occurrence of neurotonic discharges induced by mechanical irritation of the nerves being monitored. In addition, selective direct stimulation of the nerves within the surgical field with a handheld stimulator is used to differentiate the cranial nerves from each other and from non-nervous system tissue.

Posterior fossa surgery
The intracranial portions of cranial nerves VI through XII are at risk during a variety of posterior fossa surgical procedures. The most frequent procedure monitored is acoustic neuroma surgery, followed by microvascular decompression surgery for either hemifacial spasm or trigeminal neuralgia. The lower cranial nerves are monitored during surgery for lesions in the region of the jugular foramen, hypoglossal foramen, clivus, and foramen magnum.

Acoustic neuroma surgery. Cranial nerve involvement is common with acoustic neuromas, especially those over 2 cm in diameter. Hearing loss is the most frequent presenting symptom. Overall, altered facial sensation occurs in about 25% and facial weakness in 10% of cases, but in patients with tumors larger than 4 cm, 56% have loss of facial sensation and 31% have facial weakness. Electrophysiologic signs of facial nerve damage are present in an even higher proportion of patients, often without clinical symptoms or signs. The extent of abnormality is proportional to the size of the tumor and is an excellent predictor of the extent of postoperative deficit.

Facial and trigeminal nerve monitoring. As surgical techniques have improved, increasing emphasis has been placed on the preservation of facial nerve function after removal of an acoustic neuroma. The outcome depends mainly on tumor size and location and to a lesser extent on specific surgical techniques. Of patients with large tumors (over 4 cm), nearly 100% have complete facial paralysis postoperatively, even though the nerve is intact after surgery in about 10% of cases. The nerve is intact after surgery in 85% of patients with medium-sized tumors and in all of those with small (less than 2 cm) tumors. Nonetheless, 95% of patients with medium-sized tumors have some postoperative weakness, and 50% have complete paralysis. Of patients with small tumors, 20% have complete paralysis and 70% have some weakness after surgery. Fortunately, if the nerve is left anatomically intact, recovery of function eventually occurs in most patients. The trigeminal nerve suffers less damage at surgery, with only a very small percentage of patients suffering increased sensory loss over the cornea or face. Lower cranial nerve damage occurs even less frequently.

EMG and CMAP monitoring have been shown to improve the rate of facial nerve preservation after acoustic neuroma surgery. Recording electrodes are placed in facial and trigeminal muscles. Inadvertent mechanical stimulation of either nerve in the surgical field produces neurotonic discharges in these muscles. This reaction locates the nerve for the surgeon and warns of potential injury. In addition, the facial CMAP evoked by direct stimulation of the nerve by the surgeon is recorded from surface electrodes over the facial muscles. The surgeon uses the amplitude of the response to estimate the amount of damage that has occurred to the facial nerve during various stages of tumor resection.

Auditory nerve monitoring. The use of BAEP, ECoG, and NAP monitoring has improved the preservation of hearing in patients with small acoustic neuromas. In patients without hearing, monitoring is unnecessary, but if an AEP can be reliably recorded, monitoring should be attempted, even in patients with relatively poor hearing preoperatively. Should a contralateral acoustic neuroma or some other cause of hearing loss develop, even poor hearing is better than total deafness. We have found BAEP to be the most useful technique overall to monitor the auditory nerve during posterior fossa surgery. It has the advantage of monitoring the entire auditory pathway for the entire surgical procedure and does not require placement of electrodes in the surgical field. An external ear canal electrode referenced to a surface electrode at the vertex is used as the active electrode. In most patients with acoustic neuromas who have hearing preoperatively, waves I and V are readily identifiable by this method. BAEPs are recorded continuously and simultaneously with EMG monitoring once the dura is opened and the cerebellar retractor is put in place. Frequently, the latency of wave V increases at this point because of cooling of the nerve. If the amplitude of wave V begins to decrease, excess traction on the nerve is the most likely mechanism of injury early in the course of surgery. This can be corrected by having the surgeon reduce the amount of cerebellar retraction. Auditory NAPs are recorded whenever the surgical field allows reliable placement of the electrode adjacent to the eighth nerve at the brain stem and when the BAEP is too small to be followed reliably. The NAP is a much larger near-field potential, and therefore little or no averaging is required to record a well-defined potential. One disadvantage of the NAP recording is that it can only be monitored in patients with small tumors and during portions of the operation in which the auditory nerve is adequately exposed near the brain stem. In addition, the electrode can be easily dislodged or covered by cerebrospinal fluid, either circumstance causing the amplitude of the NAP to vary considerably.

SEP monitoring. Median SEPs are monitored in patients undergoing posterior fossa surgery if the function of the brain stem is at risk. This occurs in patients with large tumors that compress or infiltrate the brain stem or vascular lesions that produce ischemia of the brain stem. Changes in the SEP accurately predict brain stem injury in this situation. Unfortunately, because the SEP signal is transmitted through a relatively small area within the brain stem, significant injury can occur to ventral brain stem structures without a corresponding change in the SEP. When technically feasible, transcranial MEP provides a more reliable method to monitor motor pathways within the brain stem.

Other posterior fossa tumors. Neoplasms of the cerebellopontine angle (for example, meningiomas, epidermoid tumors, and metastatic lesions) are monitored with a protocol identical to that described for acoustic neuroma. Lesions in the region of the jugular foramen (for example, glomus tumors), foramen magnum (for example, meningioma), or clivus (for example, chordoma) may risk injury to the lower cranial nerves. The cases are reviewed preoperatively with the surgeon to judge which nerves are at risk and what types of monitoring will be performed. Often, EMG monitoring is combined with AEP monitoring and SEP monitoring in individual cases. The spinal accessory nerve is monitored by placing intramuscular wire electrodes in either the sternocleidomastoid or the trapezius muscle. The laryngeal nerves are monitored by placing electrodes in the cricothyroid or vocalis muscles. The latter technique utilizes long wires placed by the otorhinolaryngologic surgeon by direct laryngoscopy. The hypoglossal nerve is monitored with electrodes placed in the tongue through the submental approach. All the lower cranial nerves are monitored for neurotonic discharges, and direct stimulation is used to identify each nerve intraoperatively.

Microvascular decompression surgery. Microvascular decompression (MVD) is a common treatment for trigeminal neuralgia and hemifacial spasm and is sometimes used in chronic vertigo. During each of these procedures there is a slight risk of facial nerve injury and a 10% to 15% risk of hearing loss. We perform AEP and facial nerve monitoring in all cases. Neurotonic discharges are noted, especially in patients with hemifacial spasm, when the facial nerve is mechanically stimulated. As is the case with acoustic neuromas, nonspecific latency changes in wave V of the BAEP occur with nerve cooling after the dura is opened. The most common mechanism of auditory nerve injury in MVD is nerve stretch that occurs when too much traction is applied to the cerebellum. Studies have shown that AEP monitoring reduces the risk of hearing loss in patients undergoing MVD surgery.

An additional method of monitoring used in patients with hemifacial spasm helps the surgeon determine when adequate decompression of the facial nerve has been achieved. In patients with hemifacial spasm, a reflex potential can be recorded in one facial muscle in response to an antidromic stimulus applied to a different branch of the facial nerve. The response is a 100- to 200-μV CMAP that follows the stimulus by 7 to 10 msec. This response, which has been called the "lateral spread response," may arise either by ephaptic activation of adjacent facial nerve axons at the site of vascular compression outside the brain stem or by hyperexcitability of the facial nucleus within the brain stem. The lateral spread response is obtained by application of an electrical stimulus (0.1 msec duration, 5 to 15 mA) to either the mandibular or the zygomatic branch of the facial nerve. The stimulus can be applied with either surface or small subcutaneous needle electrodes. When the stimulus is applied to the lower face (mandibular branch), the reflex response is recorded from the orbicularis oculi muscle. When the stimulus is applied to the upper face, the reflex response is recorded from either the orbicularis oris or the mentalis muscle. During surgery, the same wire electrodes that are in place for EMG monitoring can be used to record the lateral spread response. The lateral spread response persists under general anesthesia but is somewhat variable from one stimulus to the next, especially in patients whose hemifacial spasm is mild and intermittent preoperatively. The response is monitored throughout surgery. When the offending vessel has been removed from the nerve, the lateral spread response disappears completely. In most cases, this occurs immediately, and when the vessel is allowed to touch the nerve again, the lateral spread response quickly returns. In patients with mild and intermittent hemifacial spasm preoperatively, the lateral spread response may disappear when the dura is opened or when cerebrospinal fluid is drained. This presumably occurs because of changes in the orientation or pressure of the vessel on the surface of the facial nerve. The absence of the lateral spread response at the end of the operation accurately predicts the absence of clinical spasms postoperatively.

Surgery is sometimes performed to section the glossopharyngeal and sensory portions of the vagus nerve in patients with intractable glossopharyngeal neuralgia. During this operation, it may be difficult for the surgeon to tell where the rootlets that constitute the glossopharyngeal and sensory vagal nerves end and those that constitute the motor vagal nerve begin. We currently monitor such cases by placing intramuscular wire electrodes in the cricothyroid or the vocalis muscle (or both), both of which are innervated by the vagus nerve. With a small electrical stimulator, the surgeon is able to identify and avoid sectioning components of the vagus nerve.

Extracranial surgery
The extracranial portions of the facial and laryngeal nerves are at risk during various types of head and neck surgery. During surgery, the facial nerve is monitored in the region of the parotid gland. Intramuscular wire electrodes are placed in the frontalis, orbicularis oculi, orbicularis oris, and mentalis muscles so that each of the major branches of the facial nerve can be monitored. The wire electrodes are inserted near the midline of the face, with the recording connections made on the side contralateral to the operation to keep the recording system away from the surgical field. EMG activity is monitored continuously for neurotonic discharges, and intermittent direct electrical stimulation is performed to help identify branches of the facial nerve.

The superior and recurrent laryngeal nerves are monitored during complicated neck dissections, such as those for recurrent thyroid cancer. Monitoring of these nerves during carotid endarterectomy has also been described. Intramuscular electrodes are placed into the cricothyroid and vocalis muscles. EMG activity is monitored continuously, and direct electrical stimulation is applied as outlined for other cranial nerves above.

Peripheral nerve monitoring
Peripheral nerve repair
EMG, NAP, CMAP, and SEP recordings are used during exploration and repair of traumatic injuries to the brachial plexus or other peripheral nerves and during the surgical release of entrapment neuropathies. Intramuscular wire electrodes placed in muscles innervated by the nerve being monitored are used to record neurotonic discharges when the nerve is

mechanically stimulated. Nerve conduction studies are performed with stimulation or recording of NAP and CMAP directly from the exposed neural elements. Short segmental stimulation can be performed in a search for areas of focal slowing of conduction or conduction block. NAP recordings made over short segments are used to detect early signs of reinnervation across traumatic areas. SEP recordings made over the brain and spinal cord after stimulation of individual nerve roots or elements help determine whether root avulsion is present in traumatic brachial plexus injury. These intraoperative studies complement preoperative nerve conduction studies and needle EMG studies. They provide information about the number, location, severity, and types of lesions affecting the peripheral nerve. The surgeon uses this information to confirm the underlying cause of the neuropathy and to guide appropriate therapy (such as release of an entrapped nerve, neurolysis, or nerve graft).

Peripheral nerve tumors
Neoplasms of the peripheral nervous system are a rare but challenging surgical problem. Metastatic and primary nerve sheath tumors invade the peripheral nerve, with tumor cells interdigitated between normal and nonfunctioning nerve fascicles. The goal of surgery is to remove as much of the tumor as possible and to preserve the normal axons traversing the area of involvement. The normal axons can be identified by stimulating individual nerve fascicles during tumor dissection and removal. The stimulation can be mechanical, which produces neurotonic discharges in distal muscles innervated by the nerve. Alternatively, an electrical stimulus is delivered by small, specially designed stimulating electrodes that can selectively activate small nerve fascicles. Electrical stimulation of a normal fascicle produces a small CMAP in a distal muscle, whereas stimulation of diseased fascicles elicits no response. The diseased fascicles are sacrificed, and, if possible, the normal fascicles are preserved.

Monitoring during spine surgery
Cervical spine
The spinal cord and cervical nerve roots are at risk during cervical spine fusion, decompressive laminectomy, removal or biopsy of spinal neoplasms, and decompression of syringomyelia. The spinal cord is monitored with upper and lower extremity SEP. The ulnar or median nerve is stimulated in the upper extremity, and the tibial nerve is stimulated in each lower extremity. Recordings are made from the cervical spinal cord through an electrode in the nasopharynx or esophagus. Cortical responses are recorded with electrodes over the scalp. In most cases, compression, contusion, or ischemia of the spinal cord occurring during surgery is indicated by a change in the amplitude and latency of the SEP. Often, the surgeon can alter the course of surgery to reverse or prevent further change in the SEP. If changes occur that cannot be reversed, new neurologic

deficits can be expected postoperatively. In general, changes in the SEP correlate well with both sensory and motor function within the spinal cord. Occasionally, motor structures within the cord are damaged without a corresponding change in the SEP. MEP would theoretically eliminate this problem by monitoring both the upper and the lower motor neurons within the spinal cord. This technique is currently under development but is not in routine use for cervical spinal cord monitoring. The function of anterior horn cells and nerve roots within the cervical spinal segments can be monitored with EMG. Intramuscular wire electrodes in upper limb muscles record neurotonic discharges when nerve roots or anterior horn cells are mechanically stimulated during surgery. This alerts the surgeon to the possibility of iatrogenic injury to these structures.

Thoracolumbar spine
The thoracic spinal cord is monitored during scoliosis surgery, removal of spinal neoplasms or vascular malformations, repair of spinal trauma, and repair of a thoracoabdominal aneurysm. SEP and MEP are used to monitor the thoracic spinal cord. For SEP, the tibial nerves are stimulated in the lower extremities with recordings made over the sciatic nerve at the buttock, the cervical spine, and the cerebral cortex. For MEP, the cervical spinal cord is stimulated with recordings of CMAPs over lower limb muscles. A constant infusion of neuromuscular blocking agent is used to minimize movement during MEP recordings. When changes occur during scoliosis surgery, alteration in the degree of spinal distraction often results in a return of normal function. In cases of trauma, arteriovenous malformations, or spinal neoplasms, the surgeon may alter the approach to surgery in an attempt to reverse any changes in the SEP or MEP that occur during surgery. Early disappearance of the MEP in thoracoabdominal aneurysm repair accurately predicts postoperative paraplegia. Sometimes shunting procedures can be performed to restore blood flow to the spinal cord while the aneurysm is being repaired.

The lumbar spinal cord is at risk during the same types of surgery listed for thoracic spine surgery. In addition, lower motor neuron elements within the spinal cord or cauda equina are at risk and can be monitored with EMG and CMAP recordings. Lesions in the region of the conus or cauda are monitored with intramuscular wire electrodes in muscles innervated by lumbosacral nerve roots, including the anal sphincter muscle. Neurotonic discharges and direct stimulation are used to identify, locate, and prevent injury to neural elements. Simultaneously, SEP and MEP are used to monitor central nervous system elements within the lumbar spinal cord. Electrical stimulation is also used to identify and prevent injury to nerve roots during the insertion of pedicle screws and other elements of spinal instrumentation in the lumbar area.

Monitoring during cerebral surgery
Stereotactic thalamotomy or pallidotomy
Stereotactic lesions are currently being placed in the thalamus and globus pallidus as adjunctive therapy to medications in selected patients with Parkinson's disease and other movement disorders. Semimicroelectrode or microelectrode recordings of neuronal activity in the thalamus and globus pallidus are used to map the somatotopic organization within and confirm the outside boundaries of the thalamus and globus pallidus. This information is vital in making sure that the lesion produces the desired effect while minimizing the risk of complications.

Cortical mapping
SEPs are used to map out the somatotopic organization of the sensory cortex and to identify the location of the rolandic fissure during epilepsy and lesion surgery involving the cerebral hemispheres. This information supplements information obtained from imaging studies and EEG recordings made from surface or depth electrodes at the time of surgery. The surgeon uses this information to plan resection of the epileptogenic area or lesion without damaging the surrounding normal areas of brain.

SECTION V: SOMATOSENSORY SYSTEM TESTING

Sensory nerve conduction studies described in Section II test the large afferent fibers of the somatosensory system in the periphery and can provide valuable evidence of peripheral nerve or dorsal root ganglion disease. However, since the central and peripheral axons of the dorsal root ganglion are independent, damage to the central segments of the somatosensory system does not result in any changes in peripheral nerve conduction studies. SEPs generated by the spinal cord and brain in response to peripheral stimulation and recorded from the surface can help identify and characterize central sensory disorders.

Averaging
The generators of the SEPs in the central nervous system give rise to lower amplitude potentials than peripheral nerves because they are at a much greater distance from the recording electrodes. SEPs are only several microvolts in amplitude, many orders of magnitude smaller than artifacts generated by overlying muscle tissue and by electrical sources. They cannot, therefore, be detected with a single stimulus. SEP recording requires applying multiple stimuli (a thousand or more) and averaging the voltage at each instant in time. This increases the signal-to-noise ratio by canceling the random noise while enhancing the time-locked SEP. Tracings from two separate averages are superimposed, and peaks that are reproducible can be used for interpretation. Sedation given before the study reduces muscle artifacts.

Nomenclature

The nerve action potential recorded from a peripheral nerve is a simple triphasic waveform. Multiple generators contribute to the SEPs recorded from the central nervous system, so that the waveform is complex with multiple peaks. The evoked potentials are named on the basis of their polarity, N (negative) or P (positive), and their time of occurrence in normal persons. The nomenclature of SEP waveforms is not yet universally agreed on.

Nerve action potentials that travel along nerves or fiber tracts are called *traveling waves*. Potentials that remain localized in areas of nuclei or synapses are called *stationary waves*. A *near-field potential* is a propagating nerve action potential recorded as the impulse passes under the recording electrodes. Routine nerve conduction studies primarily record the near-field potential. The term *far-field potential* refers to a stationary potential generated by a nerve action potential distant from the recording site. A referential montage, such as the scalp to Erb's point, preferentially detects far-field potentials.

Stimulation Methods

Mixed nerve stimulation produces the largest, most reliable potentials that can be recorded over the spine and the scalp. The nerves most often stimulated are the median and ulnar nerves at the wrist and the tibial nerve at the ankle. The low current intensities necessary for well-developed responses produce a small visible twitch of the muscle. Higher stimulus intensities are not needed and simply increase muscle artifacts. In the upper extremity, a repetition rate of 2 to 5 Hz is well tolerated, whereas in the lower extremity, rates of 1 to 2 Hz are used. Responses recorded after *cutaneous nerve stimulation* are much smaller and generally obtained only at the scalp. For example, the skin of the thigh can be stimulated to evaluate suspected entrapment of the lateral femoral cutaneous nerve. To study patients with lumbosacral and cervical radiculopathies, the examiner must stimulate peripheral nerves supplied by one nerve root, for example, the saphenous nerve for evaluation of L-4, the sural nerve for S-1, and the little finger for C-8. A patient with spinal stenosis may require multiple *dermatomal* or *segmental sensory* SEPs for full evaluation.

Origin of SEP Waveforms

The low stimulus intensities used to obtain SEPs primarily excite large myelinated fibers in the peripheral nerve, especially proprioceptive afferents. These fibers have their cell bodies in the dorsal root ganglia, and the central processes ascend in the dorsal column-medial lemniscal pathway to the ventroposterior lateral nucleus of the thalamus. Third-order neurons ascend through the internal capsule to the cerebral cortex.

The SEPs recorded after stimulation of the median and ulnar nerves include N9, generated by fibers in the brachial plexus; N11, arising from

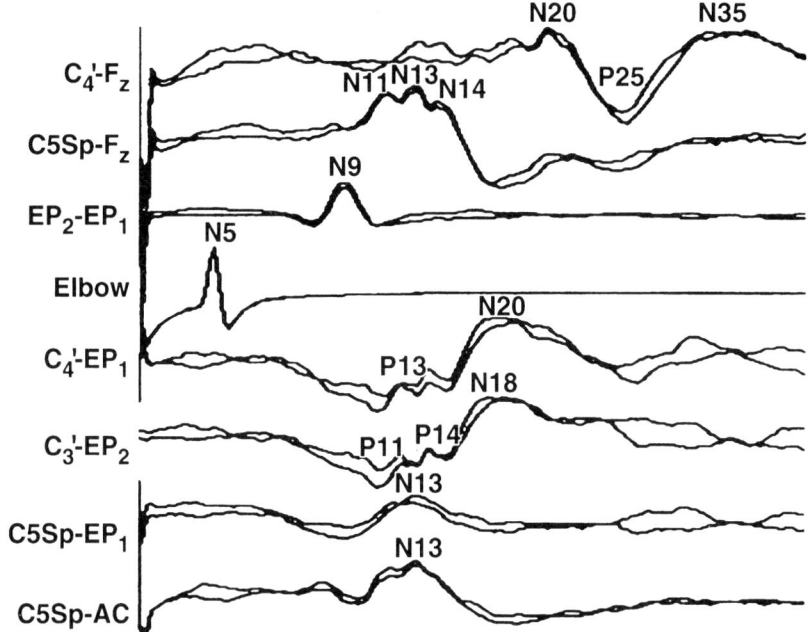

Figure 15-39
Normal left median somatosensory evoked potentials recorded from a 24-year-old woman at the elbow, supraclavicular area $(EP_2\text{-}EP_1)$, neck $(C5Sp\text{-}F_z)$, and scalp $(C_4'\text{-}F_z)$. The major peaks for clinical diagnosis are identified (N9, N11, N13, and N20). The $C_4'\text{-}EP_1$ and $C_3'\text{-}EP_2$ derivations in channels five and six use noncephalic references to further define the potential fields of the scalp potentials and to record far-field potentials P11, P13, P14, and N18. The lowest two channels record the stationary cervical N13 potential without contamination from far-field N13 and N14 potentials. C5Sp, C5 spine; EP, Erb's point; AC, anterior cervical.

fibers in the root entry zone; N13, a dorsal horn, postsynaptic potential; and N14/P14, possibly arising in the medial lemniscus (Fig. 15-39). N18 is another subcortically generated far-field potential probably reflecting postsynaptic activity from multiple generators in the brain stem. The scalp potentials N20/P25 are due to postsynaptic potentials in the primary somatosensory cortex. It should be recognized that the bipolar C_3' or C_4' to F_z montage commonly used to record the scalp potentials is probably an average of independent parietal and posterior frontal generators, each of which may be selectively eliminated. Later waves have also been named but are of little diagnostic value. Lumbar spine recordings after tibial nerve stimulation demonstrate an inconsistently seen N18 peak, a traveling wave generated by the nerve roots or cauda equina, and N22, a stationary wave from postsynaptic potentials in the

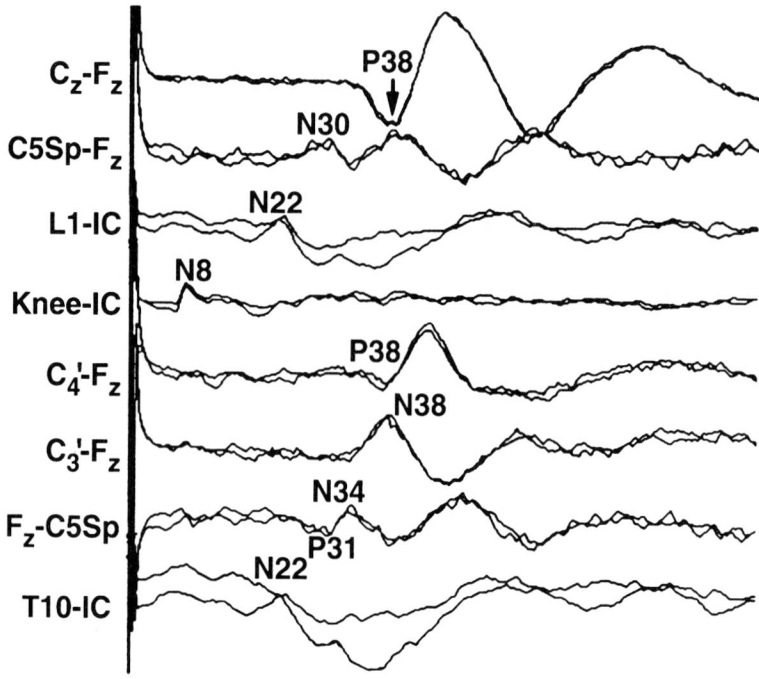

Figure 15-40
Normal tibial somatosensory evoked potentials recorded from a 30-year-old woman at the knee-iliac crest *(Knee-IC)*, lumbar spine *(L1-IC)*, cervical spine *(C5Sp-F_z)*, and scalp *(C_z-F_z)*. The major peaks for clinical diagnosis are identified *(N22, N30, and P38)*.

dorsal horn of the spinal cord (Fig. 15-40). The traveling wave in the posterior columns may be recorded as N30 at the neck. A prominent P38 waveform recorded over the scalp reflects the activity of the primary sensory cortex and is the most reliable potential to measure for central conduction with tibial stimulation.

Criteria of SEP Abnormality

Latency is the primary SEP measurement, but latencies vary significantly with body height, limb temperature, peripheral nerve conduction velocity, and age. To avoid errors of interpretation, routine median and tibial nerve conduction studies are done after the SEP study to assess the peripheral conduction velocity. *Interpeak latencies*, which measure the time intervals between successive peaks in the sensory pathway, are most useful because they are little affected by the previously mentioned variables and primarily measure central conduction times. If prolongation of *absolute latency* is used to show an abnormality, the measured latency must be compared with normal values related to height, and peripheral nerve conduction velocities must be normal. When peripheral nerve conduction is slowed, it is impossible to know whether the prolonged neck or scalp latency is due to disease in the periphery, in the central nervous system, or in both.

For purposes of interpretation, SEP waveforms are assumed to be linked in series. An exception to this rule is the loss of N13 (which arises from collaterals of the main pathway) with preservation of N20. Prolongation of interpeak latency suggests a defect between the generators of the two peaks involved. Side-to-side interpeak latency differences are also sensitive indicators of abnormality. Dispersion of the evoked potentials suggests desynchronization of the nerve action potential analogous to that found in peripheral nerve disease; however, this finding is difficult to quantify and should be interpreted cautiously. Morphologic peculiarities of waveforms with normal interpeak latencies usually have no clinical significance.

Absence of a regularly recorded peak is also significant. Loss of N13 after median nerve stimulation suggests involvement of the gray matter of the dorsal horn at C-6, C-7 and after ulnar nerve stimulation, involvement of C-8, T-1. The lumbar and cervical responses after tibial nerve stimulation are present in most normal subjects but are frequently absent in patients, particularly if they are older, are obese, or have difficulty with relaxation. The lack of superimposable tracings at these levels often represents a technical limitation rather than a patient abnormality. Bilateral simultaneous tibial nerve stimulation sometimes brings out missing lumbar and cervical potentials and allows measurement of interpeak latencies.

Decreased amplitude of SEP waveforms is helpful; however, a wide normal range in amplitude makes this measurement less useful. In addition, attenuation of scalp SEP amplitude may result from a lesion at any point along the peripheral and central pathways. A 50% or greater side-to-side difference suggests axonal loss or central conduction block.

SEP Abnormalities

SEP recording sometimes yields abnormal results in patients with peripheral nerve lesions but is not as effective as standard nerve conduction studies in identifying and characterizing the disorder. SEPs are, however, useful to evaluate the more proximal segments of nerve when slowing of conduction through the plexus or roots is suspected. For example, patients with Guillain-Barré syndrome or chronic inflammatory polyradiculoneuropathy may be studied when results of standard nerve conduction studies are normal. SEP recordings can sometimes provide an indirect measurement of peripheral conduction when no peripheral nerve action potentials can be recorded because of a severe peripheral neuropathy. The scalp SEP can still be recorded because of amplification in the central nervous system of the signals coming from a few axons. There are reports of the value of ulnar SEP recording in thoracic outlet syndrome, particularly in the neurogenic group. For cases of vascular or "disputed" thoracic outlet syndrome, SEPs are usually not helpful. After traumatic plexopathy, recordable scalp SEPs indicate continuity across the plexus and roots. Conversely, a normal Erb's point potential and lack of cervical and scalp responses suggest avulsion of the roots of the plexus. Segmental stimulation using the lateral cutaneous nerve of the forearm and digital afferents permits evaluation of nerve fibers confined to the C5-8 nerve roots. Combinations of peripheral and root damage may make interpretation of the results difficult.

Radiculopathies are most easily and reliably evaluated by routine EMG methods; however, needle EMG abnormalities reflect only dysfunction of the motor root. Dermatomal stimulation for the study of cervical and lumbosacral radiculopathies has been found useful by some authors but not by others. When magnetic resonance images show multiple levels of involvement in patients with symptoms of radiculopathy, dermatomal SEPs can help to identify which nerve roots are affected. Because they are time-consuming and can be falsely positive, dermatomal SEPs have not found widespread use.

SEPs have proven most useful in study of disease of the spinal cord, particularly multiple sclerosis, which shows the most striking changes (Fig. 15-41). In patients with clinical evidence of cranial nerve or cerebral involvement, the SEP recording may show clear signs of a clinically silent spinal cord lesion. Patients with cervical spondylotic myelopathy, arteriovenous malformations, adrenoleukodystrophy, and other spinal cord disorders also often have SEP abnormalities. Ulnar SEPs show the greatest extent of change in cervical spondylosis. A moderate or marked prolongation of the interpeak latency favors demyelinating disorders, whereas myelopathies caused by syringomyelia, spinal stenosis, and tumors usually produce mild slowing of conduction or loss of components. Despite the absence of clinical sensory involvement, mild abnormalities in central conduction time are not uncommon in amyotrophic lateral sclerosis and should not exclude the diagnosis. SEPs may also be helpful in demonstrating intact central sensory pathways in patients with sensory loss that does not have an organic basis. Patients with myoclonus arising in the cortex, such as progressive myoclonus epilepsy, can sometimes be differentiated from those with a subcortical origin by the giant SEPs found in the former. SEPs also provide evidence of residual cortical function after severe cerebral trauma or anoxia. With a multimodality evoked potential battery, including SEP recording, the prognosis for recovery of cerebral function has been predicted with an accuracy of up to 91%. Brain death results in bilateral loss of N20, whereas cervical potentials can remain intact because of the difference in blood supply between the brain and the spinal cord.

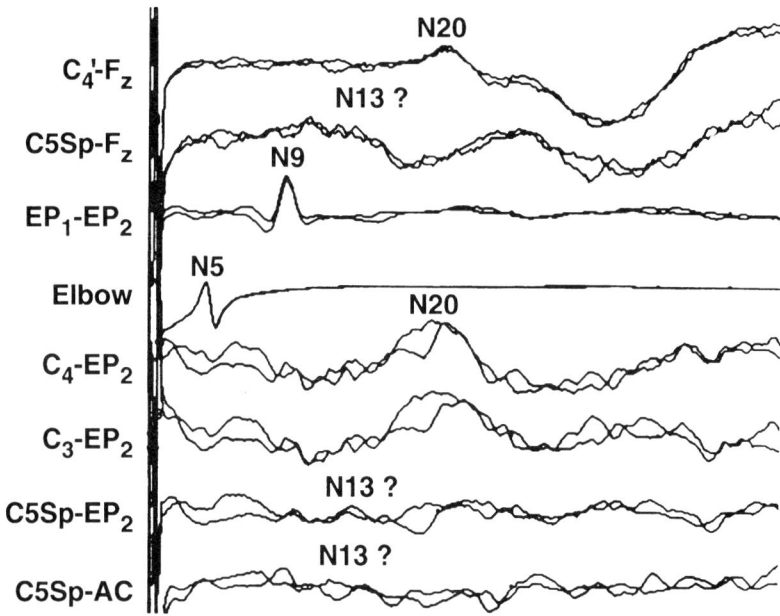

Figure 15-41
Left median somatosensory evoked potentials recorded from a 58-year-old woman with multiple sclerosis. The cervical N13 potential is absent, and the N9-N20 interpeak latency is mildly prolonged at 10.9 msec (normal, <10.6 msec).

SECTION VI: AUDITORY-VESTIBULAR SYSTEM TESTING

Physiologic testing of the function of the eighth cranial nerve and its connections can provide sensitive, quantitative measures of mild or early damage to the peripheral or central components of this system. AEPs recorded from the scalp provide the greatest diagnostic utility in central neurologic problems and can assist in preserving function during surgery in the posterior fossa. Peripheral nerve and cochlear disorders are best evaluated with audiometric testing. Electronystagmography and posturography can assess both the peripheral and the central components of the vestibular system.

Brain Stem Auditory Evoked Potentials
Stimulation and recording methods
BAEPs are a series of potentials generated by the sequential activation of the brain stem auditory pathway; they occur 10 msec after auditory stimuli. Earphones are usually used to deliver sound in outpatient, and small stimulating electrodes can be inserted into the ear canal to stimulate and record during surgery. The stimuli are rarefaction, condensation or alternating rarefaction, and condensation clicks given at 10 Hz, 65 to

70 dB above the hearing threshold. A contralateral masking noise is used to prevent bone-conducted responses from occurring in the non-stimulated ear. Low- and high-frequency filter settings of 100 and 3,000, respectively, are used in the outpatient laboratory. Two separate averages of 1,000 or more responses are superimposed to ensure reproducibility of the responses. The evoked potentials are seen as volume-conducted responses that can be recorded by surface electrodes at the vertex (CZ) and the earlobes (A_1 and A_2) or mastoid (M_1 and M_2). By convention, BAEPs are recorded positive up, which is the opposite of most electrophysiologic recording.

The normal BAEP

Five potentials, or waveforms, are usually recorded (Fig. 15-42). Wave I represents the auditory nerve potential. Wave II is a response generated at the entrance of the eighth nerve at the medullary pontine junction; it may represent a proximal response of the cochlear nucleus at this site. Wave III is generated in the lower midpontine level and may represent the activity of the ipsilateral superior olivary nucleus. Wave IV is generated at the

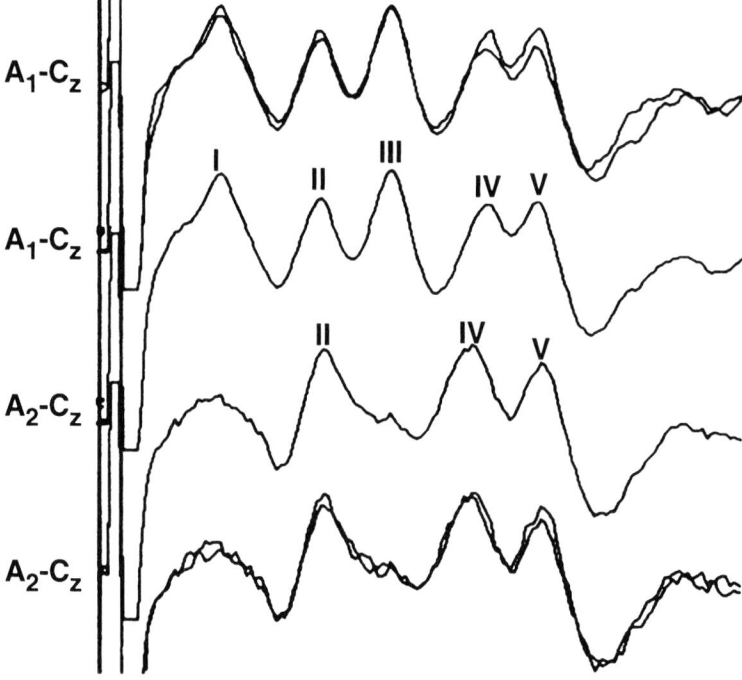

Figure 15-42
Normal brain stem auditory evoked potentials in a 32-year-old woman. Responses were obtained with rarefaction clicks of the left ear summating 2,000 responses. Channels one and four show two runs superimposed. Channels three and four show a combined average. C_z, vertex electrode; A_1, left earlobe electrode; A_2, right ear electrode.

middle to upper pontine level, possibly by the lateral lemniscal structures. Wave V is generated at the upper pontine level or by the inferior colliculus at the lower midbrain level. Waves IV and V (IV-V complex) are quite variable and may show better separation in the contralateral C_z-earlobe derivation. Waves VI and VII are variably present and not useful clinically. They are presumed to be generated by the medial geniculate body and thalamocortical pathways. BAEPs are very small potentials and usually vary in amplitude between 0.1 and 0.5 μV. This is 1/100 of the amplitude of EEG activity, which is in the range of 30 to 50 μV.

Interpretation

Although five or more waveforms are usually resolved, the most important are I, III, and V. The I to III interpeak latency is a measure of conduction of the more caudal segment of the brain stem auditory pathway, that is, the acoustic nerve and the lower pontine portion, whereas the III to V interpeak latency is a measure of the conduction in the more rostral pontine and lower midbrain portions of the pathway. The I to V interpeak latency is a measure of the total conduction time within the brain stem auditory pathway. The interpeak latency is the most important and reliable measurement. The criterion for abnormality is a prolongation of the interpeak latency beyond the 99% tolerance level in comparison with normal control values. The absolute and interpeak latencies in infants are markedly prolonged compared with those in adults. Latencies decrease with increasing age and reach adult values by 2 years. After age 60 years, there is a mild increase in latencies. The I to V normal interpeak latencies for adults in the Mayo laboratories are as follows:

Age (yr)	Female	Male
Younger than 60	4.60	4.65
60 and older	4.70	4.75

If the I to V interpeak latency difference between ears exceeds 0.4 msec, the result is considered abnormal. The amplitude of wave I and the amplitude of the IV-V complex are used to calculate the IV:V-I ratio, which is usually 0.4. The structure and amplitude of the BAEPs are highly variable and therefore are usually not useful in measurement.

Clinical applications

BAEPs may give objective evidence of an electrophysiologic disturbance within the brain stem auditory pathways when there is little or no clinical evidence of abnormality and when other laboratory test results are negative. The limitation of the test is that, although BAEPs are more sensitive to demyelinating than to axonal diseases, the test alone cannot be used to make a specific etiologic diagnosis. A normal BAEP study result does not exclude disease involving the brain stem or the auditory system. The test is best considered an extension of the neurologic examination, and the findings must be integrated with the total clinical picture before a diagnosis is made.

The major applications of BAEP testing are (1) early diagnosis of multiple sclerosis (as well as other demyelinating diseases), (2) detection of posterior fossa tumors, (3) evaluation of comatose patients, and (4) determination of brain death.

BAEPs are very sensitive to white matter disease and are useful in helping to make the diagnosis of multiple sclerosis. It should be noted, however, that pattern reversal evoked responses and SEPs are more sensitive than BAEPs in detecting abnormalities in patients with multiple sclerosis. With a demyelinating process, BAEPs can help confirm or document a lesion within the brain stem when multiple sclerosis is suspected clinically or the patient has a lesion outside the brain stem. For example, BAEP testing may be useful in the investigation of a patient who presents with optic neuritis or transverse myelitis. In addition, BAEPs may be helpful in the proper assessment of present or past symptoms that are poorly defined, such as transient diplopia. If the BAEPs are abnormal, involvement of the brain stem is suggested. The abnormalities of the BAEPs persist, so that the test can detect brain stem dysfunction when the patient's disease is in total remission. Other demyelinating processes, such as central pontine myelinosis, metachromatic leukodystrophy, and adrenoleukodystrophy, can also cause abnormalities in BAEPs. Diseases affecting the gray matter of the brain stem, such as progressive supranuclear palsy and Wernicke's encephalopathy, do not affect BAEPs. A posterior fossa tumor or mass lesion within or outside the brain stem can produce abnormal BAEPs by either direct involvement of the brain stem auditory pathways or secondary pressure on the brain stem. BAEPs are a sensitive screening test when an acoustic neuroma is suspected and may provide the first objective evidence of an abnormality. They are also quite cost-effective compared with a magnetic resonance imaging scan. The most common abnormalities are absence or abnormality of wave I and absence or delay of subsequent waveforms.

The presence or absence of abnormal BAEPs in comatose patients depends on the process and the area involved. BAEPs are relatively resistant to metabolic derangements, to anesthetic- or drug-induced coma, and to coma with a structural brain stem lesion that does not affect the auditory pathways. Coma with a structural lesion of the brain stem that involves the auditory pathways, however, is usually associated with significant BAEP abnormality.

In brain death, there is a loss of all BAEP components after wave I. If wave I is absent, no conclusion can be made about brain stem death, because the loss of wave I and the subsequent components could be due to technical factors, structural damage to the ear or the cochlea, ischemia of or damage to the auditory nerve, or preexisting deafness.

Thus, one should be cautious in interpreting the study if all waveforms are absent.

Patients with focal brain stem infarcts or embolic lesions of the brain stem may not have much abnormality of the BAEPs if the lesion spares the brain stem auditory pathways. Thus, patients with small discrete or spotty vascular lesions of the brain stem often have normal BAEPs. Patients with brain stem hemorrhages or widespread infarcts of the brain stem, on the other hand, are more likely to have abnormalities of the BAEPs. Abnormal BAEPs have been reported in a number of other conditions involving the brain stem, including degenerative disorders, such as olivopontocerebellar degeneration, Friedreich's ataxia, hereditary cerebellar ataxia, diabetes, Leigh's disease, Wilson's disease, and some cases of B_{12} deficiency. Abnormalities have also been reported in patients with hemifacial spasm.

BAEP testing may be used in screening for hearing or neurologic defects in high-risk newborns and infants. Abnormal BAEPs are seen in infants with trauma, hypoxic damage, respiratory distress syndrome, intraventricular hemorrhage, degenerative conditions involving the brain stem, and meningitis. However, special attention to the technical aspects of recording BAEPs is needed in premature and term infants, especially those with impaired hearing.

Testing Hearing

Hearing can be tested in a number of different ways. Among the most commonly used are pure tone and speech audiometry and immittance (impedance) testing.

Pure tone audiometry measures hearing sensitivity as a function of frequency. The audiogram is a graph of the level of auditory sensitivity by frequency for octave intervals from 125 Hz through 8,000 Hz. Stimulation is produced by air conduction (earphones) or bone conduction (vibrator) signals. Reliable audiometric testing requires a specially trained audiologist familiar with the equipment, handling of the patient, variability of responses, and clinical problems. For example, it is important that the ear canal be clear for testing, and if there is a large difference in sensitivity of the two ears, the sound presented in one ear must be masked with suitable noise in the opposite ear. Hearing level is defined as the loudness (decibels) required to hear and is measured by the difference from a normal standard level. With conductive hearing loss, air conduction thresholds are poorer than bone conduction thresholds. With sensorineural hearing loss, bone conduction thresholds are similar to air conduction thresholds. Although no audiometric patterns are diagnostic, noise-induced hearing loss commonly has a greater loss for a limited range of high frequencies around 4,000 Hz, producing a notched curve. Hearing loss with aging is progressively greater at higher frequencies. Meniere's syndrome shows the greatest loss at low frequencies, and congenital hearing loss has a broad loss in midrange frequencies.

Differentiation of causes of conductive hearing disorders is not possible with pure tone or speech testing. However, *acoustic immittance measures* provide valuable information on the function of the middle ear through tympanometric and acoustic reflex patterns. Tympanometry is a measure of the acoustic immittance of the ear as a function of ear canal pressure. Acoustic reflexes are measures of the change in acoustic immittance produced by the contraction of the stapedius and tensor tympani muscles in response to loud sound. These immittance subtests may be affected by middle ear disorders and abnormalities of the auditory neural and brain stem pathways, respectively. Both depend on the sound pressure reflected from the eardrum back to the test probe in the ear canal. For example, when the normally air-filled middle ear space becomes fluid-filled in otitis media, the resulting stiffness of the eardrum impedes sound transmission and greater sound pressure is reflected. If an acoustic tumor affects neural transmission to the brain stem, the corresponding acoustic reflex may be absent. Abnormalities of the tympanogram are commonly seen in otitis media, otosclerosis, and ossicular discontinuity. Testing the acoustic reflex in each ear in response to ipsilateral and contralateral sounds provides site-of-lesion testing of cochlear lesions, conductive hearing loss, auditory nerve damage, and facial nerve damage (pathway for the motor component of the reflex).

Testing Vestibular Function
Testing the function of the semicircular canals and their central vestibular connections is accomplished by *electronystagmography* (ENG), which measures eye movements electrically. ENG testing can provide information about the function of the vestibular system and, specifically, about the presence and, sometimes, location of a lesion involving this system.

The eye has a voltage difference of approximately 1 mV between the positive cornea and the negative retina. Movements of the eye can therefore be detected by electrodes placed on either side of the eyes. Standard ENG records the potential difference between a pair of electrodes at the lateral canthus of each eye and between a pair of electrodes above and below one of the eyes. Lateral movements to the right and left produce upward and downward deflections, respectively, of one of the recording pens, and upward and downward movements produce upward and downward deflections of the other pen. Disconjugate eye movements are not recognized by this recording mode but can be by use of separate sets of electrodes for each eye. Torsional rotations of the eye are not recognized by this system but would only rarely add to the information provided by the recordings of lateral and vertical movements.

Eye movements of any kind can be quantitatively measured with this recording system, but a standard set of tests has been developed and is used in most laboratories. The *saccade test* is used to calibrate the system by having the patient move the eyes laterally and vertically between two sets of points a fixed distance apart. Nystagmus is sought in the *gaze test*, in which the patient voluntarily looks to the right, to the left, up, and down. Pursuit eye movements are tested in the *tracking test*, in which the patient follows a slowly moving visual target with the eyes. *Optokinetic testing* records the eye movements in response to moving vertical stripes in both directions. In *positional testing*, eye movements in response to different head positions are recorded in search of positional nystagmus. *Caloric testing* records the eye movements in response to warm and cool air or water in the external canal.

ENG testing can be performed reliably and efficiently with a variety of stimulating and recording devices by a properly trained technician. It is important that the external ear canals and tympanic membrane be examined before the testing, but no other special preparation is required. A variety of physiologic and technical artifacts must be recognized, such as eye blinks and EMG activity.

The primary purpose of ENG is the measurement of nystagmus. Nystagmus has two components, the fast phase and the slow phase. Nystagmus on the ENG is described by the direction of the fast phase (right-beating nystagmus has its fast phase to the right) and velocity of the eyes during the slow phase. The ENG provides a quantitative measure allowing the identification of many types of nystagmus that can sometimes help in the localization and characterization of lesions of the peripheral or central vestibular system. For example, horizontal nystagmus during gaze testing and unilateral weakness with caloric testing nearly always indicate a peripheral vestibular lesion. In contrast, ocular dysmetria on saccadic testing is a sign of a cerebellar system lesion. Many features of nystagmus quantitated on the ENG can be readily recognized and used by clinical examination. Additional testing of the vestibular system can be obtained by measuring ENG during stimulation of the horizontal semicircular canals in a Bárány chair in which the patient is moved in space. *Computerized dynamic posturography* measures the change in foot pressure on sensitive plates with sudden movements of the foot plate or environment. A vestibular system dysfunction pattern is present when the patient sways or falls on conditions 5 and 6. The distortion of somatosensory cues created by sway-referencing the platform coupled with the elimination of vision (condition 5) and the distortion of vision created by sway-referencing the visual surround (condition 6) force the patient to rely on vestibular control of balance and posture.

SECTION VII: VISUAL SYSTEM TESTING

The visual system can also be tested electrophysiologically, but the testing is more limited than that for the other sensory systems. VEPs and the electroretinogram at times can detect abnormalities that are not evident clinically. The electroretinogram is used to test the retina, and VEPs are used to test central visual pathways.

Electroretinogram

The *electroretinogram* can be recorded with electrodes around the eye, but recording is best between a corneal electrode in a contact lens and a reference electrode at the lateral canthus. Diffuse flashes of light evoke a potential with components contributed by the photoreceptors and the bipolar cells. Dim, blue stimuli can isolate rod function; rapid flashes can isolate cone function. The electroretinogram is most sensitive to diffuse retinal disease, such as retinal degeneration, and may show abnormal findings before macular dysfunction is clinically detectable.

Pattern Reversal Evoked Potentials

Disorders of the central visual pathways are tested with VEPs, the cortical response to a visual stimulus. Flashes of light evoke potentials over the occipital lobes but are less sensitive to disease than responses to patterned stimuli. The most commonly used pattern is a black-and-white checkerboard shown on a video monitor in which the checks reverse color twice a second. The occipital potential evoked in response to this stimulus is called the pattern reversal evoked potential (PREP). Recordings are made with the subject seated in a chair at a distance of 1 m from the monitor screen. The patient, wearing glasses if necessary to see the checks clearly, stares at a dot in the center of the screen. One eye is stimulated at a time; the other eye is covered with a patch. When the test is done in this fashion, the PREP is most effective in detecting lesions of the prechiasmal parts of the visual pathway, but results can also be abnormal in chiasmal or retrochiasmal lesions. For evaluation of chiasmal and retrochiasmal lesions, monocular hemifield stimulation is required, but it is rarely used because of lack of sensitivity. Like other evoked potentials, PREPs are low in amplitude, requiring averages of 100 to 400 responses from electrodes over the midline of the occiput referenced to the ears or other areas of the scalp. The major positive deflection of approximately 100 msec (commonly designated "P100"), generated by occipital cortex, is most useful for clinical applications (Fig. 15-43). PREP latency varies with stimulus intensity, age, and sex. The normal P100 latencies for adults in the Mayo laboratories are as follows:

Age, yr	Female	Male
Younger than 60	<115	<120
60 and older	<120	<125

An interocular asymmetry of 10 msec or greater is abnormal.

PREPs have been most useful in the diagnosis of multiple sclerosis that produces remarkably long latency responses. In patients who have spinal cord symptoms and signs without cranial signs, PREP recording

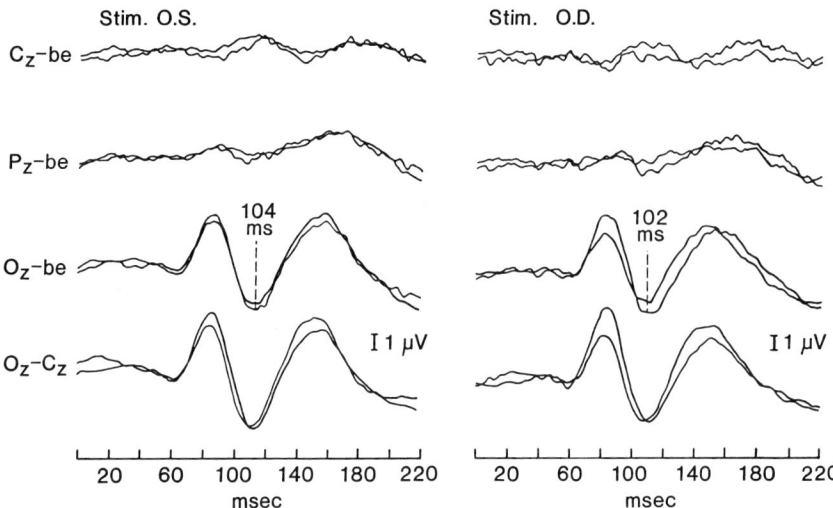

Figure 15-43
The midline scalp distribution of potentials evoked by monocular pattern reversal stimulation to the left eye and to the right eye in a 53-year-old woman are displayed in the left half and right half of the figure, respectively. In this case, the major O_z positive deflection (P100 peak) occurs with latencies of 104 msec from the left eye and 102 msec from the right eye, which are well within the normal limits of variation. C_z-be, central to ear; P_z-be, parietal to ear electrodes; O_z-be, occipital to ear electrodes; O_z-C_z, occipital to central electrodes.

may show clear signs of an optic neuropathy that is not evident clinically. More than 90% of patients with definite multiple sclerosis have abnormal PREPs. It must be remembered that PREPs are nonspecific and may also be abnormal in a variety of other disorders, such as ocular diseases, Leber's optic neuropathy, tumors compressing the optic nerve and chiasm, storage diseases, leukodystrophies, and cortical blindness. PREPs are normal in patients with hysterical blindness but can be abnormal with voluntary lack of focusing. Application of visual evoked potentials must, therefore, always take the full clinical picture into careful consideration.

SECTION VIII: EVALUATION OF PATIENTS WITH SLEEP DISORDERS

Application of the principles of sleep physiology to the results of cardiopulmonary and neurologic monitoring during sleep has allowed more precise diagnosis and treatment in patients troubled by "sleep disorders" (insomnia, excessive daytime drowsiness, sleep timing difficulty, and abnormal sleep behavior). In some instances, particularly the insomnias, sleep disorders previously viewed as having a psychiatric basis are now better explained on an organic level. Additionally, this activity has extended our knowledge of the nocturnal consequences of various neurologic disease entities previously viewed only in the daylight.

Adequate understanding of these problems requires (1) a combination of concepts derived from daytime cardiopulmonary and neuromuscular physiology; (2) knowledge of nocturnal changes in the above; (3) additional emphasis on biorhythms, sleep state and need, and drug effects (half-life, withdrawal, and tolerance phenomena); and (4) an understanding of the technical limitations of monitoring sleep. Hence, a successful approach must be multidisciplinary, incorporating skills from specialists in pulmonary medicine, psychiatry, and neurology.

Physiologic Changes With Sleep

There are two distinctly different sleep states: non-rapid eye movement (NREM) and rapid eye movement (REM) sleep. Cycling between these sleep states is linked and orderly in health but may become uncoupled in various disorders; additionally, these states follow the commands of separate central nervous system pacemakers, exerting their own pressure for occurrence and timing throughout the 24-hour cycle. Recognition of disturbances affecting either is important, since they result in unique symptoms and require different treatment approaches.

Healthy adults initially progress through four stages of NREM sleep. With sleep onset, waking background alpha activity noted on the EEG attenuates and is replaced by low-voltage, 4- to 7-Hz theta activity. This starting phase of light NREM sleep (stage 1) is also associated with slow to-and-fro rolling eye movements, as recorded by surface electro-oculography, and skeletal muscle relaxation, as seen by surface EMG, usually recorded from the submental region. A slightly deeper stage (stage 2) is characterized by specific EEG findings of 12- to 14-Hz sleep spindles, V waves, and K complexes. Although slow eye movements may persist, they usually diminish in stage 2 and deeper NREM sleep. Stages 3 and 4 NREM sleep are characterized by the appearance of delta activity of less than 2 Hz that progressively increases in amplitude and abundance. Deeper NREM sleep is associated with reduced cerebral blood flow and oxygen consumption as well as further relaxation (without total loss of surface EMG) of skeletal muscles. Systemic metabolic needs fall below those of the waking state. During NREM sleep, there is a 20- to 40-second cyclic variation in systemic blood pressure, pulmonary artery pressure, peripheral vascular resistance, heart rate, ventilation, intraventricular pressure, and EEG patterns.

REM sleep generally follows a period of NREM sleep. Profound changes occur: the most dramatic findings are the presence of rapid, irregular, phasic eye movements, for which this phase of sleep is named, and marked reduction in surface EMG. The EEG becomes "activated" and more closely approximates the cortical activity of relaxed wakefulness. Vivid dreaming occurs in REM sleep, which is not truly deeper than NREM sleep, since the tendency toward spontaneous arousal approximates that seen in stage 2 NREM sleep. Dreaming is not recalled unless the sleeper is awakened soon after an REM episode. Cerebral blood flow and oxygen consumption are greater than during wakefulness.

Sleep in adults with normal sleep architecture cycles in an orderly fashion through five or six approximately 90-minute NREM-REM periods each night, with an emphasis on deeper NREM sleep during the first third of the sleep period and on REM sleep in the last third. Since REM latency is usually greater than 75 minutes in normal young adults, REM sleep is generally not recorded in the hypnotic-induced sleep EEG performed during the day unless there is an unusual degree of REM pressure. Moreover, the first REM period is frequently less than a minute in length, and hence recording periods of at least 3 hours are required to adequately examine the phenomena of REM sleep.

NREM sleep also leads to profound changes in respiratory physiology. There is a shift from a combination of automatic (brain stem) and voluntary (supratentorial) respiratory control mechanisms during wakefulness to dependence on automatic control. There is a twofold to fourfold increase in upper airway resistance; lung volumes fall slightly. Breathing frequency remains similar to that during quiet wakefulness, and tidal volume decreases, resulting in a mild net hypoventilation with a modest fall in Pao_2 and rise in $Paco_2$. Metabolic control systems predominate, and CO_2 homeostasis maintained through medullary chemoreceptors provides the principal ventilatory drive. During the transition from wakefulness to light NREM sleep, ventilation frequently becomes unstable because there are oscillations between wakefulness and sleep. Because the setpoint for ventilation is lower during NREM sleep than during wakefulness, ventilation decreases with sleep onset. With a return to wakefulness, ventilation increases because of the enhanced ventilatory drive associated with the waking state. Consequently, these oscillations in state are responsible for the hypopneas and central apneas observed during sleep onset. These oscillations become progressively damped as the individual enters consolidated stage 2 NREM sleep. During this stage, the ventilatory response to both hypercapnia and hypoxia is reduced. As the degree of slow-wave activity increases and the individual enters stages 3 and 4 of NREM sleep, breathing becomes highly regular and the upper airway more resistant to collapse.

REM sleep is associated with atonia of the muscles of the chest wall and upper airway, with reliance on the diaphragm for the maintenance of ventilation. The ventilatory response to hypoxia and hypercapnia is further reduced from that in NREM sleep, and ventilation becomes irregular. The irregular breathing pattern that develops is considered to be due to the influence of supratentorial or cortical input during the REM sleep state. Because of the atonia of the upper airway muscles, the upper airway is at increased risk for collapse and obstruction during the REM sleep state. Patients with diaphragmatic weakness or paralysis are especially vulnerable to the development of hypoventilation and hypoxemia during REM sleep.

Polysomnography
Polysomnography consists of the continuous recording of about 6 to 8 hours of nocturnal sleep. At least four recording channels must be devoted to detection of the presence and amount of various sleep stages: two for electro-oculography, one for EEG (C_4-A_1 or C_3-A_2), and one for submental EMG. The inevitable introduction of artifacts as the recording progresses throughout the night usually demands additional, seemingly redundant, channels that can provide substitutive information if primary systems fail. Several channels are required for adequate respiratory monitoring: breathing effort can be measured only by intraesophageal pressure monitoring or intercostal surface EMG; breathing motion can be detected by rib cage and abdominal strain gauges, which also serve to reveal the paradoxical motion induced by upper airway obstruction or diaphragmatic paralysis; breathing result is usually measured by oral-nasal thermistors or CO_2 detectors; physiologic consequences are inferred from the results of electrocardiography, transcutaneous oxygen saturation, and alteration in sleep stage. A small microphone attached to the throat is of great value in detecting snoring, and position monitors can provide information relating sleep-disordered breathing events to sleeping position. Last, limb muscle activity must be monitored to exclude a sleep-related movement disorder; this requires at least one channel of EMG (usually the surface activity of the right and left anterior tibial muscles is viewed in a series) (Fig. 15-44).

Each 30-second epoch of the polysomnogram is scored according to conventional criteria as awake, stage I through IV NREM, or REM sleep. The following sleep measurements are of particular interest: sleep onset (time from "lights out" until the first evidence of sleep), REM latency (time from sleep onset until the first epoch of REM sleep), total sleep time (sum of all NREM and REM epochs), sleep efficiency (total sleep time divided by the time in bed), percentage of time spent in each NREM and REM stage, number of awakenings per hour during the total sleep period, number of arousals per hour during the total sleep period, periodic leg movements per hour of sleep, and number and type of disordered breathing events relative to various body positions and sleep stages, further qualified by an estimate of their minimum and maximum durations, sleep disruption, and oxygen desaturation. Each epoch is characterized not only as a specific sleep stage but also as a period containing a variety of events: arousal, breathing events, and movement events. An arousal is defined as a shift in EEG to al-

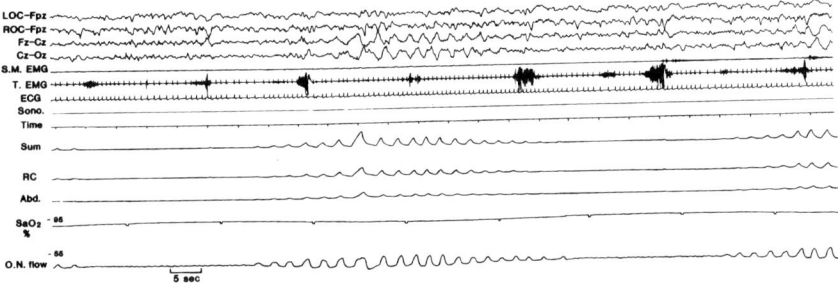

Figure 15-44
Polysomnogram illustrating Cheyne-Stokes respiration with oxygen desaturation and independent periodic movements of sleep. *LOC-Fpz*, left outer canthus to midline frontal electrode; *ROC-Fpz*, right outer canthus to midline frontal electrode; *Fz-Cz*, midline frontal to midline central electrodes; *Cz-Oz*, midline central to midline occipital electrodes. *S.M. EMG*, submental EMG; *T. EMG*, tibial EMG; *ECG*, electrocardiogram; *Sono.*, sonogram (sound detector); *Sum*, the integrated sum of rib cage and abdominal movements. *RC*, rib cage plethysmography; *Abd.*, abdominal plethysmography; SaO_2, oxygen saturation; *O.N. flow*, oral nasal airflow. *(From Fredrickson PA, Krueger BR: Insomnia associated with specific polysomnographic findings. In Kryger MH, Roth T, Dement WC, editors: Principles and practice of sleep medicine, Philadelphia, 1989, WB Saunders Co., pp 476–489. By permission of the publisher.)*

pha, fast beta, or theta rhythms lasting at least 3 seconds; in REM sleep, an increase in EMG activity is also required.

Obstructive apneas are characterized by cessation of oronasal airflow with continued thoracoabdominal movement. Obstructive hypopneas demonstrate a reduction in airflow (usually greater than 50%) with at least a 2% decrease in oxyhemoglobin saturation. They are usually accompanied by loud snoring and paradoxical movement of the chest and abdomen.

Central apneas are cessation of airflow for more than 10 seconds unassociated with evidence of breathing effort or movement. With the exception of sleep onset, they are quite rare in normal individuals, but they are common in patients with severe cardiac failure or disease of the brain stem. In practice, many apneas are mixed, starting with a central component and terminating with an obstructive component.

Periodic movements of sleep occur independently of abnormal breathing events. They are scored when there is a 0.5- to 5-second increase in baseline EMG occurring in trains of more than five stereotyped repetitions with an intermovement interval of 4 to 90 seconds. The presence or absence of EEG evidence for arousal is noted. Adequate respiratory monitoring is required to exclude sleep apnea, because leg movement may occur with each apnea-induced arousal.

A special application of polysomnography is the diagnosis of abnormal gross movements during sleep. The differential diagnosis usually lies between parasomnias, such as sleepwalking and REM sleep behavior disorder, and epileptic seizures. Additional EEG channels (preferably at least 16) and time-synchronized videotape recording of events are essential. Digital computerized recording systems are ideally suited for this type of study.

Multiple Sleep Latency Test
This test consists of four or five 20-minute attempts, once every 2 hours, to fall asleep throughout the day. Since the goal is determination of sleep latency and whether or not REM sleep is recorded during the nap, only electro-oculography, EEG, and submental EMG are usually recorded. Subjects are not allowed to sleep for more than 15 minutes on any nap to minimize distortion of subsequent sleep latencies by excessive napping during the day. Sleep onset is defined as the first 30-second epoch in which more than 15 seconds of sleep activity are present. Normal individuals have mean sleep latencies of greater than 10 minutes and fewer than two sleep onset REM periods on the multiple sleep latency test. Severe pathologic sleepiness is manifested by a mean sleep latency of less than 5 minutes, whereas a mean latency of 5 to 8 minutes indicates mild to moderate sleepiness; mean latencies of 8 to 10 minutes are in a "gray area" of uncertain significance. The occurrence of two or more sleep onset REM periods during the day is strong evidence for excessive REM pressure. This is suggestive of narcolepsy if there is no suspicion of previous REM sleep deprivation from, for example, insufficient sleep, sleep apnea, or recent withdrawal from stimulants and if one has ruled out a sleep-wake cycle disorder and major depression. Proper interpretation of the multiple sleep latency test requires direct knowledge of the previous night's sleep; hence, it usually follows polysomnography. Subjects are required to abstain from stimulants or other psychotropic agents for 2 weeks before the test and are asked to keep a sleep log documenting adequate nocturnal sleep time.

The maintenance of wakefulness test is a variant of the multiple sleep latency test in which the patient is requested to remain awake in a dark room rather than to attempt sleep. It can be useful in monitoring response to stimulant medication.

Pupillography
Increased parasympathetic tone with drowsiness leads to pupillary constriction, so that measurement of pupillary diameter over time provides an estimate of drowsiness. The subject sits in a comfortable chair in a darkened room and is instructed to remain alert while watching a target while the pupils are scanned with an infrared camera. Normal individuals are able to maintain pupillary diameters of more than 7 mm for 10

minutes without significant oscillations. Pupillography may be of value in differentiating the subjective complaints of fatigue and lack of energy from true hypersomnolence and in following the level of alertness in a narcoleptic person being treated with stimulants. However, the findings are etiologically nonspecific, and the test has been largely replaced by multiple sleep latency testing.

SECTION IX: AUTONOMIC FUNCTION TESTS

Some Tests of Distal Sympathetic Autonomic Function

Distal sudomotor and vasomotor functions can be evaluated. Four sudomotor tests in current use are the quantitative sudomotor axon reflex test (QSART), the thermoregulatory sweat test, the Silastic imprint method, and the skin potential method.

With the QSART, one population of sweat glands is stimulated by the iontophoresis of acetycholine with use of a constant current source. Impulses travel antidromically along sympathetic C fibers to a branch point and then travel orthodromically along other sympathetic C fibers to evoke a sweat response with a latency of 1 to 2 minutes. The axon-reflex-mediated sweating occupies an area of 5 to 7 cm in diameter and is measured by a sudorometer. The response may be normal, reduced, absent, excessive, or persistent and indicates the status of postganglionic sympathetic function.

Very distal sweating (fingers, feet, and toes) and areas of skin not readily studied by other techniques, such as on the forehead and trunk, can be easily tested by the thermoregulatory sweat test. This is fully described below under tests for generalized autonomic failure.

Since the postganglionically denervated eccrine sweat gland responds poorly or not at all to direct stimulation with muscarinic agents such as acetycholine and pilocarpine, the response to direct stimulation has been suggested as a suitable test to detect postganglionic sympathetic denervation. With use of a Silastic imprint, therefore, the number and sizes of sweat droplets and histograms are derived.

Recordings of skin potential or resistance have been in wide use since 1888. Recently, skin potential recordings were adapted to readily available equipment in a number of clinical electrophysiologic laboratories. The pathway of the test is a polysynaptic somatosympathetic reflex. The most effective stimuli appear to be those that activate types II and III mechanoreceptors. Commonly used stimuli are an electric shock and an inspiratory gasp. There are a spinal component, a bulbar component, and a suprabulbar component. The response depends on the integrity of these neural pathways, the eccrine sweat gland, and sweat epithelium. The response also depends on activation of the eccrine sweat gland but not on sweat secretion. The skin potential response is impaired in the peripheral and central autonomic neuropathies and is usually absent in multiple system atrophy with autonomic failure. The response rapidly habituates.

Skin vasomotor function reflexes are usually done on the toe or finger pads. Skin blood flow is measured by a laser Doppler flowmeter or by plethysmography, and the vasoconstrictor response to an autonomic maneuver is determined. Vasoconstriction can be induced by maneuvers such as inspiratory gasp, response to standing (for the finger), contralateral cold stimulus, and the Valsalva maneuver.

When venous transmural pressure is increased by 25 mm Hg (for example, by lowering the limb by 40 cm), reflex arteriolar vasoconstriction occurs, reducing blood flow by 50%. This reflex, termed the "venoarteriolar reflex," has its receptor in small veins, and its neural pathway appears to be that of the sympathetic C fiber local axon reflex. The venoarteriolar reflex has been measured in the foot of patients with diabetes and is reported to be reduced in some with diabetic neuropathy.

Tests Usually Used to Detect Generalized Autonomic Failure
Thermoregulatory sweat test

The thermoregulatory sweat test is important, especially if one does autonomic testing infrequently. The test can screen for both preganglionic and postganglionic efferent sympathetic lesions, evaluating descending pathways from hypothalamus to the thoracolumbar sympathetic outflow, sympathetic paravertebral ganglia, and postganglionic nerves to sweat glands. The test, simple to do, requires an adequate source of heat (heat cradle or cabinet, small room whose ambient temperature can be raised, and wall- or cabinet-mounted infrared heaters). The test is much more efficient and accurate if the head is also heated and the air humidity and skin temperature are controlled. The test is very sensitive, providing information on the pattern and degree of sweat loss. There are several near-diagnostic patterns. Several modifications have improved the reliability of the test. Using alizarin-red indicator powder, maintaining a relatively high humidity in the heated environment, and keeping skin temperature increased all allow for easy visualization of a maximal sweat response. Administration of anticholinergic drugs should be stopped 48 hours before the test, since they may cause anhidrosis. The patient should be well hydrated because dehydration may also impair the sweat response. Adequate end points are important. The core temperature should be raised by 1°C or to 38.0°C, whichever is higher. It is important to recognize normal and abnormal sweat patterns.

Plasma norepinephrine

Plasma norepinephrine results from a spillover of norepinephrine from sympathetic postganglionic nerve terminals. The supine value is an index of net sympathetic activity because it is affected by the rate of norepinephrine secretion and clearance. It has been used as an index to separate postganglionic from preganglionic failure. In a disorder with a preganglionic lesion, the resting supine value of norepinephrine is normal but the response to standing would be absent due to failure of activation. In a postganglionic lesion, the supine value would be reduced if the lesion were widespread.

Sustained handgrip
Sustained muscle contraction causes a rise in systolic and diastolic blood pressures and heart rate. The stimulus derived from exercising muscle is reflex in nature, and the rise in blood pressure is mediated by an increase in cardiac output and peripheral resistance. The test has been adapted as a simple test of sympathetic autonomic failure. The subject is required to maintain 30% maximal contraction for up to 5 minutes, and the diastolic blood pressure is recorded.

Baroreflex indices
The approach here is to evaluate the heart period (reciprocal of heart rate) indices to a sudden or sustained change in blood or pulse pressure, raised by phenylephrine or norepinephrine or reduced by agents such as trinitroglycerin. One approach is to determine the range of heart period by raising and lowering blood pressure and mean gain, which is the mean rate of change in heart period in response to sudden changes in pressure. An alternative approach to stimulating baroreceptors is to use a neck chamber whose pressure can be increased or decreased.

Heart period and beat-to-beat blood pressure responses
Cardiac autonomic innervation in humans is vagal-dominant, so that the heart rate responses to maneuvers such as deep breathing, the Valsalva maneuver, and standing have been used as noninvasive indices of parasympathetic function. In the response to deep breathing, the stimulus consists of lung inflation during inspiration and lung deflation during expiration, resulting in a heart period decrease during inspiration and increase during expiration. The afferent and efferent pathways are the vagus nerve, with the nucleus of tractus solitarius as the cell station. Six breaths a minute is optimal for normal subjects. The size of the response decreases linearly with age.

For the Valsalva maneuver, the stimulus is an increase in intrathoracic pressure (40 to 50 mm Hg for 15 seconds), and the response is in four phases. In phase 1, positive intrathoracic pressure by compression of the great vessels mechanically increases blood pressure, and a baroreflex-mediated reflex bradycardia results. In phase 2, continued positive intrathoracic pressure reduces venous return and results in a decrease in cardiac output and a progressive decrease in heart period (vagal withdrawal followed by sympathetic activation). Mean arterial pressure falls during early phase 2 but recovers and exceeds the baseline during late phase 2. In phase 3, the converse of phase 1, the sudden reduction in intrathoracic pressure with cessation of the maneuver results in a momentary drop in blood pressure. During the early part of phase 4, cardiac output has returned to normal but the peripheral vascular bed is still vasoconstricted, and the result is a blood pressure overshoot with reflex bradycardia. Baroreceptors are in the carotid sinus and aortic arch, and impulses travel via the vagus and glossopharyngeal nerves to the nucleus of the tractus solitarius, thence to the nucleus ambiguus, dorsal motor nucleus, and ventrolateral nucleus of the medulla, and then down the vagus to the sinoatrial node and via bulbospinal pathways to the thoracolumbar sympathetic outflow. The Valsalva ratio is the ratio of the maximum heart period divided by the minimum heart period and is impaired with cardiac parasympathetic denervation.

Chronotropic response to atropine

In humans, there is considerable vagal tone at rest, which can be blocked pharmacologically by intravenous injection of atropine. A dose of 1.2 mg is given intravenously and is followed by the same dose 5 minutes later if tachycardia does not occur. Should the second dose of atropine likewise fail to induce tachycardia, a third injection is given. If again no change in cardiac rate is obtained, efferent vagal failure may be presumed to exist.

Testing Gastrointestinal Autonomic Function

The investigation of possible gastrointestinal dysautonomia begins with a careful history and examination to uncover any coexisting neurologic disorders and to identify medications that might affect motility. Administration of drugs should be stopped at least 48 hours before autonomic testing is performed. Finding evidence of autonomic failure on testing sweating or blood pressure and heart rate responses increases the probability of gastrointestinal dysautonomia. Barium-enhanced radiologic studies are often done first to rule out mechanical obstruction by extraluminal or mucosal lesions.

Scintigraphic study of gastric emptying and determination of small intestinal and colonic transit times are commonly done to screen for motility disorders.

Continuous, simultaneous intraluminal pressure recordings from the antrum, duodenum, and jejunum can demonstrate normal and abnormal motility patterns during fasting and after a solid meal. Characteristic motility disturbances in autonomic neuropathy include postprandial antral hypomotility, uncoordinated or absent phase III of the migrating motor complex, bursts of nonpropagating segmental contractions (often with tonic elevation of baseline pressure) during fasting, and failure of conversion of fasting to fed motility.

Anorectal and esophageal manometry studies are used to assess somatovisceral reflexes that can be impaired by visceral neuropathy. Serum pancreatic polypeptide levels in response to insulin-induced hypoglycemia or sham feeding can be used to assess vagal cholinergic innervation of the viscera when the more commonly used cardiovagal tests yield borderline results or are technically unsatisfactory.

Urinary Bladder Function Tests

Because the autonomic history is frequently not sufficient to differentiate the various types of neurogenic bladders from each other and even non-neurogenic (that is, obstructive uropathy, bladder infection) causes from neurogenic ones, further testing beyond urinalysis, culture, and Gram's stain is helpful. The cystometrogram-electromyogram allows an assessment of urethral patency and pressure, of bladder capacity, and of the occurrence of uninhibited bladder contractions, urethral sphincter dyssynergia, and detrusor areflexia. Intravesical pressure and anal or urethral electromyographic signals are recorded during bladder filling with a known volume of water or carbon dioxide. Repeat instillation after injection with bethanechol provides a crude assessment of vesicle parasympathetic integrity.

Chapter 16

Examination of the Cerebrospinal Fluid

Obtaining a sample of cerebrospinal fluid (CSF) by lumbar puncture is an important part of the evaluation of many neurologic conditions. The procedure should not be undertaken lightly, as it is not without risk and is often feared by patients. When the examination is deemed necessary, it should be carried out in such a way that the maximum amount of information is provided. Careful planning and a skillful operator are essential. Transportation of the specimen to the laboratory must be rapid. The tests must be done without delay if cytologic examination and chemical analysis are to provide reliable values. For some studies, it is necessary to have a simultaneous blood sample. The CSF glucose level should be compared with the plasma level if meningeal infection or meningeal carcinoma is suspected. Similarly, for complete analysis of the CSF proteins, the serum levels must also be known.

INDICATIONS FOR CSF EXAMINATION

When any form of meningitis or encephalitis is suspected, a CSF examination is mandatory. In the evaluation of dementia, degenerative diseases of the nervous system, and suspected multiple sclerosis, it is often an important test. In suspected subarachnoid hemorrhage, a CSF examination is necessary only when the condition cannot be confirmed by computed tomography scans of the head or when there is difficulty making the differentiation from meningitis. CSF studies may provide valuable information in the evaluation of inflammatory neuropathies and polyradiculopathies. Tumor markers are sometimes detectable in the CSF, aiding in the investigation of various intracranial malignancies, including the lymphomas, primary central nervous system tumors, and metastatic lesions.

CONTRAINDICATIONS TO LUMBAR PUNCTURE

Before lumbar puncture is performed, it is essential that the possibility of raised intracranial pressure be considered. If ophthalmoscopic examination reveals papilledema, a computed tomography scan or magnetic resonance imaging scan is essential before removal of CSF. If either of these imaging techniques shows that the ventricular system is of normal size and undisplaced, and if there is no indication of a mass in the posterior fossa, lumbar puncture can be performed with little risk of tonsillar herniation or medullary compression. Patients with signs of focal intracranial dysfunction or those with signs suggesting brain-stem compression should not have a lumbar puncture before a neuroimaging examination. Patients in whom meningitis, subarachnoid hemorrhage, or a non–space-occupying lesion, such as multiple sclerosis, is suspected can undergo lumbar puncture without radiologic investigation, provided that the eye grounds have been examined to exclude papilledema.

Local sepsis, such as an infected pressure sore in the lumbar region, precludes using the lumbar route for obtaining a CSF sample. A prolonged prothrombin time, a platelet count below $50,000/mm^3$, administration of therapeutic doses of heparin, or any bleeding diathesis, such as hemophilia, should preclude lumbar puncture until the coagulation defect can be temporarily reversed, because of the risk of intraspinal bleeding with compression of the cauda equina.

A lumbar puncture should not be performed when a spinal mass is suspected unless the procedure is part of a myelogram with neurosurgical assistance readily available. A dramatic deterioration in the spinal cord or cauda equina function can occur after lumbar puncture when an intraspinal mass is present, and early surgical intervention may be required. A further reason to avoid lumbar puncture in isolation when a spinal mass is suspected is that it may be technically difficult to perform myelography for a few days after the procedure. CSF may leak into the subdural space through the original needle hole. The myelographic dye, when injected subsequently, may pass into this space rather than into the subarachnoid space, so that the procedure fails.

Queckenstedt's test, previously used to detect an intraspinal block of the CSF pathways, is outmoded and should not be performed. If a spinal mass is suspected, myelography or magnetic resonance imaging of the spine is the appropriate investigation.

TECHNIQUE OF LUMBAR PUNCTURE

Whether lumbar puncture is performed in the emergency room, in the patient's hospital room, or in a room dedicated to the procedure, strict aseptic technique is required. Organisms introduced into the subarachnoid space find an almost perfect growing environment.

Preparation and Positioning of the Patient

The natural apprehension of the patient about to undergo the test is allayed by a kindly explanation of the procedure as the subject is being positioned for it. The patient is asked to lie on the right or left side close to the edge of the bed or padded table. The side chosen depends on which position seems easier for the operator. With experience, there is no advantage of one lateral position over the other. The subject's head is supported on a small pillow, and the back is exposed from midthoracic to midgluteal region. Proper positioning of the patient is essential. Failure to do so is the commonest cause of an unsuccessful lumbar puncture. Positioning should be achieved before the back is cleansed and before the sterile drapes are applied. Maximal widening of the interspinous spaces is obtained by full flexion of the spine, which is achieved by assisting the patient in flexing the knees up toward the chin. To help assume the ideal "fetal" position, the subject can grasp the knees and pull them upward. Cooperative subjects can easily maintain this position for the few minutes it takes to perform a lumbar puncture and collect the CSF. If necessary, an attendant can help keep the spine flexed by gently holding the patient under the knees and behind the nape of the neck. For uncooperative and confused patients, a sheet can be passed behind the knees and around the nape of the neck and held firmly by the attendant to prevent sudden movements that might dislodge or even break the spinal needle. Once the flexed position is achieved, final positioning should ensure that the lumbar region of the back is at a right angle to the plane of the table or bed.

The operator should don sterile gloves after appropriate scrubbing of the hands. The sterile lumbar puncture kit should be opened by an assistant; thereafter, only the sterile equipment or the sterile drapes should be touched by the operator.

The skin of the back is prepared by swabbing with a suitable skin antiseptic; several applications are made with sterile applicator sponges. The back is then draped with sterile towels in such a way that the midline of the lower lumbar spine is left exposed.

Anesthesia

The most easily identified interspace is that between the third and fourth spinous processes. An imaginary line drawn perpendicularly from the top of the iliac crest usually passes through this interspace. The puncture can be performed at this level or at the interspace above or below this level.

A small wheal is raised at the chosen level by injection of a small quantity of lidocaine through a fine intradermal needle. It is wise to warn the patient of the impending discomfort before each step so that unexpected movements by the subject are minimized. The needle is then changed to a 2-inch-long intramuscular needle, which is inserted through the wheal and advanced slowly while the local anesthetic is injected along the anticipated tract of the spinal puncture needle.

Insertion of the Lumbar Puncture Needle

After a wait of several minutes for the local anesthetic to take effect, the lumbar puncture needle with the stylet in place is inserted through the skin. If visible, the puncture made by the local anesthetic needle can be used as the site of entry of the larger needle. For adults, a no. 20 needle is the optimal size because it is rigid enough to penetrate the tough ligamentum flavum and of large enough diameter to allow rapid collection of the specimen and accurate pressure measurements. The needle should be inserted so that the bevel splits the longitudinal fibers of the dura rather than cuts them transversely to minimize the leakage of spinal fluid into the subdural space once the needle is removed. This detail may reduce the incidence of post–spinal-tap headache. As the needle is inserted, it should be angled slightly in a cephalic direction, and care should be taken to ensure that the needle remains at right angles to the lumbar spine in the transverse plane. As the needle penetrates the ligamentum flavum, there is often a sudden decrease in resistance. A second "give" may be appreciated as the dura is perforated. When it is believed that the subarachnoid space has been entered, the stylet is removed; if no fluid emerges, the needle is rotated 180 degrees and withdrawn a few millimeters. If bone is encountered, the needle should be withdrawn to the level of the skin and redirected in a slightly different cephalocaudal direction. A common error by the inexperienced operator is to try to readjust the angle of the needle without withdrawing the tip back to the skin surface. Failure to do this results in the needle tip following the original path while the exposed portion of the needle is bent. Another error is to remove the needle completely and then insert it through a new puncture site at the same interspace. Repeated puncturing of the skin increases the risk of infection and often results in more subcutaneous bleeding. If the patient experiences a sudden stab of pain in one lower extremity, the needle is directed too far laterally and has struck a sensory nerve root on the side of the pain. The needle should be redirected more medially.

If the subarachnoid space is not reached after several attempts, it may be necessary to select a different interspace. The same procedure for administration of local anesthesia and insertion of the needle must be followed. If CSF is not obtained at the new interspace, the procedure should be abandoned or a more experienced person should be asked to attempt the puncture. In older persons with extensive hypertrophic changes of the lumbar spine, it may be very difficult to perform a lumbar puncture. Rather than persisting unreasonably, it is appropriate to request a radiologist to perform the procedure under fluoroscopic control.

Once the subarachnoid space is entered, the patient should be reassured that the additional procedures will be painless.

Pressure Studies

The opening pressure of the CSF is measured by attaching an open-ended manometer to the lumbar puncture needle by means of the right-angled adapter equipped with a stopcock. The CSF should rise rapidly, and the meniscus should show 1-mm fluctuations synchronous with the patient's pulse and somewhat larger fluctuations with respiration. If the subject coughs or strains or if the abdomen is compressed, there should be a transient increase of pressure measuring several centimeters. If there is any possibility that the needle is obstructed by a nerve root or not fully into the subarachnoid space, it should be rotated or the depth should be adjusted slightly until it is certain that the true pressure is being measured. As the pressure is measured, the patient should be encouraged to relax and breathe easily through the open mouth. The neck and hips can be gently extended from the fully flexed position. The average opening pressure, once the patient is relaxed, is in the range of 60 to 140 mm of CSF. Pressures above 200 mm are definitely high, and pressures in the 180- to 200-mm range are equivocal. The commonest cause of a high or borderline reading is poor relaxation.

After the CSF pressure has been determined, the stopcock is turned to retrieve the CSF from the manometer, which can then be disconnected while the fluid samples are collected. There is little merit in measuring the closing pressure of the fluid after the collection is completed. Finally, the needle is withdrawn without replacing the stylet, and a sterile dressing is applied to the puncture site.

BLOODY TAP

Most commonly encountered with a difficult puncture, bleeding into the CSF may occur with any spinal tap if a small subarachnoid vessel is traumatized. In traumatic bleeding, the blood may be unevenly mixed in the fluid as it emerges from the needle, and a clot may form in the hub of the needle. Furthermore, as the fluid is collected in several vials, it becomes progressively less blood-tinged. If this change is noted, it is advisable to discard the initial few milliliters and collect only the clearer fluid. If it is difficult to distinguish between blood staining due to trauma and spontaneous subarachnoid bleeding, a sample of the fluid should be promptly centrifuged. Clear supernatant fluid characterizes the traumatic puncture, whereas a xanthochromic supernatant indicates that the blood has been in contact with the CSF for several hours and, therefore, antedates the lumbar puncture. Caution is required in the interpretation of the finding of xanthochromia, because a yellow coloration occurs in CSF with a very high protein level and, conversely, the supernatant fluid can be clear if a spontaneous subarachnoid hemorrhage occurred within 1 or 2 hours of the collection of the fluid. Also, xanthrochromia may occur in traumatic lumbar punctures, with red blood cell counts exceeding 200,000/mm^3.

DRY TAP

Occasionally, the subarachnoid space is successfully entered, but no fluid emerges from the needle. The commonest cause is that the needle is blocked by a nerve root or by a wisp of arachnoid tissue. Rotation of the needle or adjustment of the depth usually resolves the difficulty. A very high protein level (several hundred milligrams per deciliter) may render the CSF so viscous that it will not flow through the needle. A very low CSF pressure is also a rare cause for a so-called dry tap. If it is suspected that the fluid will not flow through the needle, a sterile syringe can be attached and a very small negative pressure applied. This occasionally allows collection of a small sample of fluid for the most important tests, such as the cell count, protein and glucose concentrations, and culture. Excessive suction will almost certainly pull a nerve root against the needle, causing lower limb pain and defeating the collection process.

Table 16-1 Milliliters of CSF Required for Various Tests

Microbiology		Cytology	
Gram stain and/or culture	1	Cell count	1
Bacteria	2	T and B hematologic malignancy markers	5
Fungi (including cryptococcal antigen)	3	Kappa/lambda surface marker	5
Tubercle bacilli	3	Malignant cells	
Virus	3	Papanicolaou's stain	2
Counterimmune electrophoresis	1	Wright's stain	2
Polymerase chain reaction	3		
Chemistry and Serologic Tests			
Protein (total)	1	Xanthochromia	0.5
Specific proteins	1	Carcinoembryonic antigen	1
Glucose	0.5	Alpha-fetoprotein	1
β-Glucuronidase	1	Oligoclonal bands*	3
β-hCG	1	Lyme serology	0.5
CSF IgG index*	1	Anti-neuronal nuclear antibody	1
VDRL	1	Anti–Purkinje's cell antibody	4
Fluorescent treponemal antibody absorption	1	Anti-islet cell antibody	1
		Myelin basic protein	1

VDRL, Venereal Disease Research Laboratory; β-hCG, beta-human chorionic gonadotropin.
* Five milliliters of clotted blood should be obtained at the time of lumbar puncture.

AMOUNT OF CSF REQUIRED FOR TESTS

The amount of CSF removed is determined by the number and type of tests to be made. The amounts adequate for each of the various tests are shown in Table 16-1.

The characteristics of normal CSF are shown in Table 16-2.

Table 16-2 Characteristics of Normal CSF

Appearance	Clear and colorless
Cells	Fewer than 5 lymphocytes or mononuclear cells
Total protein	
Lumbar fluid	15–45 mg/dL
Cisternal fluid	10–25 mg/dL
Ventricular fluid	6–15 mg/dL
IgG	Less than 8.4 mg/dL
IgM	37–374 ng/mL
Gamma globulin	6%–13% of total protein
Oligoclonal bands	0–1 band
Myelin basic protein	0–4 ng/mL
IgM, FTA-ABS	Negative
CSF IgG index	0–0.77
CSF IgG synthesis rate	0–8 mg/24 hr
Alpha-fetoprotein	Less than 1.5 ng/mL
Glucose	45–80 mg/dL or 60%–80% of plasma glucose
VDRL	Negative
β-hCG	0.2 IU/L
β-Glucuronidase	Less than 49 mU/L
CEA	Less than 0.6 ng/mL
Anti-neuronal nuclear antibody	
Type 1 (anti-Hu)	Less than 1:2
Type 2 (anti-Ri)	Less than 1:2
Anti-islet cell antibody	Less than 1:4
Purkinje's cell antibody (anti-Yo)	Less than 1:2

FTA-ABS, fluorescent treponemal antibody absorption; VDRL, Venereal Disease Research Laboratory; β-hCG, beta-human chorionic gonadotropin; CEA, carcinoembryonic antigen.

Chapter 17

Other Laboratory Aids in Neurologic Diagnosis

CEREBROVASCULAR DISEASE

Noninvasive Neurovascular Studies
Noninvasive neurovascular techniques constitute an extension of the clinical neurovascular examination. The proper utilization of these techniques requires an understanding of the underlying disease process, the principles of the tests involved, and the advantages and limitations of each procedure.

It is useful to classify the various techniques into two major groups, indirect and direct. The indirect techniques measure physiologic hemodynamic changes in distal ophthalmic and external carotid arterial systems to provide data about the more proximal carotid system. The direct techniques provide anatomic or physiologic data about the carotid bifurcation area, the cervical intervertebral segments of the vertebral arteries, and, in the case of transcranial Doppler ultrasonography, the intracranial arterial segments at the base of the brain in both the anterior and the posterior circulations. All of these techniques have limitations. Specifically, none can reliably differentiate high-grade stenosis from occlusion or detect ulceration within lesions.

Indirect techniques
Ophthalmodynamometry (retinal artery pressures)
With this technique, the examiner applies pressure to the side of the globe with a calibrated, hand-held ophthalmodynamometer while observing the central retinal artery with an ophthalmoscope. As the intraocular pressure increases, the point at which pulsations appear is the diastolic pressure and the point at which pulsations are again eliminated is the systolic pressure. Criteria for abnormality are a 15% or greater decrease in retinal artery systolic pressure and a 50% or greater decrease in the retinal artery diastolic pressure in one eye compared with that in the other. Absolute systolic retinal artery pressure values below 40 mm Hg

are also considered abnormal in the absence of systolic hypertension. By providing a measure of central retinal artery pressure, ophthalmodynamometry yields information about pressure-significant (greater than or equal to 75% stenosis of area) ipsilateral internal carotid system lesions proximal to, and including, the central retinal artery. The procedure requires great technical expertise, and results may be subject to wide variation.

Ocular pneumoplethysmography
Ophthalmic artery systolic pressures are simultaneously measured by an air-filled system. Suction is applied to the anesthetized sclera by eyecups serving as pressure transducers, and resulting scleral displacement creates an increase in intraocular pressure that can be measured precisely. Recordings are made during continuous release of applied vacuum (300 to 500 mm Hg). The point at which ophthalmic artery pressure overcomes intraocular pressure and produces ocular pulsations represents the ophthalmic artery systolic pressure. An asymmetry in ophthalmic artery systolic pressure of 5 mm or greater indicates a pressure-significant stenosis on the side of the lower pressure proximal to the central retinal artery. The ophthalmic artery systolic pressures are also routinely expressed as fractions of brachial artery systolic pressures. When these ratios fall below calculated critical values, pressure-significant stenoses can be identified with or without asymmetries in ophthalmic artery systolic pressure. This technique may also be used for measuring collateral pressure around either carotid system by common carotid compression maneuvers performed during the ocular pneumoplethysmographic testing.

Periorbital directional Doppler ultrasonography
This technique assesses the direction and quality of periorbital Doppler blood flow and the response of these variables to various arterial compression maneuvers about the face and neck. Since the periorbital arteries are terminal branches of the ophthalmic artery, blood flow is normally directed out of the orbit and may be augmented by external compression of carotid artery branches. After locating one or more periorbital vessels near the orbital rim, the examiner positions the Doppler probe over the vessel to be studied. Reversed flow indicates extracranial collateral flow, usually resulting from a pressure-significant stenosis in the ipsilateral internal carotid system. The source of collateral flow is often better defined by sequentially compressing the superficial temporal, infraorbital, and facial arteries on each side of the head. A diminution or obliteration of periorbital flow indicates that the compressed vessel supplies collateral flow via the external carotid system. Compression of the common carotid artery may detect pressure-significant stenosis of the internal carotid system when intracranial collateral circulation from the circle of Willis

maintains periorbital blood flow in the normal direction. In such instances, periorbital blood flow is unchanged or augmented by ipsilateral compression of the common carotid artery.

Summary
All of the indirect techniques are designed to detect the presence or absence of lesions that compromise 75% or more of the luminal area somewhere within the internal carotid system proximal to and including the ophthalmic artery. None of the techniques can localize the lesion within the internal carotid system, detect mild stenosis or ulceration within lesions, or reliably differentiate high-grade stenosis from occlusion.

Direct techniques
Doppler flow velocity spectral analysis
This procedure is based on the physiologic correlation of changes in blood flow velocity with degree of stenosis. The Doppler signal is generated and recorded from a probe held directly over the distal common and proximal internal and external carotid arteries. The resulting signal is analyzed by audiofrequency or color-coding methods. A normal vessel produces a Doppler spectrum with laminar flow that has a peak frequency below 4 kHz and a readily identifiable clear area under the systolic peak. Areas of increased stenosis cause the frequency range during systole to widen. Tighter stenoses are usually associated with high peak frequencies, whereas lesser stenoses are associated with lower peak frequencies.

Real-time B-scan ultrasonic arteriography
A two-dimensional image of the vessel wall is created by sound waves generated and recorded from an ultrasonic B-mode probe. Because the sound waves are reflected differently from interfaces of different acoustic impedance, the common and proximal internal and external carotid arteries in the neck can be identified. The blood column is generally sonolucent, whereas the vessel wall and atherosclerotic deposits are comparatively dense. Both transverse and longitudinal scans are performed, allowing an estimate of percentage of stenosis in a given area in the imaging field.

Duplex scanner
The duplex scanner represents a combination of B-scan ultrasound and Doppler flow velocity analysis into the same instrument. The B-scan component allows imaging of the walls of the common carotid, internal carotid, and external carotid arteries, and a pulsed Doppler cursor can be placed within the lumen of any of these arteries to record flow velocity signals that can subsequently be analyzed by audiofrequency or color-coding methods.

Transcranial Doppler ultrasonography

Transcranial Doppler ultrasonography permits noninvasive assessment of the intracranial cerebral circulation. The most commonly used instruments have handheld 2-MHz probes that allow Doppler flow velocity analysis in the distal intracranial segments of the vertebral arteries, basilar artery, distal internal carotid artery siphon segments, middle cerebral artery M1 segments, and anterior cerebral artery A1 segments. The 2-MHz probe is of lower frequency than that commonly used in carotid ultrasound studies and permits the greater tissue penetration required for intracranial studies. The probe must be placed over the orbit or the zygomatic arch for insonation of the anterior circulation or under the inion for insonation of the posterior circulation through the foramen magnum. Transcranial Doppler ultrasonography is useful in detecting hemodynamically significant narrowing in these arteries due to atherosclerotic stenosis in patients with ischemic cerebrovascular disease or to vasospasm in patients with subarachnoid hemorrhage. The test may also be used to confirm cerebral death, to study the hemodynamic effects in feeding arteries after treatment for arteriovenous malformations, and to assess intracranial collateral patterns in patients with occlusive disease of the cervical carotid or vertebral arteries.

Magnetic resonance angiography

Magnetic resonance angiography is a relatively new technique used in conjunction with magnetic resonance brain imaging to provide anatomic imaging of the cervicocephalic vessels in the neck or the intracranial vessels at the base of the brain. This emerging technology gives images that are similar to, but not as detailed or precise as, those of conventional cerebral angiography. In particular, magnetic resonance angiography tends to overestimate the degree of stenosis in patients with cervical carotid occlusive disease and in general provides only qualitative information about the patency and presence or absence of obvious stenosis in the distal intracranial vertebral artery and basilar artery segments, the distal segments of the internal carotid artery siphons, and the middle cerebral artery M1 and anterior cerebral artery A1 segments.

Summary

These direct noninvasive tests offer the opportunity to detect hemodynamically significant lesions in the carotid bifurcation region and in the intracranial arterial segments at the base of the brain. The carotid B-scan and duplex scan techniques are particularly sensitive in detecting degrees of stenosis greater than 50%, but the results of these studies may be adversely affected by calcified plaques that prevent Doppler signal transmission and produce acoustic shadowing. Technical difficulties also often arise in carotid duplex imaging in patients who have large, short necks or very high carotid bifurcations. All ultrasound studies are technique-dependent, and accuracy may vary with the skill of the examiner.

The clinical application of noninvasive cerebrovascular studies varies widely. Although arteriography remains the most informative study of the cerebral circulation, noninvasive studies provide useful information without the risk of arteriography. The indirect and direct tests complement each other and are often used in combination, since they are providing different types of information.

Noninvasive studies of the carotid bifurcation are often used to select which patients may be the most likely to benefit from carotid arteriography and endarterectomy procedures. They may also be used repeatedly to follow the condition of the carotid circulation in patients receiving various forms of medical or surgical treatment. The results of all these tests must be interpreted in light of the clinical situation, since patients without symptoms may have positive test results and patients with symptoms may have test results that are negative.

Measurement of Cerebral Blood Flow

Regional cerebral blood flow has been measured as a clinical test in certain neurologic disorders, primarily for patients with cerebrovascular diseases and particularly for those with significant hemodynamic problems. It has also found usefulness in some patients with dementia and seizure disorders. The method that combines inhalation of xenon 133 with the external detector system can provide the actual regional flow values but has limitation in spatial resolution.

Single-photon emission tomography has offered an alternative approach. Although this method provides much better spatial resolution and yields results that can be reviewed as an actual brain image, it cannot measure the absolute blood flow values. In fact, this method displays a cerebral perfusion pattern instead of a cerebral flow pattern.

Iodine 123-isopropyl-p-iodoamphetamine hydrochloride (Iofetamine ^{123}I) is currently available for clinical use. In some institutions, a computed tomographic instrument is used in combination with inhalation of stable xenon gas. The spatial resolution is excellent, but 30% xenon gas may cause an anesthetic effect.

Although positron emission tomography can provide not only the method for measurement of regional cerebral blood flow but also the method for measurement of oxygen or glucose utilization rate, it remains unclear at this time whether positron emission tomography will become a clinical necessity or remain primarily a research instrument.

Radioisotope Cisternography

By injecting a radioisotope into the lumbar (or, occasionally, cisternal) subarachnoid space and sequentially scanning over the spinal canal and cranium, an examiner can make physiologic observations of the circulation of cerebrospinal fluid. Normally, the injected material rises and accumulates both within the ventricular system and over the convexity of the brain. Localization of the indicator within the ventricular system and failure to circulate over the brain surface after 48 hours suggest a blockage in the extraventricular cerebrospinal fluid pathways and are frequently seen in cases of communicating hydrocephalus.

ENCEPHALOPATHIES

Toxic Encephalopathies

A variety of neuropsychiatric manifestations are seen in intoxication and drug abuse. They include alteration of mood and consciousness leading to coma, confusion, hallucinations, and convulsions. Autonomic manifestations also accompany drug abuse. Many agents are accurately identified by a variety of laboratory tests. Depending on the level of sophistication of individual laboratories, various screening methods for drugs and toxic substances are available. They include thin-layer chromatography, high-performance liquid chromatography, gas chromatography, atomic absorption spectroscopy, mass spectrometry, and radioimmunoassay. Combined gas chromatography and mass spectrometry is very effective in identification of unknown toxic substances. When requesting screening tests, the clinician should understand the limits of sensitivity of the methods available in each laboratory.

A gas chromatograph or a high-performance liquid chromatograph can detect the following substances in the blood: alcohol, barbiturates, other sedatives and hypnotics, benzodiazepines, nonopiate analgesics, neuroleptics, tricyclic antidepressants, anticonvulsants, and salicylates. The toxic substance can be identified further by mass spectrometry. Many of these substances and their metabolites can also be detected in the urine by high-performance liquid chromatography, gas chromatography, and mass spectrometry. Amphetamines, opiates, including cocaine, and tetrahydrocannabinol are detected primarily with urine samples, either by immunoassays or by gas chromatography. There is currently no reliable clinical method for identification of D-lysergic acid diethylamide (LSD).

In acute *alcohol* intoxication, the blood alcohol level is often above 150 mg/dL, and coma usually occurs at 250 mg/dL. In acute *barbiturate* intoxication, it is difficult to correlate the blood concentration of barbiturate with the level of altered consciousness or incoordination, since the patient may have taken more than one dose of barbiturate, tolerance may have developed, or a combination of short-acting and long-acting barbiturates with different routes of administration may have been used. Any blood concentration greater than 10 μg/mL may be significant in the case of short-acting barbiturates, whereas a level of more than 40 to 50 μg/mL may be significant for long-acting barbiturates. Acute or subacute intoxication occurs with nonbarbiturate *anticonvulsants,* such as phenytoin, primidone, carbamazepine, and clonazepam.

Each laboratory has its own "therapeutic" and toxic ranges for blood concentration of each anticonvulsant. *Tricyclic antidepressants* have atropine-like effects, and acute intoxication may cause hyperpyrexia and hypertension. For imipramine and amitriptyline, the blood level should include the active metabolites of the drugs, desipramine and nortriptyline, respectively.

Acute *narcotic* intoxication causes fixed pinpoint pupils and respiratory depression. If the history or physical examination suggests the possibility of acute narcotic intoxication, a narcotic antagonist, such as naloxone, 0.4 mg, should be administered intravenously for both diagnostic and therapeutic reasons. This, in three repeated doses if necessary, usually produces improvement. In acute intoxication, narcotics may be detected even in the blood.

If a previously healthy infant or child suddenly becomes comatose, ingestion of a toxic substance should be considered. The child's caregivers should be questioned about accessibility of prescription drugs, toxins, and substances of abuse in the home or day-care environment. The toxicology laboratory functions most efficiently when searching for specific compounds. If there is reason to suspect aspirin or another *salicylate* preparation, this is easily ascertained by a blood sample. Toxic manifestations are likely with a serum salicylate level over 30 mg/dL.

The prominent symptoms of acute oral *arsenic* poisoning are vomiting, abdominal pain, and diarrhea followed by convulsion and coma. In acute poisoning, the urine contains more than 25 μg/24 hours. Arsenic disappears rapidly from the blood and urine after ingestion has ceased but can still be measured in hair and nails many weeks later. Acute *lead* poisoning fortunately has been relatively rare. However, this possibility should be kept in mind as the cause of sudden onset of encephalopathy with coma and convulsion in a previously healthy person. For a positive diagnosis, the concentration of lead in the blood and urine is determined. Normal persons have a blood lead level of less than 40 μg/dL and a urinary excretion of less than 80 μg/24 hours. Anything less than 150 μg/24 hours in the urine is of questionable significance. Urinary excretion of coproporphyrin and δ-aminolevulinic acid may be increased in lead intoxication.

The diagnosis of *carbon monoxide* poisoning in a comatose patient is usually apparent from the history and characteristic cherry-red skin. In doubtful cases, the determination of carboxyhemoglobin in the blood is helpful. Normally, there is less than 7% carboxyhemoglobin, but heavy smokers can have up to 15% without toxicity; a level above 20% is definitely abnormal, and severe neurologic signs occur with a level over 50%.

Metabolic Encephalopathies

Many systemic metabolic disorders affect cerebral function. Common clinical manifestations include alterations in consciousness, mentation, and personality and convulsions. Although computed tomography, magnetic resonance imaging, electroencephalography, and cerebrospinal fluid examination are helpful in ruling out other cerebral disorders and directing the diagnosis toward metabolic encephalopathies, confirmation of the cause requires specific laboratory tests for individual metabolic disorders.

In patients with acute or chronic *cardiac failure* or *pulmonary insufficiency*, encephalopathy develops in association with respiratory acidosis. Blood tests such as arterial oxygen saturation, carbon dioxide content, and acid-base balance aid the clinician. The onset of *hepatic coma* is often associated with an increased level of ammonia in the blood, but the absence of hyperammonemia does not rule out hepatic encephalopathy. Other liver function tests, such as serum enzymes (alkaline phosphatase, aspartate transaminase, γ-glutamyltransferase), prothrombin time, protein electrophoresis, and bilirubin, also may show abnormal findings. An electroencephalogram may help, particularly if triphasic waves are present. In both acute and chronic *renal insufficiency*, uremia and metabolic acidosis occur. Severe renal disease can be detected by increased serum creatinine, blood urea, metabolic acidosis, proteinuria, or hematuria.

The diagnosis of *diabetic ketoacidosis* is suspected when Kussmaul's respiration, fruity breath, and dehydration are noted and confirmed by hyperglycemia, glycosuria, and positive reactions for acetone in the blood and urine. Nonketotic coma can occur in diabetes mellitus because of a hyperglycemic hyperosmolar state or lactic acidosis. In adults, severe *hypoglycemia* is usually the result of pancreatic islet cell tumor when overdosage with insulin, an oral hypoglycemic agent, or alcohol consumption has been excluded. Laboratory tests for the study of hypoglycemia include fasting plasma glucose concentration, glucose tolerance test, prolonged fasting up to 72 hours with periodic determination of plasma glucose, and insulin levels. Significant neurologic manifestations usually occur with plasma glucose levels of less than 35 mg/dL. Hypoglycemia also occurs with liver disease, including Reye's syndrome, as well as with hypopituitarism, adrenal insufficiency, growth hormone deficiency, and retroperitoneal malignant lesions. Adequate laboratory evaluation is necessary to study these possibilities. Inborn errors of metabolism account for relatively more cases of hypoglycemia in children than in adults. Key points in elucidating the cause include the timing of hypoglycemia (after fasting or meals or unpredictably), presence of hepatomegaly, and association with lactic acidosis or ketosis. Hypoglycemia may be the presenting symptom of disorders of gluconeogenesis, glycogen breakdown, or energy generation, including fatty acid oxidation defects and oxidative phosphorylation. Laboratory testing is most likely to be helpful when the child has symptoms or is stressed by fasting or substrate loading. Potentially helpful laboratory tests include plasma lactate and pyruvate, plasma amino acids, carnitine levels, urine organic acids, and blood gases (arterial or venous).

In severe *thyrotoxicosis,* patients can present with psychotic reactions and delirium. An increased level of serum thyroxine (T_4) or, occasionally, triiodothyronine (T_3) confirms the diagnosis. In *hypothyroidism,* mental dysfunction can occur. In the congenital form (cretinism), mental retardation is associated with growth retardation. The serum T_4 value is decreased in hypothyroidism. The level of thyroid-stimulating hormone is useful in differentiating primary hypothyroidism (increased level) and hypopituitarism (decreased level). Administration of thyrotropin-releasing hormone may differentiate hypothalamic and pituitary dysfunction.

Hypercalcemia can constitute a medical emergency when the serum calcium concentration is over 15 mg/dL, the level at which neuropsychiatric symptoms develop in more than 90% of patients. In addition to hypercalcemia, these patients often have hypercalciuria. An increased serum level of parathyroid hormone confirms the diagnosis of primary hyperparathyroidism. On radiologic examination, diffuse or localized demineralization of bones, cartilaginous calcification in the joints, and nephrocalcinosis may be found. Since hypercalcemia occurs not only in patients with primary hyperparathyroidism but also in patients with metastatic carcinoma in the bones, multiple myeloma, lymphoma, leukemia, sarcoidosis, vitamin D intoxication, or, rarely, chronic renal disease and in patients who use thiazide diuretics, appropriate laboratory tests are necessary to explore these possibilities.

Hypocalcemia occurs in hypoparathyroidism, pseudohypoparathyroidism, chronic renal insufficiency, vitamin D deficiency, and various malabsorption syndromes. In newborn infants, transient hypocalcemia occurs from prematurity, maternal hyperparathyroidism, and maternal diabetes mellitus, but the classic form occurs among infants fed cow's milk. Clinical manifestations in infants consist of hyperirritability, tremor, tetany, and convulsions. In adults, alteration of mental status, grand mal or bizarre seizures, and tetany may occur. Clinical symptoms often occur when the serum calcium concentration decreases below 8 mg/dL. In addition to hypocalcemia, hypocalciuria and hypophosphaturia are present except in renal tubular insufficiency. The serum phosphorus level varies with the cause. Calcification of the basal ganglia or cerebellar nuclei may be found on roentgenography or on computed tomography in idiopathic hypoparathyroidism and pseudohypoparathyroidism. These two diseases can be distinguished by determination of the serum parathyroid hormone level, which is increased in pseudohypoparathyroidism and decreased in hypoparathyroidism.

Both the acute form (adrenal crisis) and the chronic form (Addison's disease) of *adrenocortical insufficiency* can cause altered mental status. Hyponatremia, hyperkalemia, hypercalcemia, and low levels of corticosteroids in the blood and urine are indicative of this condition. An adrenocorticotropic hormone (ACTH) stimulation test may be necessary to detect corticosteroid abnormalities in milder cases. In *Cushing's syndrome* and *Cushing's disease,* adrenocortical hyperfunction occurs and may cause psychotic reactions. Plasma corticosteroid concentration and urinary 17-hydroxy-corticosteroid excretion are increased. The urinary excretion of 17-ketosteroids varies, depending on the underlying pathologic condition. Rarely, convulsions and coma occur in *pheochromocytoma.* Increased urinary free catecholamines and metanephrine and vanillylmandelic acid excretion are helpful in establishing the diagnosis. In some patients, measurement of plasma catecholamines is useful.

Clinical manifestations of *hypopituitarism* depend on the deficiency in the target organs, the resulting picture consisting of a combination of hypothyroidism, adrenocortical insufficiency, hypogonadism, and, in children, pituitary dwarfism. Various laboratory tests already described under some of the individual target organs are useful, but direct assays of the serum levels of thyroid-stimulating hormone, ACTH, follicle-stimulating hormone, and luteinizing hormone are more confirmatory. The plasma prolactin level is often increased in patients with hypopituitarism. Several provocative tests either identify the hypothalamic causes or differentiate the hypothalamic and pituitary causes. Induction of hypoglycemia by administration of insulin, propranolol-glucagon, L-dopa, or arginine is used as a provocative test for growth hormone. Thyrotropin-releasing hormone and gonadotropin-releasing hormone are administered as provocative tests for thyrotropin and leuteinizing or follicle-stimulating hormone, respectively. Pituitary corticotropin release can be tested by insulin-induced hypoglycemia, administration of propranolol-glucagon, or administration of metyrapone.

Various types of *water and electrolyte imbalance* result in metabolic encephalopathy. Although water intoxication can occur in acute renal insufficiency, the common causes are excessive intake of water and excessive use of parenteral fluid or antidiuretic hormone. Serum hypoosmolarity and hyponatremia are helpful laboratory findings. The syndrome of inappropriate secretion of antidiuretic hormone usually results from primary central nervous system diseases but can occur in extraneural disorders, particularly in small cell carcinoma of the lung. Drugs such as carbamazepine, cyclophosphamide, and vincristine may also provoke inappropriate release of antidiuretic hormone by the pituitary gland. Findings include hyponatremia in the presence of urinary osmolarity greater than that of serum. Hyponatremia with decreased extracellular water (dehydration) occurs in gastrointestinal diseases, renal diseases with a salt-losing state, diabetic ketoacidosis, and adrenal insufficiency. Hyponatremia with increased extracellular fluid (edema) occurs in severe heart failure, liver diseases, and renal diseases. Neurologic manifestations such as lethargy, coma, and convulsion usually occur when the serum sodium level is 120 mmol/L or lower. Hypernatremia accompanies hyperosmolarity when there is too little water or too much solute. The etiologic factors are the same as those in dehydration. Neurologic manifestations such as obtundation, coma, and convulsion can occur when the serum sodium level is over 150 mmol/L. The clinician should be aware that rapid changes in electrolyte concentrations may also produce symptoms when sodium concentrations are between 120 and 150 mmol/L. Conversely, very slow changes allow some patients to tolerate sodium concentrations outside this range with comparatively mild symptoms.

Among vitamin deficiencies, metabolic encephalopathy can occur in *pellagra* (vitamin B_6 deficiency) and *pernicious anemia* (vitamin B_{12} deficiency). Vitamin B_6 deficiency can be induced by isoniazid or occur in association with Hartnup disease. The diagnosis of pellagra is established by the clinical syndrome of dementia in association with dermatitis and diarrhea. For vitamin B_{12} deficiency, gastric achlorhydria, macrocytic anemia, and a low serum level of vitamin B_{12} help confirm the diagnosis, although occasionally the Schilling test is also necessary. *Wernicke's encephalopathy* occurs among malnourished or alcoholic patients and is characterized by apathy, confusion, memory loss, and paralysis of abduction of the eyes. There is no specific laboratory test, but ocular paralysis responds to vitamin B_1 therapy.

Hereditary Metabolic Disorders

Most hereditary metabolic disorders of the nervous system are manifested in infancy and childhood. However, some disorders in this group can appear in adults with neuropsychiatric manifestations. Primary enzyme deficiencies have been identified in many hereditary metabolic disorders. Some enzyme assays are widely available, but others are performed only in a limited number of laboratories. Advances in molecular biology have led to the identification of the genes responsible for many inborn errors of metabolism. In many cases, genotype-phenotype correlations have been made, and if the gene product is unknown or not easily measured (for example, in fragile X syndrome or Huntington's disease), direct molecular analysis may be indicated as a diagnostic or predictive test. In most cases, biochemical testing remains the key to diagnosis of inborn errors of metabolism.

There is no single completely satisfying approach to classification of inborn errors of metabolism. In the following sections, the conventional mixture of groupings according to cellular organelles (for example, lysosomes and peroxisomes), accumulating compounds (for example, organic or amino acids), metabolic pathways (for example, porphyrias), and cofactors (for example, copper disorders) is used.

It is important for the clinician to have a high degree of awareness for these disorders, which are individually rare but collectively relatively common. Many inborn errors of metabolism can be managed with modification of diet or specific cofactor or drug therapy. Even when effective therapy is not available, a specific diagnosis is essential for genetic counseling.

Porphyrias

In this group of disorders, there is deficient activity of enzymes in the heme biosynthetic pathway. In North America, acute intermittent porphyria is the major hepatic porphyria with neurologic symptoms. This diagnosis should be considered in patients with neuropsychiatric disturbance, convulsions, and neuropathy, particularly if there is a history of unexplained abdominal pain and passage of reddish urine. During an acute exacerbation, urinary excretion of porphobilinogen and δ-aminolevulinic acid is markedly increased. However, the detection of a low level of erythrocytic uroporphyrinogen I synthase (porphobilinogen deaminase) confirms the diagnosis even when an acute exacerbation is absent. Up to 90% of persons with this dominantly inherited trait are asymptomatic. In variegate porphyria, there is continuous excretion of large amounts of protoporphyrin and coproporphyrin in the feces after puberty. Variegate porphyria resembles acute intermittent porphyria in neurovisceral symptoms, and definitive diagnosis requires demonstration of reduced protoporphyrinogen oxidase activity. In hereditary coproporphyria, constant and massive excretion of coproporphyrin III in the urine and feces differentiates it from the other acute porphyrias. Deficient activity of coproporphyrinogen oxidase is diagnostic.

Lysosomal storage diseases

This group includes inherited diseases marked by the accumulation of a variety of compounds within lysosomes, subcellular organelles containing hydrolases that catabolize large structural molecules in an acid environment. These have been further subclassified on biochemical and clinical grounds into the following subtypes: sphingolipidoses (accumulating compounds derived from ceramide), mucopolysaccharidoses (accumulated glycosaminoglycans), mucolipidoses (an overlap group embodying features of both sphingolipidoses and mucopolysaccharidoses), and disorders of glycoprotein structure and degradation. The neuronal ceroid lipofuscinoses share ultrastructural features with lysosomal storage diseases, but the underlying biochemical defect or defects remain unknown.

Sphingolipidoses

In most classic lipidoses in infancy and early childhood, the characteristic clinical manifestation is psychomotor regression. Extraneural manifestations, such as organomegaly, cutaneous lesions, and ocular involvement, allow more precise clinical diagnosis (Table 17-1). In most lipidoses, the diagnoses can be confirmed by demonstration of corresponding lysosomal enzyme deficiencies with use of serum, leukocytes, or cultured fibroblasts. Synthetic substrates are now widely used, including p-nitrophenol derivatives for the spectrophotometric method and 4-methylumbelliferone derivatives for the fluorometric method. The deficient enzymes and their corresponding diseases are outlined in Table 17-1.

Table 17-1 Characteristics of the Sphingolipidoses

Name	Enzyme Deficiency	Organomegaly	Ocular Findings	Other Signs	Chromosome and Gene
GM_1 gangliosidosis	β-Galactosidase	Liver and spleen	Cherry-red spot	Skeletal dysplasia, facial dysmorphism	3p21; 60 kb; 16 exons
GM_2 gangliosidosis (Tay-Sachs disease, Sandhoff's disease)	Hexosaminidase; GM_2 activator protein	Liver and spleen (Sandhoff's disease)	Cherry-red spot	"Hyperacusis"	Hex A: 15q23.4 Hex B: 5q13 GM_2A: 5q32
GM_3 gangliosidosis	N-acetylgalactosaminyl transferase	Liver and spleen	Corneal clouding	Facial dysmorphism, skeletal dysplasia	Not known
Schindler's disease	α-N-acetylgalactosaminidase (α-galactosidase)	No	Optic atrophy	Angiokeratomas (type II)	22q13; 14 kb; 9 exons
Fabry's disease	B) α-Galactosidase A	No	Cornea verticillata; cataracts; tortuous blood vessels	Angiokeratomas, autonomic dysfunction, renal failure	Xq22; 12 kb; 7 exons
Gaucher's disease	β-Glucosidase (glucocerebrosidase)	Liver and spleen	Horizontal supranuclear gaze palsy (types 2 and 3)	Neurologic signs in types 2 and 3, anemia, thrombocytopenia, bony lesions	1q21; 7 kb; 11 exons
Krabbe's disease (globoid cell leukodystrophy)	Galactocerebroside β-galactosidase	No	Optic atrophy	Irritability, fever, peripheral neuropathy	14q31; 60 kb; 17 exons
Metachromatic leukodystrophy	Arylsulfatase A	No	Optic atrophy; macular graying	Peripheral neuropathy, intermittent pain	22q13; 3.2 kb; 8 exons
Niemann-Pick disease, types A and B	Acid sphingomyelinase	Liver and spleen	Cherry-red spot (type A); macular halo (type B)	Peripheral neuropathy, pulmonary infiltrates	11p15; 5 kb; 6 exons
Niemann-Pick disease; type C	Enzyme not known; abnormal intracellular cholesterol trafficking	Liver and spleen	Vertical supranuclear gaze palsy	Gelastic cataplexy	18; gene not known

Mucopolysaccharidoses

This group of disorders is characterized by various skeletal abnormalities, facial dysmorphism, and mental retardation. Among six well-established types, type IH (Hurler), type II (Hunter), and type III (Sanfilippo A, B, C, and D) are encountered in neurologic practice because of psychomotor retardation and subsequent dementia. All are autosomal recessive except the X-linked Hunter syndrome. Urinary excretion of acid mucopolysaccharides (glycosaminoglycans) is usually increased in mucopolysaccharidoses and is detected by the cetyltrimethylammonium bromide test. Occasional patients with mucopolysaccharidosis have normal total quantities of glycosaminoglycans in the urine but an abnormal pattern on thin-layer chromatography (see below).

By chromatographic analyses, excreted mucopolysaccharides can be identified as dermatan sulfate, heparan sulfate, and keratan sulfate. In type IH (Hurler), type IS (Scheie), and type II (Hunter), both dermatan sulfate and heparan sulfate are excreted. In type III (A to D), only heparan sulfate is excreted. In type IV A and B (Morquio), keratan sulfate is excreted, whereas only dermatan sulfate is excreted in type VI (Maroteaux-Lamy). Both dermatan sulfate and heparan sulfate are accumulated in type VII (Sly). Type V is no longer used.

The key enzyme deficiency has been identified for each type of mucopolysaccharidosis. In type IH and type IS, α-L-iduronidase is deficient. Mental retardation is absent in patients with type IS. Iduronidase sulfatase is deficient in type II, which has X-linked inheritance. In type III A, B, C, and D, the enzyme deficiencies are heparan N-sulfatase, N-acetyl-α-D-glucosaminidase, acetyl-CoA:α-glucosaminide-N-acetyltransferase, and N-acetyl-α-D-glucosaminide-6-sulfatase, respectively. In type IV A, the enzyme deficiency is galactosamine-6-sulfate sulfatase, and β-galactosidase is deficient in type IV B. Arylsulfatase B (N-acetylgalactosamine-4-sulfatase) is the deficient enzyme in type VI, and β-glucuronidase is deficient in type VII.

Synthetic substrates are available for type I, type III B, type VI, and type VII for general clinical use, but other enzyme assays are available only in some specific laboratories. For those enzyme deficiencies, accumulation of [^{35}S]mucopolysaccharides in cultured skin fibroblasts supports the diagnosis.

Neuronal ceroid-lipofuscinoses

In the infantile (Haltia-Santavuori), late infantile, and juvenile (Batten's disease) forms, patients have progressive mental deterioration, visual impairment, and seizures. Patients with the adult form (Kufs' disease) have either neuropsychiatric manifestations with myoclonic seizures or dementia with cerebellar and extrapyramidal signs, but visual impairment is usually absent. The metabolic defect is not clearly elucidated, and no biochemical diagnostic test has been established, although accumulation of dolichol in the urine is used in some laboratories. This test is unreliable owing to significant numbers of both false-positive results (fever; menses; Niemann-Pick disease, type C; Hallervorden-Spatz disease; Sanfilippo's syndrome, type A) and false-negative results (in up to 15% of biopsy-proven cases). Demonstration by electron microscopy of characteristic inclusion bodies, such as granular osmiophilic deposits or curvilinear bodies and fingerprint profiles in lymphocytes, in the eccrine sweat glands of the biopsied skin specimen, or in conjunctival biopsy specimens, confirms the diagnosis. In some cases, the characteristic ultrastructural changes are found only in neurons, such as those in the myenteric plexus, accessible by rectal biopsy.

Disorders of peroxisomes

Peroxisomes are subcellular organelles with metabolic functions, including β-oxidation (of very-long-chain fatty acids and related compounds), cellular respiration, and synthesis of bile acids and plasmalogens. Three groups of disorders of these organelles have been defined:

1. Disorders of peroxisome biogenesis. Peroxisome "ghosts" are present in the cytosol, and it seems likely that normally synthesized proteins cannot be imported into the peroxisomes, resulting in general deficiency of function. The Zellweger syndrome, neonatal adrenoleukodystrophy (autosomal recessive), and infantile Refsum's disease are in this group.
2. Disorders with loss of multiple peroxisomal functions. Examples are rhizomelic chondrodysplasia punctata and "Zellweger-like" syndrome.
3. Disorders with impairment of one peroxisomal function. X-linked adrenoleukodystrophy is the best known member of this group, which also includes pseudoneonatal adrenoleukodystrophy (acyl CoA oxidase deficiency), bifunctional protein deficiency, and pseudo-Zellweger syndrome (3-oxoacyl-CoA thiolase deficiency). Refsum's disease most likely is in this group as well, although its classification has been controversial until recently.

Assay of plasma very-long-chain fatty acids is a useful screening test for many peroxisomal disorders, although findings are normal in rhizomelic chondrodysplasia punctata. Phytanic acid levels are usually increased in disorders in groups 1 and 2 but not in group 3. Precise biochemical definition may require measurement of other complex metabolites as well as direct enzyme assay.

Heredopathia atactica polyneuritiformis (Refsum's disease) is manifested by cerebellar ataxia, sensorimotor neuropathy, and atypical retinitis pigmentosa. Because of a defect in α-oxidation of β-methylated fatty acids, exogenous phytanic acid (3,7,11,15-tetramethylhexadecanoic acid) accumulates in the tissue. Increase of phytanic acid in the serum can be detected by gas chromatography.

Craniofacial dysmorphism, muscle hypotonia, sensorineural deafness, pigmentary retinopathy, hepatomegaly, and severe psychomotor retardation, reflecting abnormal neuronal migration, are the usual manifestations of Zellweger syndrome. Children with this phenotype rarely survive infancy. The absence of functional peroxisomes results in impairment of various metabolic processes, including catabolism of very-long-chain fatty acids. Increased $C_{26:0}/C_{22:0}$ fatty acid ratio can be detected in the serum or cultured skin fibroblasts. In the serum, pipecolic acid, abnormal bile acids, and phytanic acid may also be increased. The phenotypes of neonatal adrenoleukodystrophy and infantile Refsum's disease are similar to, but somewhat less severe than, the phenotype of Zellweger syndrome.

Adrenoleukodystrophy most often occurs in boys with behavioral disturbances, cortical deafness, progressive blindness, spasticity, and dementia. Adrenomyeloneuropathy is manifested by progressive spastic paraparesis and neuropathy. Both disorders have X-linked inheritance and are associated with deficient activity of very-long-chain fatty acid CoA synthetase. It has recently been found that the primary defect in these disorders is in the gene coding for the adrenoleukodystrophy protein, believed to be responsible for import of very-long-chain fatty acid CoA synthetase into the peroxisome. Very-long-chain (C_{24} and C_{26}) fatty acids accumulate in the tissue, and an increased $C_{26:0}/C_{22:0}$ fatty acid ratio can be detected in the serum or cultured skin fibroblasts.

Disorders of lipoproteins

In abetalipoproteinemia (Bassen-Kornzweig syndrome), the central nervous system manifestations, such as spinocerebellar degeneration, ophthalmoplegia, mental retardation, and retinal degeneration, as well as peripheral neuropathy, occur. Hypocholesterolemia, hypotriglyceridemia, and acanthocytosis can lead to the diagnosis. Deficiency of apolipoprotein B results in deficiency of plasma chylomicron, very-low-density lipoprotein, and low-density lipoprotein. In Tangier disease (hypoalphalipoproteinemia), sensorimotor neuropathy occurs. Hypocholesterolemia and hypertriglyceridemia are also present, high-density lipoprotein is absent, and apolipoproteins A-I and A-II are greatly reduced.

Disorders of glycoprotein metabolism

Mannosidosis, fucosidosis, sialidosis, and aspartylglycosaminuria belong to this group. Clinical manifestations are similar to those of the mucopolysaccharidoses but milder. There are two types of sialidosis. Type I is known as "cherry red spot-myoclonus syndrome," and patients do not have the somatic features of mucopolysaccharidoses. Urinary oligosaccharides are increased in mannosidosis, fucosidosis, and sialidosis, and glycoasparagines are increased in aspartylglycosaminuria and fucosidosis. The lysosomal enzyme deficiencies responsible for mannosidosis, fucosidosis, sialidosis, and aspartylglycosaminuria are α-D-mannosidase, α-L-fucosidase, α-neuraminidase, and aspartylglycosaminidase, respectively. In type II sialidosis, β-galactosidase is also reduced. These enzymes can be assayed in leukocytes and cultured skin fibroblasts.

Carbohydrate-deficient glycoprotein syndrome often is manifested in infants and young children by strokelike episodes, seizures, or coma. Characteristic features are esotropia, inverted nipples, and fat pads above the buttocks. Later, progressive cerebellar ataxia, peripheral neuropathy, and skeletal deformities become apparent. Increased liver enzymes and cerebrospinal fluid protein and abnormal results of thyroid function tests are nonspecific findings. The most useful diagnostic test is assay of carbohydrate-deficient transferrin. This is the most consistently abnormal of many affected glycoproteins in this syndrome. In carbohydrate-deficient glycoprotein syndrome, there is a shift in the proportions of the isoforms from the usually predominant tetra- and penta-sialotransferrin to a-, mono-, and di-sialotransferrin. This change can be demonstrated in blood or cerebrospinal fluid; the test is available in only a limited number of laboratories.

Aminoacidopathies

Most of the aminoacidopathies are manifested as aminoaciduria beginning in infancy. The usual clinical manifestations are mental retardation, growth retardation, convulsive disorder, and coma. Some disorders have highly suggestive phenotypes, such as homocystinuria, with its marfanoid body habitus, skin changes, and lens dislocation, and tyrosinemia type II, with palmar and plantar hyperkeratosis and corneal erosions. The aminoacidopathies are due either to the primary enzyme deficiency for metabolism of a specific amino acid or to abnormal transmembrane transport of amino acids in the intestines or kidneys. Since a fair number of aminoacidopathies can be treated with special diets, early detection is imperative. Three color reactions in the urine are traditionally used as screening tests. The ferric chloride test produces a green color in phenylketonuria, but other aminoaciduria or drug metabolites produce a variety of other colors. The dinitrophenylhydrazine test yields yellow or orange in the presence of ketoacids and is positive in phenylketonuria, tyrosinemia, and maple syrup urine disease. The sodium nitroprusside test yields red in the presence of sulfur-containing amino acids and is positive in homocystinuria, cystathioninuria, and cystinuria. Most laboratories continue to offer these tests but also perform qualitative assays of plasma and urine amino acids, proceeding to quantitation if abnormalities are detected.

Both qualitative and quantitative analyses of amino acid profiles in serum and urine by various types of chromatography, electrophoresis, and amino acid analyzer are more specific in establishing a diagnosis. Because of the relatively high incidence of phenylketonuria, the serum phenylalanine level is measured routinely in newborn infants.

Simultaneous measurement of serum tyrosine is helpful when an increased serum phenylalanine value is found. In a limited number of laboratories specializing in aminoacidopathies, the exact enzyme deficiency can be confirmed by use of liver tissue, skin fibroblasts, or leukocytes. Sometimes this is necessary, since aminoacidopathies such as phenylketonuria, ketotic hyperglycinemia, and methylmalonicacidemia result from more than one enzyme deficiency.

Because of defective membrane transport, neutral amino acids are excreted in Hartnup disease, and because of delayed intestinal absorption of tryptophan, indoles such as indoxyl sulfate and indoleacetic acid also are detected in the urine. Cystinuria is caused by a defective renal reabsorption mechanism for basic amino acids, such as cystine, lysine, arginine, and ornithine. The oculocerebrorenal syndrome (Lowe) is characterized by hypophosphatemia with renal tubular acidosis and generalized aminoaciduria with excessive excretion of lysine. Generalized aminoaciduria can also be found in Wilson's disease, galactosemia, and cystinosis.

Urea cycle disorders
The urea cycle serves to dispose of toxic nitrogen derivatives as well as providing several steps in the synthesis of arginine. An increased level of ammonia in the blood is helpful in the diagnosis of disorders of the urea cycle, including deficiency of carbamoyl phosphate synthetase (CPS), ornithine transcarbamoylase (OTC), argininosuccinic acid synthetase, and arginosuccinase. Further discrimination among these disorders may be possible by measuring citrulline (low in CPS and OTC), orotic acid (high in OTC, low in CPS), and organic acids that will separate out organic acidemias (such as methylmalonicacidemia and propionicacidemia) that may also cause hyperammonemia. The disorders outlined above typically appear between the first and the third days of life with lethargy, vomiting, hypothermia, and hyperventilation; later, atypical onsets may occur, particularly in females heterozygous for OTC (the only X-linked disorder in the group). Arginase deficiency may be confused with cerebral palsy, because the typical presentation is very slowly progressive spastic diplegia with mental retardation; hyperammonemia may be mild or absent. In all urea cycle defects, definitive diagnosis requires enzyme assay of biopsied liver tissue.

Organic acidopathies
More than 50 diseases in this category have been recognized in the past 3 decades. Organic acids accumulate in disorders of branched-chain amino acids, L-lysine, aromatic amino acids, β-oxidation, pyruvate, and carbohydrate metabolism. Common clinical manifestations are metabolic acidosis, ketosis, vomiting, hypoglycemia, seizures, and coma. Unusual odors may provide a clue to the diagnosis (for example, maple syrup

urine in branched-chain ketoaciduria, sweaty feet in isovalericaciduria). Most patients are neonates or infants with life-threatening illness; survivors are often neurologically handicapped. Some disorders are manifested as isolated neurologic deficits (for example, speech delay in 3-methylglutaconicaciduria) or progressive neurologic deterioration (glutaricaciduria, type I; mevalonicaciduria; *N*-acetylasparticaciduria [Canavan's disease]).

Investigation of organic acidopathies requires measurement of plasma electrolytes, glucose, ammonia, gases, lactate and pyruvate, and amino acids together with urine organic acids and amino acids. In selected cases, estimation of carnitine levels is useful. Specimens should be obtained fresh and processed as soon as possible. The essential diagnostic method is gas chromatography–mass spectrometry.

Although individually uncommon, collectively the organic acidurias have an incidence as high as 1:3,000 liveborn infants. Many can be successfully managed with diet, cofactor therapy, or substrate removal, and thus the clinician must be alert to the possibility of these diagnoses.

Mitochondrial cytopathies

The mitochondria play important roles in β-oxidation of fatty acids and oxidative phosphorylation. Mitochondrial DNA, 99.9% inherited through the mother, is a circular molecule containing 16,569 base pairs of double-stranded DNA that codes for 13 proteins that are subunits of the respiratory chain complexes. The approximately 70 remaining subunit proteins are coded by nuclear DNA. Although most patients with mitochondrial cytopathies have clinical evidence of myopathy and signs and symptoms attributable to the central nervous system, such as spastic hemiparesis, cerebellar ataxia, and seizures, some patients have only central nervous system manifestations. Subacute necrotizing encephalomyelopathy (Leigh) belongs to this group. The Leigh phenotype may result from several mutations, including MTATP6*NARP8993, MTTL1*MELAS3243, and MTTK*MERRF8344. These point mutations may produce the NARP (neuropathy, ataxia, and retinitis pigmentosa), MELAS (myopathy, encephalopathy, lactic acidosis, and strokelike episodes), and MERRF (myoclonus epilepsy and ragged red fibers) phenotypes in other individuals in the same kindred as the Leigh patient. Other organ systems may be involved, including the liver, kidney (renal Fanconi's syndrome complicating cytochrome-*c* oxidase deficiency), heart (Kearns-Sayre syndrome), bone marrow (Pearson's syndrome), and intestines (myoneurogastrointestinal encephalopathy).

The metabolic defects in oxidative phosphorylation and the respiratory chain are frequently multiple and are always technically difficult to demonstrate. Consequently, only a limited number of laboratories offer such testing. Detection of increased serum lactate and pyruvate levels can be used as a screening procedure. Some authorities advocate testing on arterial blood samples, because reliable results are difficult to obtain on venous blood samples drawn from struggling children. In selected cases, study of cerebrospinal fluid lactate may demonstrate increases of lactate and pyruvate that are not apparent in the blood. The yield of lactate screening procedures may be increased by glucose loading. Unfortunately, lactate does not accumulate excessively in all mitochondrial disorders, and characteristic microscopic findings (ragged red fibers) may not always be present (for example, in the NARP syndrome). In such circumstances, direct screening of mitochondrial DNA may be the most efficient means of confirming the diagnosis.

Disorders of mitochondrial β-oxidation may be manifested by sudden infant death syndrome, hypoglycemia after prolonged fasting, or myopathic symptoms. Several inborn errors of this pathway have been recognized, including long-chain, medium-chain, and short-chain acyl-CoA dehydrogenase deficiencies, defective plasma carnitine transport, and carnitine palmitoyltransferase deficiencies (I and II). In general, these patients excrete intermediates of fatty acid β-oxidation (such as dicarboxylic acids) and their acylcarnitine and acylglycine derivatives in the urine; plasma and urine carnitine levels are usually decreased. In some individuals, biochemical testing results are normal between exacerbations of illness. In these persons, loading with a variety of substrates under carefully controlled conditions may allow diagnosis. Specific enzymes can be assayed in cultured fibroblasts in a limited number of laboratories.

Galactosemia
There are three types of galactosemia: deficiency of galactokinase, deficiency of galactose 1-phosphate uridyltransferase, and deficiency of uridine diphosphate galactose 4-epimerase. The first is manifested mostly by cataract, whereas the other two syndromes are marked by vomiting, failure to thrive, hepatic impairment, and mental retardation in addition to cataract. Neonates are highly susceptible to infection by *Escherichia coli*. Benedict's test result is positive in the urine with a negative glucose oxidase test result, and the galactose and galactose 1-phosphate levels are increased in the urine and plasma. Neonatal screening for this disorder is routine in many states. Demonstration of the enzyme deficiency in erythrocytes confirms the diagnosis. The complementary DNA for galactose 1-phosphate uridyltransferase has been cloned, and a single mutation (Q188R) has been found to account for 70% of cases in white patients.

Disorders of purine and pyrimidine metabolism
Fourteen disorders of purine and pyrimidine metabolism have been recognized. The best known of those involving the nervous system is Lesch-Nyhan syndrome. This X-linked disorder is manifested by mental

retardation, choreoathetosis, and self-mutilation along with hyperuricemia, hyperuricosuria, and, in some cases, crystalluria, renal failure, and gout in the neonatal period. Plasma uric acid levels may not increase until after puberty, but excessive uric acid excretion in the urine can be demonstrated at any age. The diagnosis is confirmed by demonstrating deficiency of hypoxanthine-guanine phosphoribosyltransferase activity in lysed red cells.

The nervous system may also be involved in phosphoribosylpyrophosphate synthetase superactivity (deafness, developmental delay, hypotonia, hyperuricemia), purine-nucleoside phosphorylase deficiency (developmental delay, hypotonia, defective T-cell immunity, hypouricemia), myoadenylate deaminase deficiency (muscle cramps, myalgias), adenylosuccinase deficiency (psychomotor retardation, autistic features, seizures, cerebellar hypoplasia), dihydropyrimidine dehydrogenase deficiency (microcephaly, developmental delay, seizures, hypotonia, delayed myelination, thymine and uracil in urine), dihydropyrimidinase deficiency (seizures, spastic quadriplegia, microcephaly, chorea, urine dihydrothymine and dihydrouracil), and xanthine oxidase deficiency (crystal myopathy). Xanthine oxidase deficiency may be combined with deficient activity of sulfite oxidase when the molybdenum cofactor is absent. Children with the combined deficiency have neonatal seizures, dysmorphism, ectopia lentis, and neurodegeneration.

Disorders of copper metabolism

Copper is an essential nutrient that is an important component of several enzymes (cytochrome oxidase, superoxide dismutase, tyrosinase, dopamine β-hydroxylase, lysyl oxidase, and ceruloplasmin). When present in excess, it is toxic to the liver, kidneys, and brain.

Wilson's disease (hepatolenticular degeneration) is associated with a mutation involving a P-type adenosinetriphosphatase membrane transport gene on chromosome 13 (WD gene). Neurologic manifestations consist of a combination of tremor, dystonia, choreoathetosis, dysarthria, and behavior disorders. Kayser-Fleischer rings are almost always present by slit-lamp examination of the cornea in patients with neurologic manifestations. Liver cirrhosis may be present. The serum level of ceruloplasmin is significantly reduced in most patients, but the total concentration of copper in serum is variable, and the 24-hour urinary excretion of copper is always increased in patients with symptoms. Patients with liver impairment may have abnormalities in routine liver function tests, such as aspartate transaminase, alkaline phosphatase, bilirubin, and prothrombin time. Confirmation of the diagnosis often requires a copper kinetic study with copper 64 or copper 67 or a liver biopsy with measurement of copper concentration, if biopsy is considered safe.

Menkes' (steely-hair) disease and a milder variant, occipital horn syndrome, have been associated with mutations in a copper-transporting,

P-type adenosinetriphosphatase gene located in the Xq13 region (the MNK gene). The function of the gene product is not clearly established, but most likely it has an important role in the extrusion of copper from cells. In Menkes' disease, severe growth and mental retardation, various cerebral focal symptoms, and seizures occur, and patients have characteristic tangled grayish hair and a characteristic facies, with pudgy cheeks, sagging jowls, and unusual eyebrows. Osteoporosis, metaphyseal flaring, and fractures are common. Most children die in infancy, and most patients are boys, but fully affected girls have been described. Demonstration of pili torti by microscopic examination of hair and very low serum copper and ceruloplasmin levels help to establish the diagnosis. Excessive accumulation of copper in cultured skin fibroblasts confirms the diagnosis.

Patients with occipital horn syndrome may present with hernias, joint laxity, or complications arising from bladder diverticula. Imaging studies show dilated occipital horns of the lateral ventricles; calcification may be present. The diagnosis is established by the same criteria as those for Menkes' disease, except that changes in copper levels are usually less marked.

DISORDERS OF MUSCLE AND NEUROMUSCULAR TRANSMISSION

The cause of muscular weakness is at times most difficult to determine in spite of careful clinical and electromyographic study. Fortunately, in such cases, the pharmacologic, biochemical, and immunologic tests to be discussed may be of singular help in diagnosis.

Myasthenia Gravis

Pharmacologic tests for the diagnosis or exclusion of myasthenia gravis are based on the fact that the muscles affected in this disorder can be strengthened by the administration of an anticholinesterase drug.

Patients thought to have myasthenia gravis can be divided into two groups. The larger is composed of patients having obvious weakness detected by tests of muscle strength, and they are suitable for testing with neostigmine and edrophonium chloride. The other group is composed of patients whose complaints suggest that certain muscles become weak when fatigued but who, on tests of muscle strength, display no weakness. The nonweak group presents a greater diagnostic challenge. In this group, there is no definite weakness to be improved by neostigmine or edrophonium chloride, but single-fiber electromyography or the test for antibodies to the acetylcholine receptor in serum can help confirm the diagnosis.

At present, the most frequent errors in the diagnosis of myasthenia gravis seem to result from errors in applying and interpreting the pharmacologic tests to be described. The commonest errors may be attributed to two factors: (1) disregard of the power of suggestion and (2) dependence on subjective responses of the patient rather than on objectively measurable reactions to the drug given. Consequently, tests of muscle strength and a general survey of muscle function, as described in Chapter 8, should be carried out before the tests. Recognition of hysterical motor dysfunction (see Chapter 8) serves well in eliminating errors. Furthermore, *it is of utmost importance that the tests be performed in a neutral environment rather than in one charged with anticipation of a good or bad result.* With a thorough understanding of muscle testing and hysterical motor dysfunction, it is rarely necessary to study the effects of placebos.

Since ptosis and diplopia are the most common initial symptoms in myasthenia gravis and are present in more than 90% of cases, it is often advisable that the effect of these drugs be studied on the extraocular muscles. Consequently, the relationship of the upper eyelid to the pupil as the patient gazes straight ahead and the range of ocular rotations in all directions are carefully studied before administration of the drugs used in testing so that comparisons can be made when the effect of the drug used is at its height.

In some patients, additional quantitative assessment of the response to the drug may be desirable. In these patients, the Lancaster test for diplopia, monitoring of the vital capacity, or measurement of the arm-abduction time may be used.

Neostigmine test

Neostigmine may be administered orally or parenterally as a test for myasthenia gravis. Parenteral administration is preferred, and the subcutaneous or intramuscular route is less likely to make the patient ill than is an intravenous injection.

In testing a patient believed to have myasthenia gravis, we usually give 1.0 mg of neostigmine methylsulfate if the weight is 50 kg or more. For children, the amount administered is reduced in proportion to weight. With few exceptions, a definite increase in muscle strength, often to a surprising degree, can be recognized within 30 minutes in cases of myasthenia gravis. Should the test give equivocal results, it can be repeated 4 to 5 hours later with 1.5 to 2.0 mg, or even more. Or, if the test is being used to exclude myasthenia gravis, it is probably wise to choose a larger dose in the first place, usually 1.5 mg. With larger doses of neostigmine, particularly if it is presumed that the patient is unlikely to have myasthenia gravis, it is advisable to protect the patient against the abdominal cramping, nausea, vomiting, and even syncope that neostigmine may produce. We usually give 1/100 grain (0.65 mg) of atropine sulfate orally approximately 15 minutes before performance of the test.

Edrophonium chloride test

Edrophonium chloride is administered intravenously in a dose of 2 to 10 mg as a test for myasthenia gravis. Its strengthening action is observed within 20 to 60 seconds and persists to a significant degree for only 1 or 2 minutes. Paradoxical reactions may occur, and aggravation rather than alleviation of weakness results from higher doses. Consequently, we now give initially only 2 mg. The needle is left in place, and if no effect is observed within 1 minute, 3 mg of edrophonium is injected. The remaining 5 mg is injected 1 minute after the second injection. Aside from the possibility of a paradoxical reaction to edrophonium, the chief disadvantage of the test is the brief action of the drug; there may be inadequate time for complete appraisal of muscle strength.

Tests for autoimmunity to the acetylcholine receptor

Approximately 90% of patients with acquired autoimmune myasthenia gravis have circulating antibodies directed against the acetylcholine receptor protein. In most patients, the antibodies recognize various antigenic components of the receptor, but in some instances they are directed predominantly against its acetylcholine binding site. A negative test result for circulating antibodies to acetylcholine receptor does not exclude the diagnosis of autoimmune myasthenia gravis, because antibodies to the receptor may be bound at the motor end plate, where they cannot be detected in the serum. Antibodies bound to the acetylcholine receptor at the end plate can be revealed by appropriate immunocytochemical and immunoelectron microscopic methods performed by a few laboratories. No antibodies to the acetylcholine receptor are detected in serum or at the end plate in patients with congenital myasthenic syndromes or in patients with weakness not due to autoimmune myasthenia gravis.

Serum Creatine Kinase

Elevations of the MM fraction of serum creatine kinase (CK) usually indicate active muscle fiber necrosis and serve as an aid to the diagnosis of myopathies. Marked, even thousandfold, CK elevations occur in the course of acute rhabdomyolysis associated with myoglobinuria. Very high, such as hundredfold, CK elevations occur in the early phases of Duchenne and Becker dystrophies and in severe childhood autosomal recessive muscular dystrophy. Less marked CK increases are found in polymyositis and dermatomyositis, but in inclusion body myositis, the serum CK level can be normal or only mildly increased. Serum CK is often increased in myxedema, even without muscle fiber necrosis or weakness, but is never increased in thyrotoxic myopathy or in pure corticosteroid-induced myopathy. Trauma to muscle, intramuscular drug injections (especially of meperidine), severe voluntary exertion, or grand mal seizures can transiently increase the serum CK value. Mild elevations of the enzyme can also occur in states of neurogenic atrophy, as in amyotrophic lateral sclerosis, and are due to a myopathic process secondary to the denervation atrophy. Some patients without muscle symptoms or known injury to muscle also have increased serum CK concentration. The increase here can be caused by susceptibility to malignant hyperthermia, a preclinical myopathy, a latent metabolic myopathy, or a carrier state for muscular dystrophy.

Muscle Biopsy
The correct diagnosis of a neuromuscular disease rests on a tripod: the careful clinical history and examination, the electromyogram (including nerve conduction studies and tests for neuromuscular transmission defects), and the muscle biopsy. None of the three methods of assessing the patient is entirely adequate in itself. When used in conjunction, the three approaches yield the correct diagnosis in a very high proportion of cases.

The increasing application of light microscopic histochemistry, immunocytochemistry, electron microscopy, and biochemical and molecular genetic methods of examination to the study of the muscle biopsy has considerably enhanced its diagnostic value and has even led to the discovery of a number of new diseases.

Biopsy is made of muscles of grade -1 to -2 strength. Stronger muscles may not show diagnostic pathologic change, and in weaker muscles excessive amounts of connective tissue may obscure the basic pathologic process. Injected muscles (as is frequently the case for deltoid muscle) or muscles previously examined electromyographically are unsuitable for diagnosis.

Whenever possible, the biopsy is done under local or regional rather than general anesthesia. The anesthetic is never injected into the muscle itself. The following specimens are taken: (1) a cylinder of tissue, 2 to 3 cm long and approximately 0.1 cm wide, for electron microscopy, (2) a 0.6-cm by 0.6-cm specimen for light microscopic histochemistry, and (3) a specimen of suitable dimensions for biochemical or further histologic studies.

Before being excised, specimen 1 is tied to a segment of an applicator stick in situ with silk ligatures to hold it at constant length during fixation. This prevents objectionable contraction artifacts and facilitates subsequent orientation for longitudinal and transverse sectioning. Specimen 2 is subdivided with a razor blade into two slabs, which are then affixed to a chuck in transverse orientation with a suitable mounting medium. This specimen is then quickly frozen in isopentane chilled to -150°C by liquid nitrogen and is stored in liquid nitrogen until it is transferred to a cryostat for the preparation of fresh-frozen sections. Specimen 3 is used for immediate biochemical studies or is quickly frozen and stored under liquid nitrogen for subsequent studies.

Specimen 1 is fixed in 5% buffered ice-cold glutaraldehyde for 3 hours; it is then subdivided into numerous smaller blocks (under a dissecting microscope), which are fixed for an additional 30 minutes. After thorough rinsing with buffer, fixation with 2% ice-cold buffered osmium tetroxide for 3 hours, and dehydration with graded alcohols, the blocks are embedded in epoxy resin (Epon). At least 20 blocks are embedded for longitudinal and 10 for transverse sectioning. Sections from these blocks are used for phase-contrast and electron microscopy. They can also be stained by the periodic acid-Schiff (PAS) method and with aniline dyes (azure II and methylene blue) for examination by ordinary light microscopy.

Cryostat sections are prepared from specimen 2. Routinely, sections are stained with hematoxylin-eosin, trichrome, PAS, oil red O, and Congo red stains as well as reacted for the demonstration of oxidative enzymes (NADH dehydrogenase, succinate dehydrogenase, and cytochrome-c oxidase), lysosomal acid phosphatase, myofibrillar adenosinetriphosphatase (ATPase) (after preincubation at pH 4.3, 4.6, and 9.4), phosphorylase, cholinesterase, and nonspecific esterase. Additional stains for acid mucosubstances, phospholipids, cholesterol (free and esters), calcium, metachromatic material, lactate dehydrogenase, aldolase, phosphofructokinase, adenosine monophosphate deaminase, or others are used in selected instances.

In special cases, cryostat sections are also useful for the immunolocalization of dystrophin, dystrophin-associated proteins, utrophin, merosin, desmin and other cytoskeletal proteins, gelsolin, transthyretin, actin, α-actinin, myosin isoforms, complement components C3 and C5b9, the acetylcholine receptor, acetylcholinesterase, and mononuclear cell surface antigens. The muscle microvasculature can be readily visualized with the lectin *Ulex europaeus* agglutinin-I.

Interpretation of fresh-frozen sections
The dimension of muscle fibers in fresh-frozen sections closely approximates that in the native state. Trichromatically stained sections reveal an intermyofibrillar membranous network (composed of mitochondria and sarcoplasmic reticulum). The lipid and glycogen content of the fibers can be readily estimated by Sudan and PAS stains, the distribution of mitochondria can be inferred from the oxidative enzyme reactions, increased lysosomal activity is detected by the acid phosphatase reaction, myofibrillar integrity can be evaluated from the ATPase reaction, and the presence or absence of certain enzymes (phosphorylase, phosphofructokinase, lactate dehydrogenase, cytochrome-c oxidase, and adenosine mon-ophosphate deaminase) can be observed. In addition, each muscle fiber has a distinct histochemical profile that allows fiber typing. This is useful because all muscle fibers innervated by a single anterior horn cell have identical histochemical profiles, and, conversely, the histochemical profile of a given fiber is determined by its innervation.

Two major histochemical fiber types exist: type 1 fibers (resembling fibers in red muscles of certain animals) are more highly reactive to most oxidative enzymes, are less reactive to glycolytic enzymes, and contain less glycogen than type 2 fibers (which resemble fibers in white muscles of certain animals). The intensity of the ATPase reaction depends on the pH of the preincubating medium; thus, type 1 fibers are highly reactive after acid preincubation but not after alkaline preincubation. Type 2 fibers are highly reactive after alkaline preincubation, but some also are reactive after acid preincubation. The latter phenomenon, in turn, indicates the existence of more than two histochemical fiber types.

In the normal state, there is random intermingling of fiber types; if each fiber type is equally represented in the specimen, groups of fibers of an identical type do not arise. However, individual fiber types are not equally represented in all muscles. For example, in the anterior tibial, up to 80% of the fibers may be normally of type 1, and here grouping of type 1 fibers can normally be expected. If the normal distribution of fiber types in a muscle is known, the maximal number of fibers of a given type normally occurring in a group can be estimated. The occurrence of larger than expected groups of fibers of a given histochemical type indicates abnormal type grouping, and if abnormal type grouping is displayed by both type 1 and type 2 fibers, this is evidence for reinnervation of previously denervated muscle fibers. Data on the normal frequency of histochemical fiber types and on the size of fiber type groups that can normally be expected in different muscles are available from the literature.

The limitations of fresh-frozen sections are as follows: Artifactual spaces from ice crystals may hinder interpretations; fiber abnormalities are seen only in the transverse plane, and the three-dimensional profile of the lesions remains uncertain even after extensive serial sectioning; information can be obtained only on those components of muscle that are reactive in currently available histochemical and immunocytochemical systems; and fine structural or dimensional changes cannot be reliably assessed.

Phase-optic microscopy of epon sections

Epon sections provide resolution to 0.2 to 0.4 μm. They are unsuitable for histochemistry except for localizing PAS-reactive material. In this respect, however, they are superior to fresh-frozen sections. The main use of the phase-optic examination is selection of areas for further study by the electron microscope.

Electron microscopy

Electron microscopy is relatively time-consuming and not required for the immediate diagnosis of most biopsy material. However, it can clearly demonstrate mitochondrial abnormalities, the boundaries and contents of vacuoles, and the pathologic reactions of the sarcoplasmic reticulum and of other organelles. Some structures elude detection by light microscopy (such as the filamentous inclusions of inclusion body myositis, the nuclear inclusions in autosomal dominant oculopharyngeal dystrophy, and fingerprint bodies in fingerprint body myopathy), whereas others can be reliably identified only by electron microscopy (for example, nemaline bodies). Pathologic alterations in the surface membrane of the fiber (as in Duchenne dystrophy), in the neuromuscular junction, in intramuscular nerves, or in small blood vessels (as in dermatomyositis) are best detected by electron microscopy. Immunoelectron microscopic and electron cytochemical studies have applications in the investigation of myasthenia gravis and related syndromes. The recognition of a number of new disorders has become possible with the added use of the electron microscope in the study of the muscle biopsy.

Biochemical and molecular genetic studies

Because the biochemical basis of most neuromuscular diseases is still unknown, biochemical studies are applicable only in selected instances. Direct measurement of the muscle glycogen content, assay of glycolytic enzymes, determination of respiratory activities of mitochondria by use of different substrates, assay of the activities of complexes I, II, III, IV, I-III, and I-II of the mitochondrial respiratory chain, determination of cytochrome and coenzyme Q levels in mitochondria, assay of carnitine and of the various forms of acyl and hydroxyacyl coenzyme A dehydrogenases are examples of biochemical procedures currently used in the diagnosis of metabolic myopathies.

Molecular genetic studies are now readily available to detect large-scale deletions of the dystrophin gene (which account for about 65% of the cases of Duchenne or Becker dystrophy), the abnormal expansion of a CTG trinucleotide repeat in the 3′ untranslated region of the myotonic dystrophy gene in myotonic dystrophy, or mutations in mitochondrial DNA associated with various mitochondrial encephalomyopathies, such as the Kearns-Sayre syndrome, mitochondrial encephalopathy with stroke-like episodes and lactic acidosis, and myoclonus epilepsy with ragged red fibers.

Morphologic clues in the muscle biopsy

In many instances, the muscle biopsy does not suggest a specific disease other than indicating the presence of a myopathy or of a neurogenic disorder. In some conditions, however, it does suggest a specific diagnosis.

1. Distinctive (but not specific) morphologic abnormalities can occur in a high proportion of the muscle fibers in some congenital myopathies, such as central core disease, multicore disease, nemaline (rod or Z-disk) myopathy, myotubular myopathy and its congeners, reducing body myopathy, congenital sarcotubular myopathy,

congenital fiber-type disproportion, congenital myopathy with fingerprint bodies, and various mitochondrial myopathies.
2. Vacuolar myopathies should suggest a glycogen or lipid storage disease, inclusion body myositis, myofibrillar myopathy, exposure to chloroquine, or a type of periodic paralysis. Vacuoles highly reactive for acid phosphatase as well as positive for glycogen suggest type 2 glycogenosis (acid maltase deficiency). In this disease, many vacuoles are membrane-bound when examined with the electron microscope. In other glycogenoses, the vacuoles are usually not membrane-bound and are relatively unreactive for acid phosphatase. Massive lipid accumulation in muscle fibers can occur in muscle with carnitine deficiency, defects in β-oxidation, and neutral lipid storage disease. Chloroquine-induced vacuoles also are highly reactive for acid phosphatase and frequently associated with extensive fiber splitting. In periodic paralysis, the vacuoles are often central and show various morphologic features, depending on their stage of evolution.
3. Clusters of regenerating fibers together with isolated, or at times grouped, necrotic fibers are typically observed in Duchenne dystrophy, in severe autosomal recessive muscular dystrophy of childhood, and in some of the congenital myopathies.
4. In Duchenne dystrophy, immunostains of cryostat sections for dystrophin reveal a marked deficiency or complete absence of dystrophin from the sarcolemma of nearly all muscle fibers. In Becker dystrophy, a disorder allelic to Duchenne dystrophy, the deficiency of sarcolemmal dystrophin varies. Further confirmation of the diagnosis of Becker dystrophy may require immunoblotting of muscle extracts to show a reduced amount of dystrophin of abnormal molecular weight. Muscle specimens of some, though not all, carriers of Duchenne dystrophy reveal a mosaic of many dystrophin-positive fibers intermingled with a lesser number of dystrophin-negative fibers. Sarcolemmal dystrophin deficiency also results in a secondary deficiency of dystrophin-associated glycoproteins.
5. Mutations in the α-, β-, or γ-sarcoglycan components of the dystrophin-associated glycoprotein complex can also occur and cause autosomal recessive muscular dystrophies. Mutations in any one of the sarcoglycan components result in reduced expression of, and reduced immunostain for, all three sarcoglycans, but the immunostain for dystrophin remains normal.
6. Mutations in the α-2 chain of laminin (also known as merosin) cause a severe congenital muscular dystrophy that can be identified by immunostains for α-2 laminin.
7. Accumulation of mitochondria under the sarcolemma or within the fiber (ragged red fibers in trichrome-stained sections and

ragged blue fibers in succinate dehydrogenase–reacted sections) occur in various types of mitochondrial myopathies. Cytochrome-*c* oxidase (CCO)–negative fibers are also evidence for a mitochondrial abnormality. Many, but not all, ragged red or ragged blue fibers are CCO–negative, but not all CCO–negative fibers are ragged red or ragged blue. Mutations in the mitochondrial genome also occur in normal subjects during life, resulting in the appearance of ragged red, ragged blue, and CCO–negative fibers in old age; such fibers are often observed in elderly patients with inflammatory muscle diseases.
8. Massive degeneration with massive regeneration of muscle fibers usually signifies a recent paroxysm of rhabdomyolysis. Known biochemical causes of rhabdomyolysis (phosphorylase, phosphorylase *b* kinase, phosphofructokinase, phosphoglycerate kinase, phosphoglycerate mutase, lactate dehydrogenase, carnitine palmitoyltransferase, acyl-CoA dehydrogenase, some oxidative enzyme, and coenzyme Q deficiencies) should be ruled out.
9. Fibrinoid necrosis of arterioles with neurogenic muscle disease suggests periarteritis nodosa.
10. Extensive hyalinization of blood vessel walls and extensive proliferation of perimysial connective tissues can occur in scleroderma.
11. Concentration of degenerating, regenerating, and atrophic fibers at the periphery of several fascicles occurs in dermatomyositis at one stage in the evolution of the disease. If this characteristic alteration is absent, depletion of capillaries (demonstrated by *Ulex europaeus* agglutinin-I) and deposits of the C5b9 complement membrane attack complex on capillaries may still indicate early muscle involvement in dermatomyositis.
12. Numerous inflammatory cells, predominantly mononuclear, in perivascular and interstitial locations and in relation to degenerating fibers occur in inflammatory myopathies. However, minor degrees of inflammation can be observed in other chronic or acute myopathies as well. Invasion and destruction of nonnecrotic muscle fibers by autoaggressive mononuclear cells (T cells accompanied by macrophages) occur in polymyositis and inclusion body myositis but not in scleroderma or dermatomyositis.
13. The combination of (1) at least one muscle fiber with a rimmed vacuole per low-power field, (2) at least one group of atrophic muscle fibers per low-power field, (3) an autoaggressive inflammatory exudate, and (4) congophilic inclusions in sections stained with Congo red and viewed in the fluorescence microscope under rhodamine optics support the diagnosis of inclusion body myositis.
14. Amyloid infiltration of blood vessel walls, the endoneurium of intramuscular nerves, and the endomysium of muscle fibers can be seen in amyloidosis.

15. Numerous muscle fibers with abnormal foci of desmin, dystrophin, gelsolin, and β-amyloid precursor protein positivity as well as large congophilic deposits are present in myofibrillar myopathy.
16. Non-necrotizing granulomas with central epithelioid cells and giant cells can be found in sarcoidosis.
17. In infestations with *Trichinella* organisms, the parasites occur in muscle.
18. Selective atrophy of type 2 fibers can be seen after disuse, in cachexia, with neuromuscular transmission defects, or after exposure to corticosteroids. In corticosteroid myopathy, focal increases and decreases in mitochondria and focal myofibrillar degeneration, especially in type 1 fibers, also can occur. Selective atrophy of type 1 fibers can appear in myotonic dystrophy, in some benign congenital myopathies, and in some lipid storage myopathies.

DISORDERS OR DISEASES OF PERIPHERAL NERVES

Differential Diagnosis of Peripheral Neuropathy

Diagnosis of peripheral nerve disease rests firmly on a reliable assessment and characterization of the patient's symptoms, neurologic abnormalities, associated diseases, and test abnormalities. The history should reflect the patient's symptoms, their development with time, factors that make them better or worse, and any associated disease. Careful inquiry into family history for any neurologic disease can be very helpful. In the recording of the symptoms, use of volunteered words such as "tightness," "prickling numbness," "like a hand gone asleep," and "burning" convey a patient's experience more accurately than the medical terms "paresthesia," "hyperalgesia," and "allodynia." In the functional inquiry, questions are best organized under motor, sensory, and autonomic function. Such symptoms as "weakness" need further inquiry to decide whether tiredness, inability to perform certain motor tasks, or another symptom is meant. "Numbness" should be pursued by such nonleading replies as "tell me more" or "amplify." Numbness may mean lifelessness, absence of feeling, "asleep numbness like Novocain," or something else.

Symptoms related to neural hyperactivity (positive symptoms) must be differentiated from symptoms related to underactivity (negative symptoms). For motor neurons (axons), positive symptoms are spasms and cramps and negative symptoms are weakness and atrophy. For sensory neurons (axons), lancinating pains, paresthesia, and cold feelings are positive symptoms, whereas losses of touch-pressure, vibratory sensation, and warm and cool perception are negative. For autonomic fibers, flushing and excessive sweating are positive and loss of sweating is negative. The nature and profile of positive and negative symptoms are predictors for the physiologic class of fibers implicated, the pathologic process, and sometimes even the disease. An illustration of this point might suffice: the occurrence of true paresthesia usually implies acquired, not inherited, neuropathy.

The neurologic examination is used to determine whether nerves are affected and the localization and kind of involvement. Possible involvement may be of single or multiple cranial nerves, of single or multiple roots or segmental nerves, or of brachial, lumbar, or sacral plexus or single or multiple nerves. Partial lesions, the rule in most neuropathies, may make localization difficult.

Nerve conduction with electromyography is helpful in (1) demonstrating whether peripheral nerves are affected; (2) localizing the process to roots, plexuses, or peripheral nerves; and (3) characterizing the lesion as demyelinating or as axonal degeneration. For these purposes, the test is excellent because it is objective, sensitive, specific, and repeatable. The procedure cannot be used to imply symptoms and deficits; they must be independently assessed. The procedure is not useful for assessing severity, because the sampling is not ideal for this purpose. The procedure has little or no value in predicting positive symptoms, in assessing small fiber function or loss, or in diagnosing interstitial nerve disease.

Quantitative sensory examination and quantitative autonomic testing provide information mostly about deficits of function, information not available from electrophysiologic testing.

The specific use of the nerve biopsy in assessment of peripheral nerve disease is described later in this chapter.

A variety of tests are needed to evaluate patients with peripheral neuropathy. Since peripheral neuropathy may be a complication of diseases of internal organs, the list of tests required may be long. The following are examples, not a complete list. Neuropathy is commonly associated with primary amyloidosis, multiple myeloma, osteosclerotic myeloma, thrombocytosis, polycythemia rubra vera, and treatment of sickle cell anemia. Since neuropathy may precede other manifestations, detection and evaluation in such patients may require extensive evaluation of hematology group values, blood smears, bone marrow analysis, immunoelectrophoresis of plasma and urine, x-ray bone survey, echocardiographic heart tracing, and study of rectal, fat, or nerve biopsy tissue. For study of metabolic disorders that affect nerve, various pituitary, thyroid, adrenal, or pancreatic hormones may need to be evaluated. For detection of various rheumatologic disorders, one may need to assess antibodies to nuclear antigens, antibodies to extractable nuclear antigen, the erythrocyte sedimentation rate, and rheumatoid factor. In an assessment for the presence of various infectious agents, serologic tests for Lyme borreliosis, human immunodeficiency virus, lues, and other organisms need to be done. An increasing list of enzyme assays to detect genetic metabolic abnormalities is available.

In the following paragraphs, abbreviated patterns of involvement helpful in diagnosis and differential diagnosis are provided.

Selective motor neuron (axon) involvement: Asymmetrical: motor neuron disease (amyotrophic lateral sclerosis), poliomyelitis, multifocal motor neuropathy. Symmetrical: progressive muscular atrophy—proximal or distal, other patterns, and different patterns of inheritance.

Selective symmetrical large-diameter sensory neuron (axon) involvement: Friedreich's ataxia, other spinocerebellar degenerations, immune sensory and paraneoplastic neuropathies.

Selective symmetrical small-diameter sensory neuron (axon) involvement: Various inherited sensory and autonomic neuropathies, pandysautonomia.

Symmetrical large- and small-diameter sensory neuron (axon) involvement: Tabes dorsalis, diabetic neuropathy, uremic neuropathy, toxic and medicinal exposure, vitamin deficiency and excess (B_6), various inherited sensory and autonomic neuropathies, Sjögren's syndrome, immune sensory neuropathies, paraneoplastic neuropathies.

Symmetrical polyradiculoneuropathy: Acute (Guillain-Barré syndrome) or chronic inflammatory-demyelinating polyneuropathy, monoclonal protein-associated neuropathies, lymphoma, leukemia, paraneoplastic disease, acquired immunodeficiency syndrome.

Asymmetrical monoradiculoneuropathy or polyradiculoneuropathy: Lyme borreliosis, lymphoma, meningeal carcinomatosis, disk or tumor (primary or secondary), sarcoidosis.

Brachial or lumbosacral plexus: immune, lymphoma, bleeding, radiation, neoplastic infiltration.

Multiple mononeuropathy: Diabetes mellitus, necrotizing vasculitis of large and small arterioles (periarteritis nodosa, Churg-Strauss syndrome, Wegener's granulomatosis, hypersensitivity angiitis), necrotizing vasculitis of small nerve vessels (systemic lupus erythematosus, Sjögren's syndrome, nonsystemic vasculitis), inherited tendency to pressure palsy, multifocal motor neuropathy, sarcoidosis, lymphomatoid granulomatosis.

Distal polyneuropathy: Inherited and acquired (inflammatory-demyelinating), metabolic (diabetes, uremia, hepatic disease, acromegaly), toxic, nutritional and alcoholic, vitamin deficiency and excess, and other forms.

Quantitative Sensory Testing (QST)

There is a heightened interest in techniques and procedures to quantify cutaneous sensation because (1) detection thresholds for different kinds of sensation vary with site, age, and sex; (2) neurologists' estimates of threshold are rough at best; and (3) epidemiologic surveys and controlled clinical trials require such approaches. In clinical practice, QST is useful for the following purposes: (1) identifying whether sensory loss is or is not present, (2) characterizing the type or types of sensory loss, and (3) following the course of sensory loss with time or treatment.

QST, if properly done, is time-consuming. Repeated trials at different magnitudes of stimulus strength are needed. For these reasons, only sites for which normal results specific for site, age, and sex are known are tested. The topographic distribution of sensory loss must therefore be determined by other (clinical) approaches.

Many devices have been fabricated to evaluate touch-pressure, vibratory, cooling, warming, and pain sensations. In judging a given technique or system, one needs to consider the overall design of the device, waveform generated, reproducibility of the waveform, range of stimulus magnitudes, algorithm (the sequential steps) of testing, method of determining threshold, presentation of results, and comparison to normal (definition, number, age, sex distribution, and disease condition) values. One needs also to know whether the results are sensitive (detecting abnormality when it is present), specific (*not* detecting abnormality when it is *not* present), and relevant (measuring what is clinically meaningful). Finally, the system needs to be assessed by usefulness and cost per test.

Among QST devices, von Frey's hairs, or modifications thereof, were commonly used to test touch-pressure (tactile) detection threshold, but we consider them obsolete. The magnitude and waveform of the stimulus may vary depending on application, and the time and cost of professionals to use them may be excessive. For vibratory detection threshold, the bioesthesiometer (Chagrin Falls, OH) is commonly used. The magnitude of the stimulus is subject to damping. If it is to be used, the device should be mounted on a stand and loaded with a constant weight. The Minnesota thermal disks are useful for measuring thermal discrimination. They provide uniform cooling stimuli, have a defined surface area, and provide a constant load. The dolorimeter has been used to evaluate pain sensation.

Computer-assisted sensory examination (CASE IV, W. R. Medical Electronics, Stillwater, MN) to evaluate tactile, vibratory, cooling, and warming detection thresholds and heat-pain sensation is valuable for characterization of sensory loss, for following worsening and improvement in neuropathy, and for epidemiologic surveys and controlled clinical trials. Other semiautomatic testing devices have become available and are being used.

We suggest that QST could be offered for the evaluation of vibratory, cooling, warming, and heat-pain detection thresholds of the great toe (or dorsal part of the foot), index finger (or dorsal part of the hand), and face. Elevation of the vibratory threshold provides evidence of involvement of large afferent fibers, whereas elevation of the cooling or warming threshold indicates involvement of small afferent fibers.

Assuming that a neurologic clinic wants to establish a QST program, which approaches should it use? The major choice is between handheld devices and laboratory-based systems. The advantages of the former are lower initial cost, simpler design, and portability. The disadvantages are a less well-controlled waveform and magnitude of stimulation, extraneous stimulation because the devices are handheld, human error in testing, and physician cost of operation. It is now possible and cost-effective to use microprocessor-controlled systems that provide precise waveforms, exact magnitudes of stimulus strength, good computer algorithms of testing, and a printout of the results. If normal results are available, patient responses can be provided as a percentile value for site, age, and sex. The preprogrammed steps of testing, finding the threshold, and expressing results as a percentile for a given site can be done more quickly and accurately by a microprocessor under the supervision of a technician than by handheld devices used by a physician or psychologist. Assuming that several patients will be tested each day, the automated approach can provide better and faster results at a lower cost. Automated systems are becoming small enough that they also can be portable.

In Figure 17-1, we show the transducer of computer-assisted sensory examination IV to evaluate vibratory detection threshold. Threshold at one site can be determined accurately in from 8 to 15 minutes.

Sural Nerve Biopsy

Nerve biopsy can be used to diagnose and characterize neuropathy and especially to diagnose the underlying cause of neuropathy. These objectives may not be achieved if the patients are not wisely selected, if the techniques used are suboptimal, or if the histologic sections are assessed by physicians unfamiliar with peripheral nerve disease. For many patients with neuropathy, the side effects and costs may outweigh the possible benefits.

The main reason for biopsy is to confirm a suspected pathologic diagnosis, for example, leprosy, amyloidosis, necrotizing vasculitis (systemic and nonsystemic), sarcoidosis, lymphomatoid granulomatosis, inflammatory-demyelinating conditions, various lipid storage diseases, and other rare disorders. In some cases, the nerve may be taken to diagnose and characterize neuropathy.

Nerve biopsy is especially valuable in certain infectious and immune disorders. The sural nerve is commonly affected in lepromatous neuropathy. A Ziehl-Neelsen or Fite stain is done to identify the organism. Sural nerve biopsy may also be helpful and supportive of the clinical diagnosis in inflammatory-demyelinating disorders or sarcoidosis; however, the sural nerve often does not reveal the typical pathologic alterations. For a pathologic diagnosis of necrotizing vasculitis, necrosis of the vessel wall, especially of the tunica media, and wall inflammation must be seen. Supportive features are intimal proliferation, closure of the lumen, neovascularization, bleeding, and hemosiderin in macrophages. Increasingly, an ischemic pattern of nerve tissue injury is recognized. It may be helpful to distinguish necrotizing vasculitis of the large nerve

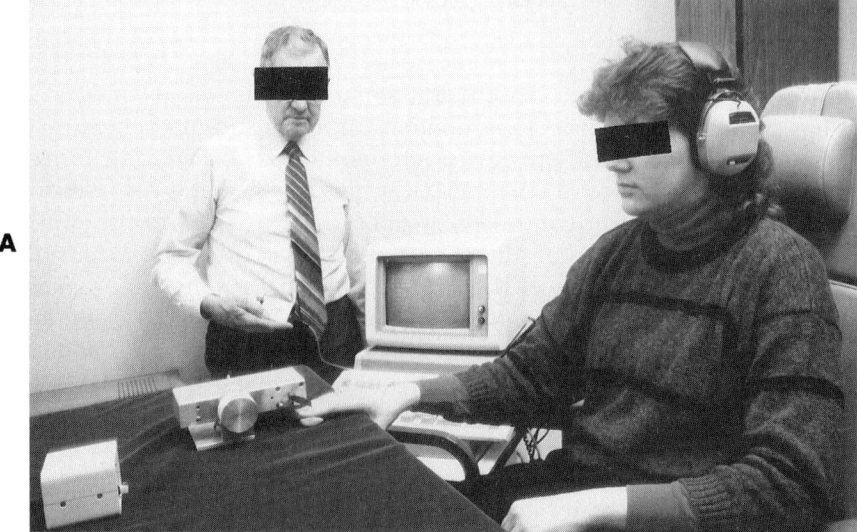

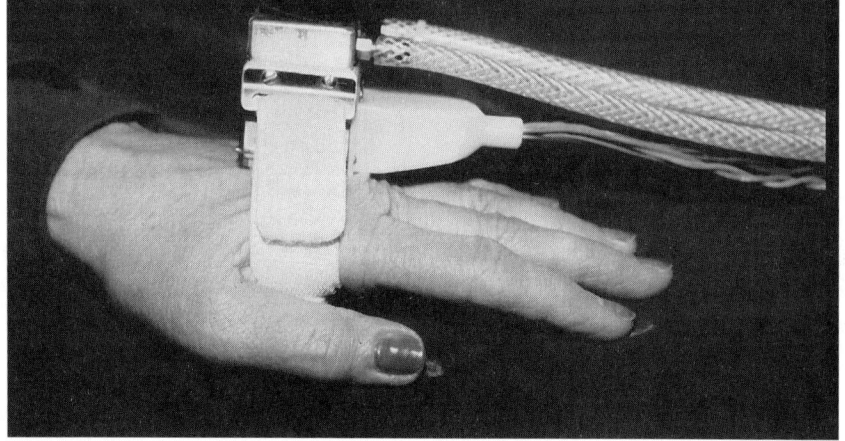

Figure 17-1
Quantitative sensory testing with the computer-assisted sensory examination, system IV. The system provides precisely described waveforms of mechanical and thermal stimuli in 25 steps of increasing magnitude. Thresholds are determined by several validated algorithms, and normal values have been determined for foot, leg, thigh, hand, forearm, shoulder, and face. **A,** The vibratory transducer is in place on the terminal phalanx of the index finger of a healthy subject. A 125-Hz auditory signal is continuously provided to ensure that the subject is not given auditory clues from the testing device. The testing program is essentially automatic, but responses are entered by the observer, and each response activates the next step in testing. Threshold is given as stimulus step, micrometers of displacement, normal deviation, and percentile for test, site, and various physical variables. **B,** Thermode, surface area of 10 cm^2, in place on the hand of a subject to test cool, warm, and heat-pain sensations. Cooling detection threshold is expressed as a step—degrees Celsius from baseline, normal deviation—and as a percentile for test, site, and various physical variables. Two levels of heat-pain (HP) responses are tested: threshold (HP, 0.5) and an intermediate degree of pain (HP, 5.0).

arterioles and of the small vessels. The first variety is associated with the clinical disorders of polyarteritis nodosa, rheumatoid arteritis, Wegener's granulomatosis, and Churg-Strauss syndrome. In the second, small arterioles, capillaries, and venules are affected. This variety is associated with nonsystemic vasculitic neuropathy and Sjögren's syndrome.

Nerve biopsy often is helpful in the diagnosis of amyloidosis. Amyloid may be recognized by its appearance (ground-glass homogeneous material in connective tissue and especially around blood vessels) and by its tinctorial properties. It stains pink in methyl violet stains and is apple green birefringent in Congo red stains under polarized light. A monoclonal protein and light chains are characteristic of primary amyloidosis. The inherited amyloidoses are point mutations on the prealbumin molecule. Not all metachromatic or apple green birefringent material in nerve is amyloid.

The characteristic pathologic features of various lysosomal and other storage disorders may require electron microscopy.

Onion bulbs are known to be characteristic of repeated demyelination and remyelination. The pattern is characteristic of various inherited neuropathies, chronic inflammatory-demyelinating polyneuropathy, and acromegaly.

The class of fibers that undergo pathologic alterations and the pathologic alterations themselves may be suggestive of a diagnosis. To illustrate, sensory fibers are spared in motor neuron disease, whereas they are selectively affected in Friedreich's ataxia. The size and functional class of sensory fibers affected distinguish various hereditary sensory and autonomic neuropathies. In inherited neuropathies, nerve fibers generally undergo chronic axonal atrophy with myelin remodeling, whereas in acquired neuropathies, axonal degeneration is commonplace. Careful assessment of teased fibers (Fig. 17-2) helps with these distinctions.

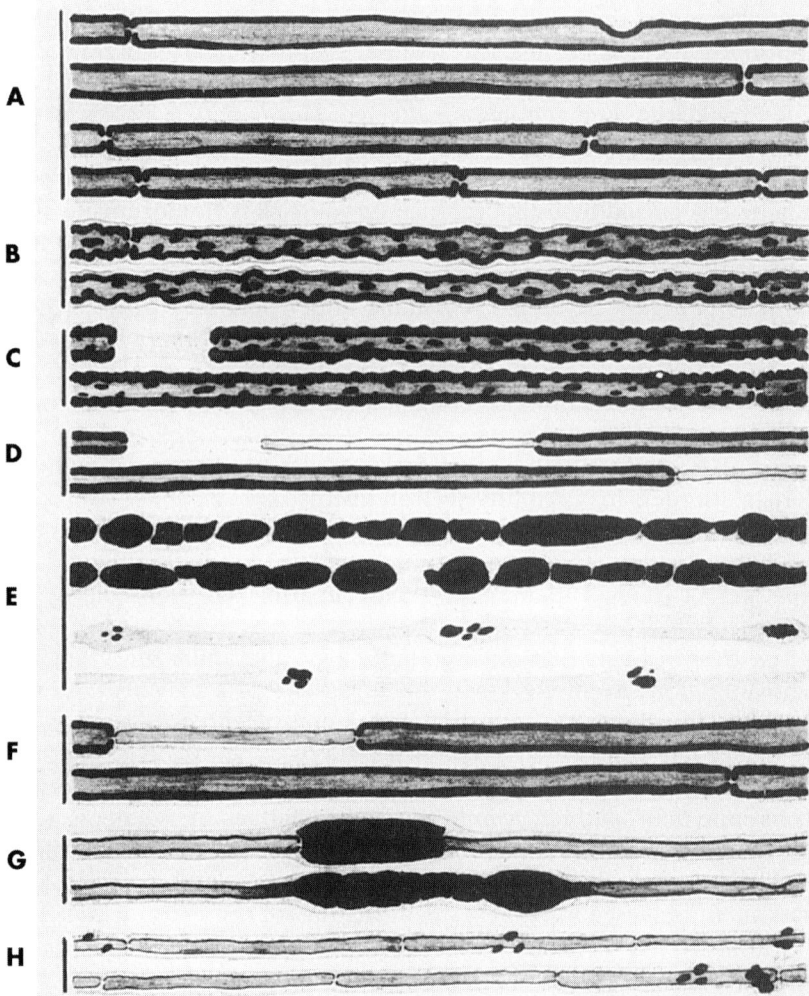

Figure 17-2
A drawing of teased fiber pathologic abnormalities encountered in sural nerve in human neuropathy. After 100 fibers are teased from systematically sampled portions of the nerve, the fibers are graded according to the conditions A through H and the percentage of each is calculated. Knowing the percentage of these conditions with age in health, one can know whether the examined nerve is abnormal and what pathologic abnormalities are present. The conditions, in brief, are **A,** normal; **B,** myelin wrinkling; **C,** demyelination; **D,** demyelination and remyelination; **E,** axonal degeneration; **F,** remyelination; **G,** myelin reduplication; and **H,** axonal regeneration. *(From Pollock M, Dyck PJ: Peripheral nerve morphometry in myotonic dystrophy, Arch Neurol 33:33–39, 1976. By permission of the American Medical Association.)*

Index

A

Abdominal reflexes, infants, 311
Abducens nerve, anatomy of, 128-129
Abductor pollicis brevis muscle, 214-215
Abductor pollicis longus muscle, 209
Abruptio placentae, 304
Abstract reasoning, 45-46
Abstraction, Short Test of Mental Status and, 48
Accessory nerve (CNXI), 101
Acetylcholine receptor, 500
Achondroplasia, 332
Acoustic nerve (CNVIII)
  anatomy of, 94-95
  clinical examination of, 95-99
  lesions of, 96
Acromegaly, 32-33, 334
Activities of daily living, 37-38
Addison's disease, 485
Adductor brevis muscle, 225
Adductor longus muscle, 225
Adductor magnus muscle, 225
Adductor pollicis muscle, 217-219
Adductor reflex, 248
Adenoma sebaceum, 32
Adie's pupil, 135
Adie's syndrome, 245
Adrenocortical insufficiency, 485
Adson's maneuver, 301-302
Agnosia, 44, 52
  tactile, 44
Akathisia, 162
Akinetic mutism, 84
Alcohol intake, seizures and, 21
Alertness, 287
  assessment of, 39
  seizures and, 20
Alexia with graphia, 84
Alexia without agraphia, 83
Allodynia, 9
  central pain syndromes and, 15
Amaurotic pupil, 134
Ambulation, of infants, 310-311
Aminoacidopathies, 493
Amplitude, 160
Amsler grid testing, 110
Anal reflex, 251
Anesthesia, lumbar puncture and, 471

Aneurysms, cerebral, angiography, 343
Angiography, cerebral, 341-344
  cerebrovascular disease, 342-343
  complications of, 342
  contrast media, 342
  craniocerebral trauma, 344
  headaches and, 19
  mass lesions, 344
  methods of, 342
Ankle reflex, infants, 311
Annulospiral fibers, 152
Anomic aphasia, 83
Anovulatory drugs, seizures and, 20
Anoxic conditions, EEG evaluation, 370-373
Antalgic gait, 174
Anterior abdominal muscles, 223
Anterior tibial muscle, 231
Antiepileptic medications, seizures and, 21
Aphasia, 24, 52, 80-81
  anomic, 83
  global, 83
  symptoms clusters in, 82-83
Apnea, sleep, syndrome, 25
Apraxia, 44, 52
  gait, 174
Apraxia of speech, 54, 68-69
  examination for, 69
  nonverbal oral, 69
Arachnoid cysts, transillumination and, 316-317
Argyll Robertson features, 136
Arterial plaques, 343
Arteriography, B-scan ultrasonic, cerebrovascular disease and, 479
Arteriovenous fistula, of cavernous sinus, 32
Arteriovenous malformation, 31
Articulation
  children and, 321-323
  spastic dysarthria and, 63
  speech examination and, 58
Asterixis, 167
Ataxia, 309
Ataxic dysarthria, 64
Ataxic gait, 171-172
Atrophy, 177-178
Atropine, chronotropic response to, 466

Attention
    assessment of, 39
    directed, 41
    language and, 71
    Short Test of Mental Status and, 48
Attention span, assessment of, 39
Auditory discrimination, children, 324-325
Auditory evoked potentials, surgical monitoring, 430-433
Auditory imperception, 83
Auditory meatus, lancinating pain in, 14
Auditory stimulation, 41
Auditory verbal agnosia, 83
Auditory-vestibular system testing, 449-455
Auditory-Vocal Sequencing Test, 324
Auscultation, neurovascular examination and, 296-297
Autonomic failure, tests for detection of, 464-466
Autonomic function, 275-286
    gastrointestinal, testing of, 466-467
    testing, 463-467
Autonomic history, 285
Autonomic nervous system function, clinical evaluation, 285-286
Axonal flare, 282

B

Babinski's reflex, 253
Back extensors, 223
Back pain, clinical examinations, 298-299
Ballismus, 166
Bárány's test, 97
Baroreflex indices, 465
Biceps reflex, 246-247
Birth, history of, 304
Bladder, 283-284
Bladder function testing, 467
Bloch-Sulzberger syndrome, 308
Blood pressure
    beat-to-beat responses, 465-466
    neurovascular examination and, 295
Bloody tap, 473-474
Brachioradialis muscle, 205
Brachioradialis reflex, 247
Brain stem auditory evoked potentials, 96
    clinical applications, 451-453
    interpretation of, 451
    monitoring during surgery, 430-433
    normal results, 450-451
    recording methods, 449-450
    stimulation methods, 449-450
Broca's aphasia, 83
Bulbocavernosus reflex, 251

C

Café au lait spots, 29, 308
Calculation performance, 46-47, 325
    Short Test of Mental Status and, 48
Caput succedaneum, 315
Carpal tunnel syndrome, 10
Cataplexy, 27
Cauda equina, 341
Cavernous sinus, arteriovenous fistula of, 32
Central midtemporal spike of childhood, 383
Central nervous system dysfunction, Moro reflex and, 312
Central pain syndromes, 14-15
Cerebellum, 151
Cerebral atrophy, transillumination and, 316-317
Cerebral blood flow, measurement of, 481
Cerebral hemisphere, lesions of, 68
Cerebrospinal fluid
    amount required for testing, 475
    bloody tap, 473-474
    dry tap, 474
    examination of, 469-475
    indications for examination, 469
    lumbar puncture and, 470-473
Cerebrovascular disease
    angiography of, 342-343
    CT analysis of, 347-348
    MRI and, 352
    noninvasive studies, 477-481
Cerebrovascular malformations, 343
Cervical disk, herniated, 31
Cervical region, pain problem diagnosis, 300-302
Chaddock's reflex, 253
Charcot-Marie-Tooth disease, 29
Chewing reflex, 254
Cheyne-Stokes respiration, 279, 291
Chiasmal lesions, 119

Children
  auditory discrimination, 324-325
  developmental milestones,
      304-307
  drawing spontaneously, 321
  EEG, abnormalities in, 382
  EEG, normal patterns of, 378-381
  examination of, 303-326, 317-327
  history-taking, 303
  lateral dominance, 32
  memory, 324-325
  praxis and, 319
  reading and spelling, 325
  sound articulation, 321-323
  sylvian seizures, 384
Chorea, 166
Choreic dysarthria, 65
Choreic gait, 173
Chvostek's sign, 169
Ciliospinal reflex, 133
Circadian rhythm abnormalities, 25
Clonus, 249
Cogan's lid twitch, 131
Cognitive disorder, history-taking
    and, 3
Cognitive tasks
  calculations, 46-47
  right-left orientation, 47
Cogwheel rigidity, 155
Coherence analysis, 388
Color vision, 109
Comatose patients
  CT of, 287
  examination of, 287-294
  Glasgow Coma Scale, 287
  level of, 289-290
  motor responses, 291
  ocular movements, 291
  pupillary abnormalities, 290-291
  respiratory patterns, 291
Comprehension, 42
Computed tomography, 345-350
  cerebrovascular disease,
      347-348
  clinical applications of, 346-350
  comatose patients, 287
  contrast enhancement, 345-346
  degenerative disorders, 34
  headaches and, 19
  hydrocephalus, 349
  infectious diseases, 349-350
  inflammatory diseases, 349-350
  intracranial trauma, 349
  metabolic disorders, 350

neoplasia of vertebral column and
    spinal cord, 336
neoplasms, 348
of skull, 336
spinal diseases, 350
theory of, 345
toxic disorders, 350
Conceptual functions, 45-46
Congenital abnormalities, MRI and,
    354
Congestive heart failure, 291
Constructional deficit, primary, 36
Constructional tasks, 44
Contraction fasciculations, 179
Contractures, muscle, 184
Convergence-retraction nystagmus,
    148
Conversation, directing of, 3
Conversion reaction, 24-25
Convulsive disorders, EEG evaluation, 375-376
Coordination, 157-159
  testing of, 158
Copper metabolism disorder,
    497-498
Corneal reflex, 250
Cornelia de Lange's syndrome, 307
Coronal synostosis, 315
Corporeal orientation, 325-326
Cortical function, 46-47
  in sensation, 256
Cortical sensory inattention, 261
Corticosteroids, 334
Cramps, 180
Cranial fossa tumor, 31
Cranial nerves
  conduction studies, 427-428
  examination of, 31
  I (olfactory), 87-89
  II, see Optic nerve
  III, see Oculomotor nerves
  infants and, 314-315
  IV, see Trochlear nerve
  IX, see Glossopharyngeal nerve
  V, see Trigeminal nerve
  VI, see Abducens nerve
  VII, see Facial nerve
  VIII, see Acoustic nerve
  X, see Vagus nerve
  XI, see Accessory nerve
Craniopharyngiomas, 336-337
Craniotomy, examination of scar,
    31-32
Cremasteric reflex, 251
  infants, 311

CSF, see Cerebrospinal fluid
CT, see Computed tomography
Cushing's disease, 486
Cushing's syndrome, 486
Cyanosis, peripheral nerves and, 33

D

Dandy-Walker syndrome, 315
Deep sensation, 256
　tests for, 263-266
Degenerative diseases/disorders
　CT and, 349
　EEG evaluation, 373-375
　MRI and, 354
Dehydration, 484
Deltoid muscle, 200-201
Dementia, 84
　CT and, 349
　retrieval failure and, 43
Demyelinating diseases, MRI and, 353-354
Dermatomes, 11
Developmental milestones, 304-307
Diabetic ketoacidosis, 484
Diagnosis, differential, determining preliminary, 3
Diaphragm muscles, 222
Digit spans, 39
Diplegia, 314
Diplopia, 141
Distal sympathetic autonomic function tests, 463-464
Doll's eye reflex, 314
Doppler flow velocity spectral analysis, cerebrovascular disease and, 479
Doppler ultrasonography
　cerebrovascular disease and, 478-479
　transcranial, cerebrovascular disease and, 480
Dorsal column lesions, pain in, 14
Down's syndrome, 307
Drug intoxication, 289
Duplex scanner, cerebrovascular disease and, 479
Dysarthria, 53-68
　examination for, 54
　mixed, 67-68
　oral mechanism, 55-57
　types of, 59-68
Dysdiadochokinesia, 160

Dystonia, 165
Dystonic dysarthria, 65
Dystonic gait, 173

E

Edinger-Westphal nucleus, 132, 276
Edrophonium chloride test, 500
Education, influence on language, 73
EEG, see Electroencephalography
Electric activity, spontaneous, EMG and, 398
Electroencephalography, 357-389
　abnormal activity, 361-364
　abnormalities in children and, 382
　abnormalities in infants and, 381
　ambulatory monitoring, 385-387
　ancillary techniques in, 376-378
　clinical correlates, 365-376
　coherence analysis, 388
　diagnostic applications of, 366-376
　headaches and, 19
　in infants and children, 378
　International 10-20 System, 359
　Mayo EEG Classification System, 361
　monitoring during surgery, 388-389
　normal activity, 359-361patient preparation, 357-359
　prolonged monitoring, 385
　recording procedure, 357-359
　special electrodes, 359
　spectral analysis, 388
　spontaneous, quantitative analysis of, 387-388
　standard report, 364-365
Electrolyte imbalance, 486
Electromyography, 389-416
　abnormalities after nerve injury and, 407-409
　abnormality criteria, 396-407
　clinical uses of, 389-391
　electric activity of muscle, 392-393
　essential components of, 391-392
　examination procedure, 393-396
　recording abnormal movements, 416
　single fiber, 411-416
　surgical monitoring, 429-430
Electron microscopy, 503-504
Electronystagmography, 97
Electroretinogram, 455-457

Embryopathies, 303
EMG, *see* Electromyography
Encephalopathy, types of, 482-498
Endocrine disorders
  facial changes and, 32-33
  roentgenography of, 338
  spine roentgenography, 334
Epilepsy, 19-25
  electrographic, 19
  MRI and, 352-353
  rolandic, of childhood, 384
Epineurium, 9
Erb-Duchenne paralysis, 307
Exophthalmic goiter, 32, 33
Exophthalmos, inspection for, 129
Extensor carpi radialis brevis muscle, 208
Extensor carpi radialis longus muscle, 205
Extensor carpi ulnaris muscle, 208
Extensor digitorum brevis, 233
Extensor digitorum communis muscle, 208-209
Extensor digitorum longus, 233
Extensor hallucis longus, 231-233
Extensor pollicis brevis muscle, 209
Extensor pollicis longus muscle, 210
Extensor toe reflex, infants, 311
Extensors of back, 223
Extensors of neck, 222
External hamstring reflex, 249
Extracorporeal space orientation, 327
Extrafusal muscle fibers, 153
Extrapyramidal system, 152
Eyelid, examination of, 130-132
Eyes, exophthalmos examination, 129

F

Fabere sign, 299-300
Facial nerve (CNVII), 91-94
  anatomy of, 91-93
  examination of, 93-94
  lesions, in flaccid dysarthria, 62
Facies, 32-33
Facioscapulohumeral dystrophy, 32
Fainters, 24
Family history, 7
Fasciculation, 178-180
  EMG and, 401-402
Fasting, seizures and, 21
Fetal abnormalities, 303-304

Fetal infection, 303
Fibrillation, 180-181
  EMG and, 399-401
Finger wiggle test, 160
Finger-nose test, 159
Fixation mechanisms, 144
Flaccid dysarthria, 59-62
Flexor carpi radialis muscle, 212
Flexor carpi ulnaris muscle, 212
Flexor digitorum profundus muscle, 214
Flexor digitorum sublimis muscle, 214
Flexor pollicis brevis muscle, 216
Flexor pollicis longus muscle, 214
Flexors of neck, 222
Fluency, 41
Foot, intrinsic muscles of, 240
Foot pat test, 161
Foraminal compression test of Spurling, 301
Friedreich's ataxia, 29
Frontal lobe functions, assessment of, 47
Frostig Developmental Test, 327

G

Gag reflex, examination of, 57
Gait, 169-175
  apraxia of, 174
  observations of, 169-171
  types of, 171-175
Galactosemia, 495
Galant's reflex, 312
Gallium radionuclide, 335
Gamma loop, 152
Gasserian ganglion cells, 89
Gastrocnemius muscle, 237
Gastrocnemius-soleus reflex, 248
Gastrointestinal tract, 284-285
Gaze palsies, 144
Gaze-evoked nystagmus, 148
Gaze-holding mechanism, 144
Genetic studies, 504
Glasgow Coma Scale, 287
Global aphasia, 83
Glossopharyngeal nerve (CNIX)
  anatomy of, 99-100
  clinical examination of, 100
Glossopharyngeal nerve injury, 14
Gluteus maximum muscles, 228-229
Glycoprotein metabolism disorders, 492-493

Goldmann fields, 110
Goldstein-Scherer Stick Test, 327
Golgi tendons, 153
Grasp reflex, 254
Gray's Reading Paragraph, 325
Growth and development, milestones of, 304-307
Guillain-Barré syndrome, 279

H

Hair growth, peripheral nerves and, 33
Hamstring muscles, 231
Headache, 15-19
  cluster, 17
  diagnostic tests/observations, 19
  history-taking, 15-17
  migraine, 16
  specific, nature of, 16-19
  tension-type, 16-19
Hearing testing, 453-454
Heel-knee test, 159
Hemifacial spasm, 169
Hemiparesis, 24
  infants, 310
Hemiplegic gait, 171
Herpes, 303
HHE syndrome, 384
Hiccup, 167
Hippocampus, 43
History-taking, 3-28, *see also* Medical history; Neurologic history
  chief complaints and, 5
  clinical problem evaluation, 4
  direct questioning, 4
  documenting, 4
  family history, 7
  headaches and, 15-17
  history of present illness and, 5-6
  infants and children, 303-307
  neurologic symptoms review, 6-7
  ordering of, 3-5
  past medical events, 6
  recording of, 4
  review of systems, 6-7
  seizure disorders and, 20-21
  sleep disorders and, 25-28
  social, 8
  time required for, 3
Hoffmann's reflex, 249
Holter monitoring, 385
Homonymous hemianopsia, 115
Horner's syndrome, 135
Hydranencephaly, transillumination and, 316-317
Hydrocephalus
  CT investigation of, 349
  gait, 174
Hydroxyamphetamine hydrobromide, 135
Hygroma, transillumination and, 316-317
Hyperalgesia, 9
  central pain syndromes and, 15
Hypercalcemia, 485
Hyperkeratosis, peripheral nerves and, 33
Hyperkinesia
  quick, 65-66
  slow, 65
Hyperkinetic dysarthria, 64-67
Hyperostosis, diffuse idiopathic skeletal, 334
Hypertrophy, 178
Hyperventilation, seizures and, 20
Hypocalcemia, 312, 485
Hypopituitarism, 486
Hypothenar muscles, 216-217
Hypothermia, 289
Hypotonicity, 155
Hysterical gait, 174
Hysterical mutism, 84

I

Iliopsoas muscle, 225
Illinois Test of Psycholinguistic Abilities, 324
Incontinentia pigmenti, 308
Incurvation reflex, 312
Infant
  ambulation, 310-311
  cranial nerve examination, 314-315
  developmental milestones, 304-307
  EEG, abnormalities in, 381
  EEG, normal patterns of, 378-381
  examination of, 303-326, 307-309
  history-taking, 303
  motor responses, 309-317
  neck control, 310
  posture, tone, muscle strength, 308-309
Infectious conditions/diseases
  CT evaluation of, 349-350
  MRI and, 354

Inflammatory conditions/diseases
  CT evaluation of, 349-350
  EEG evaluation, 373
  MRI and, 354
Infraspinatus muscle, 198
Insomnia, 25
Intellectual impairment, general, 84
Intelligence, influence on language, 73
Intercostal muscles, 222-223
Interference, resistance to, 40
Internal hamstring reflex, 248
Interossei muscles, 217
Intracranial bleeding, CT evaluation of, 349
Intradural-extramedullary lesions, myelography of, 341
Intrafusal muscle fibers, 153
Intraorbital tumor, 32
Iris, examination of, 132

J

Jaundice, neonatal, 304
Jaw reflex, 246
Junctional lesions, 119

K

Kernicterus, 312
Kernig's sign, 300
Klippel-Feil deformity, 332
Knee pat test, 158
Kohs block design, 327
Kussmaul's respiration, 484
Kyphosis, 332

L

Labyrinthine lesions, 96
Lancaster red-green test, 141
Landau reflex, 314
Language, 53-85
  assessment of, 41, 72
  children and, 323-324
  definition of, 70
  history-taking and, 72-74
  intrahemispheric organization of, 72
  localization of, 71-72
  modalities of, 70-71

Language disorders, 70-85
  definition of language, 70
  history of, 72-74
  types of, 80-85
Language examination, 72-80
  components of, 74
  observing test behavior, 74
Larynx, examination of, 57
Latissimus dorsi muscle, 198-199
Learning, Short Test of Mental Status and, 48
Learning deficits, 52
Lennox-Gastaut syndrome, 383
Lesion, determining localization of, 3
Lhermitte's sign, multiple sclerosis and, 14
Lid, see Eyelid
Light reflex, crossed/consensual, 133
Light touch, 259
Limping gait, 174
Line bisection tasks, 41
Lipoprotein disorders, 492
Listening comprehension deficits, 80
Lower extremities, clinical examinations, 298-299
Lower motor neuron disease, EMG diagnosis of, 391
Lower motor neuron lesions, EMG location of, 409
Lumbar joint testing, 300
Lumbar puncture
  anesthesia, 471
  contraindications for, 470
  needle insertion, 472
  technique of, 470-473
Lumbosacral joint testing, 300
Lysosomal storage disease, 488

M

Macrocrania, 308
Maddox rod testing, 141-144
Magnetic resonance angiography, 355
  cerebrovascular disease and, 480
Magnetic resonance imaging, 351-354
  cerebrovascular disease and, 352
  clinical applications of, 351-354
  congenital abnormalities and, 354
  demyelinating diseases, 353-354
  epilepsy, 352-353
  headaches and, 19

infectious conditions, 354
inflammatory conditions, 354
neoplasia, 352
neoplasia of vertebral column and
    spinal cord, 336
  of skull, 336
Malnutrition, 334
Marcus Gunn pupil, 134
Mayo EEG Classification System, 361
Medical history, 3
Memory
  acquisition assessment, 43
  assessment of, 42-44
  children, 324-325
  deficits, 52
  nonverbal deficits and, 43
  retention assessment, 42, 43
  retrieval assessment, 43
  seizures and, 20
  terminology, 42-44
  verbal deficits and, 43
Meningioma, 31
  of sphenoid ridge, 32
Menstrual cycle, seizures and, 20
Mental status examination, 35-52
  attention, assessment of, 39
  behavioral observations, during
    history-taking, 38
  competence vs. performance
    assessment, 35
  deviations from normal values,
    35
  final questions for, 51-52
  history of changes, 37-38
  history-taking and, 37-38
  language, assessment of, 41
  memory, assessment of, 42-44
  objectives of, 36
  onset of symptoms, 37
  routine of, 36
  Short Test of Mental Status, 36,
    48-51
Meralgia paresthetica, 10
Mesulam, three-shape test of, 43
Metabolic diseases/disorders
  CT evaluation of, 350
  EEG evaluation, 373-375
  hereditary, 487-498
  roentgenography of, 338
  spine roentgenography, 334
Metabolic encephalopathy, 483-487
Micturition reflex, 283
Migraine, *see* Headaches, migraine
Mitochondrial cytopathy, 495
Montage reformatting, 387

Moro reflex, infants, 311
Motion rate, alternate, 159-161
Motor activity, spontaneous, in
    children, 318
Motor dysfunction, hysterical, 192
Motor evoked potentials, monitoring
    during surgery, 434-435
Motor function, 151-176
  central integration, 151-176
  general survey of, 189
  specific study of muscle, 177-240
Motor nerve fibers, conduction
    studies in, 416-417
Motor nerves, conduction velocity
    of, 418
Motor responses, infants, 309-317
Motor speech, 53-85
Motor speech disorder, 53-69
  apraxia of speech, 68-69
  definition of, 53-54
  dysarthria and, 53-68
Motor unit, number estimates, 422
Motor unit action potentials, EMG
    and, 403-407
Motor unit disease, EMG detection,
    389-390
MRA, *see* Magnetic resonance
    angiography
MRI, *see* Magnetic resonance
    imaging
Mucopolysaccharidoses, 307, 490
Multiple sclerosis
  CSF examination and, 469
  Lhermitte's sign and, 14
Muscle
  biopsy, 501-502
  consistency of, 184
  contracture of, 184
  cramps, EMG and, 402
  disuse, 155
  palpation of, 183-185
  tenderness, 183
Muscle disease
  EMG diagnosis of, 390-391
  primary, differentiation of, 410-41
Muscle movements
  abnormal involuntary, 161-169
  intrinsic, 178-181
Muscle size, disorders of, 177-178
Muscle strength, 185-240
  anatomic information required for
    testing, 193-240
  examination routine, 193
  grading and recording of, 187-188
  in infants, 308-309

motor function survey and, 189
normal, 188-189
symptomatology of weakness, 185-187
testing, 190-192
Muscle tone, 154-157
disturbances of, 154-155
examination of, 155-157
in infants, 308-309
passive movement resistance and, 156
Muscle transmission disorders, 498-507
Muscle-stretch reflexes, 152, 242-249
elicitation techniques, 242-245
infants, 311-314
interpretation and grading of, 245-246
reinforcement of, 244-245
relaxation, 243
specific types, 246-249
stretch stimulus application, 244
Musician's cramp, 165
Mutism, 84
Myasthenia gravis, 498-499
facies of, 32
saccades in, 149
Myelography, 335
complications of, 339-340
general aspects of, 338-339
neoplasia of vertebral column and spinal cord, 336
pathologic findings, 340-341
Myelomeningocele, 332
Myoclonic seizures, 23
Myoclonus, 166-167
Myoedema, 182
Myokymia, 180
Myotonia, percussion, 181
Myotonic dystrophy, 32
Myxedema, 33

N

Nail growth, peripheral nerves and, 33
Naming tasks, 42
Narcolepsy, 25
Neck
extensors of, 222
flexors of, 222
muscle control in infants, 310
traction test, 301

Neonatal period, 304
history of, 304
Neoplasia
MRI and, 352
vertebral column and spinal cord, 336
Neoplasms
CT evaluation of, 348
optic nerve, 119
Neoplastic disease, 336-337
EEG evaluation, 366-369
roentgenography of, 337
Neostigmine test, 499
Nerve conduction studies, 416-428
cranial nerves, 427-428
late responses, 420-422
motor unit number estimates, 422
repetitive stimulation, 424-426
velocity of motor nerves, 418
Nerve injury, EMG, sequence of abnormalities after, 407-409
Nervi nervorum, 9
Nervous system, functional inquiry of, 5-6
Neuralgia
pain of, 14
postherpetic, 15
trigeminal, 14
Neurofibromas, 29
Neurogenic bladder dysfunction, 283
Neurologic abnormality, signs of, 151
Neurologic disease, determining, 3
Neurologic examination, 29-33
children, 317-327
facies, 32-33
infants, 303-317
order of, 30-31
patient physical condition survey, 29
peripheral nerves, 33
scalp and skull, 31-32
Neurologic history, 3-28
chief complaints, 5-6
family, 7
general aspects of, 3-8
history of present illness, 5-6
inquiry of common neurologic problems, 8-28
past medical events, 6
review of systems, 6
social, 8
symptoms review, 6
Neurologic lesion, 283
Neurologic symptoms, review of, 6-7
Neuromuscular blocking agents, 289

Neuromuscular junction transmission, EMG detection of defects in, 391
Neuromuscular system, peripheral, excitability of, 418
Neuromuscular transmission disorders, 498-507
Neuronal ceroid-lipofuscinoses, 490
Neurovascular examination, 294-298
  auscultation, 296-297
  blood pressure and, 295
  ocular fundus, 297-298
  palpation, 295-296
Nevus flammeus, 308
Nociceptive stimuli, pain and, 8
Nocturnal symptoms, 26
Nonparalytic tropia, 140
Nose-finger-nose test, 158
Nylén-Bárány test, 98
Nystagmus, 98, 146-148
  gaze-evoked, 148

O

Occupation, influence on language, 73
Ocular fundus
  examination in children, 317
  neurovascular examination and, 297-298
Ocular movement, 136-150
  examination of, 137-139
  Maddox rod testing, 141-144
  smooth pursuit and, 149
  strabismus and, 139-141
  visual axes alignment, 137
Ocular pneumoplethysmography, cerebrovascular disease and, 478
Oculomotor nerve (CNIII), anatomy of, 125-126
Oculosensory reflex, 133
Olfactory nerve (CNI), 87-89
Oligodendroglioma, 336-337
Ophthalmic artery, 103
Ophthalmodynamometry, cerebrovascular disease and, 477-478
Ophthalmoscopy, 121
Oppenheim's reflex, 253
Opponens pollicis muscle, 215-216
Optic atrophy, 124-125
Optic disk
  lesions of, 118
  ophthalmoscopy of, 121-122
Optic nerve (CNII)
  Amsler grid testing and, 110
  anatomy of, 103-104
  color vision and, 109
  field of vision and, 109
  lesions, retrobulbar, 119
  tangent screen perimetry, 110
  visual acuity and, 104-109
Optic neuropathy, anterior ischemic, 123-124
Oral mechanism examination, 55-57
Orbicularis oculi, 131
Organic acidopathy, 494
Orientation, 48
Osteomyelitis, 335
Osteoporosis, 334

P

Pacing reflex, 313
Pain, 8-15
  allodynia and, 9
  burning, 9
  central, syndromes of, *see* Central pain syndromes
  date of onset, 9
  dysesthetic, 9
  intensity/quality of, 9
  lancinating, 9
  nerve trunk, 9-10
  neuropathic, 9
  nociceptive, 8
  paresthesia, 9
  pertinent data on, elicitation of, 8-9
Pain problems, clinical examinations, 298-302
Palatal myoclonus, 167
Palatopharyngolaryngeal myoclonus, dysarthria of, 66
Pallor, peripheral nerves and, 33
Palmar responses, infants, 312
Palmaris longus muscle, 212
Palpation, neurovascular examination and, 295-296
Papilledema, 118
  ophthalmoscopy of, 122
Papillitis, ophthalmoscopy of, 122
Parachute response, 313
Parahippocampal gyri, 43
Paralytic phorias, 140
Paraphasias, 41
Paraplegia, 314
Parasomnias, 25

Paredrine, 135
Paresthesia, 9
Parkinsonian gait, 173
Parkinsonism, 155
Parkinson's syndrome, facies of, 32
Pathologic reflexes, 253-254
Pathophysiology, determining, 3
Patrick's sign, 299-300
Pattern reversal evoked potentials, 456-457
Pectoralis major muscle, 198
Pendulousness of muscle tone, 156
Perception, 287
Perceptual tasks, 44
Percussion, response to, 181-182
Performance, assessment of, 35
Perimetry
  computerized, 110
  outline, 114
Periodic alternating nystagmus, 148
Peripheral nerve lesions, pain in, 9-11
Peripheral nerves, examination of, 33
Peripheral neuropathy, 507-514
  differential diagnosis of, 507-509
  quantitative sensory testing, 509-511
  sural nerve biopsy, 511
Peroneus brevis muscle, 233
Peroneus longus muscle, 233
Peroxisome disorders, 491
Perseverance, assessment of, 40
Pes cavus, 29
Pharyngeal reflex, 250
Phonation, 57
  speech examination and, 57-58
Photic driving, 364
Photoentrainment, 364
Photomyogenic response, 364
Placenta previa, 304
Plantar grasp responses, infants, 312
Plantar reflex, 251
Plasma norepinephrine, 464-465
Polymyositis, 189
Polyneuropathy
  diabetic, 10
  peripheral, 10
Polysomnography, 460-462
Porencephaly, transillumination and, 316-317
Posterior tibial muscle, 237
Postherpetic neuralgia, 15
Postural fixation, 157
Posture, in infants, 308-309
Praxis, 319

Pregnancy, seizures and, 20
Prenatal period, history of, 303-304
Primary walking reflex, 313
Prodrome, 21
Pronation-supination test, 158-159
Pronator teres muscle, 210-212
Proptosis, 32
Pseudobulbar dysarthria, 63
Pseudoseizures, 24-25
Psoas test, 300
Psychogenic mutism, 84
Ptosis, 131
Pupil
  Adie's, 135
  amaurotic, 134
  examination of, 132-136
  Marcus Gunn, 134
Pupillary abnormalities, comatose patients, 290-291
Pupillography, 462-463
Purine metabolism disorder, 496
Pyramidal system, 151
Pyrimidine metabolism disorder, 496

Q

Quadriceps femoris muscle, 229-231
Quadriceps femoris reflex, 247
Quantitative sensory testing, 509-511

R

Radiation, ionizing, exposure during pregnancy, 303
Radioisotope cisternography, 481-482
Radionuclide imaging, 356
Reading comprehension deficits, 81
Recall
  Short Test of Mental Status and, 50
  short-term, 71
Rectal examination, 30
Reflexes, 241-254
  long latency stretch, 154
  muscle-stretch, 242
  pathologic, 241, see Pathologic reflexes
  superficial, see Superficial reflexes
Repetition tasks, 42
Resonation, speech examination and, 58
Respiration, 278-280
  sleep and, 26
  speech examination and, 57-58

Respiratory patterns, comatose
    patients, 291-292
Restless legs syndrome, 163
Retinal artery pressure,
    cerebrovascular disease and,
    477-478
Retinal embolus, 124
Retinal lesions, 117-118
Retrieval, language and, 71
Retrobulbar optic nerve lesions, 119
Review of systems, *see* Systems,
    review of
Rey-Osterrieth complex, 45
Rheumatoid arthritis, 335
Rhomboid muscles, 195
Right hemisphere lesions, language
    tasks and, 84
Righting reflexes, 313
Right-left orientation, 47
Rigidity, 155
Roentgenography
    congenital anomalies of skull,
        337-338
    endocrine disorders, 338
    inflammatory lesions, 338
    metabolic disorders, 338
    neoplastic disease, 337
    of spine, 332-336
    traumatic lesions, 337
Rolandic epilepsy of childhood, 384
Romberg sign, 175
Rooting reflex, 312
Rossolimo's reflex, 249
Rubella, 303

S

Saccades, 149
Sagittal synostosis, 315
Salaam seizures, 307
Scalp, palpation of, 31
Scalp examination, 31-32
Schmorl's nodes, 335
Scoliosis, 332
Scotomata, 24, 117
Seizures, 19-25
    absence, 23
    classification of, 21-25
    conversion reaction and, 24-25
    differentiating epileptic seizures,
        24-25
    generalized, 23-24
    history-taking from patients with,
        20-21
    myoclonic, 23
    partial, 21-23
    tonic-clonic, 23
Sensation, combined, tests for, 266
Sensory examination, 255-274
    general methods of, 257-258
    methods of, 258-268
    types of sensation, 255-257
Sensory nerve fibers, conduction
    studies, 426-427
Sensory nerve root lesions
    aggravating factors, 11-12
    pain in, 11-14
    stretching and, 12
Sensory nerves
    lesions of, 10
    pain in, 10
Sensory supply, 268-269
Serratus anterior muscle, 196
Serum creatine kinase, 500-501
Shivering, 179
Short Test of Mental Status, 36, 48-51
    scoring of, 50-51
Shoulder bracing test, 302
Shoulder hyperabduction test, 302
Similarities, interpretation of, 46
Skin atrophy, peripheral nerves and,
    33
Skin blood flow, regulation, 281-282
Skin vasomotor reflexes, 282
Skull
    depressions in, 31
    examination, 31-32
    examination, palpation of, 31
    percussion, 32
    roentgenography of, 336
Sleep
    apnea syndrome, 25
    awakening from, pain and, 12
    deprivation, seizures and, 21
    history-taking, 25-27
    initiation, 26
    maintenance, 26
    movements during, 26
    multiple latency test, 462
    paralysis, 26
    physiologic changes during,
        458-460
    termination, 26
Sleep disorders, 25-28
    assessment of, 28
    background history of patient, 27
    cataplexy and, 27
    evaluation of, 457-463
    examination of patient, 27-28

rapid eye movement behavior, 25
  sleepiness, excessive, 25
Sleepiness, excessive daytime, 27
Sleepwalking, 25
Snellen chart, 105
Social history, 8
Soleus muscle, 237
Somatosensory evoked potentials, monitoring during surgery, 433-434
Somatosensory system testing, 443-448
  abnormalities, 447-448
  averaging, 443
  criteria of abnormality, 446-447
  nomenclature, 444
  origin of waveforms, 444-446
  stimulation methods, 444
Spasms, muscle, 168-169
Spastic ataxic gait, 172
Spastic dysarthria, 63
Spastic gait, 171
Spasticity, 154-155
Speaking deficits, 81
Spectral analysis, 388
Speech
  contextual, 58
  examination, 57-59
  fluency of, children, 323
Sphingolipidosis, 488
Spina bifida, 332
Spinal column
  cervical examination, 300
  deformities of, 29-30
  traumatic lesions of, 335
Spinal cord lesions, 14
  myelography of, 339
Spinal diseases, CT evaluation of, 350
Spinal dysraphism, 332
Spinal nerves, lesions, in flaccid dysarthria, 62
Spinal stenosis, 335
  myelography, 341
Spondylolisthesis, 332
Spondylolysis, 332
Spurling, foraminal compression test of, 301
Stanford-Binet Scale, 324
Station, 175-176
Steppage gait, 172
Steppage reflex, 313
Stereognosis, 267
Stiff-man syndrome, 169
Stimulation, repetitive, 424-426

Strabismus, 139-141
Straight leg raising test, 299
Stransky's reflex, 254
Stress, seizures and, 20
Sturge-Weber syndrome, 32, 308
Sturge-Weber-Krabbe disease, 343
Subacute sclerosing panencephalitis, 384
Subdural effusion, transillumination and, 316-317
Subscapularis muscle, 202
Sucking reflex, 254, 312
Superficial abdominal reflexes, 250-251
Superficial pain, 261-262
Superficial reflexes, 250
  specific types of, 250-251
Superficial sensation, 256
  tests for, 259-263
Supinator muscle, 205
Supraspinatus muscle, 197-198
Sural nerve biopsy, 511
Surgery, EEG monitoring during, 388-389
Surgical monitoring, 428-443
  application of techniques, 435-442
  techniques of, 429-435
Sustained handgrip, 465
Sweating, peripheral nerves and, 33
Sylvian seizures of childhood, 384
Syncope, 24
Synostosis, 315
Syntax, 71
Syphilis, cytomegalic, 303
Syringomyelia, 332
Systems, review of, 6-7

T

Tabes dorsalis, 14
Tactile stimulation, 41
Tangent screen perimetry, 110
Tardive dyskinesias, 167
Temperature, 262-263
Temperature control, 280
Tenderness of muscle, 183
Teres major muscle, 200
Tetraplegia, 314
Thalamic function, in sensation, 256
Thalamic pain, 15
Thigh
  lateral rotators of, 228
  medial rotators of, 228

Thigh abductors, 227-228
Thoracic outlet syndromes, clinical tests for, 301
Tinel's sign, 9
Tingling, 24
Toe-finger test, 159
Toes, long flexors of, 240
Tongue
  examination of, 55-56
  wiggle test, 160
Tonic neck reflex, 312
Tonic-clonic seizures, 23
Toxic diseases, EEG evaluation, 373-375
Toxic disorders, CT evaluation of, 350
Toxic encephalopathy, 482-483
Toxoplasma gondii, 303
Toxoplasmosis, 303
Transient global amnesia, 24
Transient ischemic attacks, 24
Transillumination, 316-317
Trapezius muscle, 194
Traumatic conditions, EEG evaluation, 370-373
Tremor, involuntary muscle movement and, 163-164
Triceps muscle, 202
Triceps reflex, 247
Trigeminal nerve (CNI), 89-91
  lesions, in flaccid dysarthria, 62
Trigeminal neuralgia, pain and, 14
Trigger points, trigeminal neuralgia and, 14
Trochlear nerve, anatomy of, 128
Two-point discrimination, 266

U

Upper extremities, pain problem diagnosis, 300-302
Upper motor neuron dysarthria, 62-63
Urea cycle disorders, 494

V

Vagal nerve injury, 14
Vagus nerve (CNI), 100-101
Valsalva maneuver, peripheral nerve lesion pain and, 10
Vascular disease, EEG evaluation, 370
Vascular events, optic nerve and, 119
Vascular nevus, 32

Vasculitis, cerebral, angiography, 344
Vasodepressor syncope, 24
Vasomotor function, 281-283
Vasospasm, 343
Velopharynx, examination of, 56
Venoarteriolar reflex, 282
Venous occlusion, 124
Vergence movements, 149-150
Vertigo, 98
Vestibular function testing, 454-455
Vestibular system, 146
Vibration, 265-266
Visual acuity, 104-109
  color vision measurement, 104
  measuring, 104
Visual evoked potentials, monitoring during surgery, 435
Visual field, 109
  bedside testing of, 112-114
  confrontation testing, 114-115
  finger-counting, 112
  interpretation of defects, 116-120
  loss patterns, 120
  outline perimetry and, 114
  recording of observations, 115
Visual stimulation, 41
Visual system testing, 455-457
  electroretinogram and, 455-457
  pattern reversal evoked potentials, 456-457
Visuospatial tasks, 44
Voice tremor, dysarthria of, 66-67

W

Walleye, 140
Water imbalance, 486
Weber's test, 96
Wechsler Intelligence Scale for Children, 324
Wernicke's aphasia, 83
Wide Range Achievement Test, 325
Wood's lamp, 308
Wrisberg, nerve of, 92
Writer's cramp, 165
Writing deficits, 82